Apley's System of Orthopaedics and Fractures

Apley's System of Orthopaedics and Fractures

Seventh edition

A. Graham Apley
MB BS, FRCS
Consulting Orthopaedic Surgeon, St Thomas' Hospital, London Emeritus Consultant Surgeon,
Rowley Bristow Orthopaedic Hospital, Pyrford, and St Peter's Hospital, Chertsey, Surrey, Former
Editor, British Issue, *Journal of Bone and Joint Surgery*

Louis Solomon
MB ChB, MD, FRCS, FRCSEd
Professor of Orthopaedic Surgery, University of Bristol, Formerly Professor of Orthopaedic
Surgery, University of the Witwatersrand, Johannesburg

Foreword by
Henry J. Mankin
MD, FRCS(Hon)
Chief of the Orthopaedic Service, Massachusetts General Hospital, Edith M. Ashley Professor of
Orthopaedics, Harvard Medical School

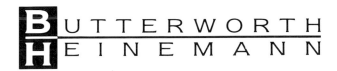

Butterworth-Heinemann Ltd
Linacre House, Jordan Hill, Oxford OX2 8DP

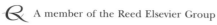 A member of the Reed Elsevier Group

OXFORD LONDON BOSTON
MUNICH NEW DELHI SINGAPORE SYDNEY
TOKYO TORONTO WELLINGTON

First published 1959
Second edition 1963
Third edition 1968
Reprinted 1970, 1972
Fourth edition 1973
Reprinted 1975, 1977
Fifth edition 1977
Reprinted 1978
Sixth edition 1982
Reprinted 1984, 1986, 1987, 1992
Seventh edition 1993
Reprinted 1993, 1994

© Butterworth-Heinemann Ltd 1993

British Library Cataloguing in Publication Data
Apley, A. Graham
    Apley's System of Orthopaedics and
    Fractures. – 7Rev.ed
    I. Title   II. Solomon, Louis
    617.3

ISBN 0 7506 0641 X

ISBN 0 7506 1606 7 Butterworth-Heinemann International Edition

Library of Congress Cataloguing in Publication Data
Apley, A. Graham (Alan Graham)
    Apley's system of orthopaedics and fractures/A.
    Graham Apley, Louis Solomon. – 7th ed.
    p.   cm.
    Includes bibliographical references and index.
    ISBN 0 7506 0641 X
    1. Orthopedics.   2. Fractures.   I. Solomon, Louis.
    II. Title.
    III. Title: System of orthopaedics and fractures.
    [DNLM: 1. Fracture Fixation.   2. Orthopedics.
    WE 168 A642s]
    RD731.A64   1993
    617.3–dc20   92–48221
                                        CIP

Composition by Genesis Typesetting, Laser Quay, Rochester, Kent
Printed and bound in Great Britain by the Bath Press, Avon

Contents

Part 3 – Fractures and Joint Injuries   **499**

Foreword

Over the decades since the remarkably durable and consummately skilful educator Alan G. Apley published his first edition of the *System of Orthopaedics and Fractures*, physicians who practise orthopaedic surgery (just as their brethren in the other specialties of medicine) have been simultaneously blessed and cursed by a veritable explosion of scientific knowledge. It was enough in our 'salad days' to be able to describe a disease, define its differential diagnosis and project a dim knowledge of which of the several procedures or even fewer non-surgical management regimens made the most sense to try. That was sufficient for the time perhaps, but hardly sufficient for our patients, for ourselves in our putative role of musculoskeletal scientists or, fortunately for the readers, for the authors of this current seventh edition of the reigning classic. Now, we not only read of the diagnostic features and principles of care, but for many of the entities we find discussions in clear and precise language (which has always been the hallmark of the *System* . . . and is responsible in part for its continued extraordinary popularity), information about the pathophysiology, the biology, the molecular genetics, the modern diagnostic tools and the technical details of management of the common and sometimes even obscure disorders. The authors are to be praised for their ability to do this and still maintain the readability of the book and keep the volume down to size. This is perhaps the ultimate test of the authors and one that they passed with flying colours – their ability to put in enough information to impart good and valid data but still maintain the interest and not exhaust the browsing reader is extraordinary; and in fact separates this volume from a host of multi-volumed, multi-authored textbooks that can only be used as references and are often left untouched on shelves.

The book is divided rather logically into three parts. The first entitled 'General Orthopaedics' is as it always has been in the past – the classic and indeed graceful entry into our specialty. Without seeming to make haste, and in remarkably readable style the authors take us through the presentation of the patient and the development of an analytic assessment technology. Once that is established the authors introduce the various basic biological entities such as infection, inflammatory joint diseases, osteoarthritis and osteonecrosis (two particularly strong offerings), metabolic and dysplastic disorders, neoplasms, neurologic entities (quite informative and updated) and a brief introduction to operative procedures.

The second part is entitled 'Regional Orthopaedics' and is just that – an exhaustive and yet practical (although still quite readable!) tour through each of the body's regions with emphasis on the diagnosis and management of the various disorders. This section is particularly well illustrated with clinical photographs supplemented with radiographs, CTs and on occasion MRIs. Periodically in this section are found short treatises entitled 'notes on applied anatomy' which are very helpful to the young student less well versed in that crucial discipline and indeed are warmly recommended as well for the older student (such as this writer!) who may need to be refreshed on some of the salient features in those sections.

The final section, 'Fractures and Joint Injuries', is a practical text, admittedly very elementary in initial approach but progressing rapidly into technical details of not only the injury, complications and pitfalls but therapeutic approaches. The illustrations in this section are particularly helpful to the reader, especially again for the young or inexperienced. This section, in this reader's opinion, stands alone as a basic text on fracture management – elemental in approach, beautifully illustrated in pictures and text and appropriately conservative in view.

I suppose it is fair in these days of burgeoning volumes of unread and unreadable literature, limited time, and diminished incomes for orthopaedists to ask why we should have another edition of *Apley's System of Orthopaedics and Fractures*. What does it give us that other books and treatises do not? Who will benefit? I think the answer is apparent to anyone who has had the experience of reading one of the prior editions; or will be to the novitiate who has the delightful experience of opening the text and reading the very first quote: 'Information consists of differences that make a difference.' He or she will know in a few sentences why this book is a treasure and can rapidly become for them what it has for all the rest of us – a dependable old friend who can be trusted to tell the truth, to counsel and to guide the way in a very special and graceful manner.

Henry J. Mankin MD, FRCS(Hon)
Chief of the Orthopaedic Service
Massachusetts General Hospital
Edith M. Ashley Professor of Orthopaedics
Harvard Medical School

Preface

Is there still a place for a general textbook of orthopaedics? If you have got as far as reading this preface you will know that we believe the answer is 'Yes: more so than ever.' Ours has been described as the age of information – facts will be delivered like fast food by hundreds of journals, free-sheets and computer networks trying bravely to disseminate news before it is obsolete. Certainly, we have to keep abreast of new ideas and techniques, but their value and significance are enormously enhanced if we can place them in a broader matrix of knowledge and understanding. This textbook aims to provide such a matrix, by emphasizing the basic skills of clinical practice and the principles on which our science and art are built.

Since the last edition much has changed. Diagnosis has been improved by newer methods of imaging (patients now ask for magnetic resonance imaging because they think it will 'show everything'). More is known of the arthritides, bone tumours, metabolic disorders and genetic syndromes. The sciences of bio-mechanics, biochemistry and immunology are making more and more impact on clinical medicine. Joint replacement has entered its fourth decade and surgeons with a philosophic turn of mind speak sagely of first, second and third generation replacements. Keyhole surgery has come to stay, with latter-day enthusiasts looking for ever smaller holes into which to insert ever smarter keys. Some of the most exciting advances have been in the field of trauma: greater awareness of the body's reaction to injury, increasing skill in resuscitating the near-dead, better understandng of the place of internal and external fixation, and recogni-tion of the need for hands-on training in the use of implants and instruments of ever-increasing sophistication.

These and many other facets of the new orthopaedics have been incorporated in this edition of the *System*. Some of it is aimed deliberately at trainees who are boning up (sic!) for higher examinations. However, we hope the book will appeal also to mature orthopaedic surgeons trying desperately to preserve a sense of proportion in the face of advancing complexity.

We have retained the familiar format that, ever since the first edition in 1959, has given the book its particular character; there is the same systematic approach and the same presentation of numerous illustrations, mostly as composites. But this seventh edition is more comprehensive than its predecessors, with extended sections on pathology and pathogenesis wherever appropriate. It is, of necessity, a good deal larger, but we have not abandoned those whose requirements are less demanding. Four years ago we anticipated this change and produced the *Concise System*, which is more closely attuned to the needs of undergraduates, junior doctors, physiotherapists, occupational therapists and other paramedicals. Any readers of that book looking for more detail will find it easily in the matching section of the present volume.

Much of what is written here we have learnt from others. Those who have taught us will recognize their influence in these pages, even if it is not always acknowledged explicitly. We thank them and pass their teaching on to a wider audience.

To those who are habitual readers we say

welcome aboard. To those who are forced to read, we owe it – at the very least – to make the process both worthwhile and as painless as possible. And for those who cannot pause long enough to read, we recall the story of the woodsman who always protested that he was so busy cutting down trees that he never had time to sharpen his axe.

A. G. A.

L. S.

Extract from preface to the sixth edition

The first outline of this book was written in 1954. The FRCS course at Pyrford was then six years old; but as it became more comprehensive the students could either pay attention or scribble notes – they could not do both. The obvious answer was to provide summaries of all the lectures. These were revised annually, but, as the course grew longer, typed notes became unmanageable (and secretaries rebellious) so in 1959 the publishers had to take over.

For the printed version the notes were converted into more readable prose, but the systematic approach was left unchanged. Students seemed to like the idea of a standard pattern of headings and welcomed the logic of a consistent sequence for describing physical signs; learning to *look*, *feel* and *move* before turning to investigations is a habit they can profitably carry over from the lecture room (via the examination hall) to the consulting room or office. We like to think that in the process they will also discover that each of these deceptively simple words conveys a meaning beyond the obvious. 'Look' says more than 'inspect'; it implies noticing and analysing what is seen. Similarly, to 'feel' is more than to palpate, and 'move' is not merely an imperative.

Illustrations were a big problem. They are so helpful that profusion is desirable – and yet the book must not become unwieldy. The answer lay in selecting, pruning and arranging; picking only good quality illustrations, excising every scrap of surplus material, and then arranging many of the figures into groups so that each 'composite' tells a story. This fits in well with something every teacher knows: that, no matter how good a single illustration may be, it is more informative when combined with others in a meaningful set. Composites are the natural way of showing stages in a process, of highlighting important clinical signs, of summing up differential diagnosis and of contrasting different methods of treatment. There are some 2240 individual photographs, x-rays and drawings arranged into just over 500 composites, which can be used by themselves for quick revision.

A. G. A.
L. S.

Acknowledgements

We have received much help from several sources and gladly acknowledge our debt to many friends and colleagues. Mr S. M. Eisenstein, Mr I. J. Leslie, Mr P. G. Stableforth, Dr Sheila Willetts, Mr P. J. Witherow and Professor P. A. Dieppe went to the trouble of reading over sections of the manuscript and offering helpful comments. We were also very fortunate in being able to call upon a number of people to provide us with illustrations to fill some of the gaps in our own collection. From the University of Bristol and the Bristol Royal Infirmary: Dr Iain Watt, Department of Diagnostic Radiology, for sundry pictures of radiographs and scans; Dr T. Wickremaratchi and Dr C. Collins, Department of Clinical Pathology, for a number of photomicrographs; Professor P. A. Dieppe for photomicrographs of crystals; Professor A. E. Goodship for photomicrographs of bone histology; Dr M. Adams for photographs of intervertebral discs; Dr S. Lawson for photomicrographs of nerve histology; Dr D. Lewis for photomicrographs of muscle histology; Mr R. M. Atkins for illustrations of haemophilia and calcaneal fractures; Mr G. C. Bannister for x-rays of elbow replacement; Mr P. G. Stableforth for x-rays of the shoulder; Mr P. J. Witherow for pictures of scoliosis and club foot; Dr Mark Cobby for MRI illustrations of the knee; and Mr R. H. Dixon for x-rays of bone tumour replacement.

Further afield in Britain, the following either supplied us with illustrations or gave us permission to copy their x-rays: Dr Barbara Ansell, Mr Malcolm Swann, Mr M. Saleh, Mrs J. M. Murray, Mr L. R. Priaulx, Mr S. M. Eisenstein, Dr V. Cassar-Pullicini, Dr W. L. Masry, Mr D. Jeffrey, Mr W. K. Pun, Mr R. Brueton and Dr R. L. Guy.

Among those of our colleagues from abroad, we are particularly indebted to the late Professor J. J. G. Craig, whose pictures of children with cerebral palsy are surely unsurpassed. Others who contributed to the collection of illustrations are: Professor K. Bose, National University Hospital, Singapore, and his staff, who have allowed us to use photographs from their teaching collection; Professor S. M. Perren, Davos, Switzerland, who gave us permission to reproduce the photomicrograph of fracture healing; Professor E. Erken, Johannesburg, who provided a photograph of bone lengthening; and Mr M Versveld, Johannesburg, who permitted us to use the x-rays of his patient with bone transport. Dr D. Pennig provided pictures of his wrist fixator and the Biomet Company and Orthofix allowed us to use some of their drawings of external fixation devices.

We are deeply grateful to Mrs M. van der Lem, Mrs P. A. Millns and Mrs A. Nelson for their enormous help in preparing the manuscript.

Most of the new photographs were produced by Miss E. Hurst of the Department of Medical Illustration at the Bristol Royal Infirmary. Many new drawings were produced by Mr Peter Cox.

We have been fortunate in having the help of our copy-editor, Miss Gillian Clarke, as well as the backing and co-operation of our publishers.

To those whose names we have inadvertently omitted, we offer our apologies and we hope they will be consoled by the fact that a part of their knowledge and experience is being passed on to others. Some of the best work in any language is written by that prolific author, Anon.

Part 1 — General Orthopaedics

Diagnosis in orthopaedics 1

Information consists of differences that make a difference.
Gregory Bateson

Orthopaedics is concerned with bones, joints, muscles, tendons and nerves – the skeletal system and all that makes it move. Conditions that affect these structures fall into seven easily remembered pairs:

1. Congenital and developmental abnormalities
2. Infection and inflammation
3. Arthritis and rheumatic disorders
4. Metabolic dysfunction and degeneration
5. Tumours and lesions that mimic them
6. Sensory disturbance and muscle weakness
7. Injury and mechanical derangement

Diagnosis in orthopaedics, as in all of medicine, is the identification of disease. It begins from the very first encounter with the patient and is gradually modified and fine-tuned until we have a picture, not only of a *pathological process* but also of the *functional loss* and the *disability* that goes with it. Understanding evolves from the systematic gathering of information from the history, the physical examination, tissue and organ imaging and special investigations. Systematic, but never mechanical; behind the enquiring head there should also be what Lawrence has called the intelligent heart. It must never be forgotten that the patient is also a person, with a mind and a personality, a job and hobbies, a family and a home; all have a bearing upon – and are in turn affected by – the disorder and its treatment.

History

Symptoms

Carefully and patiently compiled, the history can be every bit as informative as examination or laboratory tests. As we record it, certain key words will inevitably stand out: *injury, pain, stiffness, swelling, deformity, instability, weakness, altered sensibility* and *loss of function*. Each symptom is pursued for more detail: we need to know when it began, whether suddenly or gradually, spontaneously or after some specific event; how it has changed or progressed; what makes it worse; what makes it better. We consider if the story fits some pattern that we know – for we are already thinking of a diagnosis – but we should never distort it for the sake of tidiness. 'History' in this context means 'his story' (or hers), and the patient must be allowed to tell the story in his or her own words; as Trotter remarked, 'Disease reveals itself in casual parentheses'.

Pain

Pain is the most common symptom in orthopaedics. It is described in terms that range from the most boring and bland to the impossibly dramatic and bizarre. The metaphors used tell us more about the patient's psyche than about

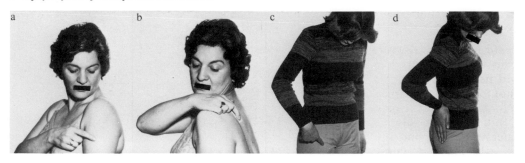

1.1 'Point to where it hurts'   In (a) and (b) the complaint would be of 'shoulder' pain; in (c) and (d) of 'hip' pain. The likely diagnoses are (a) supraspinatus tendinitis, (b) cervical spondylosis, (c) a disorder of the hip joint itself, (d) a prolapsed lumbar disc.

the pathology; yet there are clearly differences between the throbbing pain of an abscess and the aching pain of chronic arthritis, between the 'burning pain' of neuralgia and the 'stabbing pain' of a ruptured tendon.

Severity is even more subjective. High and low thresholds undoubtedly exist, but to the patient pain is as bad as it feels, and any system of 'pain grading' must take this into account. The main value of estimating severity is in assessing the progress of the disorder or the response to treatment. The following is a simple and useful system:

Grade I   Mild – pain that can easily be ignored.
Grade II   Moderate – pain that cannot be ignored, interferes with function and needs treatment from time to time.
Grade III   Severe – pain that is present most of the time, demanding constant attention.
Grade IV   Totally incapacitating pain.

Patients are often vague about the site of pain. Yet its precise location is important, and in orthopaedics it is particularly useful to ask the patient to point to where it hurts; not merely to tell us, but actually to point. But don't assume that the site of pain is always the site of pathology; 'referred' pain and 'autonomic' pain can be very deceptive.

Referred pain   Pain arising in or near the skin is usually localized accurately. Pain arising in deep structures is more diffuse and is sometimes of unexpected distribution; thus, hip disease may manifest with pain in the knee (so might an

obturator hernia). This is not because sensory nerves connect the two sites; it is due to inability of the cerebral cortex to distinguish between sensory messages from embryologically related sites. A common example is 'sciatica' – pain at various points in the buttock, thigh and leg, supposedly following the course of the sciatic nerve. Such pain is not necessarily due to pressure on the sciatic nerve; it may be 're-

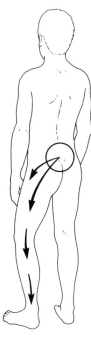

1.2 Referred pain   The pathology is in the back, but the pain may be felt in the buttock or lower down in the leg.

ferred' from any one of a number of structures in the lumbar spine and pelvis.

Autonomic pain We are so accustomed to matching pain with some discrete anatomical structure and its known sensory nerve supply that we are apt to dismiss any pain that does not fit the usual pattern as 'atypical' or 'inappropriate'. But pain can also arise in the autonomic nerves that accompany the peripheral blood vessels. This 'autonomic pain' (e.g. after operation) is much more vague, often widespread and accompanied by vasomotor and trophic abnormalities. It is poorly understood, often doubted, but none the less real.

Stiffness

Stiffness may be generalized (typically in systemic disorders such as rheumatoid arthritis and ankylosing spondylitis) or localized to a particular joint. Patients often have difficulty in distinguishing localized stiffness from painful movement; limitation of movement should never be assumed until verified by examination.

Ask when it occurs: regular early morning stiffness of many joints is one of the cardinal symptoms of rheumatoid arthritis, whereas transient stiffness of one or two joints after periods of inactivity is typical of osteoarthritis.

Locking is a special variety of stiffness. It is the sudden inability to complete one particular movement, and it suggests a mechanical block – for example, due to a loose body or a torn meniscus becoming trapped between the articular surfaces. Unfortunately, patients use the term for any painful limitation of movement; much more reliable is a history of sudden 'unlocking' when the offending body slips out of the way.

Swelling

Swelling may be in the soft tissues, the joint or the bone; to the patient they are all the same. It is important to establish whether the swelling followed an injury, whether it appeared rapidly (probably a haematoma or a haemarthrosis) or slowly (soft tissue inflammation, a joint effusion

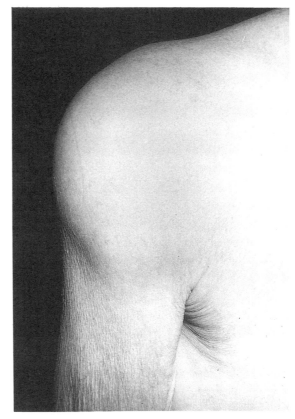

1.3 Swelling This large swelling of the shoulder appeared slowly and was the presenting symptom. Is it in the muscle, the bone or the joint?

or a tumour), whether it is painful (acute inflammation, infection – or a tumour), whether it is constant or comes and goes, and whether it is continuing to enlarge.

Deformity

The common deformities are well described in terms such as round shoulders, spinal curvature, knock knees, bow legs, pigeon toes and flat feet. Deformity of a single bone or joint is less easily described and the patient may simply declare that the limb is 'crooked'.

Some deformities are merely variations of the normal (e.g. short stature or wide hips); others disappear spontaneously with growth (e.g. flat feet or bandy legs in an infant). However, if the deformity is *progressive* it may be serious.

Weakness

Generalized weakness is a feature of all chronic illness. However, true muscular weakness – especially if it is confined to one limb or to a single muscle group – is much more specific and suggests some neurological or muscle disorder. Patients sometimes say that the limb is 'dead' when it is actually weak, and this can be a source of confusion. Questions should be framed to discover precisely which movements are affected, for this may give important clues, if not to the exact diagnosis at least to the site of the lesion.

Instability

The patient may complain of 'giving way'. This may be due to muscle weakness or to ligamentous deficiency from laxity or rupture. If there is a history of injury its precise nature is important.

Change in sensibility

Tingling or numbness signifies interference with nerve function – pressure from a neighbouring structure (e.g. a prolapsed intervertebral disc), local ischaemia (e.g. nerve entrapment in a fibro-osseous tunnel) or a peripheral neuropathy. It is important to establish its exact distribution; from this we can tell whether the fault lies in a peripheral nerve or in a nerve root. We should also ask what makes it worse or better; a change in posture might be the trigger, thus focusing attention on a particular site.

Loss of function

Functional disability is more than the sum of individual symptoms and its expression depends upon the needs of the patient. The patient may say 'I can't sit for long' rather than 'I have backache', or 'I can't put my socks on' rather than 'my hip is stiff'. Moreover, what to one patient is merely inconvenient may, to another, be incapacitating. Thus a lawyer or a teacher may readily tolerate a stiff knee provided it is painless and does not impair walking;

but to a plumber or a parson the same disorder might spell economic or spiritual disaster. One question should elicit the important information: 'What can't you do that you used to be able to do?'

Past history

Patients often forget to mention previous illnesses or accidents, or they may simply not appreciate their relevance to the present complaint. They should be asked specifically about childhood disorders, periods of incapacity and old injuries. A 'twisted ankle' many years ago may be the clue to the onset of osteoarthritis in what is otherwise an unusual site for this condition. Gastrointestinal disease, which in the patient's mind 'has nothing to do with bones', may be important in the later development of ankylosing spondylitis or osteoporosis. Similarly, rheumatic disorders may be suggested by a history of eye, skin or urogenital disease. Patients should also be asked about previous medication; many drugs, and especially corticosteroids, have long-term effects on bone. Alcohol and drug abuse are important, and we must not be afraid to ask about them.

Family history

Patients often wonder (and worry) about inheriting a disease or passing it on to their children. To the doctor, information about musculoskeletal disorders in the patient's family may help with both diagnosis and counselling.

Social background

No history is complete without enquiry about the patient's background: details about work, travel, recreation, home circumstances and the level of support by family and friends. These always impinge on the assessment of disability; occasionally a particular activity (at work, on the sportsfield, or in the kitchen) is responsible for the entire condition.

Examination

In 'A Case of Identity' Sherlock Holmes has the following conversation with Dr Watson.

Watson: You appeared to read a good deal upon [your client] which was quite invisible to me.
Holmes: Not invisible but unnoticed, Watson.

Examination begins from the moment we set eyes on the patient; we should be observing his appearance, his posture, gait and general attitude. Are his movements smooth and rhythmic, or has he learnt to substitute an unusual action for one that is now too difficult? Does he walk with a symmetrical swing or does he have a limp?

Gait and limp

The gait cycle (the sequence of events in each step) consists of four parts: heel strike; stance phase; toe off; and swing phase. A limp is simply an abnormal gait. Its possible causes range from a tight shoe to a 'tight' person, but the orthopaedic causes (fortunately more limited) are best analysed by noticing the point in the gait cycle at which the abnormality occurs (though if the patient is incoordinate or is wearing a prosthesis his limp may be obvious at more than one point in the cycle).

1. Heel strike

The patient with heel pain steps on the toes rather than the heel. A slapping movement (and sound) immediately after heel strike is characteristic of foot drop.

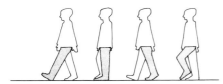

1.4 The gait cycle This oddly dressed individual's left leg shows the stages: 'heel strike' is followed by the 'stance phase'; next is 'toe off' (almost) and finally the 'swing phase'.

2. Stance phase

Limp at this point results from pain, shortening or instability. If there is pain on weightbearing, the patient hurries off the leg (the so-called antalgic gait). With shortening, the ipsilateral shoulder merely droops. With instability at the hip it also swings sideways over the weightbearing leg (this, a Trendelenburg gait, is the dynamic equivalent of Trendelenburg's sign). Instability at the knee is usually self-evident, and may result from muscle weakness (e.g. polio), bony incongruity (e.g. following rheumatoid arthritis) or ligamentous injury. Fixed flexion of the knee also is easily spotted and may result from mechanical obstruction (a locked knee) or from old inflammatory disease.

3. Toe off

At this point fixed flexion of the hip becomes apparent in that the heel lifts off too soon; and with a stiff straight knee the whole body is heaved up to provide clearance.

4. Swing phase

Foot drop now becomes obvious and, to avoid tripping, the patient adopts a high-stepping gait. If bilateral, this must be distinguished from the gait of a tabetic: here the foot does not drop but the patient lifts it too high because he lacks position sense. Abnormality in the swing phase may also result from stiffness (usually of the hip or knee, but sometimes of the back or foot) or from spasticity. A severely painful knee is held stiff, even though passive movement may be good.

Examination of the affected parts

When we proceed to the structured examination, the patient must be suitably undressed; no mere rolling up of a trouser leg is sufficient. If one limb is affected, both must be exposed so that they can be compared.

We examine the good limb, then the bad. There is a great temptation to rush in with both hands – a temptation that must be resisted.

Only by proceeding in a purposeful, orderly way can we avoid missing important signs. The system we use is simple but comprehensive:

First we LOOK
Then we FEEL
Then we MOVE

However, this is a guide, not a law carved on tablets of stone. Sometimes we need to look while we move (e.g. a spinal deformity may become apparent only when the patient bends forwards); or we may have to move a joint (especially one that is swollen) before we can feel exactly where it is! Our purpose in emphasizing the discipline – LOOK, FEEL, MOVE – is to encourage the habit of systematic thought which alone ensures that no important detail will be neglected or forgotten.

● LOOK

Skin We should look first at the skin – not merely looking *at* it, but looking *for* specific features: scars, colour and creases. Scars are an accurate record of the past – the surgical archaeology so to speak. Colour may indicate the present state – for example, the blueness of cyanosis or bruising and the redness of inflammation. Abnormal creases, unless due to underlying fibrosis, suggest underlying deformity such as scoliosis or spondylolisthesis; shiny skin with no creases suggests oedema or trophic change.

Shape Next we look at the shape. Is there swelling, or is there wasting (one often enhances the appearance of the other)? Or is there a definite lump? And is a normally straight bone bent?

Position A joint is three dimensional and it is important, at every joint, to look for deformity in three planes. In many joint disorders and in most nerve lesions the limb assumes a characteristic attitude.

Deformity

The word 'deformity' may be applied to a person, a bone or a joint. Shortness of stature is a kind of deformity; it may be due to shortness of the limbs or of the trunk, or both. An individual bone also may be abnormally short; this is rarely important in the upper limbs, but it is in the lower.

If a limb appears to be crooked, it is important to establish whether the deformity is in the bone or in the joint.

A joint may be held in an unnatural position either because of faulty alignment or because it lacks full movement. The more common deformities are designated by special terms.

VARUS AND VALGUS It seems pedantic to replace 'bow legs' and 'knock knees' with 'genu varum' and 'genu valgum'. But comparable colloquialisms are not available for deformities of the

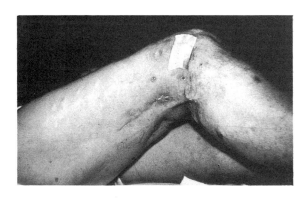

1.5 Scars Scars are a map of the past. The original operation wound on the thigh has faded. The infection that followed needed another operation (more posteriorly) and has left the scars of sinuses, one of them still draining.

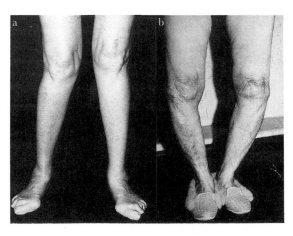

1.6 Valgus and varus (a) Valgus deformity in rheumatoid arthritis; (b) varus with osteoarthritis.

elbow, hip or big toe; and, besides, the formality is justified by the need for clarity and consistency. *Varus* means that the part distal to the joint is displaced towards the midline, *valgus* away from it.

KYPHOSIS AND LORDOSIS   Seen from the side, the spine has a series of curves – convex posteriorly in the dorsal region (kyphosis), and convex anteriorly in the cervical and lumbar regions (lordosis). Excessive curvature constitutes kyphotic or lordotic deformity.

SCOLIOSIS   Seen from behind, the spine is straight. Any curvature in this (coronal) plane is called a scoliosis.

'FIXED' DEFORMITY   This does not mean that the joint is unable to move; it means that a particular movement cannot be completed. Thus, the knee may flex fully but not extend fully – at the limit of its extension it is still 'fixed' in a certain amount of flexion. In the spine a fixed deformity is called a *structural deformity*; it differs from a *postural deformity* which the patient himself can, if properly instructed, correct it by his own muscular effort.

Causes of joint deformity

There are three basic causes of joint deformity:

1. *Contracture of the overlying soft tissues,* pulling the joint into an abnormal position. This is seen typically with severe scarring (e.g. after a burn) or after ischaemic necrosis of muscles.
2. *Muscle imbalance,* usually the result of a neurological disorder. Other signs of motor disturbance will be present.

> ### SIX CAUSES OF JOINT DEFORMITY
>
> 1. Skin contracture (e.g. burn)
> 2. Fascial contracture (e.g. Dupuytren's)
> 3. Muscle contracture (e.g. Volkmann's)
> 4. Muscle imbalance (e.g. asymmetrical paralysis)
> 5. Joint instability (e.g. torn ligament, or dislocation)
> 6. Joint destruction (e.g. arthritis)

3. *Chronic arthritis* (of any kind) resulting in articular destruction, capsular fibrosis or joint instability.

Causes of bone deformity

Bone deformity in a child may be the result of distorted growth due to injury or disease (perhaps a genetic disorder) of the physis; rickets, once common, is now rarely seen.

In adults the more likely causes are malunion of a fracture, Paget's disease and bone tumours.

● FEEL

The skin   Is it warm or cold; moist or dry; and is sensation normal?

The soft tissues   Is there a lump; if so, what are its characteristics? Are the pulses normal?

The bones and joints   Are the outlines normal? Is the synovium thickened? Is there excessive joint fluid?

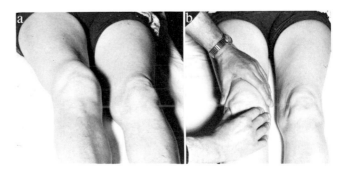

1.7 Fluid in the knee   (a) The suprapatellar pouch is bulging and the thigh wasted; (b) cross-fluctuation (see p. 433).

SIX CAUSES OF BONE DEFORMITY

1. Congenital disorders (e.g. pseudarthrosis)
2. Bone softening (e.g. rickets, osteomalacia)
3. Dysplasia (e.g. multiple exostosis)
4. Growth plate injury (e.g. epiphyseal separation)
5. Fracture malunion
6. Paget's disease

Tenderness   This is always important, and if localized is often diagnostic. If we know precisely *where* it is, we can often work out *what* it is. It is essential to watch the patient's face while eliciting tenderness.

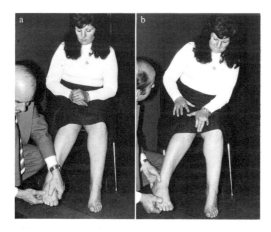

1.8 Feeling for tenderness   (a) How not to do it. It is better to watch the patient's face (b), and to stop the moment she feels pain.

Bony lumps

A bony lump may be due to faulty development, injury, inflammation or a tumour. Although x-ray examination is essential, the clinical features can be highly informative.

SIZE   A large lump attached to bone, or a lump that is getting bigger, is nearly always a tumour.

SITE   A lump near a joint is most likely to be a tumour (benign or malignant); a lump in the shaft may be fracture callus, inflammatory new bone or a tumour.

MARGIN   A benign tumour has a well-defined margin; malignant tumours, inflammatory lumps and callus have a vague edge.

CONSISTENCY   A benign tumour feels bony hard; malignant tumours often give the impression that they can be indented.

TENDERNESS   Lumps due to active inflammation, recent callus or a rapidly growing sarcoma are tender.

MULTIPLICITY   Multiple bony lumps are uncommon: they occur in hereditary multiple exostosis and in Ollier's disease.

● MOVE

Active   Ask the patient to move the joint. Is the movement smooth and rhythmic, or hesitant and painful? Any limitation implies that examining passive movements needs to be cautious and gentle.

Passive   Record the range of movement in each physiological plane.

Abnormal   Is the joint unstable? To assess joint stability the limb is held above and below the joint which is then deliberately (but gently) stressed across the normal anatomical planes of movement. With a history of injury the bone should be examined to see if there is movement at an old fracture site.

Normal movement

The range of joint movement is recorded in degrees, starting from zero, which is always the neutral or anatomical position of the joint. The eye soon acquires sufficient accuracy to estimate joint angles and a goniometer is needed only for special purposes.

The common planes of movement are the following.

Flexion/extension   These are movements in the sagittal plane; for example, at the knee, elbow, ankle and the joints of the fingers and toes.

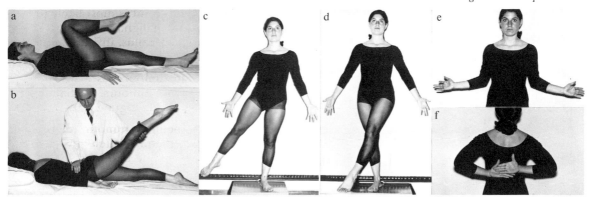

1.9 Active movements   (a) Flexion, (b) extension, (c) abduction and (d) adduction at the hip; (e) external (lateral) and (f) internal (medial) rotation at the shoulder.

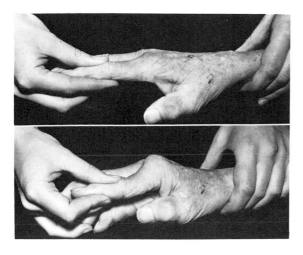

1.10 Passive movement   Stability is tested by moving the joint passively across the normal planes of action – in this case by thrusting the entire finger volarwards, thus demonstrating abnormal movement at the metacarpophalangeal joint.

Adduction/abduction   These are movements in the coronal plane, towards or away from the midline.

External rotation/internal rotation   These are rotational movements around a longitudinal axis. Strictly speaking they should be called lateral and medial rotation.

Pronation/supination   These, too, are rotatory movements, but the terms are applied only to movements of the forearm and the foot.

Circumduction   This is a composite movement made up of a rhythmic sequence of all the other movements. It is possible only for ball-and-socket joints (hip, shoulder).

Certain specialized movements, such as opposition of the thumb, lateral flexion and rotation of the spine, and inversion or eversion of the foot, will be described under the relevant regions.

While testing movement, feel for crepitus: *joint crepitus* is usually coarse and fairly diffuse; *tendon crepitus* is fine and precisely localized to the affected tendon sheath.

Joint stiffness

The term 'stiffness' covers a variety of limitations of movement. We consider three types of stiffness in particular: (1) all movements absent; (2) all movements limited; (3) one or two movements limited.

ALL MOVEMENTS ABSENT
A fixed joint has no movement, yet there may be such good function that the restriction goes unnoticed until the joint is examined. Surgical fusion is called 'arthrodesis'; pathological fusion is called 'ankylosis'. Acute suppurative arthritis typically ends in bony ankylosis; tuberculous arthritis heals by fibrosis and causes fibrous ankylosis – not strictly a 'fusion' because there may still be a small jog of movement.

ALL MOVEMENTS LIMITED

With active inflammation of synovium, extremes of all movements are limited and the joint is said to be 'irritable'. With acute arthritis there is joint rigidity, spasm preventing all but a few degrees of movement.

Tuberculous arthritis heals by fibrosis, leading to an unsound joint; that is, one in which forced movement causes spasm or pain, and deformity may increase with time. The term 'fibrous ankylosis' is used when fibrous tissue across the joint is so short that only a few degrees of movement exist. With longer fibrous tissue and more movement, the term 'ankylosis' is best avoided; 'long fibrous joint' is better.

In osteoarthritis the capsule fibroses and as the fibrous tissue matures it shrinks, limiting movement. In rheumatoid arthritis, movement at several joints may be limited by pain; subsequent fibrosis may perpetuate the limitation.

After severe injury, especially compound fractures near a joint, movement in all directions may be limited as a result of oedema, infection, adhesions or loss of muscle extensibility.

SOME MOVEMENTS LIMITED

When movement in at least one direction is full and painless the cause of any limitation is usually mechanical. Thus a torn and displaced meniscus may prevent extension of the knee but not flexion.

Again, if one group of muscles acting on a joint is paralysed, the opposing group eventually loses the ability to stretch fully.

Bone deformity may alter the arc of movement, such that it is limited in one direction (loss of abduction in coxa vara is an example) but movement in the opposite direction is full or even increased.

These are all examples of 'fixed deformity'.

Joint laxity

Children's joints are much more mobile than adults; their greater flexibility allows them to adopt postures that would be impossible for their parents. An unusual degree of mobility can, of course, be attained in dancers and athletes, but when the exercises are stopped mobility soon reverts to the normal range.

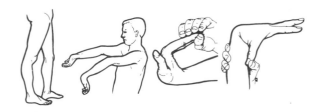

1.11 Generalized joint hypermobility Being double-jointed is not an unmixed blessing. Recurrent dislocation and painful joints are possible sequels. (Redrawn from *Journal of Bone and Joint Surgery* vol. 25B, p. 704, by courtesy of Miss R. Wynne-Davies, and the Editor.)

Persistent generalized joint hypermobility occurs in about 5% of normal people and is inherited as a simple mendelian dominant. The knees and elbows can be hyperextended, and the hands and feet can attain unusual positions. Such hypermobile joints are not necessarily unstable – as witness the controlled performances of acrobats and the legendary skill of Paganini – but they do have a tendency to recurrent dislocation (e.g. of the shoulder or patella). They also have a tendency to unexplained joint pains (arthralgia). There is, however, no convincing evidence that hypermobility by itself predisposes to degenerative arthritis; only if the joint becomes unstable is this likely to develop.

Generalized hypermobility is not usually associated with any obvious disease; but severe laxity is a feature of certain rare connective tissue disorders such as Marfan's syndrome, Ehlers–Danlos syndrome, Larsen's disease and osteogenesis imperfecta.

Neurological examination

If the symptoms include weakness or incoordination or a change in sensibility, or if they point to any disorder of the neck or back, a complete neurological examination of the related part is mandatory.

Once again we follow a systematic routine, first looking at the *general appearance*, then assessing *motor function* (muscle tone, power and reflexes) and finally testing for *sensory function* (both skin sensibility and deep sensibility).

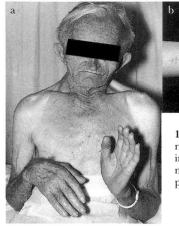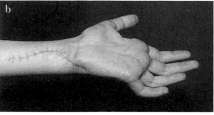

1.12 Deformities   (a) The drop wrist of a radial nerve palsy due to carcinomatous infiltration of the supraclavicular lymph nodes. (b) The claw hand of an ulnar nerve palsy.

Appearance

Some neurological disorders result in postures that are so characteristic as to be diagnostic at a glance: the claw hand of an ulnar nerve lesion; drop wrist following radial nerve palsy; or the 'waiter's tip' deformity of the arm in brachial plexus injury. Usually, however, it is when the patient moves that we can best appreciate the type and extent of motor disorder: the dangling arm following a brachial plexus injury; the flail lower limb of poliomyelitis; the symmetrical paralysis of spinal cord lesions; the characteristic drop-foot gait following sciatic or peroneal nerve damage; and the jerky, 'spastic' movements of cerebral palsy.

Concentrating on the affected part, we look for trophic changes that signify loss of sensibility: the smooth, hairless skin that seems to be stretched too tight; atrophy of the fingertips and the nails; scars that tell of accidental burns; and ulcers that refuse to heal. Muscle wasting is important; if localized and asymmetrical, it may suggest dysfunction of a specific motor nerve.

Tone and power

Tone in individual muscle groups is tested by moving the nearby joint to stretch the muscle. Increased tone (spasticity) is characteristic of

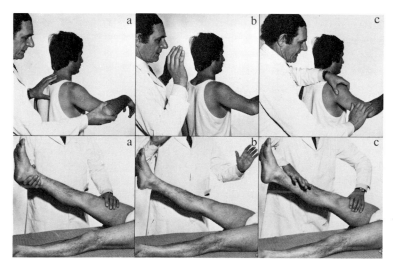

1.13 Testing muscle power The sequence is always the same, no matter whether the deltoid, quadriceps or any other muscle is being examined. (a) 'Let me lift it.' (b) 'Hold it there.' (c) 'Keep it there.'

upper motor neuron disorders such as cerebral palsy and stroke. It must not be confused with rigidity (the 'lead-pipe' or 'cogwheel' effect) which is seen in Parkinson's disease. Decreased tone (flaccidity) is found in lower motor neuron lesions; for example, poliomyelitis. Muscle power is diminished in all three states; it is important to recognize that a 'spastic' muscle may still be weak.

Testing for power is not as easy as it sounds; few patients have studied anatomy, and we must make ourselves understood. The easiest way is shown in Fig. 1.13. The sequence is important: you place the limb – he holds it – you try to force movement, asking him to resist while you feel the muscle. The normal limb is examined first, then the affected limb and the two are compared. Finer muscle actions, such as those of the thumb and fingers, may be reproduced by first demonstrating the movement yourself, then testing it in the unaffected limb, and then in the affected one. We may learn even more about composite movements by asking the patient to perform specific tasks, such as holding a pen or gripping a rod.

Muscle power is usually graded on the Medical Research Council scale:

Grade 0 – no movement
Grade 1 – only a flicker of movement
Grade 2 – movement with gravity eliminated
Grade 3 – movement against gravity
Grade 4 – movement against resistance
Grade 5 – normal power

It is important to recognize that muscle weakness may be due to muscle disease rather than nerve disease. In muscle disorders the weakness is usually symmetrical and sensation is normal.

Tendon reflexes

A deep tendon reflex is elicited by rapidly stretching the tendon near its insertion. A sharp tap with the tendon hammer does this well; but all too often this is performed with a flourish and with such force that the finer gradations of response are missed. It is better to employ a series of taps, starting with the most forceful and reducing the force with each successive tap until there is no response. Comparing the two

sides in this way, we can pick up fine differences showing that a reflex is 'diminished' rather than 'absent'. In the upper limb we test biceps, triceps and supinator and in the lower limb the patellar and Achilles tendons.

The tendon reflexes are monosynaptic segmental reflexes; that is, the reflex pathway takes a 'short cut' through the spinal cord at the segmental level. Depression or absence of the reflex signifies interruption of the pathway at the posterior nerve root, the anterior horn cell, the motor nerve root or the peripheral nerve. It is a reliable pointer to the segmental level of dysfunction: thus, a depressed biceps jerk suggests pressure on the fifth or sixth cervical (C5 or 6) nerve roots while a depressed ankle jerk signifies a similar abnormality at the first sacral level (S1). An unusually brisk reflex, on the other hand, is characteristic of an upper motor neuron disorder (e.g. cerebral palsy, a stroke or injury to the spinal cord); the lower motor neuron is released from the normal central inhibition and there is an exaggerated response to tendon stimulation. This may manifest as *ankle clonus*: a sharp upward jerk on the foot (dorsiflexion) causes a repetitive, 'clonic' movement of the foot; similarly, a sharp downward push on the patella may elicit patellar clonus.

Superficial reflexes

The superficial reflexes are elicited by stroking the skin at various sites to produce a specific muscle contraction; the best known are the abdominal (T7-T12), cremasteric (L1, 2) and anal (S4, 5) reflexes. These are corticospinal (upper motor neuron) reflexes. Absence of the reflex indicates an upper motor neuron lesion (usually in the spinal cord) above that level.

The plantar reflex

Forceful stroking of the sole normally produces flexion of the toes (or no response at all). An extensor response (the big toe extends while the others remain in flexion) is characteristic of upper motor neuron disorders. This is the Babinski sign – a type of withdrawal reflex which is present in young infants and normally disappears after the age of 18 months.

Sensibility

Sensibility to touch and to pinprick may be increased (*hyperaesthesia*) in certain irritative nerve lesions. More often, though, it is diminished (*hypoaesthesia*) or absent (*anaesthesia*), signifying pressure on or interruption of a peripheral nerve, a nerve root or the sensory pathways in the spinal cord. The area of sensory change can be mapped out on the skin and compared with the known segmental or dermatomal pattern of innervation. If the abnormality is well defined it is an easy matter to establish the level of the lesion, even if the precise cause remains unknown.

Brisk percussion along the course of an injured nerve may elicit a tingling sensation in the distal distribution of the nerve (*Tinel's sign*). The point of hypersensitivity marks the site of abnormal nerve sprouting: if it progresses distally at successive visits this signifies regeneration; if it remains unchanged this suggests a local neuroma.

Tests for *temperature recognition* and *two-point discrimination* (the ability to recognize two touch-points a few millimetres apart) are sometimes used in the assessment of peripheral nerve injuries.

Deep sensibility can be examined in several ways. In the *vibration test* a sounded tuning-fork is placed over a peripheral bony point (e.g. the medial malleolus or the head of the ulna); the patient is asked if he can feel the vibrations and to say when they disappear. By comparing the two sides, differences can be noted. *Position sense* is tested by asking the patient to find certain points on the body with the eyes closed – for example, touching the tip of the nose with the forefinger. The *sense of joint posture* is tested by grasping the big toe and placing it in different positions of flexion and extension. The patient is asked to say whether it is 'up' or 'down'. *Stereognosis*, the ability to recognize shape and texture by feel alone, is tested by giving the patient (whose eyes are closed) a variety of familiar objects to hold and asking him to name each object.

The pathways for deep sensibility run in the posterior columns of the spinal cord. Disturbances are, therefore, found in peripheral neuropathies and in spinal cord lesions such as posterior column injuries or tabes dorsalis. The *sense of balance* is also carried in the posterior columns. This can be tested by asking the patient to stand upright with his eyes closed; excessive body sway is abnormal (Romberg's sign).

Cortical and cerebellar function

A staggering gait may imply an unstable knee – or a disorder of the spinal cord or cerebellum. If there is no musculoskeletal abnormality to account for the sign, a full examination of the central nervous system will be necessary.

Diagnostic imaging

The map is not the territory
Alfred Korzybski

Plain film radiography

Plain film x-ray examination is almost 100 years old. Notwithstanding the extraordinary technical advances of the last few decades, it remains the most useful method of diagnostic imaging. Whereas other methods may define an inaccessible anatomical structure more accurately, or may reveal some localized tissue change, the plain film provides information simultaneously on the size, shape, tissue 'density' and bone architecture – characteristics which, taken together, will usually suggest a diagnosis, or at least a range of possible diagnoses.

How to read an x-ray

The process of reading x-ray films should be as methodical as clinical examination. It is seductively easy to be led astray by some flagrant anomaly; systematic study is the only safeguard. A convenient sequence for examination is: *patient – soft tissues – bone – joint – diagnostic associations*; but before starting it is important to stand well back from the viewing screen – proximity breeds tunnel vision.

The patient

Make sure that the name on the film is that of your patient; mistaken identity is a potent source of error. Then try to 'look through' the film and to visualize the living person, especially the age, build and sex.

The soft tissues

Unless examined early, these are liable to be forgotten. Look for variations in shape and variations of density.

SHAPE   Muscle planes are often visible and may reveal wasting or swelling. Bulging outlines around a hip, for example, may suggest a joint effusion; and soft-tissue swelling around interphalangeal joints may be the first radiographic sign of rheumatoid arthritis.

DENSITY   Increased density in the soft tissues follows calcification in a tendon, a blood vessel, a haematoma or an abscess; often the shape and site suggest which is involved. The radiographic density of a metallic foreign body is, of course, unmistakable; but even wood or glass may show in suitable films. Slight variations are often seen best by viewing the film tangentially. The

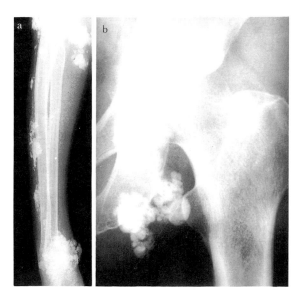

1.14 Calcification in soft tissues   (a) In dermatomyositis. (b) In a bursa.

precise localization of foreign bodies necessitates multiple views.

Decreased density of soft tissues is due either to fat (the most radiolucent tissue) or to gas. The recognition of gas bubbles may be crucial in the early diagnosis of gas gangrene.

The bones

When studying the bones and joints, establish a search pattern based on the local anatomy. Thus, for the spine, look at the overall vertebral alignment, then at the disc spaces, and then at each vertebra separately, moving from the body to the pedicles, the facet joints and finally the spinous appendages. For the pelvis, see if the shape is symmetrical with the bones in their normal positions, then look at the sacrum, the two innominate bones, the pubic rami and the ischial tuberosities, then the femoral heads and the upper ends of the femora, always comparing the two sides.

Throughout this search we record abnormalities of shape, 'density' and architecture (internal structure). The bone as a whole may be bent, or it may be unduly wide – as in Paget's disease. A localized deformity or swelling may be due to bulging from within (a cyst or other radiolucent lesion) or to excessive new bone formation (perhaps a tumour). Examine carefully *the periosteal surface* (periosteal new bone is characteristic of infection, fracture or malignancy), the *cortex* (for evidence of destruction) and the *endosteum* (is it sharp and clear, or fuzzy and excavated?). Note whether the 'density' is increased (sclerosis) or diminished (osteoporosis or replacement by abnormal tissue). The trabecular structure is usually visible: is it regular? is it disarranged? or even absent? Remember that 'vacant areas' are not necessarily cysts; any tissue that is radiolucent looks 'cystic'.

The joint

The radiographic 'joint' consists of the articulating bones and the 'space' between them. The 'joint space' is, of course, illusory; it is occupied by a film of synovial fluid plus radiolucent articular cartilage which varies in thickness from 1 mm or less (the carpal joints) to 6–8 mm (the knee). It looks much wider in children than in adults because much of the epiphysis is still cartilaginous and therefore radiolucent.

Note the general orientation of the joint and the congruity of the bone ends (the sub-articular bone plates), if necessary comparing the abnormal with the normal opposite side. Then look for narrowing or asymmetry of the

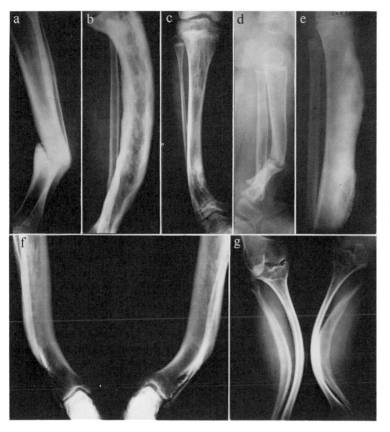

1.15 Bent tibiae Unilateral: (a) mal-united fracture; (b) Paget's disease; (c) dyschondroplasia; (d) congenital pseud-arthrosis; (e) syphilitic sabre tibia.

Bilateral: (f) old rickets; (g) osteogenesis imperfecta.

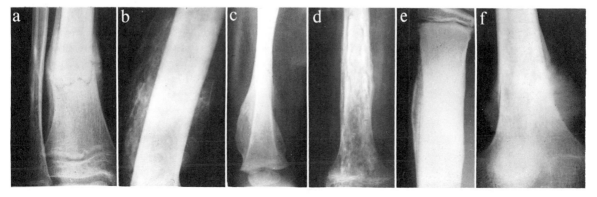

1.16 'Visible periosteum' Ossification just outside the cortex is seen when periosteum has been lifted away from the bone. It may have been lifted by blood, as in (a) callus, (b) myositis ossificans and (c) scurvy; or by inflammatory material, as in (d) chronic osteomyelitis and (e) syphilitic periostitis; or by tumour material, as in (f) osteosarcoma.

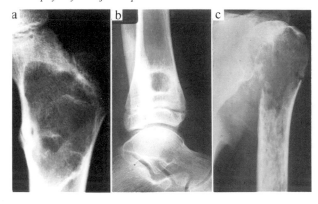

1.17 Rare areas in bone   This may represent a true cyst (a), but any radiolucent lesion can look 'cystic' – as with the abscess in (b) and the metastatic tumour in (c).

joint 'space', which could signify loss of articular cartilage thickness – a classic sign of arthritis. Further stages of joint destruction are revealed by interruption of the subarticular bone plates and radiolucent bone cysts or periarticular erosions. Bony outgrowths from the joint margins (osteophytes) are typical of osteoarthritis.

Lines of increased density within the articular space may be due to calcification of the cartilage or menisci (chondrocalcinosis). Loose bodies, if they are radio-opaque, appear as rounded or irregular patches overlying the normal structures.

Diagnostic associations

However carefully the individual x-ray features are observed, the diagnosis will not leap ready-made off the x-ray plate. Even a fracture is not always obvious. It is the pattern of abnormalities that counts: if you see one feature that is suggestive, look for others that are commonly associated. Narrowing of the joint space + subarticular cysts + osteophytes = osteoarthritis. Narrowing of the joint space + osteoporosis + periarticular erosions = inflammatory arthritis. Bone destruction + periosteal new-bone formation = infection or malignancy until proven otherwise.

The search for associated abnormalities, or clarification of some poorly observed feature in the plain film, may call for further examination by one of the other imaging techniques.

X-rays using contrast media

Substances that alter x-ray attenuation characteristics can be used to produce images which contrast with those of the normal tissues. The contrast media used in orthopaedics are mostly iodine-based liquids which can be injected into

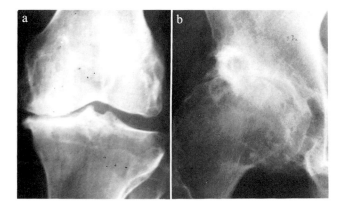

1.18 Joint x-rays   (a) The lateral compartment of this knee is normal; in the medial compartment some articular cartilage has worn away and the joint 'space' is therefore reduced. (b) In this osteoarthritic hip the superior joint space is virtually obliterated and there are subarticular cysts.

sinuses, joint cavities or the spinal theca. Air or gas also can be injected into joints to produce a 'negative image' outlining the joint cavity.

Oily iodides are not absorbed and maintain maximum concentration after injection. However, because they are non-miscible, they do not penetrate well into all the nooks and crannies. They are also tissue irritants, especially if used intrathecally. Ionic, water-soluble iodides permit much more detailed imaging and, although also somewhat irritant and neurotoxic, are rapidly absorbed and excreted. Metrizamide, a non-ionic iodide, is the least toxic and least irritant.

SINOGRAPHY

Sinography is the simplest form of contrast radiography. The medium (usually one of the ionic water-soluble compounds) is injected into an open sinus; the film shows the track and whether or not it leads to the underlying bone or joint.

ARTHROGRAPHY

Arthrography is a particularly useful form of contrast radiography. Intra-articular loose bodies will produce filling defects in the opaque contrast medium. In the knee, torn menisci, ligament tears and capsular ruptures can be shown. In children's hips, arthrography is a useful method of outlining the cartilaginous (and therefore radiolucent) femoral head. In adults with avascular necrosis of the femoral head, arthrography may show up torn flaps of cartilage. After hip replacement, loosening of a prosthesis may be revealed by seepage of the contrast medium into the cement/bone interface. In the ankle, wrist and shoulder, extrusion of the injected contrast medium may disclose tears in the capsular structures. In the spine, contrast radiography can be used to diagnose disc degeneration (discography) and abnormalities of the small facet joints (facetography).

MYELOGRAPHY

Myelography was used extensively in the past for the diagnosis of disc prolapse and other spinal canal lesions. It has been largely replaced by non-invasive methods such as computed tomography (CT) and magnetic resonance imaging (MRI). However, it is still indicated for the investigation of cervical nerve root lesions and as an adjunct to other methods in patients with back pain.

The oily media are no longer used, and even with the ionic water-soluble iodides there is a considerable incidence of complications, such as low-pressure headache (due to the lumbar puncture), muscular spasms or convulsions (due to neurotoxicity, especially if the chemical is allowed to flow above the mid-dorsal region) and arachnoiditis (which is attributed to the

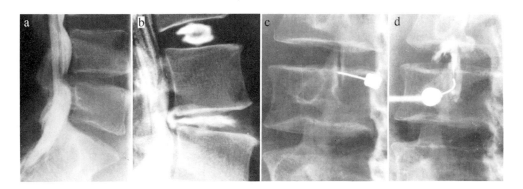

1.19 Contrast radiography (a) Myelography outlines the spinal theca; the contrast medium has been indented by a bulging disc. (b) Contrast material can be injected into the disc itself; in this discogram the upper disc is normal, but the lower is degenerate, allowing injected material to escape. (c) Under x-ray control a needle can be inserted into the small facet joints; (d) this facetogram shows escape of contrast material from an abnormal joint (the injection reproduced the patient's pain).

hyperosmolality of these compounds in relation to cerebrospinal fluid). Precautions, such as keeping the patient sitting upright after myelography, must be strictly observed.

Metrizamide has low neurotoxicity and at working concentrations it is more or less isotonic with cerebrospinal fluid. It can therefore be used throughout the length of the spinal canal; the nerve roots are also well delineated (radiculography). A bulging disc, an intrathecal tumour or narrowing of the bony canal will produce characteristic distortions of the opaque column in the myelogram.

Xeroradiography

Xeroradiography uses conventional x-ray exposure, but the recording plate registers the activity as an electric charge density pattern which is then transferred to plastic-coated paper as a 'positive' image. Its advantage over plain x-ray negatives is that the photoelectric process is particularly sensitive to changes in tissue density (the 'edge effect'); also, fuzzy outlines (e.g. subperiosteal erosions or faint soft-tissue calcification) are more easily displayed. Some soft-tissue shadows show well and the early stages of cartilage calcification (chondrocalcinosis) appear before they are visible on plain x-rays.

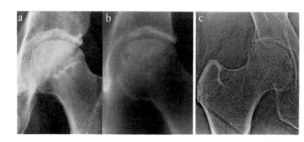

1.20 Tomography and xeroradiography (a) The plain x-ray of this hip shows only doubtful increase in density, suggestive of avascular necrosis; but (b) the tomograph confirms the diagnosis and clearly demonstrates the triangular segment. (c) Xeroradiography, as in this patient, is often the best way to show calcification of articular cartilage (chondrocalcinosis).

Tomography

Tomography provides an image 'focused' on a selected plane. By moving the tube and the x-ray film in opposite directions on an imaginary pivot during the exposure, images on either side of the pivotal plane are deliberately blurred out. When several 'cuts' are studied, lesions obscured in conventional x-rays may be revealed. The method is useful for diagnosing segmental bone necrosis and depressed fractures in cancellous bone (e.g. of the vertebral body or the tibial plateau); these defects are often obscured in the plain x-ray by the surrounding intact mass of bone. Small radiolucent lesions, such as osteoid osteomas and bone abscesses, can also be revealed.

A good standby in former years, conventional tomography has been largely supplanted by computed tomography.

Computed tomography (CT)

Like simple tomography, CT produces 'cutting' images through selected tissue planes – but with much greater resolution. A further advance over conventional tomography is that the images are transaxial (like transverse anatomical sections), thus exposing anatomical planes that are never viewed in plain film x-rays. A general (or 'localization') view is obtained, the region of interest is selected and a series of cross-sectional images is produced. Slices through the larger joints or tissue masses may be 5–10 mm apart; those through the small joints or intervertebral discs have to be much thinner.

Because it achieves such excellent contrast resolution, CT is able to display the size and shape of bone and soft-tissue masses in transverse planes. This makes it particularly useful in the assessment of tumour size and spread, even if it is unable to characterize the tumour type. Other common applications are in the diagnosis of spinal disorders (especially intervertebral disc prolapse), joint abnormalities and pelvic lesions. It is invaluable – sometimes indispensable – in the assessment of complex fractures, or indeed any fractures in sites not normally accessible to plain x-rays (e.g. verte-

Magnetic resonance imaging (MRI)

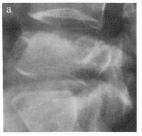
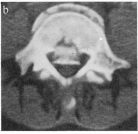

1.21 Computed tomography   The plain x-ray (a) shows a fracture of the vertebral body, but one cannot tell precisely how the bone fragments are displaced. The computed tomograph (b) shows clearly that they are dangerously close to the cauda equina.

Unlike x-ray imaging, MRI relies upon radio-frequency emissions from atoms and molecules in tissues exposed to a static magnetic field. The images produced by these signals are similar to those of CT scans, but with even better contrast resolution and more refined differentiation of tissues. Moreover, the sectional images can be obtained in almost any plane, and can be reconstituted to give a three-dimensional picture, thus adding even further to the information available.

All atomic nuclei with an odd number of protons possess the property of magnetic resonance, but, because it is so abundant in human tissues and so easily detectable, the hydrogen nucleus is the one currently employed for MR imaging. The intensity of the MR signal depends partly on the density of hydrogen nuclei in the tissue scanned and partly on the spin characteristics and relaxation rates following proton excitation. This phenomenon of relaxation is defined by two independent time constants, T_1 and T_2, thus giving rise to two simultaneous signals.

bral bodies, tibial condyles, tarsal and carpal bones, and the sacroiliac joints), and the detection of intra-articular bone fragments.

The value of CT can be extended in several ways. Intravascular, intra-articular or intrathecal contrast media can be used to highlight blood vessels or cavity outlines and show their relationship to adjacent masses. With suitable equipment transaxial images can be reconstructed to give sagittal or coronal images, or even three-dimensional images of bones with complicated shapes, like the vertebrae. CT is also used to assess bone density in selected sites, although this is now better achieved by other techniques.

Tissues containing abundant hydrogen (fat, cancellous bone and marrow) emit high-intensity signals and produce the brightest images; those containing little hydrogen (cortical bone, ligament, tendon and air) appear black; intermediate in the grey scale are cartilage, spinal canal and muscle. In producing the

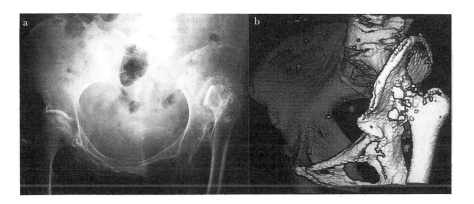

1.22 Reconstructed CT images   (a) The plain x-ray shows an old untreated congenital dislocation on the left. (b) The three-dimensional image reveals just how far the femoral head is from the anatomical socket, information that is important in planning hip surgery.

1.23 MRI   (a, b) T_1-weighted and (c) STIR (short tau inversion recovery) sequences of the torso and thigh areas, showing the contrasting definition and brightness of the various structures and tissues.

images, either the T_1 or the T_2 characteristics of the tissue may be enhanced or 'weighted' to give complementary information. The T_1-weighted images show greater definition and provide almost 'anatomical' pictures; the T_2-weighted images tell more about the physiological characteristics of the tissue. Other pulse sequences often used are proton density and short tau inversion recovery (STIR), which suppresses the signal from fat and increases the contrast for water-containing tissues.

By selecting the most appropriate anatomical plane, coil type, slice thickness, magnification and pulse sequence, different tissues and organs can be displayed with extraordinary clarity. Bone tumours can be shown in their transverse and longitudinal extent, and extraosseous spread can be accurately assessed. Moreover, there is the potential for characterizing the actual tissue, thus allowing a pathological as well as an anatomical diagnosis.

Other areas of usefulness are in the early diagnosis of bone ischaemia and necrosis, the investigation of backache and spinal disorders, and the elucidation of cartilage and soft-tissue injuries. Because MRI is so versatile, and free of the risks of ionizing radiation, it is tempting to overindulge its use. It is well to remember that it is still only one diagnostic method among many.

Diagnostic ultrasound

High-frequency sound waves, generated by a transducer, can penetrate several centimetres into the soft tissues; as they pass through the tissue interfaces some of these waves are reflected back (like echoes) to the transducer, where they are registered as electrical signals and displayed as images on a screen or plate. With modern equipment, tissues of varying density can be 'imaged' in gradations of grey that allow reasonable definition of the anatomy. Real-time display on a monitor gives a dynamic image, which is more useful than the usual static images on transparent plates. One big advantage of this technique is that the equipment is simple and portable and can be used almost anywhere. Another is that it produces no harmful side effects.

Depending on their structure, different tissues are referred to as highly echogenic, mildly echogenic or echo-free. Fluid-filled cysts are echo-free; fat is highly echogenic; and semi-solid organs manifest varying degrees of 'echogenicity' which permits their spatial identification.

Because of the marked echogenic contrast between cystic and solid masses, ultrasonography is particularly useful for identifying hidden 'cystic' lesions such as haematomas, abs-

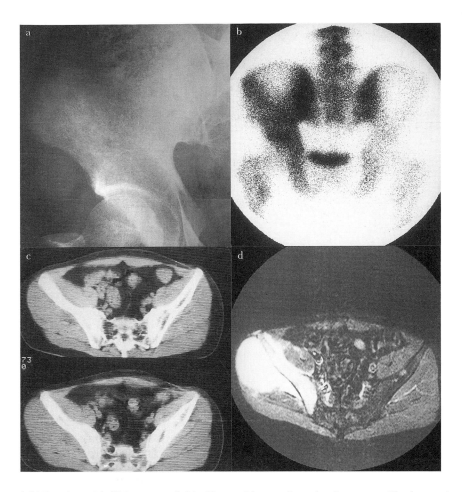

1.24 Imaging   (a) Plain x-rays of this 40-year-old man showed only non-specific destructive changes in the right innominate bone. (b) The radioisotope scan revealed diffuse activity throughout the ilium and also in the ischium. (c) CT studies added further information: there is increased bulk in the glutei and the iliacus. (d) The MRI (STIR sequence) shows the full extent of the lesion – a large tumour involving the whole of the iliac blade with soft-tissue masses in the glutei and iliacus. Note also the metastatic deposit in the opposite iliac blade. Biopsy revealed a non-Hodgkin's lymphoma.

cesses, popliteal cysts and arterial aneurysms. It is also capable of detecting intra-articular fluid and may be used to diagnose a synovial effusion or to monitor the progress of an 'irritable hip'. More recently it has come into its own as a means of screening newborn babies for congenital dislocation (or dysplasia) of the hip; the cartilaginous femoral head and the acetabular labrum can be clearly identified, and their relationship to each other shows whether the hip is normal or abnormal. Ultrasound has also been used to diagnose rotator cuff tears of the shoulder, though the interpretation of these images can be difficult.

Radionuclide imaging

Photon emission by radionuclides taken up in specific tissues can be recorded by either a simple rectilinear scanner or a gamma camera, to produce an image which reflects current

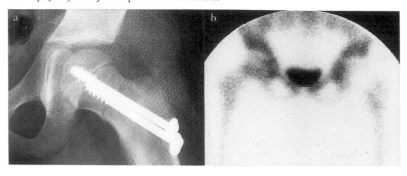

1.25 Radionuclide imaging (a) This fractured femoral neck in a child has resulted in loss of the blood supply, as shown by (b) the void in the left hip on the technetium scan.

activity in that tissue or organ. The ideal isotope for this purpose is technetium-99m (^{99m}Tc): it has the appropriate energy characteristics for gamma-camera imaging, it has a relatively short half-life (6 hours) and it is rapidly excreted. The low background activity means that any site of increased uptake is readily visible. When ^{99m}Tc is linked to a bone-seeking phosphate compound, it is selectively concentrated in skeletal tissues.

Bone-seeking isotopes

In current practice, technetium-labelled hydroxymethylene diphosphosphonate (^{99m}Tc-HDP) is injected intravenously and its activity is recorded at two stages: (1) shortly after injection, while it is still in the blood stream or the perivascular space (the *perfusion* or *bloodpool phase*), and (2) 3 hours later when the isotope has been taken up in bone (the *bone phase*). Normally, in the early perfusion phase the vascular soft tissues around the joints produce the darkest (most active) image; 3 hours later this activity has faded and the bone outlines are shown more clearly, the greatest activity appearing in the cancellous tissue at the ends of the long bones.

Changes in radioactivity are most significant when they are sharply localized or asymmetrical. Four types of abnormality are seen, described below.

Increased activity in the perfusion phase, due to increased soft-tissue blood flow – one of the cardinal features of inflammation (e.g. acute or chronic synovitis).

Decreased activity in the perfusion phase This is much less common and signifies local vascular insufficiency.

Increased activity in the bone phase This could be due either to excessive isotope uptake in the osseous extracellular fluid or to more avid incorporation into newly forming bone tissue; either would be likely in a fracture, infection, a local tumour or healing after necrosis, and nothing in the bone scan itself distinguishes between these conditions.

Diminished activity in the bone phase is due to an absent blood supply (e.g. in the femoral head after a fracture of the femoral neck) or to replacement of bone by pathological tissue.

The clinical applications are manifold and include: (1) the diagnosis of stress fractures (or other undisplaced fractures) that do not appear on the plain x-ray; (2) the detection of a small bone abscess, or an osteoid osteoma; (3) the investigation of loosening or infection around prostheses; (4) the diagnosis of femoral head ischaemia in Perthes' disease or avascular necrosis in adults; (5) the early detection of bone metastases. The scintigraphic appearances in these conditions are described in the relevant chapters. In most cases the isotope scan serves chiefly to pinpoint the site of abnormality and it should always be read in conjunction with other modes of imaging.

Other radionuclide compounds

Technetium-labelled sulphur colloid (^{99m}Tc-S$_c$) is taken up by phagocytes in the reticuloendothelial system and is therefore a better indicator of marrow vascularity than the bone-seeking compounds. Its use may permit early diagnosis of femoral head ischaemia, but the method is not sensitive enough to justify its routine use in hip fractures or suspected femoral head necrosis.

Gallium-67 (^{67}Ga) concentrates in inflammatory cells and has been used to identify sites of hidden infection; for example, in the investigation of prosthetic loosening after joint replacement. However, it is arguable whether it gives any more reliable information than the ^{99m}Tc bone scan.

Indium-111-labelled leucocytes can also be used as markers for infection. Leucocytes from the patient's own blood are labelled with ^{111}In and then reinjected into the blood stream. Areas of increased activity show where they are concentrated.

Blood tests

Non-specific blood tests

Non-specific blood abnormalities are common in bone and joint disorders; their interpretation hinges on the clinical and x-ray findings.

Hypochromic anaemia is usual in rheumatoid arthritis; but it may also be a consequence of gastrointestinal bleeding due to the anti-inflammatory drugs.

Leucocytosis is generally associated with infection; but a mild leucocytosis is not uncommon in rheumatoid arthritis and during an attack of gout.

The *erythrocyte sedimentation rate* (ESR) is usually increased in acute and chronic inflammatory disorders and after tissue injury. However, patients with low-grade infection may have a normal ESR and this should not be taken as a reassuring sign. The ESR is strongly affected by the presence of monoclonal immunoglobulins; a high ESR is almost mandatory in the diagnosis of myelomatosis.

C-reactive protein (and other acute phase proteins) may be abnormally increased in chronic inflammatory arthritis and (temporarily) after injury. The test is often used to monitor the progress and activity of rheumatoid arthritis.

Plasma gamma-globulins can be measured by protein electrophoresis. Their precise characterization is helpful in the assessment of certain rheumatic disorders, and more particularly in the diagnosis of myelomatosis.

Rheumatoid factor tests

Rheumatoid factor is an autoantibody (or antiglobulin) which is often present in patients with rheumatoid arthritis (RA). However, it is not diagnostic of RA and some patients remain 'seronegative'. Rheumatoid factor is also absent in patients with ankylosing spondylitis, Reiter's disease or psoriatic arthritis; these disorders have been grouped together as the 'seronegative spondarthritides'.

Tissue typing

HLA antigens can be detected in white blood cells and they are used to characterize individual tissue types. The seronegative spondarthritides are closely associated with the presence of HLA-B27 on chromosome 6; this is frequently used as a confirmatory test in patients suspected of having ankylosing spondylitis or Reiter's disease, but it should not be regarded as a specific test because it is positive in about 8% of normal Caucasians.

Biochemistry

Biochemical tests are essential in monitoring patients after any serious injury. They are also used routinely in the investigation of rheumatic disorders and abnormalities of bone metabolism. Their significance is discussed under the relevant conditions.

Synovial fluid analysis

Arthrocentesis is a much-neglected diagnostic procedure; given the correct indications it can often yield valuable information. It should always be considered in the following conditions.

Acute joint swelling after injury The distinction between synovitis and bleeding may not be obvious; aspiration will settle the question immediately.

Suspected infection Careful examination and laboratory investigations may provide the answer, but they take time. Aspiration is essential for early diagnosis.

Acute synovitis in adults Synovial fluid analysis may be the only way to distinguish between infection, gout and pseudogout.

Chronic synovitis Here joint aspiration is less urgent, and is only one of many diagnostic procedures in the investigation of suspected tuberculosis or atypical rheumatic disorders.

Technique

The joint should be aspirated under strict aseptic conditions. Even a small quantity of fluid (less than 0.5 ml) is enough for diagnostic analysis.

Gross examination

The volume of fluid and its appearance are immediately noted. Normal synovial fluid is clear and slightly yellow. A cloudy or turbid fluid is due to the presence of cells, usually a sign of inflammation. Blood-stained fluid may be found after injury, but is also seen in acute inflammatory disorders and in pigmented villonodular synovitis.

Microscopic examination

A single drop of fresh synovial fluid is placed on a glass slide and examined through the microscope. Blood cells are easily identified; abundant leucocytes may suggest infection. Crystals may be seen, though this usually requires a careful search; they are better characterized by polarized light microscopy (see Fig. 4.3).

Dry smears are prepared with heparinized fluid; more concentrated specimens can be obtained if the fluid is centrifuged. After suitable staining (Wright's and Gram's), the smear is examined for pus cells and organisms. Remember, though, that *negative findings do not exclude infection.*

Laboratory tests

If enough fluid is available, it is sent for full laboratory investigation (cells, biochemistry and bacteriological culture). A simultaneous blood specimen allows comparison of synovial and blood glucose concentration; a marked reduction of synovial glucose suggests infection.

A high white cell count (more than $100\,000/mm^3$) is usually indicative of infection,

Table 1.1 Examination of synovial fluid

Suspected condition	Appearance	Viscosity	Cells	Crystals	Biochemistry	Bacteriology
Normal	Clear yellow	High	Few	–	As for plasma	–
Septic arthritis	Purulent	Low	White cells +++	–	Glucose low	+
Tuberculous arthritis	Turbid	Low	White cells +	–	Glucose low	+
Rheumatoid arthritis	Cloudy	Low	White cells ++	–	–	–
Gout	Cloudy	Normal	White cells ++	+ urate	–	–
Pseudogout	Cloudy	Normal	White cells +	+ pyrophosphate	–	–
Osteoarthritis	Clear yellow	High	Few	Often +	–	–

but a moderate leucocytosis is also seen in gout and other types of inflammatory arthritis.

Bacteriological culture and tests for antibiotic sensitivity are essential in any case of suspected infection.

Bone biopsy

Bone biopsy is often the crucial means of making a diagnosis or distinguishing between local conditions that closely resemble one another. Confusion is most likely to occur when the x-ray or MRI discloses an area of bone destruction that could be due to a compression fracture, to a destructive bone tumour or to infection (e.g. a collapsed vertebral body). In other cases it is obvious that the lesion is a tumour – but what type of tumour? Benign or malignant? Primary or metastatic? Radical surgery should never be undertaken for a suspected neoplasm without first confirming the diagnosis histologically – no matter how 'typical' or 'obvious' the x-ray appearances may be.

In bone infection, the biopsy permits not only histological proof of acute inflammation but also bacteriological typing of the organism and tests for antibiotic sensitivity.

The investigation of metabolic bone disease is, likewise, seldom complete without a biopsy to show (1) the type of abnormality (osteoporosis, osteomalacia, hyperparathyroidism) and (2) the severity of the disorder.

Open or closed?

Open biopsy, with exposure of the lesion and excision of a sizeable portion of the bone, seems preferable, but it has several drawbacks. (1) It requires an operation, with the attendant risks of anaesthesia and infection. (2) New tissue planes are opened up, predisposing to spread of infection or tumour. (3) The biopsy incision may jeopardize subsequent wide excision of the lesion. (4) The more inaccessible lesions (e.g. a tumour of the acetabular floor) can be reached only by dissecting widely through healthy tissue.

A carefully performed 'closed' biopsy, using a needle or trephine of appropriate size to ensure the removal of an adequate sample of tissue, is the procedure of choice except when the lesion cannot be accurately localized or when the tissue consistency is such that a sufficient sample cannot be obtained. Solid or semi-solid tissue is removed intact by the cutting needle or trephine; fluid material can be aspirated through the biopsy needle.

Precautions

The appropriate size of biopsy needle or cutting trephine should be selected. A soft tumour, or focus of infection, can be sampled with a comparatively thin needle (1–2 mm diameter); an iliac crest biopsy for histomorphometry in metabolic bone disease requires a trephine at least 5 mm in diameter.

The biopsy site and approach should be carefully planned with the aid of x-rays or other imaging techniques. Small bone-forming lesions (e.g. an osteoid osteoma) can be localized by giving an intravenous injection of ^{99m}TC-HDP 3 hours beforehand and then 'finding' the lesion with a sterilized radiation probe during open operation.

The procedure is carried out in an operating theatre, under anaesthesia (local or general) and with full aseptic techniques. For deep-seated lesions, fluoroscopic control of the needle insertion is essential.

It goes without saying that a knowledge of the local anatomy, and of the likely consistency of the lesion, is important. Large blood vessels and nerves must be avoided; potentially vascular tumours may bleed profusely and the means to control haemorrhage should be readily to hand. More than one surgeon has plunged a wide-bore needle into an aneurysm which he has mistaken for a soft-tissue tumour or an abscess!

Finally, the tissue obtained at the biopsy should be suitably processed. If infection is suspected, the material should go into a culture tube and be sent to the laboratory as soon as possible. A smear may also be useful. Whole tissue is transferred to a jar containing formalin, without damaging the specimen or losing any material. Aspirated blood should be allowed to clot and can then be preserved in formalin for later paraffin embedding and sectioning. Tissue thought to contain crystals should not be placed in formalin as this may destroy the crystals; it should either be kept unaltered for immediate examination or stored in saline.

No matter how careful the biopsy, there is always the risk that the tissue will be too scanty or too unrepresentative for accurate diagnosis. Close consultation with the radiologist and pathologist beforehand will minimize this possibility. In the best hands, needle biopsy has yielded an accuracy rate of over 94% (Murphy, Destouet and Gilula, 1981).

Arthroscopy

Arthroscopy is commonly performed for diagnostic and therapeutic reasons. Almost any joint can be reached but the procedure is most usefully employed in the knee, the shoulder and the wrist. It is a very useful method of diagnosing intra-articular pathology; moreover, if the lesion is amenable to surgery, this can often be carried out at the same time by a 'closed' operation. However, arthroscopy is an invasive procedure and its mastery requires skill and practice; it should not be used simply as an alternative to clinical examination and imaging.

Technique

The instrument is basically a rigid telescope fitted with fibreoptic illumination. Tube diameter ranges from about 2 mm (for small joints) to 4–5 mm (for the knee). It carries a lens system that gives a magnified image. The eyepiece allows direct viewing by the arthroscopist, but it is far more convenient to fit a small, sterilizable solid-state television camera which produces a picture of the joint interior on a television monitor.

The procedure is best carried out under general anaesthesia; this gives good muscle relaxation and permits manipulation and open-

ing of the joint compartments. The joint is distended with fluid and the arthroscope is introduced percutaneously. Various instruments (probes, curettes and forceps) can be inserted through other skin portals; they are used to help expose the less accessible parts of the joint, or to obtain biopsies for further examination. Guided by the image on the monitor, the arthroscopist explores the joint in a systematic fashion, manipulating the arthroscope with one hand and the probe or forceps with the other. At the end of the procedure the joint is washed out and the small skin wounds are sutured. The patient is usually able to return home later the same day.

Diagnosis

The appearance of the synovium and the articular surfaces usually allow differentiation between inflammatory and non-inflammatory, destructive and non-destructive lesions. In the knee joint, meniscal tears can be diagnosed and treated immediately by removal of partially detached segments; cruciate ligament deficiency is also clearly visible.

Arthroscopy of the shoulder is more difficult, but the articular surfaces and glenoid labrum can be adequately explored.

Arthroscopy of the wrist is useful for diagnosing a torn triradiate cartilage.

Complications

Diagnostic arthroscopy is safe but not entirely free of complications, the commonest of which are haemarthosis, thrombophlebitis, infection and joint stiffness.

Electrodiagnosis

Nerve and muscle function can be studied by various electrical methods. This information on physiological activity is invaluable in the diagnosis of neuromuscular disorders, but it must be used to supplement – not replace – the systematic clinical examination. Two types of investigation are employed: nerve conduction studies and electromyography.

Motor nerve conduction

Electrical stimulation of a motor nerve normally produces contraction of the muscles supplied by that nerve. The stimulus is applied to the skin over the nerve, and the motor unit response is measured by a concentric needle electrode inserted into the muscle; the electrical discharge, or *motor action potential* (MAP), is amplified and displayed on an oscilloscope.

The time interval between stimulation of the nerve and the appearance of the MAP is the *latency*. If the test is repeated at two points a measured distance apart along the nerve, and the latency values obtained are subtracted from one another, the conduction velocity between those two points can be determined. Normal values are about 40–60 metres per second (m/s).

Conduction velocity is slowed in peripheral nerve damage or compression, and the site of the lesion can be established by taking measurements in different segments of the nerve (e.g. in the diagnosis of nerve entrapment syndromes). With more severe demyelination, the amplitude of the MAP is also diminished.

If the nerve is completely divided, from the 14th day after injury there is no response to either faradic or galvanic stimulation of the nerve, and there is an abnormal response from galvanic stimulation of the muscle (the 'reaction of degeneration'). By plotting the strength of current against the duration of stimulus necessary to produce contraction, a *strength/duration curve* can be obtained, which reflects the degree of denervation and progressive changes in nerve function over time. Other lower motor neuron disorders produce characteristic changes in latency and motor action potentials.

Sensory nerve conduction

If a sensory nerve is stimulated distally, the *sensory nerve action potential* (SNAP) can be recorded at a proximal site. Here again, by measuring the distance between stimulating and recording electrodes, and the time lapse between stimulus and response, the sensory nerve conduction velocity can be calculated. In compression or entrapment of a mixed nerve, sensory conduction is often affected before motor conduction, so it is useful to measure both.

A special application of this test is in the recording of *somatosensory evoked potentials* (SEPs). Percutaneous electrical stimulation of a peripheral nerve (for convenience usually the median nerve at the wrist or the posterior tibial nerve at the ankle) produces a response that can be recorded by electrodes placed on the spinal cord, on the skin over one of the vertebrae or on the scalp over the cerebral cortex. This is useful in monitoring the integrity of the spinal cord during operative correction of severe spinal deformities. A significant fall in signal amplitude or an increase in latency is regarded as a sign of danger, and tension on the cord can be released before irreversible damage occurs.

The same principle is used in the diagnosis of sensory neuropathies such as Friedreich's ataxia, and in the investigation of brachial plexus injuries where the anatomy makes it impossible to carry out the more usual nerve conduction studies.

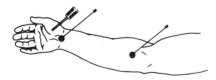

1.26 Electrodiagnosis Electrodes at different levels are used to stimulate the median nerve and one in the thenar muscle records contraction. If the distance between the electrodes is measured and the time interval (from stimulation to muscle contraction) is recorded, conduction velocity can be calculated.

Electromyography

Electromyography (EMG) does not involve electrical nerve stimulation. Instead, a concentric needle in the muscle is used to record motor unit activity at rest and when attempts are made to contract the muscle.

Normally there is no electrical activity at rest. However, spontaneous discharges may occur after partial or complete denervation, with pressure on spinal nerve roots, with anterior horn cell degeneration (e.g. in progressive muscular atrophy) and in various muscle disorders. This is thought to be due to increased sensitivity of the denervated (or abnormal) muscle fibres to circulating acetylcholine.

On voluntary muscle contraction, characteristic oscilloscope patterns appear. The number, shape, amplitude and duration of these action potentials make up a pattern that can distinguish between neuropathic and myopathic disorders. In myopathies the action potentials are smaller; in neuropathies they are abnormally large and extended. Mapping denervation activity in peripheral muscles can give important information on the exact levels of nerve and spinal cord lesions.

Interpretation and diagnosis

Electromyography is not a print-out of disease; it should always be considered in conjunction with clinical findings, x-ray, biochemical tests, nerve conduction studies and – if necessary – muscle biopsy before a diagnosis is reached. With the development of computer-assisted analysis, electrodiagnosis will have considerably wider application in the future.

References and further reading

Hoppenfeld, S. (1976) *Physical Examination of the Spine and Extremeties*, Appleton-Century-Crofts, Norwalk

Kimura, J. (1983) *Electrodiagnosis in Diseases of Nerve and Muscle: Principles and Practice*, F. A. Davis, Philadelphia

Murphy, W. A., Destouet, J. M. and Gilula, L. A. (1981) Percutaneous skeletal biopsy: a procedure for radiologists – results, review and recommendations. *Radiology* **139**, 545–549

Resnick, D. and Niwayama, G. (1988) *Diagnosis of Bone and Joint Disorders*, vol. 1, *Diagnostic Techniques*, 2nd edn, W. B. Saunders, Philadelphia

Watt, I. (1988) Musculoskeletal system. In *Nuclear Medicine: Applications to Surgery* (eds. E. R. Davies and W. E. G. Thomas), Castle House Publ., Tunbridge Wells, pp. 219–253

Infection

2

Infection may reach the bones and joints via the *blood stream* from a distant site, or by *direct invasion* from a skin puncture, operation or an open fracture. Depending on the type of organism, the site of infection and the host response, the result may be a pyogenic osteomyelitis or arthritis, a chronic granulomatous reaction (classically seen in tuberculosis), or an indolent response to an unusual organism (e.g. a fungal infection). Parasitic lesions such as hydatid disease also are considered in this chapter, although these are infestations rather than infections.

Acute haematogenous osteomyelitis

Acute osteomyelitis is almost invariably a disease of children. When adults are affected it may be because their resistance is lowered by debility, disease or drugs. An association with diabetes has long been recognized, whilst immunosuppression, either acquired or induced, is increasingly encountered as a predisposing factor. Trauma may determine the site of infection, possibly by causing a small haematoma or fluid collection in a bone.

The causal organism is usually *Staphylococcus aureus*, less often one of the other Gram-positive cocci, such as *Streptococcus pyogenes* or *S. pneumo-niae*. In children under 4 years of age the Gram-negative *Haemophilus influenzae* is a fairly common pathogen, the quoted incidence varying from 5 to 50%. Other Gram-negative organisms (e.g. *Escherichia coli*, *Pseudomonas aeruginosa*, *Proteus mirabilis* and the anaerobic *Bacteroides fragilis*) occasionally cause acute bone infection. Unusual organisms are more likely to be found in heroin addicts and as opportunistic pathogens in patients with compromised immune defence mechanisms. Curiously, patients with sickle-cell disease are prone to infection by *Salmonella*.

The blood stream is invaded, perhaps from a minor skin abrasion, a boil, a septic tooth or – in the newborn – from an infected umbilical cord. In adults the source of infection may be a urethral catheter, an indwelling arterial line or a dirty needle and syringe.

Organisms usually settle in the metaphysis, most often at the proximal end of the femur. This predilection for the metaphysis has been attributed to the peculiar arrangement of the blood vessels in that area: the non-anastomosing terminal branches of the nutrient artery twist back in hairpin loops before entering the large network of sinusoidal veins; the relative vascular stasis favours bacterial colonization. In young infants, in whom there is still a free anastomosis between metaphyseal and epiphyseal blood vessels, infection can just as easily lodge in the epiphysis. In adults, haematogenous infection is more common in the vertebrae than in the long bones.

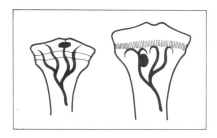

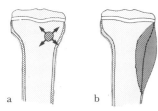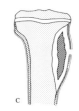

2.1 Acute osteomyelitis (1) In babies infection may settle near the very end of the bone; joint infection and growth disturbance easily follow. In children, metaphyseal infection is usual; the growth disc acts as a barrier to spread.

2.2 Acute osteomyelitis (2) (a) Infection in the metaphysis may spread towards the surface, to form a subperiosteal abscess (b). Some of the bone may die, and is encased in periosteal new bone as a sequestrum (c). The encasing involucrum is sometimes perforated by sinuses.

Pathology

The pathological picture varies considerably, depending on the patient's age, the site of infection, the virulence of the organism and the host response. However, underlying the variations there is a characteristic pattern marked by *inflammation, suppuration, necrosis, reactive new bone formation* and, ultimately, *resolution and healing.*

INFLAMMATION   The earliest change is an acute inflammatory reaction with vascular congestion, exudation of fluid and infiltration by polymorphonuclear leucocytes. The intraosseous pressure rises rapidly, causing intense pain, obstruction to blood flow and intravascular thrombosis. Even at an early stage the tissues are threatened by impending ischaemia.

SUPPURATION   By the second or third day, pus forms within the bone and forces its way along the Volkmann canals to the surface where it produces a subperiosteal abscess. From there the pus spreads along the shaft, to re-enter the bone at another level or burst into the surrounding soft tissues. In infants, infection often extends through the physis into the epiphysis and thence into the joint. In older children the physis is a barrier to direct spread but where the metaphysis is partly intracapsular (e.g. at the hip, shoulder or elbow) pus may discharge through the periosteum into the joint. In adults the abscess is more likely to spread within the medullary cavity. Vertebral infection may spread through the end-plate and the intervertebral disc into the adjacent vertebral body.

NECROSIS   The rising intraosseous pressure, vascular stasis, infective thrombosis and periosteal stripping increasingly compromise the blood supply; by the end of a week there is usually evidence of bone death. Bacterial toxins and leucocytic enzymes also may play their part in the advancing tissue destruction. In infants the growth disc is often irreparably damaged and the epiphysis may undergo avascular necrosis. With the gradual ingrowth of granulation tissue the boundary between dead and living bone becomes defined. Pieces of dead bone separate as sequestra varying in size from mere spicules to large necrotic segments. Macrophages and lymphocytes arrive in increasing numbers and the debris is slowly removed by a combination of phagocytosis and osteoclastic resorption. However, the larger sequestra remain entombed in cavities of bone, inaccessible to either final destruction or repair.

NEW BONE FORMATION   New bone forms from the deep layers of the stripped periosteum. This is typical of pyogenic infection and is usually obvious by the end of the second week. With time the new bone thickens to form an involucrum enclosing the infected tissue and sequestra. If the infection persists, pus may continue to discharge through perforations (cloacae) in the involucrum and track by sinuses to the skin surfaces; the condition is now established as a chronic osteomyelitis.

RESOLUTION   Once common, chronic osteomyelitis following on acute is nowadays seldom seen. If infection is controlled and intraosseous pressure released at an early stage, this dire progress can be aborted. The bone around the zone of infection is at first osteoporotic (probably due to hyperaemia). With healing, there is fibrosis and appositional new bone formation; this, together with the periosteal reaction, results in sclerosis and thickening of the bone. In some cases, remodelling may restore the normal contours; in others, though healing is sound, the bone is left permanently deformed.

Clinical features

The patient, *usually a child*, presents with severe pain, malaise and a fever; in neglected cases, toxaemia may be marked. The parents will have noticed that the child refuses to use one limb or to allow it to be handled or even touched. There may be a recent history of infection – a septic toe, a boil, a sore throat or a discharge from the ear.

Typically the child looks ill and feverish. The limb is held still and there is acute 'fingertip' tenderness near one of the larger joints. Even the gentlest manipulation is painful and joint movement is restricted. Local redness, swelling, warmth and oedema are later signs and signify that pus has escaped from the interior of the bone. Lymphadenopathy is common but non-specific. It is important to remember that all these features may be attenuated if antibiotics have been administered.

In infants, and especially in the newborn, the constitutional disturbance can be misleadingly mild; the baby simply fails to thrive and is drowsy but irritable. Suspicion should be aroused by a history of birth difficulties or umbilical artery catheterization. Metaphyseal tenderness and resistance to joint movement can signify either osteomyelitis or septic arthritis; indeed, both may be present, so the distinction hardly matters. Look for other sites – multiple infection is not uncommon.

In adults the commonest site of infection is the thoracolumbar spine. There may be a history of some urological procedure followed by a mild fever and backache. Local tenderness is not very marked and it may take weeks before x-ray signs appear; when they do appear the diagnosis may still need to be confirmed by fine-needle aspiration and bacteriological culture.

Other bones are occasionally involved, especially if there is a background of diabetes, malnutrition, drug addiction, immunosuppressive therapy or debility. In the very elderly, and in those with immune deficiency, systemic features are mild and the diagnosis is easily missed.

DIAGNOSTIC IMAGING During the first few days the plain x-ray shows no abnormality of the bone. Displacement of the fat planes signifies soft-tissue swelling, but this could as well be due to a haematoma or soft-tissue infection. By the end of the second week there may be periosteal new bone formation. This is the classic x-ray sign of pyogenic osteomyelitis, but treatment

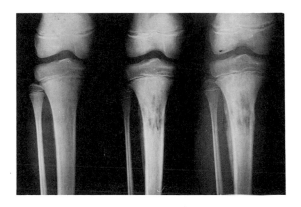

2.3 Acute osteomyelitis (3) The first x-ray, 2 days after symptoms began, is normal – it always is; metaphyseal mottling and periosteal changes were not obvious until the second film, taken 14 days later; eventually much of the shaft was involved.

ACUTE OSTEOMYELITIS

Pain
Fever   } Unless modified
Inflammation   by antibiotics
Acute tenderness
X-RAYS NORMAL DURING FIRST 10 DAYS

should not be delayed while waiting for it to appear. Later there is patchy rarefaction of the metaphysis, and later still the ragged appearance of bone destruction.

An important late sign is the combination of regional osteoporosis with a localized segment of apparently increased density (e.g. in the femoral head). Osteoporosis is a feature of metabolically active, and thus living, bone; the segment that fails to become osteoporotic is metabolically inactive and possibly dead.

Radioscintigraphy with ^{99m}Tc-HDP reveals increased activity in both the perfusion phase and the bone phase. This is a highly sensitive investigation, even in the very early stages, but it has relatively low specificity and other inflammatory lesions can show similar changes. In doubtful cases, scanning with ^{67}Ga-citrate or ^{111}In-labelled leucocytes may be more revealing.

MRI, which is able to distinguish between pus and blood, is particularly helpful in atypical cases.

INVESTIGATIONS   The most certain way to confirm the clinical diagnosis is to aspirate pus from the metaphyseal subperiosteal abscess or the adjacent joint. Even if no pus is found, a smear of the aspirate is examined immediately for cells and organisms; a simple Gram stain may help to identify the type of infection and assist with the initial choice of antibiotic. A sample is also sent for detailed bacteriological examination and tests for sensitivity to antibiotics.

The white cell count is usually high and the haemoglobin concentration diminished; the ESR is raised and often remains somewhat elevated even after the infection subsides. However, in the very young and the very old these tests are less reliable and may show values within the range of normal. Blood culture is positive in only about half the cases of proven infection.

Antistaphylococcal antibody titres may be raised. This test is most useful in atypical cases where the diagnosis is in doubt.

Osteomyelitis in an unusual site or with an unusual organism should alert one to the possibility of heroin addiction, deficient host defence mechanisms or sickle-cell disease. *Salmonella* may be cultured from the faeces.

Differential diagnosis

CELLULITIS   This is often mistaken for osteomyelitis. There is widespread superficial redness and lymphangitis. The source of skin infection may not be obvious and should be searched for (e.g. on the sole or between the toes).

ACUTE SUPPURATIVE ARTHRITIS   Tenderness is diffuse, and all movement at the joint is abolished by muscle spasm. In infants the distinction between osteomyelitis and septic arthritis is somewhat theoretical, as both usually coexist.

ACUTE RHEUMATISM   The pain tends to flit from one joint to another, and there may be carditis, rheumatic nodules or erythema marginatum.

SICKLE-CELL CRISIS   The patient may present with features indistinguishable from those of acute osteomyelitis. In areas where *Salmonella* is endemic it would be wise to treat such patients with suitable antibiotics until infection is definitely excluded.

GAUCHER'S DISEASE   Pseudo-osteitis may occur with features closely resembling osteomyelitis. The diagnosis is made by finding other stigmata of the disease, especially enlargement of the spleen and liver.

Treatment

There are four important aspects to the management of acute osteomyelitis: (1) supportive treatment for pain and dehydration; (2) splintage of the affected part; (3) antibiotic therapy; and (4) surgical drainage.

GENERAL SUPPORTIVE TREATMENT   The distressed child needs to be comforted and treated for pain. Analgesics should be given at repeated intervals without waiting for the patient to ask for them. Septicaemia and fever can cause severe dehydration and it may be necessary to give fluid intravenously.

SPLINTAGE   Some type of splintage is desirable, partly for comfort but also to prevent joint contractures. Simple skin traction may suffice and, if the hip is involved, this also helps to prevent dislocation. At other sites a plaster slab or half-cylinder may be used but it should not obscure the affected area.

ANTIBIOTICS Blood and, if possible, aspiration material are sent immediately for culture, but the prompt administration of antibiotics is so vital that treatment should not await the result. Initially the choice of antibiotics is based on the findings from direct examination of the pus smear and a 'best guess' at the most likely pathogen; a more appropriate drug can be substituted once the organism is identified and its antibiotic sensitivity is known. Factors such as the patient's age, general state of resistance, renal function, degree of toxaemia and previous history of allergy must be taken into account. The following recommendations are offered as a guide rather than a specific policy.

Older children and previously fit adults, who probably have a staphylococcal infection, are started on flucloxacillin and fusidic acid, intravenously for the first 3 or 4 days and then – once their condition begins to improve – orally for another 3–6 weeks. Fusidic acid is preferred to benzylpenicillin (1) because of the increasing prevalence of penicillin-resistant staphylococci and (2) because it is well concentrated in bone. However, for a streptococcal infection benzyl penicillin is probably better.

In children under 4 years (who have a high incidence of haemophilus infection) and in any case in which *Gram-negative organisms* are seen in the smear, it is advisable to start with one of the second-generation cephalosporins (cefuroxime or cephamandole). This is effective against both staphylococci and Gram-negative bacteria; it can be given intravenously or orally and reaches high concentrations in bone. A good alternative is amoxycillin combined with clavulanic acid (a β-lactamase inhibitor).

Patients with sickle-cell disease, who may have a salmonella infection, can be treated with either co-trimoxazole or amoxycillin combined with clavulanic acid.

Heroin addicts and immunocompromised patients often have unusual infections (e.g. pseudomonas, proteus or bacteroides). When the background is known, it is wise to start with one of the newer cephalosporins or with gentamicin and flucloxacillin.

DRAINAGE If antibiotics are given early, drainage is often unnecessary. However, if there are signs of deep pus (swelling, oedema, fluctuation), or if pyrexia, toxaemia and local tenderness fail to improve within 36 hours of starting antibiotic treatment, the abscess should be drained by open operation under general anaesthesia. If pus is found – and released – there is little to be gained by drilling into the medullary cavity. If there is no obvious abscess, it is reasonable to drill one or two holes into the bone; however, there is no evidence that widespread drilling has any advantage and it may do more harm than good. The wound is closed without a drain and the splint (or traction) is reapplied. At present about one-third of patients with confirmed osteomyelitis are likely to need an operation; adults with vertebral infection seldom do.

Once the signs of infection subside, movements are encouraged and the child is allowed to walk with the aid of crutches. Full weight-bearing is usually possible after 3–4 weeks.

Complications

A lethal outcome from septicaemia is nowadays extremely rare; with antibiotics the child nearly always recovers and the bone may return to normal. But morbidity is common, especially if treatment is delayed or the organism is insensitive to the chosen antibiotic.

METASTATIC INFECTION This is sometimes seen – generally in infants – and may involve other bones, joints, serous cavities, the brain or lung. In some cases the infection may be multifocal from the outset. It is easy to miss secondary sites of infection when attention is focused on one particular area; it is important to be alert to this complication and to examine the child all over and repeatedly.

SUPPURATIVE ARTHRITIS This may occur: (1) in very young children, in whom the growth disc is not an impenetrable barrier; (2) where the metaphysis is intracapsular, as in the upper femur; or (3) from metastatic infection. In infants it is so common as almost to be taken for granted, especially with osteomyelitis of the femoral neck. Ultrasound will help to demonstrate an effusion, but the definitive diagnosis is given by joint aspiration.

ALTERED BONE GROWTH   In infants, physeal damage may lead to arrest of growth and shortening of the bone. In older children, however, the bone occasionally grows too long because metaphyseal hyperaemia has stimulated the growth disc.

CHRONIC   OSTEOMYELITIS   Despite improved methods of diagnosis and treatment, acute osteomyelitis sometimes fails to resolve and the patient is left with a chronic infection and a draining sinus. This may be due to neglect but is also seen in debilitated patients and in those with compromised defence mechanisms.

Subacute haematogenous osteomyelitis

This condition is no longer rare, and in some countries the incidence is almost equal to that of acute osteomyelitis. Its relative mildness is presumably due to the organism being less virulent or the patient more resistant (or both). It is more variable in skeletal distribution than acute osteomyelitis, but the distal femur and the proximal and distal tibia are the favourite sites (Jones, Anderson and Stiles, 1987).

Pathology

Typically there is a well-defined cavity in cancellous bone, containing glairy seropurulent fluid (rarely pus). The cavity is lined by granulation tissue containing a mixture of acute and chronic inflammatory cells. The surrounding bone trabeculae are often thickened.

Clinical features

The patient is usually a child or young adolescent who has had pain near one of the larger joints for several weeks or even months. He may have a limp and often there is slight swelling, muscle wasting and local tenderness. The temperature is usually normal and there is little to suggest an infection. The white cell count may be normal but the ESR is often raised.

DIAGNOSTIC IMAGING   The typical radiographic lesion is a circumscribed, round or oval 'cavity' 1–2 cm in diameter; most often it is seen in the tibial or femoral metaphysis, but it may occur in the epiphysis or in one of the cuboidal bones (e.g. the calcaneum). Sometimes the 'cavity' is surrounded by a halo of sclerosis (the classic Brodie's abscess); occasionally it is less well defined, extending into the diaphysis. Metaphyseal lesions cause little or no periosteal

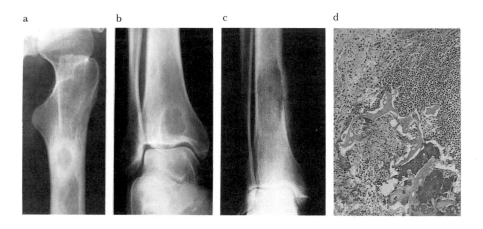

a   b   c   d

2.4 Subacute osteomyelitis   (a, b) The classic Brodie's abscess looks like a small walled-off cavity in the bone with little or no periosteal reaction; (c) sometimes rarefaction is more diffuse and there may be cortical erosion and periosteal reaction. (d) The histology shows islands of dead bone; the marrow spaces are infiltrated by plasma cells and lymphocytes – a characteristic feature of low-grade infection.

reaction; diaphyseal lesions may be associated with periosteal new bone formation and cortical thickening.

The radioisotope scan shows markedly increased activity.

Diagnosis

The clinical and x-ray appearances are often similar to those of an osteoid osteoma; occasionally they mimic a malignant bone tumour. The diagnosis often remains in doubt until a biopsy is performed. If fluid is encountered, it should be sent for bacteriological culture; this is positive in about half the cases – the organism almost always is *Staphylococcus aureus*.

Treatment

Treatment may be conservative if the diagnosis is not in doubt; immobilization and antibiotics (flucloxacillin and fusidic acid) for 6 weeks usually result in healing, though this may take another 6–12 months. If the diagnosis is in doubt, an open biopsy is needed and the lesion may be curetted at the same time. Curettage is also indicated if the x-ray shows that there is no healing after conservative treatment; this is always followed by a further course of antibiotics (Ross and Cole, 1985).

Sclerosing osteomyelitis (Garre's non-suppurative osteomyelitis

In this condition there is no abscess cavity in the bone, only a diffuse area of sclerosis in either the metaphysis or the diaphysis of one of the tubular bones. The patient is usually an adolescent or young adult with a long history of low-grade pain and slight swelling over the bone. Occasionally there are recurrent attacks of more acute pain accompanied by malaise and slight fever.

X-rays show increased bone density and cortical thickening, but no central cavity.

Diagnosis can be difficult. If a small segment of bone is involved, it may be mistaken for an osteoid osteoma. If there is marked periosteal layering of new bone, the lesion resembles a Ewing's sarcoma. At operation the bone is thickened but there is no pus. The biopsy will disclose an inflammatory lesion with reactive sclerosis.

Treatment is by operation: the abnormal area of bone is excised and the exposed surface thoroughly curetted.

Recurrent multifocal osteomyelitis

This rare disorder was first described by Bjorksten et al. in 1978. It is a subacute inflammatory condition which occurs in children and adolescents. It is characterized by the insidious appearance of pain and swelling near the end of one of the tubular bones, usually the distal femur or the proximal or distal tibia. Over the course of several years multiple sites are affected, sometimes symmetrically; with each exacerbation the child is slightly feverish and may have a raised ESR.

X-ray changes are characteristic. There are small lytic lesions in the metaphysis, usually closely adjacent to the physis. Some of these 'cavities' are surrounded by sclerosis; others

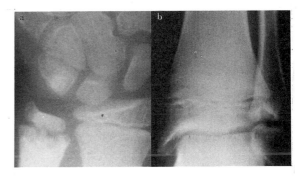

2.5 Multifocal osteomyelitis The small lesions at the junction of metaphysis and physis in (a) the ulna and (b) the fibula are typical of multifocal osteomyelitis.

show varying stages of healing. If the spine is affected, it may lead to collapse of a vertebral body or vertebra plana (Yu et al., 1989).

The ^{99m}Tc-HDP bone scan always shows increased activity.

Biopsy of the lytic focus shows the typical histological features of acute or subacute inflammation. In long-standing lesions there is a chronic inflammatory reaction with lymphocyte infiltration. Bacteriological cultures are invariably negative (Bjorksten and Boquist, 1980).

Treatment is entirely palliative; antibiotics have no effect on the disease. The prognosis is good and the lesions eventually heal without complications.

Post-traumatic osteomyelitis

Open fractures are always contaminated and are therefore prone to infection. The combination of tissue injury, vascular damage, oedema, haematoma, dead bone fragments and an open pathway to the atmosphere must invite bacterial invasion even if the wound is not contaminated with particulate dirt. This is the most common cause of osteomyelitis in adults.

Staphylococcus aureus is the usual pathogen, but other organisms such as *E. coli, Proteus* and *Pseudomonas* are sometimes involved. Occasionally, anaerobic organisms (clostridia, anaerobic streptococci or *Bacteroides*) appear in contaminated wounds.

Clinical features

The patient is feverish and develops pain and swelling over the fracture site; the wound is inflamed and there may be a seropurulent discharge. Blood tests reveal a leucocytosis and an increased ESR. A wound swab should be examined and cultured for organisms.

Treatment

The essence of treatment is prophylaxis: thorough cleansing and debridement of open fractures, the provision of drainage by leaving the wound open, and antibiotics. In most cases a combination of benzylpenicillin and flucloxacillin, given 6-hourly for 48 hours, will suffice. If the wound is clearly contaminated, it is wise also to give metronidazole for 4 or 5 days to control both aerobic and anaerobic organisms.

Pyogenic wound infection, once it has taken root, is difficult to eradicate. The presence of necrotic soft tissue and dead bone, together with a mixed bacterial flora, conspire against effective antibiotic control. Treatment calls for regular wound dressing and repeated excision of all dead and infected tissue. Loose or ineffectual implants should be removed; stable implants are left undisturbed until the fracture has united. If the fracture is unfixed, or if it becomes unstable, an external fixator can be applied.

If these measures fail, the management is essentially that of chronic osteomyelitis.

Postoperative osteomyelitis

Osteomyelitis can occur after any operation on bone, but especially after implanting foreign material for internal fixation of fractures (metal nails, plates and screws) or joint replacement (plastic, ceramic, metal and acrylic cement).

Organisms may be introduced directly into the wound from the atmosphere, the instruments, the patient or the surgeon; or indirectly by haematogenous spread from a distant focus.

The resulting infection is sometimes obvious within days, but it may not occur until months or even years later. The basis of Charnley's (1979) classification of infection after joint replacement is as follows.

A. Early infection
   1. Superficial
   2. Deep
   3. Both superficial and deep
B. Late infection
   1. Following early infection
   2. Covert infection appearing later
   3. Following a long period of normality

Whatever the 'cause' of this infection, and whether 'early' or 'late', the *foreign implant* is both a predisposing factor and an important element in its persistence. Bacteria as well as human tissue cells have an affinity for molecules on the surface of the implant. Both compete for occupancy of the same surface – the tissue cells by adaptation and integration, the bacteria by adhesion and colonization. This contest has been aptly called 'the race for the surface' (Gristina, 1988). If the tissue cells win, the implant is incorporated as an 'inert' biomaterial. If the bacteria win, the resulting infection usually persists until the implant is removed.

The organisms in postoperative osteomyelitis are usually a mixture of pathogenic bacteria (*Staphylococcus aureus, Proteus, Pseudomonas*) and others that are not normally pathogenic (e.g. *Staph. epidermidis*) but may become so in the presence of the implant. Factors that favour bacterial invasion are: (1) soft-tissue damage and bone death; (2) poor contact between implant and bone; (3) loosening of the implant; (4) corrosion of the implant; and (5) fragmentation of polymeric material such as polyethylene and methylmethacrylate. Patients with poor host defences are always at greater risk than others.

Clinical features

Early postoperative infection (within 3 months) is usually fairly obvious. With a purely superficial infection the symptoms are minimal, but if the infection is deep, the patient complains of persistent pain and may have a fever. The skin over the implant is inflamed, and there may be a purulent discharge from the wound. Often there is tenderness and pain on moving the limb. The ESR and white cell count are elevated, and blood culture may be positive. Bacteriological examination of the wound discharge will help to identify the organism and establish the antibiotic sensitivity.

Initially the infection usually appears to be superficial. This is no cause for optimism, for the bone may be involved from the outset. Plain x-rays and MRI are unlikely to be helpful, as they cannot distinguish between the tissue changes due to the operation and those associated with infection.

Rarely (e.g. in patients on immunosuppressive therapy) there may be a fulminant postoperative infection with septicaemia and toxaemia.

Late postoperative infection is much more difficult to diagnose. Pain usually starts insidiously and may never become acute. Often there is no more than a low-grade inflammatory reaction, little different from that due to aseptic loosening of the implant; this is especially true of cemented joint prostheses. Local examination, x-ray signs of bone resorption and increased activity on radionuclide scanning may equally fail to distinguish between aseptic loosening and infection. However, if there is marked periosteal new bone formation and cortical destruction, with increased scintigraphic activity in both the perfusion phase and the bone phase, the likelihood of infection is greatly increased. The MRI may show a localized area of high signal activity due to pus.

Blood investigations are seldom helpful. The ESR is always elevated after joint replacement and may not return to normal for 6 months or longer.

Final confirmation of the diagnosis is obtained by aspirating purulent material from the area, or by culturing the organism in washings taken after attempted aspiration.

Prevention

'Prevention is better than cure.' This adage applies with greater force to postoperative infection than to any other variety. The risk of implant-mediated infection can be reduced by: (1) avoiding operations on immune-depressed patients; (2) eliminating any focus of infection before operating; (3) insisting on optimal operative sterility; (4) giving prophylactic antibiotics; (5) using high-quality implant materials; (6) ensuring close fit and secure fixation of the implant; (7) preventing or counteracting later intercurrent infection.

Antibiotics and clean air The introduction by Charnley of the ultra-clean air operating enclosure and special operating suits with body exhausts brought a substantial reduction in his incidence of wound infection (especially 'early' infection) after hip replacement. Significant

reductions have also been achieved with prophylactic antibiotics: e.g. one of the cephalosporins, 1 g given intravenously shortly before and then 8-hourly for two further doses
after operation. Wearing impervious operative
clothing also is of value. Using all methods
combined, the sepsis rate can be reduced to
below 0.2% (Lidwell, 1986).

Treatment

OPERATIONS WITHOUT IMPLANTS Postoperative
infection in these cases is similar to post-
traumatic infection – with the advantage of less
tissue damage. Treatment follows the same
lines.

INFECTION AFTER INTERNAL FIXATION OF FRAC-
TURES Appropriate antibiotics, given intravenously and in large doses, are the first line of
defence. If there is an abscess, it should be
drained and the wound left open until it is
clean. These measures alone may suffice. If they
fail, excision of infected and necrotic material
followed by intermittent antibiotic irrigation
and suction drainage may yet control the
infection and prevent it from becoming an
intractable chronic osteomyelitis. If at all possible the fixation device should be retained until
the fracture has united; even worse than a septic
fracture is a septic unstable fracture! If the
implant has to be removed in order to achieve
adequate debridement, the fracture should be
held securely with an external fixator.

INFECTION FOLLOWING JOINT REPLACEMENT Early
postoperative infection is treated as above, by
antibiotics and local drainage with excision of
dead and avascular tissue. However, even if the
wound heals, there remains the risk of recurrent late infection.

The variability of presentation of late infection calls for a flexible strategy. As a general
rule, unless there is pus which needs drainage,
it is the stability of the prostheses rather than
the presence of bacteria that dictates treatment.
If the prosthesis is secure and the patient not in
discomfort, there is no absolute indication for
operation. A draining sinus which requires
dressing once a day is less of a hazard than
revision surgery for an infected prosthesis. Skin
irritation can be treated with colostomy paste.

If the prosthesis is loose, or painful, the
choice of treatment is determined by the
patient's general condition.

Those who are unfit for the very extensive
operation that will be necessary are better
treated with long-term antibiotics and restriction of activities (Hughes, Nixon and Dash,
1981). Those who are fit can be offered a
'revision arthroplasty' – i.e. meticulous removal
of the infected prosthesis, acrylic cement and
infected bone, followed by the insertion of a
new prosthesis. If a frank abscess is encountered, the revision is done in two stages, with a
period of 4–6 weeks of intermittent irrigation
and suction of the entire infected field between
removal of the old and insertion of the new
implant. If there is no abscess, a one-stage
revision is carried out, using either antibiotic-
impregnated acrylic cement or no cement at all
(Buchholz et al., 1981).

The alternative (especially with infected hip
replacements) is simply to remove the implant
and acrylic cement, leaving an unstable joint.
The infection may heal but function is not very
satisfactory.

Chronic osteomyelitis

This used to be the dreaded sequel to acute
haematogenous osteomyelitis; nowadays it
more frequently follows an open fracture or
operation.

The usual organisms (and with time there is
always a mixed infection) are *Staphylococcus
aureus, Escherichia coli, Streptococcus pyogenes, Proteus* and *Pseudomonas*; in the presence of foreign
implants *Staph. epidermidis*, which is normally
non-pathogenic, is the commonest of all.

Pathology

Bone is destroyed or devitalized, in a discrete
area at the focus of infection or more diffusely
along the surface of a foreign implant. Cavities
containing pus and pieces of dead bone (sequestra) are surrounded by vascular tissue, and

beyond that by areas of sclerosis – the result of chronic reactive new bone formation. The sequestra act as substrates for bacterial adhesion in much the same way as foreign implants, ensuring the persistence of infection until they are removed or discharged through draining sinuses. Sinuses may seal off for weeks or even months, giving the appearance of healing, only to reopen (or appear somewhere else) when the tissue tension rises. Bone destruction, and the increasingly brittle sclerosis, may occasionally result in a pathological fracture. The histological picture is one of chronic inflammatory cell infiltration around areas of acellular bone or microscopic sequestra.

Clinical features

The patient presents because pain, pyrexia, redness and tenderness have recurred (a 'flare'), or with a discharging sinus. In longstanding cases the tissues are thickened and often puckered or folded in where a scar or sinus is attached to the underlying bone. There may be a seropurulent discharge and excoriation of the surrounding skin. In post-traumatic osteomyelitis the bone may be deformed or ununited.

X-RAY   The classic picture is one of bone resorption – either as a patchy loss of density or as frank excavation around an implant – with thickening and sclerosis of the surrounding bone. However, there are marked variations: there may be no more than localized loss of trabeculation, or an area of osteoporosis, or periosteal thickening; sequestra show up as unnaturally dense fragments, in contrast to the surrounding vascularized bone; sometimes the bone is crudely thickened and misshapen, resembling a bone tumour. A *sinogram* may help to localize the site.

RADIOISOTOPE SCANNING ^{99m}Tc-HDP scans show increased activity in both the perfusion phase and the bone phase. Scanning with ^{67}Ga-citrate or ^{111}In-labelled leucocytes is said to be more specific for osteomyelitis; such scans are useful for showing up hidden foci of infection.

CT AND MRI   are invaluable in planning operative treatment: together they will show the extent of bone destruction and reactive oedema, hidden abscesses and sequestra.

INVESTIGATIONS   During acute flares the ESR and blood white cell count may be increased; these non-specific signs are helpful in assessing the progress of bone infection but they are not diagnostic.

Antistaphylococcal antibody titres may be elevated – a valuable sign in the diagnosis of hidden infections and in tracking progress to recovery.

Organisms cultured from discharging sinuses should be tested repeatedly for antibiotic sensitivity; with time, they often change their characteristics and become resistant to treatment.

Treatment

ANTIBIOTICS   Chronic infection is seldom eradicated by antibiotics alone. Yet bactericidal drugs are important (1) to stop the spread of infection to healthy bone and (2) to control acute flares. The choice of antibiotic depends on bacteriological studies, but the drug must be capable of penetrating sclerotic bone and should be non-toxic with long-term use. Fusidic acid, clindamycin and the cephalosporins are good examples (Hughes, Nixon and Dash, 1981).

LOCAL TREATMENT   A sinus may be painless and need dressing simply to protect the clothing.

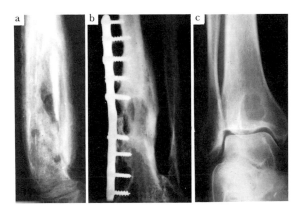

2.6 Chronic osteomyelitis   Chronic bone infection, with a persistent sequestrum, may be a sequel to acute osteomyelitis (a). More often it follows an open fracture or operation (b). Occasionally it presents as a Brodie's abscess (c).

Colostomy paste can be used to stop excoriation of the skin. An acute abscess may need urgent incision and drainage, but this is only a temporary measure.

OPERATION   A waiting policy, punctuated by spells of bed rest and antibiotics to control flares, may have to be patiently endured until there is a clear indication for radical surgery, i.e. significant symptoms, combined with the clear evidence of a sequestrum or dead bone.

Under antibiotic cover all infected soft tissue and all dead or devitalized bone must be excised; dead material can be identified by the preoperative injection of sulphan blue which stains all living tissues green, leaving dead material unstained; the patient and his visitors should be warned that the skin will (temporarily) look green. Double-lumen tubes are laid in the resulting cavity and the tissues are closed with the tubes emerging through separate stab wounds. An appropriate antibiotic solution is instilled 4-hourly and cleared shortly before the next instillation by low-pressure suction. (This is much more tidy than continuous irrigation, which normally fails after a few days due to leakage from the wound.) Cavity injection and drainage should be continued until the effluent is sterile (usually 3–6 weeks); the tubes are then gradually withdrawn as the cavity diminishes in size. The method needs meticulous care and supervision.

As an alternative, porous gentamicin-impregnated beads may be used to 'sterilize' the cavity (Vecsei and Barquet, 1981). This is easier, but less successful; moreover, if the beads are not taken out by 2–3 weeks they are extremely difficult to remove.

Another way of preventing recurrent infection and encouraging healing is to fill completely the dead space left after excision of necrotic tissue with living – or potentially living – material. The best-tried methods are the Papineau technique and muscle flap transfer. With the *Papineau technique* (Papineau et al., 1979) the cavity is packed with small cancellous bone grafts (preferably autogenous) mixed with an antibiotic and a fibrin sealant. Where possible, the area is covered by adjacent muscle and the skin wound is sutured without tension (Lack, Bosch and Arbes, 1987). With *muscle flap transfer*, in suitable sites a large wad of muscle, with its blood supply intact, can be mobilized and laid into the cavity; the surface is later covered with a split-skin graft (Fitzgerald et al., 1985). In areas with too little adjacent muscle (e.g. the distal part of the leg), the same thing can be achieved by transferring a myocutaneous island flap on a long vascular pedicle (Yoshimura et al., 1989).

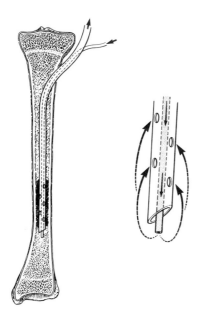

2.7 Chronic osteomyelitis – treatment The surest way of delivering antibiotics to the site of infection is by one or more double-lumen tubes. A narrow catheter is threaded (like an intravenous line) into the wider suction tube; antibiotic solution is run in through the catheter and sucked out through the drainage tube. (Courtesy of Mr C. Lautenbach, Johannesburg General Hospital.)

AFTERCARE   Success is difficult to measure; a minute focus of infection might escape the therapeutic onslaught, only to flare into full-blown osteomyelitis many years later. Prognosis should always be guarded; local trauma must be avoided and any recurrence of symptoms, however slight, should be taken seriously and investigated. The watchword is 'cautious optimism' – a 'probable cure' is better than no cure at all.

Acute suppurative arthritis

A joint can become infected (1) by direct invasion through a penetrating wound, intra-articular injection or arthroscopy; (2) by eruption of a bone abscess; or (3) by blood spread from a distant site. The causal organism is usually *Staphylococcus aureus*; however, in infants *Haemophilus influenzae* is an important pathogen. Occasionally other organisms, such as *Streptococcus*, *Escherichia coli* and *Proteus*, are encountered.

In infants it is often difficult to tell whether the infection started in the bone and spread to the joint or vice versa. In practice it hardly matters and in advanced cases it should be assumed that the entire joint and the adjacent bone ends are involved.

Pathology

The infection usually starts in the synovial membrane; there is an acute inflammatory reaction with a serous or seropurulent exudate and an increase in synovial fluid. As pus appears in the joint, articular cartilage is eroded and destroyed, partly by bacterial enzymes and partly by enzymes released from synovium, inflammatory cells and pus. In infants the epiphysis, which is still largely cartilaginous, may be destroyed; in older children, vascular occlusion may lead to necrosis of the epiphyseal bone. In adults the effects are usually confined to the articular cartilage.

If the infection goes untreated, it will spread to the underlying bone or burst out of the joint to form abscesses and sinuses.

With healing there may be: (1) complete resolution and a return to normal; (2) partial loss of articular cartilage and fibrosis of the joint; (3) loss of articular cartilage and bony ankylosis; or (4) bone destruction and permanent deformity of the joint.

Clinical features

The clinical features differ somewhat according to the age of the patient.

In newborn infants   the emphasis is on septicaemia rather than joint pain. The baby is irritable and refuses to feed; there is a rapid pulse and sometimes a fever. Infection is usually suspected, but it could be anywhere! The joints should be carefully felt and moved to elicit the local signs of warmth, tenderness and resistance to movement. The umbilical cord should be examined for a source of infection.

In children   the usual features are acute pain in a single large joint – commonly the hip – and reluctance to move the limb ('pseudoparesis'). The child is ill, with a rapid pulse and a swinging fever. The skin looks red and in a superficial joint swelling may be obvious. There is local warmth and marked tenderness. All movements are restricted, and often completely

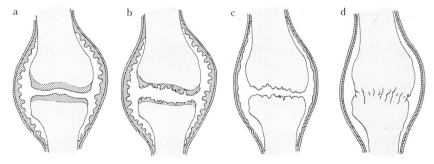

2.8 Acute suppurative arthritis   In the early stage (a) there is an acute synovitis with a purulent joint effusion. (b) Soon the articular cartilage is attacked by bacterial and cellular enzymes. If the infection is not arrested, the cartilage may be completely destroyed (c); healing then leads to bony ankylosis (d).

abolished, by pain and spasm. It is essential to look for a source of infection – a septic toe, a boil or a discharge from the ear.

In adults it is often a superficial joint (knee, wrist or ankle) that is painful, swollen and inflamed. There is warmth and marked local tenderness, and movements are restricted. The patient should be questioned and examined for evidence of gonococcal infection or drug abuse.

DIAGNOSTIC IMAGING Early on the x-ray is usually normal but ultrasound shows a joint effusion. In children the joint 'space' may seem to be widened (because of fluid in the joint) and there may be slight subluxation of the joint. With *E. coli* infections there is sometimes gas in the joint. Later there may be osteoporosis and narrowing or irregularity of the joint space.

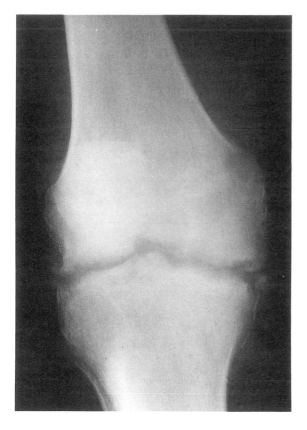

2.9 Suppurative arthritis Acute suppurative arthritis has severely damaged the articular cartilage, resulting in narrowing and irregularity of the joint space.

INVESTIGATIONS The white cell count and ESR are raised and blood culture may be positive. However, special investigations take time and it is much quicker (and usually more reliable) to aspirate the joint and examine the fluid. It may be frankly purulent – but beware! – in early cases the fluid may look clear. A white cell count and Gram stain should be carried out immediately: Gram-positive cocci are probably *S. aureus*; Gram-negative cocci are either *H. influenzae* (in children) or *Gonococcus* (in adults). A sample of fluid is also sent for full bacteriological examination and tests for antibiotic sensitivity.

Differential diagnosis

ACUTE OSTEOMYELITIS In young children, osteomyelitis may be indistinguishable from septic arthritis; often one must assume that both are present.

TRAUMA Traumatic synovitis or haemarthrosis may be associated with acute pain and swelling. A history of injury does not exclude infection. Diagnosis may remain in doubt until the joint is aspirated.

IRRITABLE JOINT At the onset the joint is painful and lacks some movement. But the child is not really ill and there are no signs of infection.

HAEMOPHILIC BLEED An acute haemarthrosis closely resembles septic arthritis. The history is usually conclusive, but aspiration will resolve any doubt.

RHEUMATIC FEVER Typically the pain flits from joint to joint, but at the onset one joint may be misleadingly inflamed. However, there are no signs of septicaemia.

GOUT AND PSEUDOGOUT In adults, acute crystal-induced synovitis may closely resemble infection. On aspiration the joint fluid is often turbid, with a high white cell count; however, microscopic examination by polarized light will show the characteristic crystals.

GAUCHER'S DISEASE In this rare condition acute joint pain and fever can occur without any organism being found ('pseudo-osteitis'). Because of the predisposition to true infection, antibiotics should be given.

Treatment

The first priority is to aspirate the joint and examine the fluid. Treatment is then started without further delay and follows the same lines as for acute osteomyelitis.

GENERAL SUPPORTIVE CARE   Analgesics are given for pain and intravenous fluids for dehydration.

SPLINTAGE   The joint must be rested either on a splint or in a widely split plaster. With hip infection, the joint should be held abducted and 30 degrees flexed, on traction to prevent dislocation.

ANTIBIOTICS   The initial choice of antibiotics is based on judgement of the most likely pathogens; a more appropriate drug can be substituted after full bacteriological investigation.
  Older children and adults are given flucloxacillin and fusidic acid, intravenously for 2–4 days and then orally for another 3 weeks.
  Children under 4 years, in whom there is a high incidence of haemophilus infection, should be treated with ampicillin or one of the newer cephalosporins from the outset.

DRAINAGE   Under anaesthesia pus is drained from the joint. It is usually recommended that this be done by a small incision into the joint. This is the safest policy and is certainly advisable (1) in very young infants, (2) when the hip is involved and (3) if the aspirated pus is very thick. Some, however, advocate repeated closed aspiration of the joint for 24–48 hours.

AFTERCARE   Once the patient's general condition is satisfactory and the joint is no longer painful or warm, further damage is unlikely. If articular cartilage has been preserved, gentle and gradually increasing active movements are encouraged. If articular cartilage has been destroyed the aim is to keep the joint immobile while ankylosis is awaited. Splintage in the optimum position is therefore continuously maintained, usually by plaster, until ankylosis is sound.

Complications

BONE DESTRUCTION   and, at the hips, dislocation of the joint are serious threats if infection is not rapidly controlled. The x-ray sometimes gives a misleadingly pessimistic picture: the femoral head may seem to have disappeared, but as the condition resolves and the bone recalcifies the true state of affairs becomes apparent.

CARTILAGE DESTRUCTION   may lead to either fibrous or bony ankylosis. In adults, partial destruction of the joint will result in secondary osteoarthritis.

GROWTH DISTURBANCE   may occur, presenting either as a localized deformity or as shortening of the bone.

Spirochaetal infection

Although rarely seen in northern countries, spirochaetal bone infection is still quite common in some parts of the world.

Early congenital syphilis

Treponema pallidum can cross the placental barrier and infect the fetus during the latter half of pregnancy. However, bone changes do not usually appear until several weeks after birth (Rasool and Govender, 1989).
  The infant is sick and irritable. The commonest clinical features are hepatosplenomegaly. Serological tests are usually positive in both mother and child.
  The first signs of skeletal involvement may be joint swelling and 'pseudoparalysis' – the child refuses to move a painful limb. Several sites may be involved, often symmetrically, with slight swelling and tenderness at the ends or along the shafts of the tubular bones.

X-RAYS   The characteristic changes are of two kinds: (1) 'periostitis' – diffuse periosteal newbone formation along the diaphysis, usually of mild degree but sometimes producing an 'onion-peel' effect; and (2) 'metaphysitis' – trabecular erosion in the juxtaepiphyseal region, showing first as a lucent band near the physis and later as frank bone destruction.

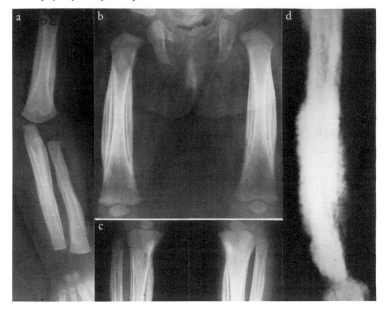

2.10 Syphilis   (a, b, c) Congenital syphilis – with diffuse periostitis of many bones; (d) acquired syphilitic periostitis of the femur.

DIAGNOSIS   The condition must be distinguished from scurvy (rare in the first 6 months of life), multifocal osteomyelitis, the battered baby syndrome and Caffey's disease.

INFANTILE CORTICAL HYPEROSTOSIS (CAFFEY'S DISEASE)

Caffey's disease is a type of 'periostitis' affecting infants aged less than 6 months. It presents with malaise, fever and painful swelling of long bones, the mandible and scapulae. X-rays show marked periosteal new-bone formation. The disorder is easily mistaken for osteomyelitis or scurvy, but, unlike these conditions, it always resolves spontaneously.

TREATMENT   Penicillin, given for 10–14 days, is highly effective. The bone lesions usually heal leaving no trace of the ominous pathology.

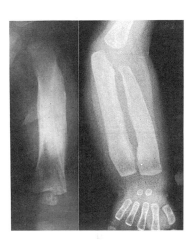

2.11 Caffey's disease   In this infant with Caffey's disease, subperiosteal bone was laid down over a wide area of many bones.

Late congenital and acquired syphilis

Bone lesions in older children and adults are usually manifestations of tertiary disease, the result of gumma formation and endarteritis.

Gummata appear either as discrete, punched-out radiolucent areas in the medulla or as more extensive destructive lesions in the cortex. The surrounding bone is thick and sclerotic. Sometimes the dense endosteal and periosteal new-bone formation is the predominant feature, affecting almost the entire bone (the classic 'sabre tibia').

TREATMENT   Antibiotics are ineffectual in tertiary syphilis. An operation is occasionally needed if the gumma breaks down or if there is a pathological fracture.

Yaws

Yaws is a non-venereal spirochaetal infection caused by *Treponema pertenue*. It is seen mainly in the tropics, and usually in children, presenting with features resembling those of syphilis. The characteristic bone changes are periosteal new-bone formation and cortical rarefaction or destruction. Sclerosis is less marked than in syphilis. Active infection is treated with pencillin.

Tuberculosis

In contrast to pyogenic infection, tuberculosis causes a granulomatous reaction which is associated with tissue necrosis and caseation. *Mycobacterium tuberculosis* (usually human, sometimes bovine) enters the body via the lung (droplet infection) or the gut (swallowing infected milk products) or, rarely, through the skin.

Pathology

PRIMARY COMPLEX The initial lesion in lung, pharynx or gut is a small one with lymphatic spread to regional lymph nodes; this combination is the primary complex. Usually the bacilli are fixed in the nodes and no clinical illness results, but occasionally the response is excessive, with enlargement of glands in the neck or abdomen.

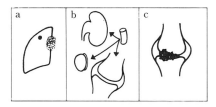

2.12 The tuberculous process The primary infection is usually arrested in the local lymph glands (a); secondary spread is by the blood stream (b); the term 'tertiary' can be used for the local destructive lesion (c).

Even though there is usually no clinical illness, the initial infection has two important sequels: (1) within nodes which are apparently healed or even calcified, bacilli may survive for many years, so that a reservoir exists; (2) the body has been sensitized to the toxin (a positive Heaf test being an index of sensitization) and, should reinfection occur, the response is quite different, the lesion being a destructive one which spreads by contiguity.

SECONDARY SPREAD If resistance to the original infection is low, widespread dissemination via the blood stream may occur, giving rise to miliary tuberculosis or meningitis. More often, blood spread occurs months or years later and bacilli are deposited in extrapulmonary tissues. Some of these foci develop into destructive lesions to which the term 'tertiary' may be applied.

TERTIARY LESION Bones or joints are affected in about 5% of patients with tuberculosis. There is a predilection for the vertebral bodies and the large synovial joints. Multiple lesions occur in about one-third of patients. In established cases it is difficult to tell whether the infection started in the joint and then spread to the adjacent bone or vice versa; synovial membrane and subchondral bone have a common blood supply and they may, of course, be infected simultaneously.

Once the bacilli have gained a foothold, they elicit a chronic inflammatory reaction. The characteristic microscopic lesion is the tuberculous granuloma – a collection of epithelioid and multinucleated giant cells surrounding an area of necrosis, with round cells (mainly lymphocytes) around the periphery.

Within the affected area, small patches of caseous necrosis appear. These may coalesce into a larger yellowish mass, or the centre may break down to form an abscess containing pus and fragments of necrotic bone.

Bone lesions tend to spread quite rapidly. Epiphyseal cartilage is no barrier to invasion and soon the infection reaches the joint. Only in the vertebral bodies, and more rarely in the greater trochanter of the femur or the small bones of the hands or feet, does the infection persist as a pure chronic osteomyelitis.

If the synovium is involved, it becomes thick and oedematous, giving rise to a marked

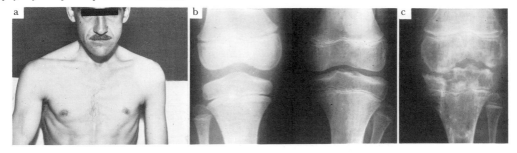

2.13 Tuberculosis   A characteristic feature of tuberculosis is wasting of muscle (a). The knees in (b) show osteoporosis on the left, due to synovitis. This often resolves with treatment, but, if cartilage and bone are destroyed (c), healing is by fibrosis.

effusion. A pannus of granulation tissue may extend across the joint and articular cartilage is slowly destroyed, though the rapid and complete destruction elicited by pyogenic organisms does not occur in the absence of secondary infection. At the edges of the joint, along the synovial reflections, there may be active bone erosion. In addition, the increased vascularity causes local osteoporosis.

If unchecked, caseation and infection extend into the surrounding soft tissues to produce a 'cold' abscess ('cold' only in comparison to a pyogenic abscess). This may burst through the skin, forming a sinus, or it may track along the tissue planes to point at some distant site. Secondary infection by pyogenic organisms is common.

If the disease is arrested at an early stage, healing may be by resolution to apparent normality. If articular cartilage has been damaged, healing is by fibrosis and incomplete ankylosis, with progressive joint deformity. Within the fibrocaseous mass, mycobacteria may remain imprisoned, retaining the potential to flare up into active disease many years later.

Clinical features

There may be a history of previous infection or recent contact with tuberculosis. The patient, usually a child or young adult, complains of pain and (in a superficial joint) swelling. In advanced cases there may be attacks of fever or lassitude and loss of weight. Relatives tell of 'night cries': the joint, splinted by muscle spasm during the day, relaxes with sleep and the damaged tissues are stretched or compressed, causing sudden episodes of intense pain. Muscle wasting is characteristic and synovial thickening is often striking. Movements are limited in all directions. As articular erosion progresses the joint becomes stiff and deformed.

In tuberculosis of the spine, pain may be deceptively slight – often no more than an ache when the spine is jarred. Consequently the patient may not present until there is a visible abscess (usually in the groin or the lumbar region to one side of the midline) or until collapse causes a localized kyphosis. Occasionally the presenting feature is weakness or loss of sensibility in the lower limbs.

Multiple foci of infection are sometimes found, with bone and joint lesions at different stages of development (Kumar and Saxena, 1988). This is more likely in people with lowered resistance.

X-RAY   Soft-tissue swelling and periarticular osteoporosis are characteristic. The bone ends take on a 'washed-out' appearance and the articular space is narrowed. In children the epiphyses may be enlarged, probably the result of long-continued hyperaemia. Later on there is erosion of the subarticular bone; characteristically this is seen *on both sides of the joint,* indicating an inflammatory process starting in the synovium. Cystic lesions may appear in the adjacent bone ends but there is little or no periosteal reaction. In the spine the characteristic appearance is one of bone erosion and

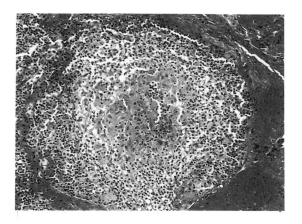

2.14 Tuberculosis A typical tuberculous granuloma, with central necrosis and scattered giant cells surrounded by lymphocytes and histiocytes.

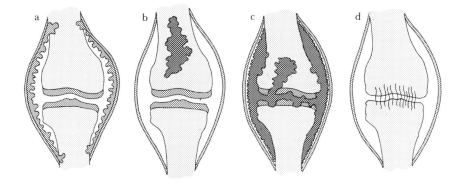

2.15 Tuberculous arthritis The disease may begin as synovitis (a) or osteomyelitis (b), both of which can resolve. From either it may extend to become a true arthritis (c); not all the cartilage is destroyed, and healing is usually by fibrous ankylosis (d).

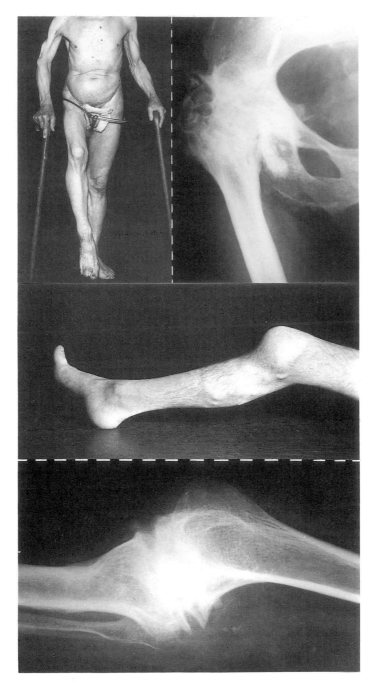

2.16 The aftermath of tuberculous arthritis Joint destruction and deformity: flexion and adduction at the hip; flexion, lateral rotation and backward subluxation at the knee.

collapse around an intervertebral disc space; the soft-tissue shadows may define a paravertebral abscess.

INVESTIGATIONS The ESR is increased and there may be a relative lymphocytosis. The Mantoux or Heaf test will be positive: these are sensitive but not specific tests; i.e. a negative Mantoux virtually excludes the diagnosis, but a positive test merely indicates tuberculous infection, now or at some time in the past.

If synovial fluid is aspirated, it may be cloudy, the protein concentration is increased and the white cell count is elevated.

Acid-fast bacilli are identified in synovial fluid in 10–20% of cases, and cultures are positive in over half. A synovial biopsy is more reliable; sections will show the characteristic histological features, and acid-fast bacilli may be identified; cultures are positive in over 80% of cases.

Diagnosis

Except in areas where tuberculosis is common, diagnosis is often delayed simply because the disease is not suspected. Features that should trigger more active investigation are:

- a long history
- involvement of only one joint
- marked synovial thickening
- marked muscle wasting
- periarticular osteoporosis
- a positive Mantoux test

Synovial biopsy for histological examination and culture is often necessary.

Joint tuberculosis must be differentiated from the following.

TRANSIENT SYNOVITIS This is fairly common in children. At first it seems no different from any other low-grade inflammatory arthritis; however, it always settles down after a few weeks' rest in bed. If the synovitis recurs, further investigation (even a biopsy) may be necessary.

MONARTICULAR RHEUMATOID ARTHRITIS Occasionally, rheumatoid arthritis starts in a single large joint. This is clinically indistinguishable from tuberculosis and the diagnosis may have to await the results of synovial biopsy.

SUBACUTE ARTHRITIS Diseases such as amoebic dysentery or brucellosis are sometimes complicated by arthritis. The history, clinical features and pathological investigations usually enable a diagnosis to be made.

HAEMORRHAGIC ARTHRITIS The physical signs of blood in a joint may resemble those of tuberculous arthritis. If the bleeding has followed a single recent injury, the history and absence of marked wasting are diagnostic. Following repeated bleeding, as in haemophilia, the clinical resemblance to tuberculosis is closer, but there is also a history of bleeding elsewhere.

PYOGENIC ARTHRITIS In long-standing cases it may be difficult to exclude an old septic arthritis.

Treatment

REST H. O. Thomas long ago urged that tuberculosis should be treated by rest – which had to be prolonged, uninterrupted, rigid and enforced. This often involved splintage of the joint and traction to overcome muscle spasm and prevent collapse of the articular surfaces. With modern chemotherapy this is no longer mandatory; rest and splintage are varied according to the needs of the individual patient. Those who are diagnosed and treated early are kept in bed only until symptoms subside, and thereafter are allowed restricted activity until the joint changes resolve (usually 6 months to a year). Those with progressive joint destruction may need a longer period of rest and splintage to prevent ankylosis in a bad position; however, as soon as symptoms permit, movements are again encouraged.

CHEMOTHERAPY The most effective treatment is a combination of antituberculous drugs, which should always include rifampicin and isoniazid. A recommended regimen is rifampicin, isoniazid and ethambutol (or pyrazinamide) for 8 weeks, and thereafter rifampicin and isoniazid for a further 6–12 months. Streptomycin and ethambutol are more toxic and should not be used for long-term treatment.

OPERATION Operative drainage or clearance of a tuberculous focus is seldom necessary nowadays. However, a cold abscess may need draining.

Once the condition is controlled and arthritis has completely subsided, normal activity can be resumed, though the patient must report any renewed symptoms. If, however, the joint is painful and the articular suface is destroyed, replacement arthroplasty may be considered, but the longer the period of inactivity, the less the risk of reactivation of the disease. There is always some risk and it is essential to give chemotherapy before and after the operation.

If there is severe deformity, osteotomy may be useful. In joints where mobility can be sacrificed, arthrodesis is the safest option.

Brucellosis

Brucellosis is an unusual but none the less important cause of subacute or chronic granulomatous infection in bones and joints. Three species of organism are seen in humans: *Brucella melitensis, B. abortus* (from cattle) and *B. suis* (from pigs). Those infected are usually farmers (or others in contact with farm animals) – mainly in countries around the Mediterranean and in certain parts of Africa and India.

The organism enters the body with infected milk products or, occasionally, directly through the skin or mucosal surfaces. It is taken up by the lymphatics and then carried by the blood stream to distant sites.

Pathology

Foci of infection may occur in bones (usually the vertebral bodies) or in the synovium of the larger joints. The characteristic lesion is a chronic inflammatory granuloma with round-cell infiltration and giant cells. There may be central necrosis and caseation leading to abscess formation and invasion of the surrounding tissues.

Clinical features

The patient usually presents with fever, headache and generalized weakness, followed by joint pains and backache. The initial illness may be acute and alarming; more often it begins insidiously and progresses until the symptoms localize in a single large joint (usually the hip or knee) or in the spine. The joint becomes painful, swollen and tender; movements are restricted in all directions. If the spine is affected, there is usually local tenderness and back movements are restricted.

The systemic illness follows a fluctuating course, with alternating periods of fever and apparent improvement (hence the older term 'undulant fever'). Diagnosis is often delayed and may not be resolved until destructive changes are advanced.

X-RAYS   show the features of a subacute arthritis, with loss of articular space, slowly progressive bone erosion and periarticular osteoporosis. In the spine there may be destruction and collapse of adjacent vertebral bodies with obliteration of the disc.

INVESTIGATIONS   A positive agglutination test (titre above 1/80) is diagnostic. Joint aspiration or biopsy may allow the organism to be cultured and identified.

Diagnosis

Diagnosis is usually delayed while other types of subacute arthritis are excluded.

Tuberculosis   and brucellosis have similar clinical and radiological features. The distinction is often difficult and may have to await the results of agglutination tests, synovial biopsy and bacteriological investigation.

Reiter's disease   and other forms of reactive arthritis often follow an initial systemic illness. However, fever is not so marked and joint erosion is usually late and mild.

Treatment

ANTIBIOTICS   The infection usually responds to a combined onslaught with tetracycline and streptomycin for 3–4 weeks.

OPERATION   An abscess will need drainage, and necrotic bone and cartilage should be meticulously excised. If the joint is destroyed, arthrodesis or arthroplasty may be necessary once the infection is completely controlled.

Mycotic infections

Mycotic or fungal infection causes an indolent granulomatous reaction, often leading to abscess formation, tissue destruction and ulceration. When the musculoskeletal system is involved, it is usually by direct spread from the adjacent soft tissues. Occasionally, however, a bone or joint may be infected by haematogenous spread from a distant site.

These disorders are conveniently divided into 'superficial' and 'deep' infections (Hoffman and Sentochnik, 1989).

THE 'SUPERFICIAL' MYCOSES are primarily infections of the skin or mucous surfaces, which spread into the adjacent soft tissues and bone. The more common examples are the *maduromycoses* (a group consisting of several species), *Sporothrix* and various species of *Candida*.

The *actinomycoses* are usually included with the superficial fungal infections. The causal organisms, of which *Actinomyces israelii* is the commonest in humans, are not really fungi but anaerobic bacilli with fungus-like appearance and behaviour.

THE 'DEEP' MYCOSES comprise infections by *Blastomyces, Histoplasma, Coccidioides, Cryptococcus, Aspergillus* and other rare fungi. The organisms, which occur in rotting vegetation and bird droppings, gain entry through the lungs and, in humans, may cause an influenza-like illness. Bone or joint infection is uncommon except in patients with compromised host defences.

Maduromycosis

This chronic fungal infection is usually seen in northern Africa and the Indian subcontinent. The organisms usually enter through a cut in the foot; from there they spread through the subcutaneous tissues and along the tendon sheaths. The bones and joints are infected by direct invasion; local abscesses form and break through the skin as multiple sinuses. The patient may present at an early stage with a tender subcutaneous nodule (when the diagnosis is seldom entertained); more often he is seen when the foot is swollen and indurated,

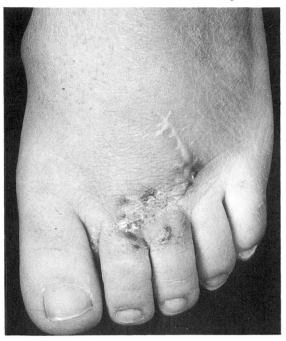

2.17 Maduromycosis This Mediterranean market-worker was perpetually troubled by tiny abscesses and weeping sinuses in her foot. X-rays showed that bone destruction had already spread to the tarsal bones, and after 2 years of futile treatment the foot had to be amputated.

with discharging sinuses and ulcers. X-rays may show multiple bone cavities or progressive bone destruction. The organism can be identified in the sinus discharge or in tissue biopsies.

Treatment is unsatisfactory as there is no really effective chemotherapy. Intravenous amphotericin B is advocated, but it is fairly toxic and causes side effects such as headaches, vomiting and fever.

Necrotic tissue should be widely excised. Even then it is sometimes difficult to stop further invasion, and amputation is sometimes necessary.

Actinomycosis

Infection is usually by *Actinomyces israelii*, an anaerobic Gram-positive bacillus. Although rare, it is important that it should be diagnosed because the organism is sensitive to antibiotics.

The most common site of infection is the mandible (from the mouth and pharynx), but bone lesions are also seen in the vertebrae (spreading from the lung or gut) and the pelvis (spreading from the caecum or colon). Peripheral lesions may occur by direct infection of the soft tissues and later extension to the bones. There may be a firm, tender swelling in the soft tissues, going on to form an abscess and one or more chronic discharging sinuses. X-rays may show cyst-like areas of bone destruction. The organism can be readily identified in the sinus discharge, but only on anaerobic culture.

Treatment by large doses of penicillin G, tetracycline or erythromycin, has to be continued for several months.

The deep mycoses

Histoplasmosis, blastomycosis and coccidioidomycosis are rare causes of bone infection, but they should always be considered in patients on immunosuppressive therapy. Diagnosis is usually delayed and often involves specialized microbiological investigations to identify the organism.

Treatment with intravenous amphotericin B is moderately effective. Operation may be necessary to drain an abscess or to remove necrotic tissue.

Hydatid disease

Hydatid disease is caused by the tapeworm *Echinococcus.* Parasitic infestation is common among sheep farmers, but bone lesions are rare.

The organism, a cestode worm, has a complicated life-cycle. The definitive host is the dog or some other carnivore that carries the tapeworm in its bowel. Segments of worm and ova pass out in the faeces and are later ingested by one of the intermediate hosts – usually sheep or cattle or man. Here the larvae are carried via the portal circulation to the liver, and occasionally beyond to other organs, where they produce cysts containing numerous scolices. Infested

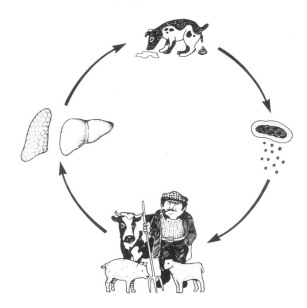

2.18 Hydatid disease The life-cycle of the tapeworm which causes hydatid disease; the sheep-farmer's pipe is no protection.

meat is then eaten by dogs (or humans), giving rise to a new generation of tapeworm.

Scolices carried in the blood stream occasionally settle in bone and produce hydatid cysts that slowly enlarge with little respect for cortical or epiphyseal boundaries. The bones most commonly affected are the vertebrae, pelvis, femur and ribs.

Clinical features

The patient may complain of pain and swelling, or may present for the first time with a pathological fracture or compression of the spinal cord. The diagnosis is more likely if the patient comes from a sheep-farming district.

X-RAYS show solitary or multiloculated bone cysts, but only moderate expansion of the cortices. In the spine, hydatid disease may involve adjacent vertebrae, with large cysts extending into the paravertebral soft tissues; these features are often best seen on CT scans or MRI.

INVESTIGATIONS Casoni's (complement fixation) test may be positive. The diagnosis can be confirmed by carrying out a needle biopsy.

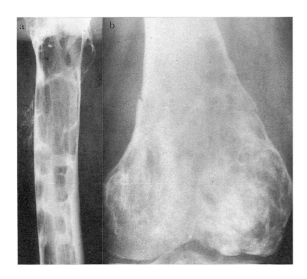

2.19 Hydatid disease of bone Two examples of hydatid involvement of bone: there is no expansion of the cortex in (a) and very little in (b).

Treatment

The anthelminthic drug albendazole is moderately effective in destroying the parasite. However, the bone cysts do not heal and may require curettage and bone grafting to lessen the risk of pathological fracture. At operation the cavity can be further 'sterilized' with copious amounts of hypertonic saline.

References and further reading

Bjorksten, B. and Boquist, L. (1980) Histopathological aspects of chronic recurrent multifocal osteomyelitis. *Journal of Bone and Joint Surgery* **62B**, 276–380

Bjorksten B., Gustavson, K.-H., Eriksson, B., Lindholm, A. and Nordstrom, S. (1978) Chronic recurrent multifocal osteomyelitis and pustulosis palmoplantaris. *Journal of Pediatrics* **93**, 227–231

Blockey, N.J. and McAllister, T.A. (1972) Antibiotics in acute osteomyelitis in children. *Journal of Bone and Joint Surgery* **54B**, 299–309

Buchholz, H.W., Elson, R.A., Engelbrecht, E., Lodenkamper, H., Rottger, J. and Siegel, Q. (1981) Management of deep infection of total hip replacement. *Journal of Bone and Joint Surgery* **63B**, 342–353

Charnley, J. (1979) *Low Friction Arthroplasty of the Hip*, Springer, Berlin

Fitzgerald, R.H., Ruttle, P.E., Arnold, P.G., Kelly, P.J. and

Irons, G.B. (1985) Local muscle flaps in the treatment of chronic osteomyelitis. *Journal of Bone and Joint Surgery* **67A**, 175–185

Gristina, A.G. (1988) Biomaterial-centred infection: microbial adhesion versus tissue integration. *Science* **237**, 437–451

Hoffman, G.S. and Sentochnik, D.E. (1989) Mycobacterial and fungal infections. In *Textbook of Rheumatology*, 3rd edn (eds. W.N. Kelley, E.D. Harris, S. Ruddy and C.B. Sledge), W.B. Saunders, Philadelphia, pp. 1586–1601

Hughes, S.P.F., Nixon, J. and Dash, C.H. (1981) Cephaloxin in chronic osteomyelitis. *Journal of the Royal College of Surgeons of Edinburgh* **26**, 335–339

Jones, N.S., Anderson, D.J. and Stiles, P.J. (1987) Osteomyelitis in a general hospital. *Journal of Bone and Joint Surgery* **69B**, 779–783

Kumar, K. and Saxena, M.B.L. (1988) Multifocal osteoarticular tuberculosis. *International Orthopaedics* **12**, 135–138

Lack, W., Bosch, P. and Arbes, H. (1987) Chronic osteomyelitis treated by cancellous homografts and fibrin adhesion. *Journal of Bone and Joint Surgery* **69B**, 335–337

Lidwell, O.M. (1986) Clean air at operation and subsequent sepsis in the joint. *Clinical Orthopaedics and Related Research* **211**, 91–102

Lindenbaum, S. and Alexander, H. (1984) Infections simulating bone tumours; a review of subacute osteomyelitis. *Clinical Orthopaedics and Related Research* **184**, 193–203

Nade, S. (1983) Acute haematogenous osteomyelitis in infancy and childhood. *Journal of Bone and Joint Surgery* **65B**, 109–119

Papineau, L.J., Alfageme, A., Dalcourt, J.P. and Pilon, L. (1979) Ostéomyélite chronique: excision et greffe de spongieaux à l'air libre après mises à plat extensives. *International Orthopaedics* **3**, 165–176

Rasool, M.N. and Govender, S. (1989) The skeletal manifestations of congenital syphilis. *Journal of Bone and Joint Surgery* **71B**, 752–755

Ross, E.R.S. and Cole, W.G. (1985) Treatment of subacute osteomyelitis in childhood. *Journal of Bone and Joint Surgery* **67B**, 443–448

Schwartz, J. (1984) What's new in mycotic bone and joint disease? *Pathology Research and Practice* **178**, 617–634

Szypryt, E.P., Morris, D.L. and Mulholland, D.L. (1987) Combined chemotherapy and surgery for hydatid bone disease. *Journal of Bone and Joint Surgery* **69B**, 141–144

Vecsei, V. and Barquet, A. (1981) Treatment of chronic osteomyelitis by necrectomy and gentamicin-PMMA beads. *Clinical Orthopaedics and Related Research* **159**, 201–207

Waldvogel, F.A. and Vasey, H. (1980) Osteomyelitis: the past decade. *New England Journal of Medicine* **303**, 360–370

Wroblewski, M. (1986 One-stage revision of infected cemented total hip arthroplasty. *Clinical Orthopaedics and Related Research* **211**, 103–107

Yoshimura, M., Shimada, T., Matsuda, M. Hosokawa, M. and Imura, S. (1989) Treatment of chronic osteomyelitis of the leg by peroneal myocutaneous island flap transfer. *Journal of Bone and Joint Surgery* **71B**, 593–596

Yu, L., Kasser, J.R., O'Rourke, E. and Kozakewich, H. (1989) Chronic recurrent multifocal osteomyelitis. *Journal of Bone and Joint Surgery* **71A**, 105–112

Rheumatic disorders

3

'Rheumatic disorder' is a descriptive term linking a number of diseases that cause chronic pain, stiffness or swelling around joints and tendons. Many common conditions, such as influenza, are associated with painful muscles and joints, but the rheumatic disorders are distinguished by (1) their chronicity and (2) the appearance of local and systemic features of inflammation. Many – perhaps all – result from a faulty immune reaction.

Rheumatoid arthritis

Rheumatoid arthritis (RA) is the commonest cause of chronic inflammatory joint disease. The most typical features are a symmetrical polyarthritis and tenosynovitis, morning stiffness, elevation of the ESR and the appearance of anti-IgG globulins (rheumatoid factors) in the serum. However, changes can be widespread in the tissues of the body and the condition should really be called rheumatoid *disease*.

It affects about 3% of the population, usually starting in the fourth decade, and is three times as common in women as in men. Both the prevalence and the clinical expression vary between populations; it is more common (and generally more severe) in the urban communities of Europe and North America than in the rural populations of Africa (Solomon et al., 1975).

Cause

The exact cause is unknown. The condition is a type of chronic inflammatory disease in which abnormal immunological reactions are prominent. These include the production of antibodies (both IgG and IgM) to the body's own IgG. Such 'autoantibodies' appear as serum rheumatoid factors (RF) in 60–80% of patients with RA, and they can also be demonstrated in the synovium.

How this comes about is unclear, and whether or not the RFs and the immune complexes that they can form are directly pathogenic remains unknown. The final common pathway of synovial inflammation is associated with immune events including massive T-cell infiltration as well as B-cell reactivity.

The condition appears to require genetic susceptibility and environmental trigger factors to initiate the chronic inflammation. Genetic susceptibility resides in the HLA-DR regions (DR4 in Caucasians) of chromosome 6, and depends on subtle abnormalities of antigen-presenting complexes. The trigger factors could be multiple, but infective agents seem the most likely culprits.

There is no simple screening test for susceptibility or for the disease. Most HLA-DR4 people will not develop RA and many patients with RA do not produce rheumatoid factors.

Susceptibility is affected by age and sex (young women are at greatest risk), hormones (RA often subsides during pregnancy) and possibly diet and psychological stress.

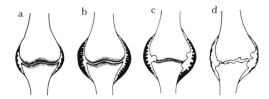

3.1 Pathology of rheumatoid arthritis (a) The normal joint. (b) Stage 1 – synovitis and joint swelling. (c) Stage 2 – early joint destruction with periarticular erosions. (d) Stage 3 – advanced joint destruction and deformity.

Pathology

The condition is widespread, but the brunt of the attack falls on synovium. The constant and characteristic feature is a chronic inflammation; an inconstant but pathognomonic lesion is the rheumatoid nodule.

JOINTS AND TENDONS
The pathological changes, if unchecked, proceed in three stages.

Stage 1: synovitis Early changes are vascular congestion, proliferation of synoviocytes and infiltration of the subsynovial layers by polymorphs, lymphocytes and plasma cells. There is thickening of the capsular structures, villous formation of the synovium and a cell-rich effusion into the joints and tendon sheaths. Though painful, swollen and tender, these structures are still intact and mobile, and the disorder is potentially reversible.

Stage 2: destruction Persistent inflammation causes joint and tendon destruction. Articular cartilage is eroded, partly by proteolytic enzymes, partly by vascular tissue in the folds of the synovial reflections, and partly due to direct invasion of the cartilage by a pannus of granulation tissue creeping over the articular surface. At the margins of the joint, bone is eroded by granulation tissue invasion and osteoclastic resorption.

Similar changes occur in tendon sheaths, causing tenosynovitis, invasion of the collagen bundles and, eventually, partial or complete rupture of tendons.

A synovial effusion, often containing copious amounts of fibrinoid material, produces swelling of the joints, tendons and bursae.

Stage 3: deformity The combination of articular destruction, capsular stretching and tendon rupture leads to progressive instability and deformity of the joints. By this time the inflammatory process may have subsided; the emphasis is now on the mechanical and functional effects of joint and tendon disruption.

EXTRA-ARTICULAR TISSUES
The rheumatoid nodule is a small granulomatous lesion consisting of a central necrotic zone surrounded by a radially disposed palisade of local histiocytes, and beyond that by inflammatory granulation tissue. Nodules occur under the skin (especially over bony prominences), in the synovium, on tendons, in the sclera and in many of the viscera.

Lymphadenopathy can affect not only the nodes draining inflamed joints, but also those at a distance such as the mediastinal nodes. This, and a mild *splenomegaly*, is due to hyperactivity of the reticuloendothelial system. *Vasculitis*, more usually associated with disseminated lupus, may be fairly widespread. *Muscle weakness* may be due to a rheumatoid myopathy or neuropathy, but it can also result from spinal cord involvement or cervical spine displacement. *Sensory changes* may be part of a neuropathy, but isolated symptoms can result from nerve compression by thickened synovium. *Visceral disease* can occur in the lungs, heart, kidneys, brain and gastrointestinal tract.

Clinical features

In the early stages the picture is mainly that of a polysynovitis, with soft-tissue swelling and stiffness. Typically, a woman of 30–40 years complains of pain, swelling and loss of mobility in the proximal joints of the fingers. There may be a previous history of 'muscle pain', tiredness, loss of weight and a general lack of well-being. As time passes the symptoms 'spread' to other joints – the wrists, feet, knees and shoulders in order of frequency. Another classic feature is generalized stiffness after periods of inactivity, and especially after rising from bed in the early morning.

Physical signs may be slight, but usually there is symmetrically distributed swelling and tenderness of the metacarpophalangeal joints, the proximal interphalangeal joints and the wrists. Tenosynovitis is common in the extensor compartments of the wrist and the flexor sheaths of the fingers; it is diagnosed by feeling thickening, tenderness and crepitation over the back of the wrist or the palm while passively moving the fingers. If the larger joints are involved, local warmth, synovial hypertrophy and intra-articular effusion may be more obvious. Movements are often limited but the joints are still stable and deformity is unusual.

In the later stages joint deformity becomes increasingly apparent and the acute pain of synovitis is replaced by the more constant ache of progressive joint destruction. The combination of joint instability and tendon rupture produces the typical 'rheumatoid' deformities: ulnar deviation of the fingers, radial and volar displacement of the wrists, valgus knees, valgus feet and clawed toes. Joint movements are restricted and often very painful. About a third of all patients develop pain and stiffness in the cervical spine. Function is increasingly disturbed and patients may need help with grooming, dressing and eating.

EXTA-ARTICULAR FEATURES are often seen in patients with severe disease. The most characteristic is the appearance of *nodules*. They are usually found as small subcutaneous lumps, rubbery in consistency, at the back of the elbows, but they also develop in tendons (where they may cause 'triggering' or rupture), in the viscera and the eye. They are pathognomonic of RA, but occur in only 25% of patients.

Less specific features include *muscle wasting, lymphadenopathy, scleritis, nerve entrapment syndromes, skin atrophy or ulceration* and *peripheral sensory neuropathy*. Marked *visceral disease*, such as pulmonary fibrosis, is rare. *Vasculitis* of some degree is almost ubiquitous and may account for many of the features listed here.

X-rays

Early on, x-rays show only the features of synovitis: soft-tissue swelling and periarticular osteoporosis. The later stages are marked by the appearance of marginal bony erosions and narrowing of the articular space, especially in the proximal joints of the hands and feet.

In advanced disease, articular destruction and joint deformity are obvious. Flexion and extension views of the cervical spine often show subluxation at the atlantoaxial or mid-cervical levels; surprisingly, this causes few symptoms in the majority of cases.

Blood investigations

Normocytic, hypochromic anaemia is common and is a reflection of abnormal erythropoiesis due to disease activity. It may be aggravated by chronic gastrointestinal blood loss caused by anti-inflammatory drugs.

In active phases the ESR is raised, C-reactive protein may be present and mucoprotein levels are high.

Serological tests for rheumatoid factor are positive in about 80% of patients and antinuclear factors are present in 30%. Neither of these tests is specific and neither is required for a diagnosis of rheumatoid arthritis.

Synovial biopsy

Synovial tissue may be obtained by needle biopsy, via the arthroscope, or by open operation. Unfortunately, most of the histological features of rheumatoid arthritis are non-specific and the report is more likely to read 'consistent with' rather than 'diagnostic of'.

Diagnosis

The usual criteria for diagnosing rheumatoid disease are the presence of a bilateral, symmetrical polyarthritis involving the proximal joints of the hands or feet, and persisting for at least 6 weeks. If there are subcutaneous nodules or x-ray signs of periarticular erosions, the diagnosis is certain. *A positive test for rheumatoid factor in the absence of the above features is not sufficient evidence of rheumatoid arthritis, nor does a negative test exclude the diagnosis if the other features are all present.* The chief value of the rheumatoid factor

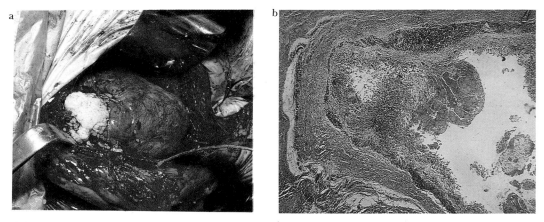

3.2 Rheumatoid synovitis (a) The macroscopic appearance of rheumatoid synovitis with fibrinoid material oozing through a rent in the capsule. (b) Histology shows proliferating synovium with round-cell infiltration and fibrinoid particles in the joint cavity. (×120).

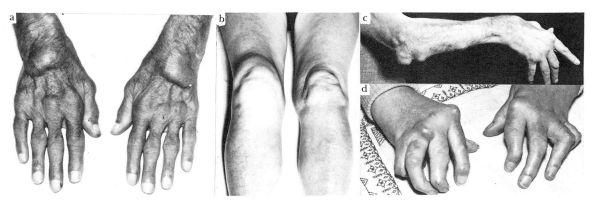

3.3 Rheumatoid arthritis – clinical features Spindling of the fingers and synovitis of the wrists. (b) Sometimes rheumatoid arthritis starts with monarticular synovitis. (c) Rheumatic nodules. (d) Typical late deformities.

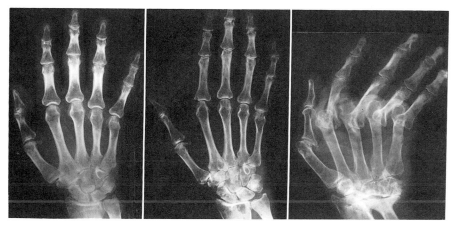

3.4 Rheumatoid arthritis – sequence of changes The progress of disease is well shown in this patient's x-rays. First there was only soft-tissue swelling and periarticular osteoporosis; later juxta-articular erosions appeared; ultimately the joints became unstable and deformed, with four of the metacarpophalangeal joints dislocated.

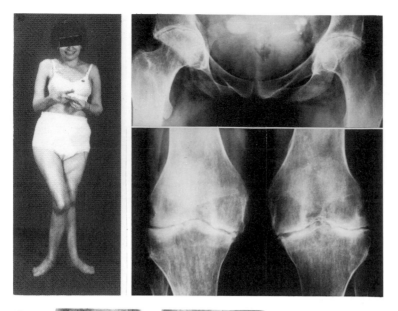

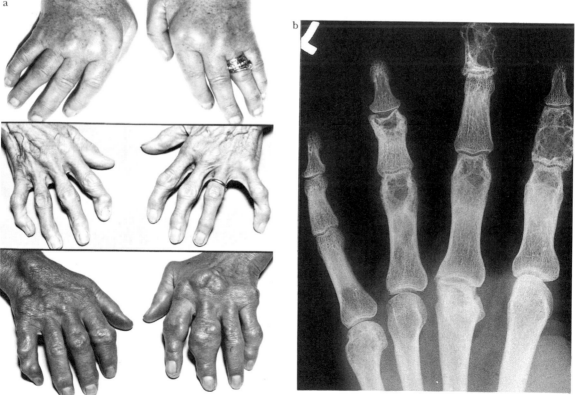

3.5 Rheumatoid arthritis The acute phase is over, but the patient is left with secondary osteoarthritis of the hips and knees.

a

b

3.6 Rheumatoid arthritis – differential diagnosis (a) These three patients all presented with painful swollen finger joints. In the upper figure it is the proximal joints which are enlarged and deformed (rheumatoid arthritis); in the middle figure the distal joints are the worst (Heberden's osteoarthritis); while in the lower the asymmetrical nodules are actually large tophi (gout). (b) Stiff hands and swollen fingers suggested rheumatoid arthritis, but the x-ray showed the classic bubbly 'cysts' of sarcoidosis in the phalanges.

tests is in the assessment of prognosis: persistently high titres herald more serious disease.

Atypical forms of presentation are not uncommon. The early stages may be punctuated by long spells of quiescence, during which the diagnosis is doubted, but sooner or later the more characteristic features appear. Occasionally, in older people, the onset is explosive, with the rapid appearance of severe joint pain and stiffness; paradoxically these patients have a relatively good prognosis. Now and then (more so in young women) the disease starts with chronic pain and swelling of a single large joint and it may take months or years before other joints are involved.

In the differential diagnosis of polyarthritis several disorders must be considered.

SERONEGATIVE POLYARTHRITIS is a feature of a number of conditions vaguely related to rheumatoid arthritis: psoriatic arthritis, juvenile chronic arthritis (Still's disease), systemic lupus erythematosus and other connective-tissue diseases. These are considered in later sections.

ANKYLOSING SPONDYLITIS may involve the peripheral joints, but it is primarily a disease of the sacroiliac and intervertebral joints, causing back pain and progressive stiffness.

REITER'S DISEASE usually affects the larger joints and the lumbosacral spine. There is a history of urethritis or colitis and often also conjunctivitis.

POLYARTICULAR GOUT affects large and small joints, and tophi may be mistaken for rheumatic nodules. On x-ray the erosions are quite different from those of rheumatoid arthritis; the diagnosis can be clinched by finding birefringent crystals in the joint fluid or the 'nodule'.

CALCIUM PYROPHOSPHATE DEPOSITION DISEASE is usually seen in older people. Typically it affects large joints, but it may occur in the wrist and metacarpophalangeal joints as well. X-ray signs are fairly characteristic and crystals may be identified in synovial fluid or synovium.

HEBERDEN'S ARTHROPATHY affects the *distal* interphalangeal joints, and causes a nodular arthritis with radiologically obvious osteophytes – all of which are absent in the erosive arthritis of rheumatoid disease.

SARCOIDOSIS may present with a symmetrical small-joint polyarthritis and no bone involvement; erythema nodosum and hilar lymphadenopathy are clues to the diagnosis. The condition usually subsides spontaneously within 6 months. Another form of the disease, with chronic granulomatous infiltration of bone, synovium and other organs, is more common in Negroes. In addition to polyarthritis and tenosynovitis, x-rays show punched-out 'cysts' and cortical erosions in the bones of the hands and feet. The ESR is raised and the Kveim test may be positive. Treatment with non-steroidal anti-inflammatory drugs (NSAIDs) may be adequate but in more intractable cases corticosteroids are necessary.

POLYMYALGIA RHEUMATICA occurs mostly in middle-aged or elderly women, causing marked post-inactivity stiffness and weakness. Pain is most severe around the pectoral and pelvic girdles; tenderness is in muscles rather than joints. The ESR is almost always remarkably high. This is a form of giant-cell arteritis and carries the risk of temporal arteritis resulting in blindness. Corticosteroids (as little as 10 mg a day) provide rapid and dramatic relief of all symptoms, and this response is often used as a diagnostic test.

Treatment

There is no cure for rheumatoid arthritis. This must be explained to the patient, who also needs to be reassured that it is not necessarily a crippling disease, that much can be done to alleviate symptoms and delay progression, and that there is every chance of a useful and active life despite some undoubted functional limitations.

Management is guided by four simple injunctions:
(1) *stop the synovitis*; (2) *prevent deformity*; (3) *reconstruct*; and (4) *rehabilitate*. A multidisciplinary approach is needed from the beginning: the physician, surgeon, physiotherapist, occupational therapist, orthotist and social worker must co-operate as a team.

● STOP THE SYNOVITIS

REST is one of the oldest and still one of the most effective methods of reducing joint pain and swelling. During a flare-up of polyarthritis, bed rest for 2–3 weeks will allow the acute inflammation to settle. Gentle active and passive exercises are given to maintain joint mobility, and care should be taken to prevent postural deformities. Continuous splintage (e.g. for·the knees, elbows or wrists) is equally effective during acute exacerbations. Night splints can be used intermittently for pain at any stage of the disease.

NON-STEROIDAL ANTI-INFLAMMATORY DRUGS (NSAID) are used in almost all cases. The oldest of these is aspirin; it is still used in some clinics but, because of the frequency of side effects, it has been largely replaced by indomethacin and the newer acetic acid and propiónic acid derivatives. They are not curative, do not influence the progress of erosions and do not lower the ESR, but they do control pain and stiffness (probably through their anti-prostaglandin activity) and therefore improve function. Side effects are common (rashes, gastrointestinal symptoms, peptic ulceration) but usually reversible.

DISEASE-MODIFYING DRUGS Gold, penicillamine, hydroxychloroquine and immunosuppressive drugs such as methotrexate have a direct action on the immunopathological process and can control disease progress. However, they all have unpredictable – and potentially lethal – side effects on the kidney, liver and haemopoietic system. They are, therefore, usually introduced only when other measures have failed; but in severe cases with florid synovitis, high ESR and strongly positive rheumatoid factor tests (when simpler measures are likely to fail) they may be used much earlier. Their effects must always be monitored by regular blood tests and by liver and renal function tests. Dosage should be adjusted with great caution; the rule is: 'Start low, go slow'. It may take 6–12 weeks before the patient improves.

SYSTEMIC CORTICOSTEROIDS relieve joint pain and stiffness so effectively that their use is a constant temptation; a temptation to be resisted, however, because of their serious side effects (osteoporosis, hypertension, diabetes, predisposition to infection). With experience and discipline they can be used (1) during severe, incapacitating exacerbations, to help weather the storm while waiting for gold or penicillamine to start acting; (2) when no other treatment helps; and (3) in the rare instance of fulminating disease.

INTRASYNOVIAL INJECTIONS Cortiscosteroids and cytotoxic drugs such as nitrogen mustard are highly effective when injected into inflamed joints or tendon sheaths. Local pain and swelling may be relieved for weeks or even months. Some of this improvement may be due to a systemic effect; even the so-called depot steroids are absorbed to some extent. It is sometimes feared that repeated infections may harm the

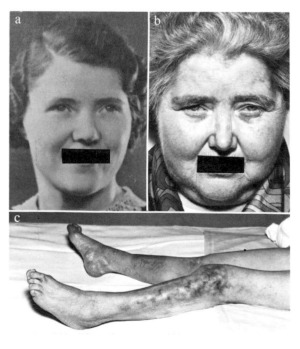

3.7 Treatment of rheumatoid arthritis – (1) control the synovitis Anti-inflammatory drugs are necessary – but can be harmful. (a) This young woman on corticosteroids became (b) severely cushingoid. (c) This patient had multiple ecchymoses which, combined with tissue-paper skin, increase the risk of limb surgery.

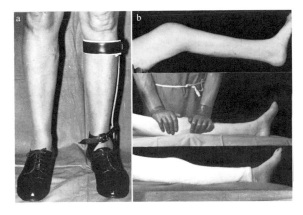

3.8 Treatment of rheumatoid arthritis – (2) prevent deformity (a) Splintage to rest inflamed joints may, if started early, halt the progress of deformity. (b) An early fixed deformity of the knee can be corrected by gentle manipulation and temporary plaster splintage.

joint; animal experiments have shown that intra-articular corticosteroids can induce deposition of hydroxyapatite crystals in articular cartilage (Ohira and Ishikawa, 1986). However, there is little evidence that intra-articular injections in humans are harmful, provided they are used sparingly and with full precautions against infection.

Intra-articular radiocolloids have been used to produce synovial irradiation – another way of counteracting inflammation. Yttrium-90 can be injected on an outpatient basis, provided the limb is splinted for a day or two to reduce absorption of the isotope.

SYNOVECTOMY Even at an early stage of the disease, if all other measures fail, synovectomy is worth while; in the knee this should be done arthroscopically. Synovectomy is particularly useful for rheumatoid tenosynovitis.

● PREVENT DEFORMITY

SPLINTAGE may be used to prevent an anticipated deformity, especially during a flare-up in disease activity where joints are painful and swollen.

PHYSIOTHERAPY, usually in the form of active exercises, is important both to maintain a good range of movement and to strengthen muscle power. Continuous passive motion (CPM) is effective in preventing fixed deformity of the knee.

POSTURAL TRAINING is equally important; patients are taught to avoid postures that would favour the development of deformities.

OPERATION Tendon rupture and joint instability lead to progressive deformity. They should be looked for and treated whenever they occur – either by permanent splintage or by operation. Ruptured tendons – quite common around the wrist or ankle – can be sutured or replaced. Soft-tissue stabilization of the wrist or finger joints can prevent increasing destruction and deformity. Excision of the radial head or the distal end of the ulna is a simple method of relieving local pain and stiffness.

● RECONSTRUCT

Advanced joint destruction, instability and deformity are clear indications for reconstructive surgery, often combined with synovectomy of the joint or tendons. Arthrodesis, osteotomy and replacement all have their place and are considered in the appropriate chapters.

● REHABILITATE

Rehabilitation should not be seen as a rearguard action; it accompanies all stages of treatment from the start, and includes functional assessment, special training, social integration and psychological adjustment. A full understanding of the patient's specific needs must influence treatment. Some patients are well motivated and crave to return to work and domestic independence; others are passive and dependent. For the one group mechanical aids, special utensils, adjustment of home and work space are essential adjuncts to medical and surgical treatment; for the other the support of family and friends may be all that is wanted.

Complications

FIXED DEFORMITIES The perils of rheumatoid arthritis are often the commonplace ones resulting from ignorance and neglect. Early assessment and planning should prevent postural deformities which will result in joint contractures.

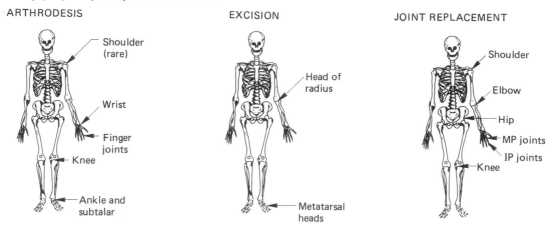

3.9 Treatment of rheumatoid arthritis – (3) reconstruct   Sites where each operation may be useful.

MUSCLE WEAKNESS   Even mild degrees of myopathy or neuropathy, when combined with prolonged inactivity, may lead to profound muscle wasting and weakness. This should be prevented by physiotherapy and pain control, if possible; if not, the surgeon must be forewarned of the difficulty of postoperative rehabilitation.

JOINT RUPTURE   Occasionally the joint lining ruptures and synovial contents spill into the soft tissues. Treatment is directed at the underlying synovitis – i.e. splintage and injection of the joint, with synovectomy as a second resort.

INFECTION   Patients with rheumatoid arthritis – and even more so those on corticosteroid therapy – are susceptible to infection. Sudden clinical deterioration, or increased pain in a single joint, should alert one to the possibility of septic arthritis and the need for joint aspiration.

SPINAL CORD COMPRESSION   is a rare complication of cervical spine instability. The onset of weakness and upper motor neuron signs in the lower limbs is suspicious. If they occur, immobilization of the neck is essential and spinal fusion should be carried out as soon as possible.

SYSTEMIC VASCULITIS   is a rare but potentially serious complication. High doses of corticosteroids and intravenous plasma volume expanders may be called for.

AMYLOIDOSIS   is another rare but potentially lethal complication of long-standing rheumatoid disease. The patient presents with proteinuria and progressive renal failure. The diagnosis is made by finding amyloid in a rectal or renal biopsy. There is no specific treatment.

Prognosis

Rheumatoid arthritis runs a variable course. When the patient is first seen it is difficult to predict the outcome, but high titres of rheumatoid factor, periarticular erosions, rheumatoid nodules, severe muscle wasting, joint contractures and evidence of vasculitis are bad prognostic signs. About 10% of patients improve steadily after the first attack of active synovitis; 60% have intermittent phases of disease activity and remission, but with a slow downhill course over many years; 20% have severe joint erosion, often requiring multiple operations; and 10% end up completely disabled.

Ankylosing spondylitis

Like rheumatoid arthritis, this is a generalized chronic inflammatory disease – but its effects are seen mainly in the spine and sacroiliac joints. It is characterized by pain and stiffness of the back, with variable involvement of the hips and shoulders and (more rarely) the peripheral joints. Its prevalence is about 0.2% in western Europe, but is much lower in Japanese and Negroid peoples. Males are affected more frequently than females (estimates vary from 2:1 to 10:1) and the usual age at onset is between 15 and 25 years. There is a strong tendency to familial involvement.

Cause

Genetic predisposition is important. The disease is much more common in family members than in the general population, and HLA-B27 is present both in patients and in half of their first-degree relatives. But, as only a fraction of people with HLA-B27 develop ankylosing spondylitis, there must be some additional trigger. Since classic ankylosing spondylitis is sometimes associated with genitourinary or bowel infection, and disorders such as Reiter's disease and ulcerative colitis cause vertebral and sacroiliac changes indistinguishable from those of ankylosing spondylitis, it is thought that lymphatic drainage to the spine may be important.

Pathology

There are two basic lesions: synovitis of diarthrodial joints and inflammation at the fibro-osseous junctions of syndesmotic joints and tendons. The preferential involvement of the insertion of tendons and ligaments (the entheses) has spawned the somewhat unwieldy term *enthesopathy.*

Synovitis of the sacroiliac and vertebral facet joints causes destruction of articular cartilage and periarticular bone. The costovertebral joints also are frequently involved, leading to diminished respiratory excursion. When peripheral joints are affected the same changes occur.

Inflammation of the fibro-osseous junctions affects the intervertebral discs, sacroiliac ligaments, symphysis pubis, manubrium sterni and the bony insertions of large tendons. Pathological changes proceed in three stages: (1) an inflammatory reaction with round-cell infiltration, granulation tissue formation and erosion of adjacent bone; (2) replacement of the granulation tissue by fibrous tissue; and (3) ossification of the fibrous tissue, leading to ankylosis of the joint.

Ossification across the surface of the disc gives rise to small bony bridges or *syndesmophytes* linking adjacent vertebral bodies. If many vertebrae are involved the spine may become absolutely rigid.

Clinical features

The disease starts insidiously: a teenager or young adult complains of backache and stiffness recurring at intervals over a number of years. This is often diagnosed as 'back strain'; but typically the symptoms are worse in the early morning and after inactivity. Referred pain in the buttocks and thighs may appear as 'sciatica' and some patients are mistakenly treated for intervertebral disc prolapse. Gradually pain and stiffness become continuous and other symptoms begin to appear: general fatigue, pain and swelling of joints, tenderness at the insertion of the tendo Achillis, 'foot strain', or intercostal pain and tenderness.

Early on there is little to see apart from slight flattening of the lower back and limitation of extension in the lumbar spine. There may be diffuse tenderness over the spine and sacroiliac joints, or (occasionally) swelling and tenderness of a single large joint.

In established cases the posture is typical: loss of the normal lumbar lordosis, increased thoracic kyphosis and a forward thrust of the neck; upright posture and balance are maintained by standing with the hips and knees slightly flexed, and in late cases these may become fixed deformities.

Spinal movements are diminished in all directions, but loss of extension is always the earliest and the most severe disability. It is revealed dramatically by the 'wall test': the

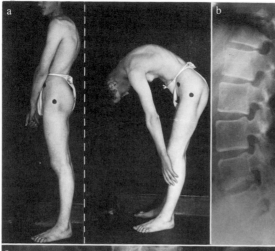

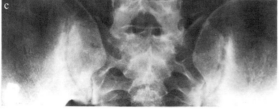

3.10 Ankylosing spondylitis – early   The early features are (a) a stiff spine, (b) 'squaring' of the lumbar vertebrae and (c) bilateral sacroiliac erosion.

and loss of mobility. There may also be tenderness of the ligament and tendon insertions close to a joint or under the heel.

EXTRASKELETAL MANIFESTATIONS   Prostatitis is common but it is usually asymptomatic. Uveitis and conjunctivitis occur in about 20% of patients. Other extraskeletal disorders, such as aortic valve disease, carditis and pulmonary fibrosis, are rare and occur very late in the disease.

X-rays

The cardinal sign – and often the earliest – is erosion and fuzziness of the sacroiliac joints. Later there may be periarticular sclerosis, especially on the iliac side of the joint, and finally bony ankylosis.

The earliest vertebral change is flattening of the normal anterior concavity of the vertebral body ('squaring'). Later, ossification across the intervertebral discs produces delicate syndesmophytes spanning the gaps between adjacent vertebrae. Bridging at several levels gives the appearance of a 'bamboo spine'.

Peripheral joints may show erosive arthritis or progressive bony ankylosis.

Special investigations

The ESR is usually elevated during active phases of the disease. HLA-B27 is present in 90% of cases. Serological tests for rheumatoid factor are negative.

Diagnosis

Diagnosis is easy in patients with spinal rigidity and typical deformities, but it is often missed in those with early disease or unusual forms of presentation. In over 10% of cases the disease starts with an asymmetrical inflammatory arthritis – usually of the hip, knee or ankle – and it may be several years before back pain appears. Atypical onset is more common in women, who may show less obvious changes in the sacroiliac joints.

patient is asked to stand with his back to the wall; heels, buttocks, scapulae and occiput should all be able to touch the wall simultaneously. If extension is seriously diminished the patient will find this impossible. In the most advanced stage the spine may be completely ankylosed from occiput to sacrum – sometimes in positions of grotesque deformity. Marked loss of cervical extension may restrict the line of vision to a few paces.

Chest expansion, which should be at least 7 cm in young men, is often markedly decreased. In old people, who may have pulmonary disease, this test is unreliable.

Peripheral joints (usually shoulders, hips and knees) are involved in over a third of the patients; they show the features of inflammatory arthritis – swelling, tenderness, effusion

MECHANICAL DISORDERS A number of conditions in young adults (spondylolisthesis, facet joint instability, disc disorders) cause chronic low back pain, and because they are so common they are the first to be thought of. They differ from ankylosing spondylitis in several ways: the onset is more acute, stiffness is less pronounced and symptoms are eased rather than aggravated by inactivity. Tenderness is also more localized and the peripheral joints are normal.

ANKYLOSING HYPEROSTOSIS (FORESTIER'S DISEASE) This is a fairly common disorder, predominantly of older men, characterized by widespread ossification of ligaments and tendon insertions. X-rays show pronounced but asymmetrical intervertebral spur formation and bridging throughout the dorsolumbar spine. Although it bears a superficial resemblance to ankylosing spondylitis, it is not an inflammatory disease, spinal pain and stiffness are seldom severe, the sacroiliac joints are not eroded and the ESR is normal.

THE SERONEGATIVE SPONDARTHRITIDES A number of disorders are associated with vertebral and sacroiliac lesions indistinguishable from those of ankylosing spondylitis. They are Reiter's disease, psoriatic arthritis, ulcerative colitis, Crohn's disease, Whipple's disease and Behçet's syndrome (Moll et al., 1974). In each there are certain characteristic features: the rash or nail changes of psoriasis, intestinal ulceration in enterocolitis, genitourinary and ocular inflammation in Reiter's disease, buccal and genital ulceration in Behçet's syndrome. Yet there is considerable overlap between them; all show some familial aggregation and all are associated with the histocompatibility antigen, HLA-B27. Patients with one of these disorders (including ankylosing spondylitis) often have close relatives with another, or with a positive HLA-B27.

Treatment

The disease is not nearly as damaging as rheumatoid arthritis and most patients continue to lead an active life. In the absence of a specific agent, treatment consists of (1) general measures to maintain satisfactory posture and

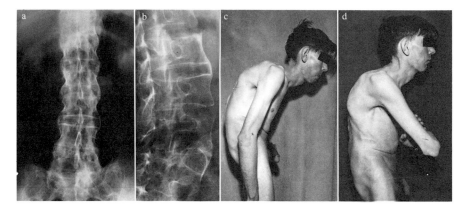

3.11 Ankylosing spondylitis – late (a, b) Bony bridges (syndesmophytes) between the vertebral bodies convert the spine into a rigid column ('bamboo spine'); note that the sacroiliac joints have fused. Spinal osteotomy may be necessary at this stage: (c) before operation this man could see only a few paces ahead; (d) after osteotomy his back is still rigid, but his posture, function and outlook are vastly improved.

preserve movement, (2) anti-inflammatory drugs to counteract pain and stiffness, and (3) operations to correct deformity or restore mobility.

GENERAL MEASURES   Patients are encouraged to remain active and follow their normal pursuits as far as possible. They should be taught how to maintain satisfactory posture and urged to perform spinal extension exercises every day. Swimming, dancing and gymnastics are ideal forms of recreation. Rest and immobilization, effective in other inflammatory joint diseases, are contraindicated because they tend to increase muscle wasting, osteoporosis and ankylosis.

NON-STEROIDAL ANTI-INFLAMMATORY DRUGS   It is doubtful whether these drugs prevent or retard the progress to ankylosis, but they do control pain and counteract soft-tissue stiffness, thus making it possible to benefit from exercise and activity. Indomethacin is often used but other, less powerful, drugs may be adequate; they usually have to be continued for many years.

OPERATION   Stiffness of the hips can be treated by joint replacement, though this seldom provides more than moderate mobility. Moreover, the incidence of infection is higher than usual and patients may need prolonged rehabilitation.

Deformity of the spine may be severe enough to warrant lumbar or cervical osteotomy. These are difficult and potentially hazardous procedures; fortunately, with improved activity and exercise programmes, they are seldom needed. If spinal deformity is combined with hip stiffness, hip replacements (permitting full extension) often suffice.

Reiter's syndrome and reactive arthritis

The syndrome described by Hans Reiter in 1916 (and 100 years before that by Benjamin Brodie) is a clinical triad of *urethritis, arthritis* and *conjunctivitis* occurring some weeks after either *dysentery* or *venereal infection*. It is now recog-

nized that this is one of the classic forms of reactive arthritis, i.e. an aseptic inflammatory arthritis associated with non-specific urogenital or bowel infection.

Its prevalence is difficult to assess, but it is probably the commonest type of large-joint polyarthritis in young men. It is thought to occur in 1–3% of all people who develop either non-specific urogenital infection or *Shigella* dysentery, but its incidence may be as high as 25% in those who are HLA-B27 positive (Calin and Fries, 1976). Men are affected more often than women (the ratio is about 10:1), but this may simply reflect the difficulty of diagnosing the venereal infection in women. The usual age at onset is between 20 and 40 years, but children are affected too – perhaps after an episode of diarrhoea.

Cause

Familial aggregation, overlap with other forms of seronegative spondarthritis in first-degree relatives and a close association with HLA-B27 point to a genetic predisposition, the bowel or urogenital infection acting as a trigger. Dysenteric organisms include *Shigella flexneri, Salmonella, Campylobacter* species and *Yersinia enterocolitica. Lymphogranuloma venereum* and *Chlamydia trachomatis* have been implicated as sexually transmitted infections.

Pathology

The pathological changes are essentially the same as those in ankylosing spondylitis, with the emphasis first on subacute large-joint synovitis and later tending towards sacroiliitis and spondylitis.

Clinical features

The acute phase of the disease is marked by an asymmetrical inflammatory arthritis of the lower limb joints – usually the knee and ankle but often the tarsal and toe joints as well. The joint may be acutely painful, hot and swollen with a tense effusion, suggesting gout or infection. Tendo Achillis tenderness and plantar fasciitis (evidence of enthesopathy) are common, and the patient may complain of backache even in the early stage. Conjunctivitis, urethritis and bowel infections are often mild and easily missed; the patient should be carefully questioned about symptoms during the previous few weeks. Cystitis and cervicitis may occur in women.

Less frequent, but equally characteristic, features are a vesicular or pustular dermatitis of the feet (keratoderma blennorrhagica), balanitis and mild buccal ulceration.

a

b

c

3.12 Reiter's syndrome The classic triad of Reiter's syndrome – urethritis (sometimes colitis), conjunctivitis and arthritis. Tenderness of the tendo Achillis and the plantar fascia is also common.

The acute disorder usually lasts for a few weeks or months and then subsides, but most patients have either recurrent attacks of arthritis or other features of chronic disease.

The chronic phase is more characteristic of a spondarthropathy. Over half of the patients with Reiter's disease complain of mild, recurrent episodes of polyarthritis (including upper limb joints). About half of those again develop sacroiliitis and spondylitis with features resembling those of ankylosing spondylitis. Uveitis is also fairly common and may give rise to posterior synechiae and glaucoma.

X-RAYS are at first normal, but after many months may show an erosive arthritis. Sacroiliac and vertebral changes are similar to those of ankylosing spondylitis.

SPECIAL INVESTIGATIONS Tests for HLA-B27 are positive in 75% of patients with sacroiliitis. The ESR may be high in the active phase of the disease. The causative organism can sometimes be isolated from urethral fluids or faeces, and tests for antibodies may be positive.

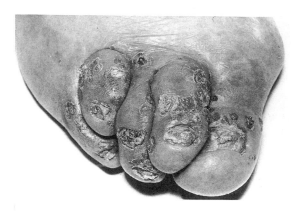

3.13 Reiter's disease – other features The characteristic pustular dermatitis of the feet – keratoderma blennorrhagica.

Diagnosis

The diagnosis should be considered in any young adult who presents with an acute or subacute arthritis in the lower limbs. It is more likely to be missed in women, in children and in those with very mild (and often forgotten) episodes of urogenital or bowel infection. Some patients never develop the full syndrome and one should be alert to the *formes fruste* with large-joint arthritis alone.

GOUT OR INFECTIVE ARTHRITIS may be mistaken for Reiter's disease. Examination of synovial fluid for organisms and crystals will exclude these disorders.

ENTEROPATHIC ARTHRITIS Ulcerative colitis and Crohn's disease may be associated with subacute synovitis, causing pain and swelling of one or more of the peripheral joints. These subside when the intestinal disease is controlled.

GONOCOCCAL ARTHRITIS takes two forms: (1) bacterial infection of the joint; and (2) a reactive arthritis with sterile joint fluid. A history of venereal infection further complicates the distinction from Reiter's disease, and diagnosis may depend on identifying the organism or gonococcal antibodies.

Treatment

There is no specific treatment for Reiter's disease; even if the triggering infection is identified, treating it will have no effect on the reactive arthritis. However, many people advocate giving tetracycline 1 g daily for 5–10 days if there is persistent or recurrent urethral infection.

Acute arthritis or tendinitis may benefit from local injection of corticosteroids and a period of splintage. Topical steroids are also used for severe uveitis.

For the rest, treatment is palliative and supportive. Patients may need long-term non-steroidal anti-inflammatory and analgesic therapy. If spinal and sacroiliac changes are marked, treatment is the same as for ankylosing spondylitis.

Psoriatic arthritis

Polyarthritis and psoriasis are often seen together. Usually this is simply a chance concurrence of two fairly common disorders. In some cases, however, the patient has a true psoriatic arthritis – a distinct entity characterized by seronegative polysynovitis, erosive (sometimes very destructive) arthritis, and a significant incidence of sacroiliitis and spondylitis.

The prevalence of psoriasis is 1–2%; only about 5% of those affected will develop psoriatic arthritis. The sex ratio is reported as 1 : 1 and the usual age at onset 30–50 years (much later than the skin lesions).

Cause

As with the other seronegative spondoarthritides, there is a strong genetic component: patients often give a family history of psoriasis; there is a significantly increased incidence of other spondarthritides in close relatives; and 60% of those with psoriatic spondylitis or sacroiliitis have HLA-B27.

Psoriatic skin lesions may well be a reactive phenomenon, and the joint lesions a form of 'reactive arthritis'. However, no specific trigger agent has thus far been identified.

Pathology

The joint changes are similar to those in rheumatoid arthritis – chronic synovitis with round-cell infiltration and exudate, going on to fibrosis. Cartilage and bone destruction may be unusually severe ('arthritis mutilans'). However, rheumatoid nodules are not seen.

Sacroiliac and spine changes, which occur in about 30% of patients, are similar to those in ankylosing spondylitis.

Clinical features

The patient usually presents with a comparatively mild, asymmetrical polyarthritis affecting some of the interphalangeal joints of the fingers or toes. The condition progresses slowly and may become quiescent. Sometimes (particularly in women) joint involvement is more symmetrical, and in these cases the condition may be indistinguishable from seronegative rheumatoid arthritis.

Sacroiliitis and spondylitis are seen in about one-third of patients, and occasionally this is the predominant change with a clinical picture resembling ankylosing spondylitis.

In the worst cases both the spine and the peripheral joints may be involved. Fingers and toes are severely deformed due to erosion and instability of the interphalangeal joints (arthritis mutilans).

Psoriasis of the skin or nails usually precedes the arthritis, but hidden lesions (in the natal cleft or umbilicus) are easily overlooked.

Ocular inflammation occurs in about 30% of patients.

X-RAYS show destruction of the distal and/or proximal interphalangeal joints; changes in the large joints are similar to those of rheumatoid disease. Sacroiliac erosion is fairly common; if the spine is involved the appearances are identical to those of ankylosing spondylitis.

SPECIAL INVESTIGATIONS Tests for rheumatoid factor are almost always negative. HLA-B27 occurs in 50–60%, especially in those with overt sacroiliitis.

Diagnosis

The main difficulty is to distinguish 'psoriatic arthritis' from 'psoriasis with seronegative RA'. The important distinguishing features of psoriatic arthritis are: (1) asymmetrical joint distribution; (2) involvement of distal finger joints; (3) the presence of sacroiliitis or spondylitis; and (4) the absence of rheumatoid nodules.

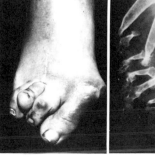
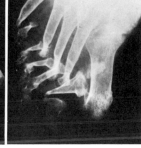

3.14 Psoriatic arthritis (1) (a) Psoriasis of the elbows and forearms; (b) typical finger deformities, and (c) x-rays show *distal* joint involvement – so clearly the disease is not simply rheumatoid arthritis in a patient with psoriasis.

3.15 Psoriatic arthritis (2) The feet also may be affected, and this patient first presented at an orthopaedic clinic.

Treatment

GENERAL TREATMENT aims at controlling the skin disorder with topical preparations, and alleviating joint symptoms with non-steroidal anti-inflammatory drugs. In resistant forms of arthritis, immunosuppressive agents (azathioprine and methotrexate) have proved effective.

LOCAL TREATMENT consists of judicious splintage to avoid undue deformity, and surgery for unstable joints. Arthrodesis of the distal interphalangeal joints may greatly improve function.

Enteropathic arthritis

Both Crohn's disease and ulcerative colitis may be associated with either peripheral arthritis or sacroiliitis and spondylitis.

PERIPHERAL ARTHRITIS is fairly common, occurring in about 15% of patients with inflammatory bowel disease. Typically one or perhaps a few of the larger joints are involved. Pain and swelling appear quite suddenly and may last for 2–3 months before subsiding. Synovitis is usually the only feature and joint erosion is rare. Men and women are affected with equal frequency and there is no particular association with HLA-B27. Treatment is directed at the underlying disorder: attacks of arthritis are triggered by a flare-up of bowel disease and when the latter is brought under control the arthritis disappears. Anti-inflammatory drugs are useful if synovitis is marked; they have not been shown to have any deleterious effect on the bowel disease.

SACROILIITIS AND SPONDYLITIS are seen in about 10% of patients with inflammatory bowel disease, and in half of these patients the clinical picture closely resembles that of ankylosing spondylitis. HLA-B27 is positive in 60% and there is an increased incidence of ankylosing spondylitis in close relatives. Unlike the peripheral arthritis, sacroiliitis shows no temporal relationship to gastrointestinal inflammation and its course is unaffected by treatment of the bowel disease. Management is the same as that of ankylosing spondylitis.

Complications

In addition to spondarthritis, there are several unusual but important complications of inflammatory bowel disease that may confuse the clinical picture.

Septic arthritis of the hip arises by direct spread of infection from the bowel. The patient presents with a fever and pain in the groin. Hip movements are limited and there may be swelling due to an abscess. Treatment is by antibiotics and operative drainage.

Psoas abscess In Crohn's disease a posterior fistula may track into the psoas sheath. The patient complains of back pain and may develop a typical psoas abscess with pain in the hip, limitation of movement and a tender mass in the groin. Treatment is by operative drainage of the abscess.

Avascular necrosis Pain in the hip may be due to 'idiopathic' avascular necrosis of the femoral head following treatment of the bowel disease with corticosteroids. Occasionally, other joints (hip or shoulder) are involved. The clinical features and treatment are described in Chapter 6.

Osteopenia Patients with chronic bowel disease often develop osteoporosis and osteomalacia – partly due to malabsorption and partly as a consequence of treatment with corticosteroids. Compression fractures of the spine may cause severe back pain. Treatment is futile if the patient has to remain on cortisone.

Juvenile chronic arthritis

Juvenile chronic arthritis (JCA) is the preferred term for non-infective inflammatory joint disease of more than 3 months' duration in children under 16 years of age. It embraces a group of disorders in all of which pain, swelling and stiffness of the joints are common features. The prevalence is about 1 per 1000 children, and boys and girls are affected with equal frequency.

The cause is probably similar to that of rheumatoid disease: an abnormal immune response to some antigen in children with a particular genetic predisposition. However, rheumatoid factor is usually absent.

The pathology, too, is like that of rheumatoid arthritis: primarily a synovial inflammation leading to fibrosis and ankylosis. Stiffening tends to occur in whatever position the joint is allowed to assume; thus flexion deformities are a common and characteristic feature. Chronic inflammation and alterations in the local blood supply may affect the epiphyseal growth plates, leading to both local bone deformities and an overall retardation of growth. However, cartilage erosion is less marked than in rheumatoid arthritis and severe joint instability is uncommon.

Clinical features

Children with JCA present in several characteristic ways. About 15% have a *systemic illness,* and arthritis only develops somewhat later; the majority (60–70%) have a *pauciarticular arthritis* affecting a few of the larger joints; about 10% present with *polyarticular arthritis,* sometimes closely resembling RA; the remaining 5–10% develop a *seronegative spondarthritis.*

Systemic JCA This, the classic Still's disease, is usually seen below the age of 3 years and affects boys and girls equally. It starts with intermittent fever, rashes and malaise; during these episodes, which occur almost daily, the child appears to be quite ill but after a few hours the clinical condition improves again. Less constant features are lymphadenopathy, splenomegaly and hepatomegaly. Joint swelling occurs some weeks or months after the onset; fortunately, it usually resolves when the systemic illness subsides but it may go on to progressive seronegative polyarthritis, leading to permanent deformity of the larger joints and fusion of the cervical apophyseal joints. By puberty there may be stunting of growth, often abetted by the earlier use of corticosteroids.

Pauciarticular JCA This is by far the commonest form of JCA. It usually occurs below the age of 6 years and is much more common in girls; occasionally older children are affected. Only a few joints are involved and there is no systemic illness. The child presents with pain and swelling of medium-sized joints (knees, ankles, elbows and wrists); sometimes only one joint is affected. Rheumatoid factor tests are negative. A serious complication is chronic iridocyclitis, which occurs in about 50%. The arthritis often goes into remission after a few years but by then the child is left with asymmetrical deformities and growth defects that may be permanent.

Polyarticular JCA Polyarticular arthritis, typically with involvement of the temporomandibular joints and the cervical spine, is usually seen in older children, mainly girls. The hands and wrists are often affected, but the classic deformities of rheumatoid arthritis are uncommon and rheumatoid factor is usually absent. In some cases, however, the condition is indistinguishable from adult rheumatoid arthritis, with a positive rheumatoid factor test; these probably warrant the designation 'juvenile rheumatoid arthritis'.

Seronegative spondarthritis In older children – usually boys – the condition may take the form of sacroiliitis and spondylitis; hips and knees are sometimes involved as well. Tests for HLA-B27 are often positive and this should probably be regarded as 'juvenile ankylosing spondylitis'.

x-rays In early disease non-specific changes such as soft-tissue swelling may be seen, but x-ray is mainly useful to exclude other painful disorders. Later there may be signs of progressive joint erosion and deformity.

investigations The white cell count and ESR are markedly raised in systemic JCA, less so in the other forms. Rheumatoid factor tests are positive only in juvenile RA.

Joint aspiration and synovial fluid examination may be essential to exclude infection or haemarthrosis.

Diagnosis

In the early stages, before chronic arthritis is fully established, diagnosis may be difficult. Systemic JCA may start with an illness resembling a *viral infection*. Pauciarticular JCA, especially if only one joint is involved, is indistinguishable from *Reiter's disease* or *septic arthritis* (if the signs are acute) or *tuberculous synovitis* (if they are more subdued).

Other conditions that need to be excluded are *rheumatic fever*, one of the *bleeding disorders* and *leukaemia*.

In most cases the problem is resolved once the full pattern of joint involvement is established, but blood investigations, joint aspiration and synovial biopsy may be required to clinch the diagnosis.

Complications

ANKYLOSIS Whilst most patients recover good function, some loss of movement is common. Hips, knees and elbows may be unable to extend fully, and in the spondylitic form of JCA the spine, hips and knees may be almost rigid. Temporomandibular ankylosis and stiffness of the cervical spine can make general anaesthesia difficult and dangerous.

GROWTH DEFECTS There is a general retardation of growth, aggravated by prolonged corticosteroid therapy. In addition, epiphyseal disturbances lead to characteristic deformities: external torsion of the tibia, dysplasia of the distal ulna, underdevelopment of the mandible, shortness of the neck and scoliosis.

FRACTURES Children aged under 5 years with chronic joint disease may suffer osteoporosis and they are prone to fractures.

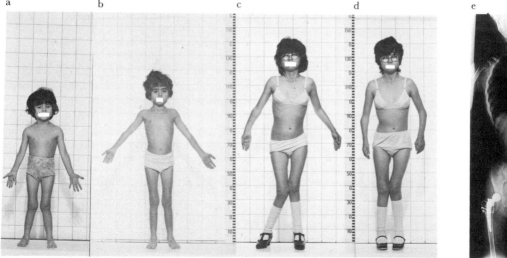
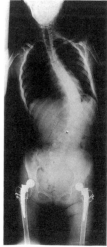

3.16 Juvenile chronic arthritis (a–d) This young girl developed JCA when she was 5 years old. Here we see her at 6, 9 and 14 years of age. The arthritis has become inactive, leaving her with a knee deformity which was treated by osteotomy. Her eyes, too, were affected, by iridocyclitis. (Courtesy of Mr Malcolm Swann and Dr Barbara Ansell.) (e) X-ray of another young girl who required hip replacements at the age of 14 and, later, surgical correction of her scoliosis.

IRIDOCYCLITIS This is most common in pauciarticular disease; untreated it may lead to blindness.

AMYLOIDOSIS In children with long-standing active disease there is a serious risk of amyloidosis, which may be fatal.

Treatment

GENERAL TREATMENT is similar to that of rheumatoid arthritis, including the use of gold or penicillamine for those with seropositive juvenile RA. Corticosteroids should be used only for severe systemic disease and for chronic iridocyclitis unresponsive to topical therapy.

LOCAL TREATMENT aims to prevent stiffness and deformity. Night splints are useful for the wrists, hands, knees and ankles; prone lying for some period of each day may prevent flexion contracture of the hips. Between periods of splinting, active exercises are encouraged; these are started by the physiotherapist but the parents must be taught how to continue the programme.

Fixed deformities may need correction by serial plasters or by a spell in hospital on a CPM machine; when progress is no longer being made, joint capsulotomy may help. For painful eroded joints, useful procedures include custom-designed arthroplasties of the hip and knee (even in children), and arthrodesis of the wrist or ankle (Ansell and Swann, 1983).

SUPPORT Children and parents alike need sympathetic counselling to help them cope with the difficulties of social adjustments, education and training.

Prognosis

Fortunately, most children with JCA recover from the arthritis and are left with only moderate deformity and limitation of function. However, 5–10% (and especially those with juvenile rheumatoid arthritis) are severely crippled and require treatment throughout life.

A significant number of children with JCA (about 3%) still die – usually as a result of renal failure due to amyloidosis, or following overwhelming infection.

The systemic connective tissue diseases

'Systemic connective tissue disease' is a collective term for a group of closely related conditions that have features which overlap with those of rheumatoid disease. Like RA, these are 'autoimmune disorders', probably triggered by viral infection in genetically predisposed individuals.

SYSTEMIC LUPUS ERYTHEMATOSUS is the best known. It occurs mainly in young females and may be difficult to differentiate from RA. Although joint pain is usual, it is often overshadowed by systemic symptoms such as malaise, anorexia, weight loss and fever. Characteristic clinical features are skin rashes (especially the 'butterfly rash' of the face), Raynaud's phenomenon, peripheral vasculitis, splenomegaly, and disorders of the kidney, heart, lung, eye and central nervous system. Anaemia, leucopenia and elevation of the ESR are common. Tests for antinuclear factor are always positive.

Corticosteroids are indicated for severe systemic disease and may have to be continued for life. Progressive joint deformity is unusual and the arthritis can almost always be controlled by anti-inflammatory drugs, physiotherapy and intermittent splintage.

A curious complication of systemic lupus is avascular necrosis (usually of the femoral head). This may be due in part to the corticosteroid treatment, but the disease itself seems to predispose to bone ischaemia.

References and further reading

Ansell, B.M. and Swann, M. (1983) The management of chronic arthritis of children. *Journal of Bone and Joint Surgery* **65B**, 536–543

Calin, A. and Fries, J.F. (1976) An 'experimental' epidemic of Reiter's syndrome revisited. *Annals of Internal Medicine* **84**, 564–566

Moll, J.M.H., Haslock, I., Macrae, I.F. and Wright, V. (1974) Associations between ankylosing spondylitis, psoriatic arthritis, Reiter's disease, the intestinal arthropathies and Behçet's syndrome. *Medicine* **53**, 343–364

Ohira, T. and Ishikawa, K. (1986) Hydroxyapatite deposition in articular cartilage by intra-articular injections of methylprednisolone. *Journal of Bone and Joint Surgery* **68A**, 509–520

Solomon, L. (1979) Surgery of the major joints in arthritis. *Medicine* **12**, 600

Solomon, L. and Berman, L. (1979) Rheumatic disorders of the lumbar spine. In *Disorders of the Lumbar Spine* (eds. A.J. Helfet and D.M.G. Lee), Lippincott, Philadelphia

Solomon, L., Beighton, P., Valkenburg, H.A., Robin, G. and Soskolne, G.L. (1975) Rheumatic disorders in the South African Negro. *South African Medical Journal* **49**, 1292–1296

Crystal deposition disorders 4

The crystal deposition disorders are a group of conditions characterized by the presence of crystals in and around joints, bursae and tendons. Although many different crystals are found, three clinical conditions in particular are associated with this phenomenon: gout, calcium pyrophosphate dihydrate (CPPD) deposition disease and hydroxyapatite deposition. Characteristically, in each of the three conditions, crystal deposition has three distinct consequences: (1) it may be totally inert and asymptomatic; (2) it may induce an acute inflammatory reaction; or (3) it may result in slow destruction of the affected tissues.

Gout

This is a disorder of purine metabolism characterized by hyperuricaemia and recurrent attacks of acute synovitis. It is due to deposition of monosodium urate monohydrate crystals. Late changes include cartilage degeneration. It is much more common in males (20:1) and is rarely seen before the menopause in females. Two forms are recognized: (1) *primary* (95%), an inherited disorder with overproduction or underexcretion of uric acid; and (2) *secondary* (5%), resulting from acquired conditions that cause uric acid overproduction (e.g. myeloproliferative disorders) or underexcretion (e.g. renal failure). This division is somewhat artificial; people with an initial tendency to 'primary' hyperuricaemia may develop gout only when secondary factors are introduced – for example, obesity, alcohol abuse, or treatment with diuretics or salicylates which increase tubular reabsorption of uric acid.

Although the risk of developing gout increases with increasing levels of hyperuricaemia, only a fraction of those with hyperuricaemia develop gout. Local factors (including trauma) may be important in triggering crystal formation.

Pathology

Urate crystals are deposited in minute clumps in connective tissue, including articular cartilage. For months, perhaps years, they remain inert. Then, possibly as a result of local trauma, crystals are dispersed into the joint and the surrounding tissues where they excite an acute inflammatory reaction. Individual crystals may be phagocytosed by synovial cells and polymorphs or may float free in the synovial fluid.

With the passage of time, urate deposits may build up in joints, periarticular tissues, tendons and bursae; common sites are around the metatarsophalangeal joints of the big toes, the Achilles tendons, the olecranon bursae and the pinnae of the ears. These clumps of chalky material, or tophi (L. *tophus* = porous stone), vary in size from less than 1 mm to several centimetres in diameter. They may ulcerate through the skin or destroy cartilage and periarticular bone.

Clinical features

Patients are usually men over the age of 30 years; women are seldom affected until after the menopause. Often there is a family history of gout.

The gouty stereotype is obese, rubicund, hypertensive and fond of alcohol. However, many patients have none of these attributes and some are nudged into an attack by the uncontrolled administration of diuretics or aspirin.

THE ACUTE ATTACK   The sudden onset of severe joint pain which lasts for a week or two before resolving completely is typical of acute gout. The attack usually comes out of the blue but may be precipitated by minor trauma, operation, intercurrent illness, unaccustomed exercise or alcohol. The commonest sites are the metatarsophalangeal joint of the big toe, the ankle and finger joints, and the olecranon bursa. Occasionally, more than one site is involved. The skin looks red and shiny and there is considerable swelling. The joint feels hot and extremely tender, suggesting a cellulitis or septic arthritis. Sometimes the only feature is acute pain and tenderness in the heel or the sole.

Hyperuricaemia is present at some stage, though not necessarily during an acute attack. However, whilst a low serum uric acid makes gout unlikely, hyperuricaemia is not 'diagnostic' and is often seen in normal middle-aged men.

The true diagnosis can be established beyond doubt by finding the characteristic negatively birefringent urate crystals in the synovial fluid. A drop of fluid on a glass slide is examined by polarizing microscopy. Crystals may be sparse but if the fluid specimen is centrifuged a concentrated pellet may be obtained for examination.

CHRONIC GOUT   Recurrent acute attacks may eventually merge into polyarticular gout. Joint erosion causes chronic pain, stiffness and deformity; if the finger joints are affected, this may be mistaken for rheumatoid arthritis. Tophi may appear around joints over the olecranon, in the pinna of the ear and – less frequently – in almost any other tissue. A large tophus can ulcerate through the skin and discharge its chalky material. Renal lesions include calculi, due to uric acid precipitation in the urine, and parenchymal disease due to deposition of monosodium urate from the blood.

X-rays

During the acute attack x-rays show only soft-tissue swelling. Chronic gout may result in joint space narrowing and secondary osteoarthritis. Tophi appear as characteristic punched-out 'cysts' or deep erosions in the para-articular bone ends; these excavations are larger and slightly further from the joint margin than the typical rheumatoid erosions. Occasionally, bone destruction is more marked and may resemble neoplastic disease (see Fig. 9.2).

Differential diagnosis

INFECTION   Cellulitis, septic bursitis, an infected bunion or septic arthritis must all be excluded, if necessary by immediate joint aspiration. Remember that crystals and sepsis may coexist, so always send fluid for both culture and crystal analysis.

REITER'S DISEASE   This may present with acute pain and swelling of a knee or ankle, but the history is more protracted and the response to anti-inflammatory drugs less dramatic.

PSEUDOGOUT   Pyrophosphate crystal deposition may cause an acute arthritis indistinguishable from gout – except that it tends to affect large rather than small joints and is somewhat more common in women than in men. Articular calcification may show on x-ray. Demonstrating the crystals in synovial fluid establishes the diagnosis.

RHEUMATOID ARTHRITIS   Polyarticular gout affecting the fingers may be mistaken for rheumatoid arthritis, and elbow tophi for rheumatoid nodules. In difficult cases biopsy will establish the diagnosis. RA and gout seldom occur together.

Treatment

The acute attack should be treated by resting the joint and giving large doses of one of the

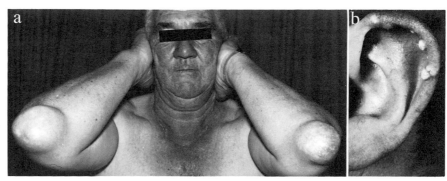

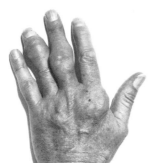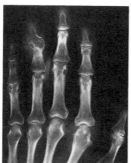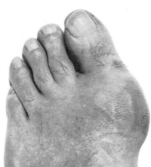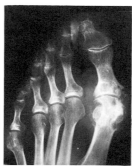

4.1 Gout This man with chronic gout declares his diagnosis at a glance, with his rubicund face, bulging olecranon bursae and tophi.

4.2 Gout In both the hand and the foot, joints are asymmetrically swollen; x-rays show large periarticular excavations, which are filled with uric acid deposits. The joints felt curiously 'pulpy'.

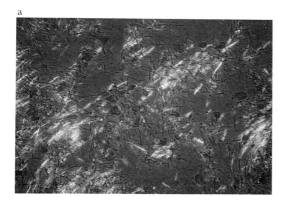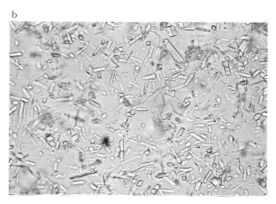

4.3 Crystals In polarized light, crystals appear bright on a dark background. If a compensator is added to the optical system, the background appears in shades of mauve and the birefringent crystals as yellow or blue, depending on their spatial orientation. In these two specimens (obtained from crystal deposits in cartilage) there are differences in shape, size and type of birefringence of the crystals. (a) Urate crystals are needle-like, 5–20 μm long and exhibit strong negative birefringence. (b) Pyrophosphate crystals are rhomboid-shaped, slightly smaller than urate crystals and show weak positive birefringence. (Courtesy of Professor P. A. Dieppe.)

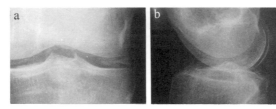

4.4 Chondrocalcinosis Calcium pyrophosphate crystals may be deposited in cartilage, causing (a) calcification of menisci and (b) a thin, dense line within the articular cartilage. Usually no specific cause is found, but chondrocalcinosis may be associated with metabolic disorders such as hyperparathyroidism and haemochromatosis.

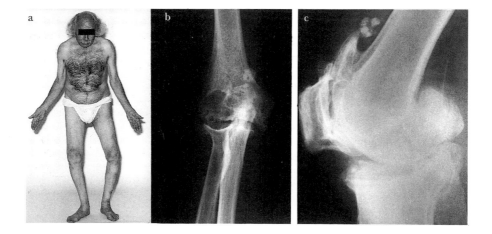

4.5 Pyrosphate arthropathy (a, b) A middle-aged man who presented with osteoarthritis in several of the larger joints, including unusual sites such as the elbow and ankle. (c) The left knee was the worst and x-ray showed the characteristic features of articular calcification, loose bodies in the joint and large trailing osteophytes around the patellofemoral joint.

non-steroidal anti-inflammatory drugs. Colchicine is less effective and may cause diarrhoea, nausea and vomiting. A tense joint effusion may require aspiration and local injection of hydrocortisone.

Between attacks, attention should be given to simple measures such as losing weight, cutting out alcohol and eliminating diuretics. Interval therapy is indicated if acute attacks recur at frequent intervals, if there are tophi or if renal function is impaired. Asymptomatic hyperuricaemia does not call for treatment. Uricosuric drugs (probenecid or sulphinpyrazone) can be used if renal function is normal. Allopurinol, a xanthine oxidase inhibitor, is usually preferred. *These drugs should never be started during an acute attack, and they should always be covered by an anti-inflammatory preparation or colchicine*, otherwise they may actually precipitate an acute attack.

In chronic tophaceous gout, and in all patients with renal complications, allopurinol is the drug of choice. With prolonged administration, adjusted to maintain a normal serum uric acid level (less than 0.4 mmol/l), tophi may gradually dissolve. Ulcerating tophi that fail to heal with conservative treatment can be evacuated by curettage; the wound is left open and dressings are applied until it heals.

Calcium pyrophosphate dihydrate (CPPD) deposition

The term 'CPPD deposition' encompasses three overlapping conditions: (1) *chondrocalcinosis* – the appearance of calcific material in cartilage; (2) *pseudogout* – a crystal-induced synovitis; and (3) *chronic pyrophosphate arthropathy* – a type of degenerative joint disease. Any one of these conditions may occur on its own or in any combination with the others (McCarty, Kohn and Faires, 1962; Dieppe et al., 1982). In contrast to classic gout, serum biochemistry shows no consistent abnormality.

CPPD crystal deposition is known to occur in certain metabolic disorders (e.g. hyperparathyroidism and haemochromatosis) that cause a critical change in ionic calcium and pyrophosphate equilibrium in cartilage. The rare familial forms of chondrocalcinosis are probably due to a similar biochemical defect (Lust et al., 1981). However, in the vast majority of cases chondrocalcinosis follows some local change in the cartilage due to ageing, degeneration, enzymatic degradation or trauma.

Pathology

Pyrophosphate is probably generated in abnormal cartilage by enzyme activity at chondrocyte surfaces; it combines with calcium ions in the matrix where crystal nucleation occurs on collagen fibres. The crystals grow into microscopic 'tophi', which appear as nests of amorphous material in the cartilage matrix. Chondrocalcinosis is most pronounced in fibro-cartilaginous structures (e.g. the menisci of the knee, triangular ligament of the wrist, pubic symphysis and intervertebral discs) but may also occur in hyaline articular cartilage, tendons and periarticular soft tissues.

From time to time CPPD crystals are extruded into the joint where they excite an inflammatory reaction similar to gout. The long-standing presence of CPPD crystals also seems to influence the development of osteoarthritis in joints not usually prone to this condition (e.g. elbows and ankles). Characteristically, there is a hypertrophic reaction with marked osteophyte formation but sometimes, for reasons that are poorly understood, the joint shows severe destructive changes.

Clinical features

CPPD crystal deposition disease occurs in several forms, all of them appearing with increasing frequency in relation to age. The majority of patients are women over the age of 60 years.

ASYMPTOMATIC CHONDROCALCINOSIS Calcification of the menisci is common in elderly people and is usually asymptomatic. When it is seen in association with osteoarthritis, this does not necessarily imply cause and effect. Both are common in elderly people and they are bound to be seen together in some patients; x-rays may reveal chondrocalcinosis in other, asymptomatic, joints.

GOUT AND PSEUDOGOUT

Gout
Smaller joints
Intense pain
Inflammation
Hyperuricaemia
Uric acid crystals

Pseudogout
Large joints
Moderate pain
Swelling
Chondrocalcinosis
Calcium pyrophosphate crystals

Chondrocalcinosis in patients under 50 years of age should suggest the possibility of an underlying metabolic disease or a familial disorder.

ACUTE SYNOVITIS (PSEUDOGOUT) The patient, typically a middle-aged woman, complains of acute pain and swelling in one of the larger joints – usually the knee. Sometimes the attack is precipitated by a minor illness or operation. The joint is tense and inflamed, though usually not as acutely as in gout. Untreated the condition lasts for a few weeks and then subsides spontaneously. *X-rays* may show signs of chondrocalcinosis, and the diagnosis can be confirmed by finding *positively birefringent crystals* in the synovial fluid.

CHRONIC PYROPHOSPHATE ARTHROPATHY The patient, usually an elderly woman, presents with polyarticular 'osteoarthritis' affecting the larger joints (hips, knees) and – much more helpfully – *unusual joints*, such as the ankles, shoulders, elbows and wrists where osteoarthritis is seldom seen. There are the usual features of pain, stiffness, swelling, joint crepitus and loss of movement. It is often diagnosed, simply, as 'generalized osteoarthritis', but the x-ray features are distinctive.

Sometimes alternating bouts of acute synovitis and chronic arthritis may mimic rheumatoid disease. Occasionally joint destruction is so marked as to suggest neuropathic joint disease.

X-rays

The characteristic x-ray features arise from a combination of (1) intra-articular and peri-articular calcification, and (2) degenerative arthritis in distinctive sites (Resnick and Resnick, 1982).

Calcification is usually seen in and around the knees, wrists, shoulders, hips, pubic symphysis and intervertebral discs; it is often bilateral and symmetrical. In articular cartilage it appears as a thin line parallel to the joint. In the fibro-cartilaginous menisci and discs it produces cloudy, irregular opacities. Less common sites are the joint synovium, capsule, ligaments, tendons and bursae.

Degenerative changes are similar to those of straightforward osteoarthritis but notably involving unusual sites such as the non-weight-bearing joints, the isolated patellofemoral compartment in the knee and the talonavicular joint in the foot. In advanced cases joint destruction may be marked, with the formation of loose bodies.

Diagnosis

PSEUDOGOUT must be distinguished from other acute or subacute inflammatory conditions.

ACUTE GOUT usually occurs in men, and typically in smaller joints or in the olecranon bursa. The final word often lies with joint aspiration and identification of the characteristic crystals.

POST-TRAUMATIC HAEMARTHROSIS can be misleading; pseudogout, too, is often precipitated by trauma. A clear history and aspiration of blood-stained fluid will solve the problem.

INFECTION, too, can be excluded by joint aspiration; fluid should be submitted with a request for both crystal analysis and bacteriological culture.

REITER'S DISEASE, which can start in a single large joint, is suspected if there are signs of urethritis, colitis or conjunctivitis.

CHRONIC CPPD ARTHROPATHY poses an entirely different set of diagnostic problems.

OSTEOARTHRITIS and joint calcification are both common in older people; the two together do not necessarily make it a CPPD arthropathy. The distinctive x-ray features, and especially the involvement of unusual joints, point to a CPPD disorder rather than a simple concurrence of two common conditions.

INFLAMMATORY POLYARTHRITIS usually involves the smaller joints as well, and systemic features of inflammation are more marked.

METABOLIC DISORDERS, such as hyperparathyroidism, haemochromatosis and alkaptonuria, occasionally present with joint pain, osteoporosis and chondrocalcinosis. An important feature distinguishing these conditions from CPPD deposition disease is the generalized osteoporosis; however, the pattern of joint involvement is also helpful.

HAEMOCHROMATOSIS is an uncommon disorder of middle-aged people (usually men), resulting from chronic iron overload. Clinical features are those of cirrhosis and diabetes, with a typical bronze pigmentation of the skin. About half of those patients develop joint pain and stiffness (particularly in the hands and fingers);

some also have chronic backache. X-rays reveal chondrocalcinosis and a destructive arthropathy similar to that of CPPD deposition disease, most commonly in the metacarpophalangeal joints. The spine is usually osteoporotic. The plasma iron and iron-binding capacity are raised.

ALKAPTONURIA* is a rare heritable metabolic disorder characterized by the appearance of homogentisic acid in the urine, dark pigmentation of the connective tissues (*ochronosis*) and calcification of hyaline and fibrocartilage. The inborn error is an absence of homogentisic acid oxidase in the liver and kidney. Those affected usually remain asymptomatic until the third or fourth decade when they present with pain and stiffness of the spine and (later) larger joints. There may also be dark pigmentation of the ear cartilage and the sclerae, and clothes may become stained by homogentisic acid in the sweat. X-rays reveal narrowing and calcification of the intervertebral discs at multiple levels, and spinal osteoporosis. At a later stage the large peripheral joints may show chondrocalcinosis and severe osteoarthritis. A curious feature – and one that gives the condition its name – is that the urine turns dark brown when it is alkalinized or if it is left to stand for some hours.

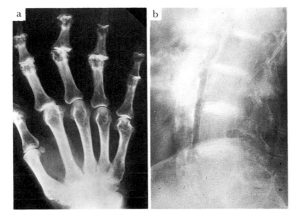

4.6 Haemochromatosis and alkaptonuria (a) Haemochromatosis: the degenerative arthritis of the proximal finger joints is typical. (b) Alkaptonuria: the intervertebral discs are calcified – this man has backache.

Treatment

The treatment of pseudogout is the same as that of acute gout: rest and appropriate anti-inflammatory therapy. In elderly patients joint aspiration and intra-articular corticosteroid injection is the treatment of choice as these patients are more vulnerable to the side effects of non-steroidal anti-inflammatory drugs.

Chronic chondrocalcinosis appears to be irreversible. Fortunately it usually causes few symptoms and little disability. When it is associated with progressive joint degeneration the treatment is essentially that of osteoarthritis with progressive joint destruction.

*Gout strikes the small joints, pseudogout the large joints, and alkaptonuria the spine.

Calcium hydroxyapatite (HA) deposition disorders

Crystalline calcium hydroxyapatite is a normal component of bone mineral. It also occurs abnormally in dead or damaged tissue. Minute deposits in joints and periarticular tissues can give rise to either an acute reaction or a chronic, destructive arthropathy.

Prolonged hypercalcaemia or hyperphosphataemia, of whatever cause, may result in widespread metastatic calcification. However, by far the most common cause of HA crystal deposition in and around joints is local tissue damage – torn ligaments, tendon attrition and cartilage damage or degeneration.

Pathology

The minute (less than 1 μm) HA crystals are deposited around chondrocytes in articular cartilage and in relatively avascular or damaged parts of tendons and ligaments – most notably around the shoulder and knee. The deposits grow by crystal accretion and eventually may be detectable by x-ray in the periarticular tendons or ligaments. Sometimes the calcific deposit has a creamy consistency but in long-standing cases it is more like chalk. The mini-tophus may be completely inert; but in symptomatic cases it is surrounded by an acute vascular reaction and inflammation. Crystal shedding into joints may give rise to synovitis. More rarely this is complicated by the development of a rapidly destructive, erosive arthritis.

Clinical features

Two clinical syndromes are associated with HA crystal deposition: (1) an acute or subacute periarthritis, and (2) a chronic destructive arthritis.

ACUTE OR SUBACUTE PERIARTHRITIS   This is by far the commonest form of HA crystal deposition disorder affecting joints. The patient, usually an adult between 30 and 50 years, complains of pain close to one of the larger joints – most commonly the shoulder or the knee. Symptoms may start suddenly, perhaps after minor trauma, and rise to a crescendo during which the tissues around the joint are swollen, warm and exquisitely tender – but tender *near* the joint in relation to a tendon or ligament, rather than *in* the joint. At other times the onset is more gradual and it is easier to localize the area of tenderness to one of the periarticular structures. Both forms of the condition are seen most commonly in the rotator cuff lesions of the shoulder. Symptoms usually subside after a few weeks or months; sometimes they are aborted only when the calcific deposit is removed or the surrounding tissues are decompressed. In acute cases, operation may disclose a tense globule of creamy material oozing from between the frayed fibres of tendon or ligament.

CHRONIC DESTRUCTIVE ARTHRITIS   HA crystals are sometimes found in association with a chronic erosive arthritis; whether they cause the arthritis or modify a pre-existing disorder remains uncertain.

A more dramatic type of rapidly destructive arthritis of the shoulder is occasionally seen in elderly patients with rotator cuff lesions. This was described in 1981 by McCarty and his colleagues from Milwaukee and has acquired the sobriquet 'Milwaukee shoulder'. Similar conditions affect the hip and knee. They have been attributed to HA crystal (or mixed HA and CPPD crystal) shedding but there remains

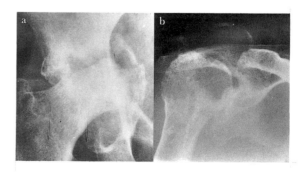

4.7 Rapidly destructive OA Two patients with rapidly destructive OA of a large joint, (a) the hip in one and (b) the shoulder in the other. Common features are rapid progression to joint disruption, crumbling of the subarticular bone and periarticular ossification.

some doubt about the true association with crystal deposition.

X-rays

With periarthritis, calcification may be seen in tendons or ligaments close to the joint, most commonly in the rotator cuff around the shoulder.

Articular cartilage and fibrocartilaginous menisci and discs never show the type of calcification seen in CPPD deposition disease, but 'loose bodies' may be seen in synovial joints.

Erosive arthritis causes loss of the articular space, with little or no sclerosis or osteophyte formation. In destructive arthritis, subchondral bone is severely eroded or excavated.

Investigations

There is little help from special investigations. Serum biochemistry is usually normal, except in those patients with hypercalcaemia or hyperphosphataemia. Synovial fluid examination may reveal high counts of polymorphonuclear leucocytes, but this hardly serves to distinguish the condition from other types of subacute synovitis. HA crystals can be identified only by electron probe or transmission electron microscopy.

Treatment

Acute periarthritis should be treated by rest and non-steroidal anti-inflammatory drugs. Resistant cases may respond to local injection of corticosteroids; they should be used only to weather the acute storm – repeated injections for lesser pain may dampen the repair process in damaged tendons or ligaments and thus predispose to recurrent attacks. Persistent pain and tenderness may call for operative removal of the calcific deposit or 'decompression' of the affected tendon or ligament.

Erosive arthritis is treated like osteoarthritis. However, rapidly progressive bone destruction calls for early operation: in the case of the shoulder, synovectomy and soft-tissue repair; for the hip, usually total joint replacement.

References and further reading

Dieppe, P.A., Alexander, G.J.M., Jones, H.E. et al. (1982) Pyrophosphate arthropathy: a clinical and radiological study of 105 cases. *Annals of the Rheumatic Diseases* **41**, 371–376

Ishikawa, K., Masuda, I., Ohira, T. and Yokoyama, M. (1989) A histological study of calcium pyrophosphate dihydrate crystal-deposition disease. *Journal of Bone and Joint Surgery* **71A**, 875–886

Lust, G., Faure, G., Netter, P. et al. (1981) Evidence of a generalized metabolic defect in patients with hereditary chondrocalcinosis. *Arthritis and Rheumatism* **24**, 1517–1521

McCarty, D.J., Kohn, N.N. and Faires, J.S. (1962) The significance of calcium phosphate crystals in the synovial fluid of arthritis patients: the 'pseudogout syndrome'. I. Clinical aspects. *Annals of Internal Medicine* **56**, 711–745

McCarty, D. J., Halverson, P.B., Carrera, G.F., Brewer, B.J. and Kozin, F. (1981) 'Milwaukee shoulder' – association of microspheroids containing hydroxyapatite crystals, active collagenase and neutral protease with rotator cuff defects. *Arthritis and Rheumatism* **24**, 464–473

Resnick, C.S. and Resnick, D. (1983) Crystal deposition disease. *Seminars in Arthritis and Rheumatism* **12**, 390–403

Osteoarthritis and related disorders 5

Osteoarthritis

Osteoarthritis (OA) is a chronic joint disorder in which there is progressive softening and disintegration of articular cartilage accompanied by new growth of cartilage and bone at the joint margins (osteophytes) and capsular fibrosis. These changes result from a variety of abnormalities that predispose to mechanical failure of the hyaline articular cartilage.

OA is designated *primary* when no cause is obvious, and *secondary* when it follows a demonstrable abnormality. However, in most cases both 'primary' and 'secondary' factors are important, the former determining who is likely to develop OA and the latter specifying when and where it occurs.

In general it is a disease of advancing years but young people can develop OA if articular cartilage is damaged or subjected to abnormal stress from an early age. It is more common in some joints (the hip, knee and spine) than in others (the elbow and ankle). Moreover, individual joints are affected with differing frequency in men and women (terminal interphalangeal OA chiefly affects postmenopausal women), and in different ethnic groups (OA of the hip is rare in Africans but common in southern European women who have a high incidence of acetabular dysplasia). Prevalence is also related to body build (OA of the knees is more common in obese people) and occupational factors (OA of the hands in manual workers) (Lawrence, 1961; Felson et al., 1987).

Despite these differences, OA is a truly universal disorder: everyone will get it somewhere if they live long enough. Usually only one or two joints are symptomatic, though others may show minor changes; a common variant is the generalized OA of postmenopausal women, affecting the terminal joints of the fingers as well as the knees.

Cause

From the foregoing it is clear that many things conspire to cause OA: genetic predisposition, metabolic and hormonal influences on cartilage, patterns of joint usage, local mechanical stresses, pre-existing joint disease and specific incidents of cartilage damage. Is there a unifying theory that accommodates these variable influences?

The most obvious thing about OA is that it increases in frequency with age. This does not mean that it is an expression of senescence; it simply shows that OA takes many years to develop. To be sure, cartilage ageing does occur, resulting in splitting and flaking of the surface, diminished cellularity, reduction of the proteoglycan ground substance, and loss of elasticity with a concomitant decrease in breaking strength. But, although these changes are qualitatively similar to those of early OA, they differ from it in two important respects: they are not progressive, and they occur in areas that seldom manifest as clinical OA (Byers, Contepomi and Farkas, 1970).

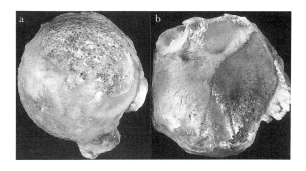

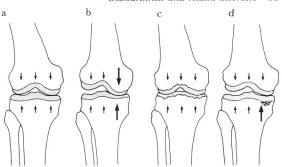

5.1 Osteoarthritis – limited and progressive (a) End-on view of the femoral head showing complete loss of cartilage (eburnation) superiorly, as well as non-progressive changes inferiorly. (b) Undersurface of the patella: the medial facet shows only the limited changes due to 'wear and tear', but the lateral facet shows advanced osteoarthritis with complete loss of cartilage.

5.2 Osteoarthritis – causal factors In the normal joint (a) the forces are evenly distributed. The remaining diagrams show the three ways in which cartilage may be damaged: (b) deformity increases the stress in a localized area by concentrating the load at this point; (c) cartilage which has been weakened by some preceding disorder is unable to bear even normal loads; (d) if the subarticular bone is abnormal it may be unable to support the cartilage adequately.

We distinguish, therefore, between two types of cartilage deterioration: (1) *limited cartilage loss*, seen mainly away from loadbearing areas and probably due to 'wear and tear'; and (2) *progressive cartilage destruction*, which is always maximal in the major loadbearing area and is associated with symptomatic OA.

There is no single cause of OA; it results from a disparity between the stress applied to articular cartilage and the ability of the cartilage to withstand that stress. This may be due to increased stress, weak cartilage or abnormal support by subchondral bone.

INCREASED STRESS Stress is load per unit area. It may increase because of *increased load* (e.g. in deformities that affect the lever system around a joint) or because of *decreased contact area* (e.g. due to joint incongruity or instability). Both factors operate in varus deformity of the knee and in acetabular dysplasia – common precursors of OA.

WEAK CARTILAGE There is normally a loss of cartilage tensile strength with age; add to this any disorder that stiffens the cartilage, making it less resilient (e.g. ochronosis), or softens the cartilage (e.g. chronic inflammation), and progressive destruction may ensue. Crystal deposition has been implicated as a cause of OA (Ali, 1980), but the evidence is still incomplete.

Polyarticular osteoarthritis and Heberden's arthritis are more likely due to a generalized cartilage defect than to mechanical dysfunction.

ABNORMAL SUPPORT The subchondral bone may be abnormally fragile (e.g. in osteonecrosis), providing inadequate support for the articular cartilage, or abnormally dense (e.g. following fracture healing), and so a poor shock absorber. In either case the overlying cartilage is exposed to damaging stresses.

Pathogenesis

The initial stages of OA have been studied in animal models with induced joint instability (Moskowitz et al., 1973; McDevitt and Muir, 1976) and may not be representative of all types of OA.

The earliest changes, while the cartilage is still morphologically intact, are an increase in water content of the cartilage and easier extractability of the matrix proteoglycans; similar findings in human cartilage have been ascribed to failure of the internal collagen network that normally restrains the matrix gel (Freeman, 1975; Maroudas, 1976). At a slightly later stage there is loss of proteoglycans and defects

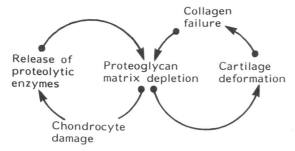

appear in the cartilage. As the cartilage becomes less stiff, secondary damage to chondrocytes may cause release of cell enzymes and further matrix breakdown. Cartilage deformation may also add to the stress on the collagen network, thus amplifying the changes in a cycle that leads to tissue breakdown.

Articular cartilage has an important role in distributing and dissipating the forces associated with joint loading. When it loses its integrity these forces are increasingly concentrated in the subchondral bone. The result – focal trabecular degeneration and cyst formation, as well as increased vascularity and reactive sclerosis in the zone of maximal loading.

What cartilage remains is still capable of regeneration, repair and remodelling. As the articular surfaces become increasingly malapposed and the joint unstable, cartilage at the edges of the joint reverts to the more youthful activities of growth and endochondral ossification, giving rise to the bony excrescences, or osteophytes, that so clearly distinguish osteoarthritis (once called 'hypertrophic arthritis') from 'atrophic' disorders such as rheumatoid disease.

Pathology

The cardinal features are: (1) progressive cartilage destruction; (2) subarticular cyst formation, with (3) sclerosis of the surrounding bone; (4) osteophyte formation; and (5) capsular fibrosis.

Initially the cartilaginous and bony changes are confined to one part of the joint – the most heavily loaded part. There is softening and fraying, or fibrillation, of the normally smooth and glistening cartilage. (The term 'chondromalacia' [Greek = cartilage softening] seems apt for this stage of the disease, but it is used only of the patellar articular surfaces where it features as one of the causes of anterior knee pain in young people.)

With progressive disintegration of cartilage, the underlying bone becomes exposed and some areas may be polished, or burnished, to ivory-like smoothness (eburnation). Sometimes small tufts of fibrocartilage may be seen growing out of the bony surface. At a distance from the damaged area the articular cartilage looks relatively normal, but at the edges of the joint there are bony excrescences covered by thin, bluish cartilage – the osteophytes.

When the subarticular bone is cut through, additional features come to light. Beneath the damaged cartilage the bone is dense and sclerotic. Often within the area of subchondral sclerosis, and immediately subjacent to the surface, are one or more *cysts* containing thick, gelatinous material.

The *joint capsule* usually shows thickening and fibrosis, sometimes of extraordinary degree. The *synovial lining*, as a rule, looks only mildly inflamed; sometimes, however, it is thick and red and covered by villi.

The histological appearances vary considerably, according to the degree of destruction. Early on, the cartilage shows small irregularities or splits in the surface, while in the deeper layers there is patchy loss of metachromasia (obviously corresponding to the depletion of matrix proteoglycans). Most striking, however, is the increased cellularity, and the appearance of clusters, or clones, of chondrocytes – 20 or more to a batch. In later stages, the clefts become more extensive and in some areas cartilage is lost to the point where the underlying bone is completely denuded. The biochemical abnormalities corresponding to these changes were described by Mankin et al. (1971).

The subchondral bone is thickened and may show marked osteoblastic activity, especially on the deep aspect of any cyst. The cyst itself contains amorphous material; its origin is mysterious: it could arise from stress disintegration of small trabeculae, from focal areas of osteonecrosis or from the forceful pumping of synovial fluid through cracks in the subchondral bone plate. As in all types of arthritis, small areas of osteonecrosis are quite common.

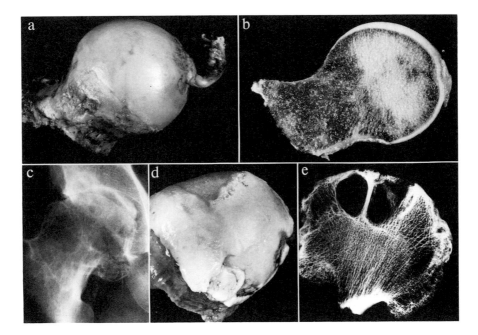

5.3 Osteoarthritis – pathology (a) Normal ageing causes slight degeneration of the articular surface, but the coronal section (b) shows that the cartilage thickness is well preserved even in old age. By contrast, in progressive osteoarthritis (lower row) the weightbearing area is severely damaged: the x-ray (c) shows cartilage loss at the superior pole and cysts in the underlying bone; the specimen (d) shows that the top of the head was completely denuded of cartilage; and a fine-detail x-ray of the specimen (e) shows that the subchondral bone plate has been perforated.

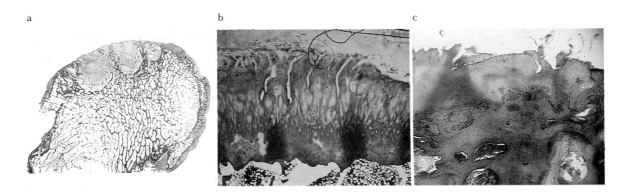

5.4 Osteoarthritis – histology (a) Destructive changes (loss of articular cartilage and cyst formation) are most marked where stress is greatest; reparative changes are represented by sclerosis around the cysts and new bone formation (osteophytes) in less stressed areas. (b) In this high-power view, the articular cartilage shows loss of metachromasia and deep clefts in the surface (fibrillation). Attempts at repair result in (c) subarticular sclerosis and buds of fibrocartilage mushrooming where the articular surface is destroyed.

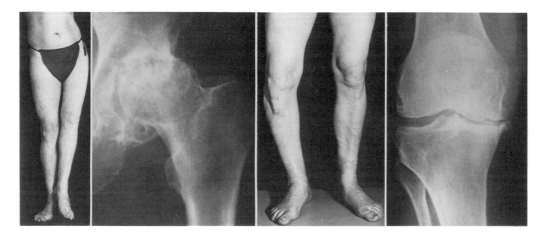

5.5 Osteoarthritis – clinical   Deformity and diminished joint space at the hip and the knee.

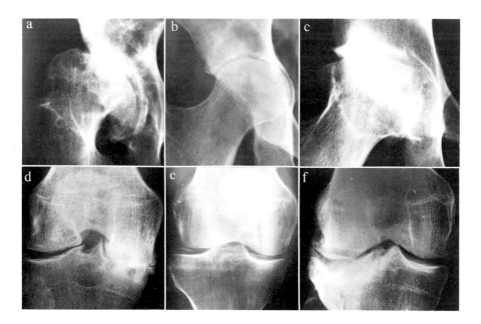

5.6 Osteoarthritis – x-rays   The three types of osteoarthritis are shown in the hip (a, b, c) and the knee (d, e, f). In type I mechanical overload has damaged a localized area of cartilage – the upper pole in this hip (a) and the medial compartment in this knee (d). In type II the articular cartilage was already abnormal – following an inflammatory arthritis of the hip (b) and chondrocalcinosis of the knee (e), so that even normal loads damaged the surfaces. In type III the underlying bone was defective – either too weak as in osteonecrosis of the hip (c) or too sclerotic, as in this old tibial plateau fracture (f) – causing breakdown of the covering cartilage.

The osteophytes are seen to arise from the edge of the articular surface as bony outgrowths covered by hyaline cartilage.

The capsule and synovium are often thickened but cellular activity is slight; however, sometimes there is marked inflammation or fibrosis of the capsular tissues.

A feature of OA, which is difficult to appreciate from the morbid anatomy, is the marked vascularity and venous congestion of the subchondral bone (Arnoldi, Linderholm and Mussbichler, 1972). This may be shown by angiographic studies and the demonstration of increased intraosseous pressure. It is also apparent from the intense activity around osteoarthritic joints on radionuclide scanning.

Clinical features

Patients usually present after middle age. Joint involvement follows several different patterns: symptoms centre either on one or two of the large weightbearing joints (hip or knee), on the interphalangeal joints (especially in women) or on any joint that has suffered a previous affliction (e.g. congenital dysplasia, osteonecrosis or intra-articular fracture). A family history is common in patients with polyarticular OA.

Pain is the usual presenting symptom. It is often quite widespread, or it may be referred to a distant site – for example, pain in the knee from OA of the hip. It usually starts insidiously and increases slowly over months or years. It is aggravated by exertion and relieved by rest, although with time relief is less and less complete. The worst is pain in bed at night, when the patient has difficulty finding any position of comfort. There are several possible causes of pain: capsular fibrosis, with pain on stretching the shrunken capsule; muscular fatigue; and, perhaps most important of all, bone pressure due to vascular congestion and intraosseous hypertension.

Stiffness is common; characteristically it occurs after periods of inactivity, but with time it becomes constant and progressive.

Swelling may be intermittent (suggesting an effusion) or continuous (with capsular thickening or large osteophytes).

Deformity may result from capsular contracture or joint instability; but beware, it may have preceded and contributed to the onset of OA.

Loss of function, though not the most dramatic, is often the most distressing symptom. A limp, difficulty in climbing stairs, restriction of walking distance, or progressive inability to perform everyday tasks or enjoy recreation may eventually drive the patient to seek help.

Typically, the symptoms of OA follow an *intermittent course*, with periods of remission sometimes lasting for months.

Although the patient complains of only one or two joints, examination may show that others are affected in varying degrees.

Swelling and *deformity* may be obvious in peripheral joints; at the hip, deformity is usually masked by postural adjustments of the pelvis and spine. In long-standing cases there is *muscle wasting*. Tell-tale scars denote previous abnormalities. Local *tenderness* is common, and in superficial joints *fluid, synovial thickening* or *osteophytes* may be felt.

Movement is always restricted, but is often painless within the permitted range; it may be accompanied by *crepitus*. Some movements are more curtailed than others; thus, at the hip extension, abduction and internal rotation are usually the most severely limited.

In the late stages joint *instability* may occur for any of three reasons: loss of cartilage and bone; asymmetrical capsular contracture; and muscle weakness.

PLAIN X-RAYS are so characteristic as to make other imaging studies unnecessary. The four cardinal signs are *asymmetric narrowing of the joint space, sclerosis* of the subchondral bone under the area of cartilage loss, *cysts* close to the joint surface and *osteophytes* at the margins of the joint. In addition there may be evidence of *previous disorders* (congenital defects, old fractures, rheumatoid arthritis, chondrocalcinosis).

RADIONUCLIDE SCANNING with ^{99m}Tc-HDP shows increased activity during the bone phase in the subchondral regions of affected joints. This says something about vascularity and new bone formation; it may also have some diagnostic value in imaging otherwise obscure areas such as the vertebral apophyseal joints.

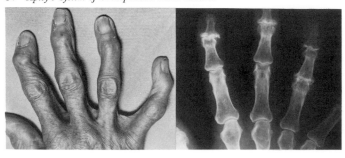

5.7 Heberden's nodes Osteoarthritis of the terminal interphalangeal joints is common. The pain always improves, but the knobbly deformities remain.

Diagnosis

A diagnosis of 'OA' is never an end in itself; there are always underlying causes and influences to be unravelled. In this, the patterns of joint involvement and progression are most helpful.

MONARTICULAR AND PAUCIARTICULAR OA

In its 'classic' form, OA presents with pain and dysfunction in one or two of the large weight-bearing joints. There may be an obvious underlying abnormality: acetabular dysplasia, old Perthes' disease or slipped epiphysis, a previous fracture or damage to ligaments or menisci. In the majority, however, the abnormality is more subtle and one may question whether its discovery will influence subsequent treatment.

POLYARTICULAR (GENERALIZED) OA

This is far and away the most common form of OA, though most of the patients never consult an orthopaedic surgeon. The patient is usually a middle-aged woman who presents with pain, swelling and stiffness of the finger joints. The first carpometacarpal and the big toe metatarsophalangeal joints, or the knees and lumbar facet joints, may be affected as well.

The changes are most obvious in the hands. The interphalangeal joints become swollen and tender, and in the early stages they often appear to be inflamed. Over a period of years osteophytes and soft-tissue swelling produce a characteristic knobbly appearance of the distal interphalangeal joints (*Heberden's nodes*) and, less often, the proximal interphalangeal joints (*Bouchard's nodes*); pain may disappear but stiffness and deformity can be disturbing. Some patients present with painful knees or backache and the knobbly fingers are noticed only in passing.

There is a strong association with carpal tunnel syndrome and isolated tenovaginitis.

X-rays show the characteristic features of OA, usually maximal in the distal interphalangeal joints of the fingers.

OA IN UNUSUAL SITES

OA is uncommon in the shoulder, elbow, wrist, metacarpophalangeal joints, ankle and the lesser toes. If these joints are affected, certain associations come to mind, as follow.

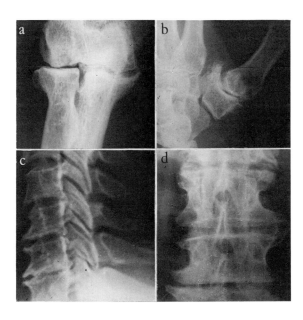

5.8 Primary generalized osteoarthritis The most obvious feature may be deformity of the fingers; but x-rays often show that other joints also are affected – in this case (a) the elbow (where symptoms are rare) and (b) the carpometacarpal thumb joint (where they are common). Often the spine shows marked disc degeneration and large bony spurs (c, d).

Local disorders, such as intra-articular fractures, dislocation, recurrent instability, osteochondritis dissecans or avascular necrosis may affect any joint. The tell-tale signs of past events should be sought in the x-rays.

General disorders, and in particular the *crystal arthropathies,* may be associated with destructive changes indistinguishable from OA. This is particularly likely with OA of the shoulder, the elbow or the isolated patellofemoral joint. X-rays may reveal chondrocalcinosis or calcification of ligaments or tendons.

Congenital disorders (e.g. multiple epiphyseal dysplasia) sometimes go undiagnosed until the patient presents with OA later in life. The general features and x-ray signs are diagnostic.

ENDEMIC OA

Osteoarthritis occasionally occurs as an endemic disorder affecting entire communities. It may be due either to some environmental factor peculiar to that region or to an underlying generalized dysplasia in a genetically isolated community.

Kashin–Beck disease is seen in the northern parts of Russia and China; in some areas it is thought to affect over 8% of the population (Sokoloff, 1985). It usually manifests as a generalized osteoarthritis of the finger joints, elbows, knees and ankles. Shortness of stature is common, suggesting that the condition starts in childhood. It remains uncertain whether the widespread bone deformity and cartilage degeneration are due to a genetic disorder, an unusual dietary deficiency or the ingestion of mycotoxins in spoiled wheat.

Mseleni joint disease is found among the Tsonga people along the eastern seaboard of southern Africa. Osteoarthritis of the hips is common but numerous other joints are affected as well, leading to crippling deformities in older adults. At least two underlying disorders have been identified – a genetically determined form of multiple epiphyseal dysplasia in both sexes and progressive protrusio acetabuli of unknown aetiology in the women (Solomon et al., 1986).

It is important to recognize endemic disorders of this kind as it may be possible to reduce the prevalence of OA by appropriate public health measures and genetic counselling.

RAPIDLY DESTRUCTIVE OA (see also p. 78)

Every so often a patient with apparently straightforward osteoarthritis shows rapid and startling progression of bone destruction, quite out of keeping with the usual slow progress of OA. Usually it is the hip that is affected, but similar changes may be seen in other joints. Names such as *analgesic arthropathy* and *indomethacin hip* reflect the belief that it is due to the pain-dampening effect of strong anti-inflammatory drugs (Solomon, 1976; Newman and Ling, 1985). These drugs also suppress prostaglandin synthesis and they might, theoretically, inhibit healing of microfractures in osteoarthritic joints. Alternative explanations are that the condition is a form of *crystal arthropathy* – crystal deposition being quite common in OA (Doherty et al., 1986) or that it is due to osteoporosis and bone necrosis supervening on pre-existing OA. The fact that most of the patients are elderly women favours the latter hypothesis.

NEUROPATHIC JOINT DISEASE (CHARCOT'S DISEASE)

The most destructive arthropathy is that associated with lack of pain sensibility and position sense. There is evidence that lack of position sense is the more important feature, and indeed some Charcot joints are painful. Neuropathic joints lack the normal reflex safeguard against abnormal stress or injury and the subchondral bone disintegrates with alarming speed. The patient complains of weakness, instability, swelling and progressive deformity. The joint is neither warm nor particularly tender, but swelling is marked, fluid is greatly increased and bits of bone may be felt everywhere. There is always some instability and in the worst cases the joint is flail. The appearances suggest that movement would be agonizing and yet it is often painless. The paradox is diagnostic.

X-rays show gross bone erosion and irregular calcified masses in the capsule.

The underlying neurological conditions include tabes dorsalis, syringomyelia, myelomeningocele and peripheral neuritis (usually diabetic). Leprosy and congenital indifference to pain are other possibilities.

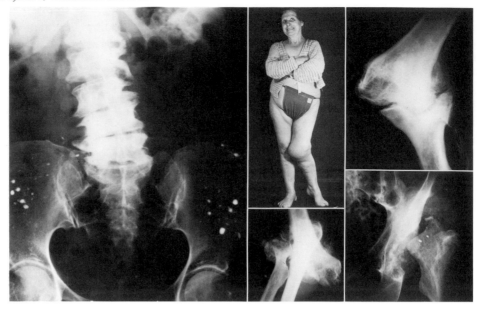

5.9 Charcot's disease   The vertebrae are distorted and dense, the buttocks show the radio-opaque remains of former injections; the knee, elbow and hip joints look grotesque. Moral: 'If it's bizarre, do a WR'. Note also the happy smile (though not all Charcot joints are tabetic, nor are they always painless).

Differential diagnosis of OA

A number of conditions may mimic OA, some presenting as a monarthritis and some as a polyarthritis affecting the finger joints.

AVASCULAR NECROSIS   'Idiopathic' necrosis causes joint pain and local effusion. Typically the x-ray shows preservation of the joint space (articular cartilage) in the face of progressive bone collapse and deformity.

RHEUMATOID ARTHRITIS   Pain, stiffness and swelling in a single joint may herald the onset of rheumatoid disease. X-rays show an erosive arthritis with minimal or no osteophytes. Sooner or later other joints are affected and systemic features appear.

More often it is polyarticular OA that is confused with RA, especially in the early phase when the finger joints are painful and inflamed. Mistakes should not arise because RA hardly ever affects the terminal interphalangeal joints and OA seldom occurs in the metacarpophalangeal joints.

PSORIATIC ARTHRITIS   This does involve the terminal finger joints but is an erosive arthritis causing marked destruction and no osteophytes.

GOUT   Chronic polyarticular gout produces knobbly finger joints, but the bumps are due to tophi and x-rays reveal periarticular bone destruction.

DIFFUSE IDIOPATHIC SKELETAL HYPEROSTOSIS (DISH)   This is a fairly common disorder of middle-aged people, characterized by bone proliferation at the ligament and tendon insertions around peripheral joints and the intervertebral discs (Resnick, Shaul and Robins, 1975). On x-ray examination the large bony spurs are easily mistaken for osteophytes, and indeed OA is quite commonly associated with DISH. But

DISH is not OA: the bone spurs are symmetrically distributed, especially along the pelvic apophyses and throughout the vertebral column; sometimes changes are confined to the spine (ankylosing hyperostosis or Forestier's disease). In itself DISH is usually asymptomatic but any associated OA will need treatment.

Treatment of OA

In planning treatment, three observations should be borne in mind: (1) symptoms characteristically wax and wane, and pain may subside spontaneously for long periods; (2) some forms of OA (e.g. Heberden's nodes) actually become less painful with the passage of time and the patient may need no more than reassurance and a prescription for pain killers; (3) at the other extreme, the recognition (from serial x-rays) that the patient has a rapidly progressive type of OA may warrant an early move to reconstructive surgery before bone loss compromises the outcome of any operation.

EARLY

There are three principles in the treatment of early osteoarthritis: (1) relieve pain; (2) increase movement; and (3) reduce load.

PAIN RELIEF Analgesics and non steroidal anti-inflammatory agents may control pain for many years. But overmedication with powerful anti-inflammatory drugs must be avoided; there is some evidence that it may accelerate articular destruction (Newman and Ling, 1985; Rashad et al., 1989). Measures to provide local warmth usually give only short-lived relief. Rest periods and modification of activities may be necessary.

MOBILIZATION A programme of exercises is important. Early on, pain is felt mainly at the extremes of movement, and so increasing the range (by exercise or gentle manipulation) reduces capsular strain.

LOAD REDUCTION Commonsense measures to reduce joint load include weight loss, the use of a walking stick, avoidance of unnecessary stress (such as jogging or climbing stairs) and even intermittent periods of complete rest.

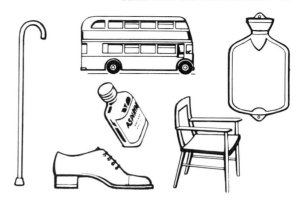

5.10 Osteoarthritis – conservative treatment Simple measures to relieve pain in osteoarthritis of the hip: analgesics, warmth, a raised heel and a stick; 'don't stand when you can sit, don't walk when you can ride'.

INTERMEDIATE

If symptoms and signs increase, then at some joints (chiefly the hip and knee) realignment osteotomy should be considered. It must be done while the joint is still stable and mobile and x-rays show that a major part of the joint space is preserved. Pain relief is often dramatic and is ascribed to (1) vascular decompression of the subchondral bone, and (2) redistribution of loading forces towards less damaged parts of the joint. After femoral osteotomy, fibrocartilage may grow to cover exposed bone.

LATE

Progressive joint destruction, with increasing pain, instability and deformity (particularly of one of the weightbearing joints), usually requires reconstructive surgery. Arthrodesis is indicated if the stiffness is acceptable and neighbouring joints are not likely to be prejudiced. With arthroplasty, timing is essential. Too early, and the odds against a durable result lengthen in proportion to the demands of strenuous activity and time; too late, and bone destruction, deformity, stiffness and muscle atrophy make the operation more difficult and the results more unpredictable. In neuropathic joint disease the underlying condition may need treatment, but the affected joints cannot recover. They should be stabilized by external splintage (e.g. a caliper or brace). Operation is seldom advised.

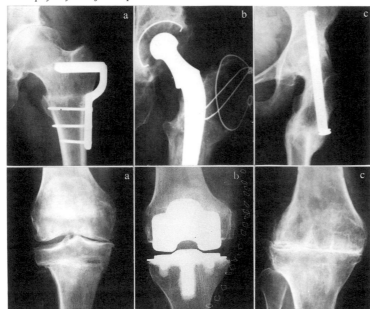

5.11 Operative treatment   The three basic operations: (a) osteotomy, (b) arthroplasty, (c) arthrodesis:
at the hip

at the knee

Haemophilic arthropathy

Recurrent intra-articular bleeding may lead to chronic synovitis and progressive articular destruction. Clinically this is seen only in classic haemophilia, in which there is a deficiency of clotting factor VIII, and Christmas disease, due to deficiency of factor IX. Both are X-linked recessive disorders manifesting in males but carried by females. Their incidence is about 1 per 10 000 male births. Plasma-clotting factor levels above 40% of the normal are compatible with normal control of haemorrhage. Patients with clotting factor levels above 5% ('mild haemophilia') may have prolonged bleeding after injury or operation; those with levels below 1% ('severe haemophilia') have frequent spontaneous joint and muscle haemorrhages.

Pathology

Haemorrhage into the joint causes synovial irritation, inflammation and subsynovial fibrosis. Haemosiderin appears in the synovial cells and macrophages, and after repeated bleeds the synovium becomes thick and heavily pigmented. A vascular pannus creeps over the articular surface and the cartilage is gradually eroded. The subchondral bone may be exposed and penetrated, and occasionally large cysts develop at the bone ends. These changes are attributed to cartilage-degrading enzymes released by the proliferative synovitis and by cells that have accumulated iron, but an additional factor may be the interference with normal cartilage nutrition due to prolonged or repeated joint immobilization.

Bleeding into muscles is less common but equally harmful. Increased tension may lead to muscle necrosis, reactive fibrosis and joint contractures. Sometimes nerves are compressed, causing a neurapraxia; temporary weakness may contribute further to the development of joint deformity.

Cysts and pseudotumours are rare phenomena. A large soft-tissue haematoma may become encapsulated before it is absorbed, and may then draw in more fluid by osmosis to produce a slowly expanding 'cyst'. A subperiosteal haematoma occasionally stimulates cystic resorption of bone resembling a tumour.

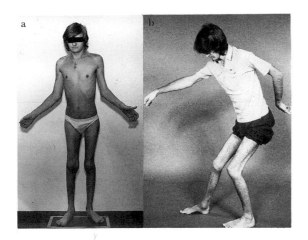

5.12 Haemophilic arthropathy – clinical features (a) Recurrent haemarthrosis and chronic synovitis led to contractures of the elbow joints and deformities of the knees and ankles. (b) This man, with contractures of the knees and ankles, had difficulty staying upright, let alone walking, without support.

Clinical features

Only males are affected and in severe haemophilia joint bleeds usually begin when the child starts to walk. The clinical picture depends on the severity of the disorder, the site of bleeding and the efficacy of long-term treatment. The commonest features are acute bleeding into joints or muscles, chronic arthritis and joint contractures. The sites most frequently involved are the knees, ankles, elbows, shoulders and hips.

ACUTE BLEEDING INTO A JOINT OR MUSCLE With trivial injury a joint (usually the knee, elbow or ankle) may rapidly fill with blood. Pain, warmth, boggy swelling, tenderness and limited movement are the outstanding features. The resemblance to a low-grade inflammatory joint is striking, but the history is diagnostic.

Acute bleeding into muscles (especially the forearm, calf or thigh) is less common. A painful swelling appears and movement of the related joint is resisted. The distinction from a haemarthrosis may be difficult (e.g. with groin pain due to iliopsoas haemorrhage); usually only those movements that stretch the affected muscles are painful, whereas in haemarthrosis all movements are painful.

Pressure on a peripheral nerve may cause temporary loss of power and sensation.

Following effective treatment, the haematoma is usually resorbed within 10–14 days but full movement may take longer to return.

JOINT DEGENERATION This, the sequel to repeated bleeding, usually begins before the age of 15 years. Chronic synovitis is followed by cartilage degeneration. An affected joint shows wasting, limitation of movement, and fixed deformity not unlike a tuberculous or rheumatoid joint. In long-standing cases, articular destruction may lead to instability.

On x-ray several stages can be identified (Arnold and Hilgartner, 1977): I, soft-tissue swelling; II, osteoporosis and epiphyseal overgrowth; III, slight narrowing of the joint space and squaring of the patella and femoral condyles; IV, marked narrowing of the joint space and joint disorganization; and V, joint disintegration.

Cysts and pseudotumours are rare complications (see above).

5.13 Haemophilic arthritis (a) At first there is blood in the joint but the surfaces are intact; (b) later the cartilage is attacked and the joint 'space' narrows; (c) bony erosions appear and eventually the joint becomes deformed and unstable; in (d) early subluxation is obvious.

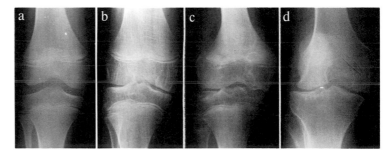

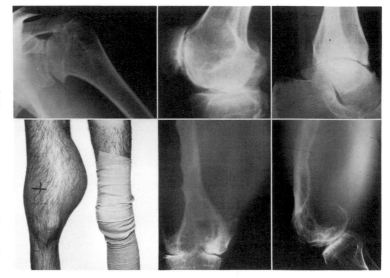

5.14 Haemophilia Top row: degeneration in several joints after repeated bleeding.

Bottom row: since it threatened the integrity of the femur, this large pseudo-tumour was extirpated; at the same time massive bone grafts were inserted – no light undertaking in a haemophilic.

Treatment

The most important aspect of treatment is to provide the patient with the means to counteract the haemorrhage as soon as it occurs. Patients are taught to recognize the early symptoms of bleeding and to administer the appropriate clotting factor concentrate themselves.

It is important to establish the precise diagnosis; factor VIII or IX is effective only for the specific disorder. Frozen cryoprecipitate is sometimes used instead but is much less effective. Fresh-frozen plasma is no longer used.

The acute bleed is treated by immediate factor replacement. Analgesics are given for pain and the limb is immobilized in a splint – but not for more than a day or two; once the acute episode has passed, movement is encouraged, under continuing cover with factor concentrate. Aspiration is avoided unless distension is severe or there is strong suspicion of infection. Nerve palsy may require intermittent splintage and physiotherapy until the neurapraxia recovers, and during this time the skin must be protected from injury.

Chronic arthropathy requires continual treatment to prevent the development of joint contractures, stiffness and progressive muscle weakness. Under cover of factor infusions the patient is given physiotherapy, and impending contractures are managed by intermittent splintage and, if necessary, traction or passive correction by an inflatable splint (Atkins, Henderson and Duthie, 1986).

Operative treatment has become safer since the introduction of factor concentrates. However, patients who develop antifactor antibodies are unsuitable for any form of surgery. It is also important to screen patients for hepatitis B virus and HIV antibodies, as their presence demands special precautions during the operation. Useful procedures are tendon lengthening (to correct contractures), osteotomy (for established deformity) and arthrodesis of the knee or ankle (for painful joint destruction). Synovectomy is sometimes performed but the benefits are somewhat dubious. Total hip replacement is technically feasible, but tissue dissection should be kept to a minimum and meticulous haemostasis is advisable. Continuous factor replacement is, of course, essential.

References and further reading

Ali, S.Y. (1980) Mineral-containing matrix vesicles in human osteoarthrotic cartilage. In *The Aetiopathogenesis of Osteoarthosis* (Ed. G. Nuki), Pitman Medical, Tunbridge Wells, pp. 105–116

Arnold, W.D. and Hilgartner, M.W. (1977) Hemophilic arthropathy. *Journal of Bone and Joint Surgery* **59A**, 287–305

Arnoldi, C.C., Linderholm, H. and Mussbichler, H. (1972) Venous engorgement and intraosseous hypertension in osteoarthritis of the hip. *Journal of Bone and Joint Surgery* **54B**, 409–421

Atkins, R.M., Henderson, N.J. and Duthie, R.B. (1986) Joint contractures in the haemophilias. *Clinical Orthopaedics and Related Research* **219**, 97–106

Byers, P.D., Contepomi, C.A. and Farkas T.A. (1970) A post mortem study of the hip joint including the prevalence of features on the right side. *Annals of the Rhematic Diseases* **29**, 15–31

Doherty, M., Holt, M., MacMillan, P. et al. (1986) A reappraisal of 'analgesic hip'. *Annals of the Rheumatic Diseases* **45**, 272–276

Felson, D.T., Anderson, J.J., Naimack, A. et al. (1987) Obesity and symptomatic knee osteoarthritis. *Arthritis and Rheumatism* **30**, S130

Freeman, M.A.R. (1975) The fatigue of cartilage in the pathogenesis of osteoarthrosis. *Acute Orthopaedica Scandinavica* **46**, 323–328

Lawrence, J.S. (1961) Rheumatism in cotton operatives. *British Journal of Industrial Medicine* **18**, 270–276

McDevitt, C.A,. and Muir, H. (1976) Biochemical changes in the cartilage of the knee in experimental and natural osteoarthritis in the dog. *Journal of Bone and Joint Surgery* **58B**, 94–101

Mankin, H.J., Dorfman, D.D., Lippiello, L. and Zarins, A. (1971) Biochemical and metabolic abnormalities in articular cartilage from osteoarthritic human hips. II. Correlation of morphology with metabolic data. *Journal of Bone and Joint Surgery* **53A**, 523–537

Maroudas, A. (1976) A balance between swelling pressure and collagen tension in normal and degenerate cartilage. *Nature* **260**, 808–809

Moskowitz, R.W., Davis, W., Sammarco, J. et al. (1973) Experimentally induced degenerative joint lesions following partial meniscectomy in the rabbit. *Arthritis and Rheumatism* **16**, 297–405

Newman, N.M. and Ling, R.S.M. (1985) Acetabular bone destruction related to non-steroidal anti-inflammatory drugs. *Lancet* **2**, 11–14

Rashad, S., Revell, P., Hemingway, A. et al. (1989) Effect of non-steroidal anti-inflammatory drugs on the course of osteoarthritis. *Lancet* **2**, 519–522

Resnick, D., Shaul, S.R. and Robins, J.M. (1975) Diffuse idiopathic skeletal hyperostosis (DISH): Forestier's disease with extraspinal manifestations. *Radiology* **115**, 513–524

Sokoloff, L. (1985) Endemic forms of osteoarthritis. *Clinics in Rheumatic Diseases* **11**, 187–202

Solomon, L. (1976) Patterns of osteoarthritis of the hip. *Journal of Bone and Joint Surgery* **58B**, 176–183

Solomon, L., McLaren, P., Irwig, L. et al. (1986) Distinct types of hip disorder in Mseleni joint disease. *South African Medical Journal* **69**, 15–17

Osteonecrosis – bone death – is due either to impaired blood supply or to severe marrow and bone cell damage. Osteochondritis is a poorly defined condition in which bone damage and necrosis follow trauma or repetitive stress.

Ischaemic necrosis (avascular necrosis)

Circumscribed bone necrosis is a definitive feature in a variety of conditions: Perthes' disease, certain fractures, epiphyseal infection, sickle-cell disease, caisson disease, Gaucher's disease, alcohol abuse and high-dosage corticosteroid administration. Certain sites are peculiarly susceptible to ischaemic necrosis: the femoral head, femoral condyles, head of humerus, capitulum, scaphoid, lunate and talus. The vulnerability of the femoral head has been attributed to its relatively poor collateral circulation (Sevitt and Thompson, 1965). In a sense, though, the other sites (all of them convex bone ends or small cuboidal bones) are somewhat compromised in that they are largely enclosed by avascular cartilage, allowing limited access of blood vessels to the subchondral bone; if the main (nutrient) supply is cut off, the bone furthest from the collateral supply may not survive.

Pathogenesis

Cuboidal bones and long-bone ends consist of a honeycomb of cancellous bone packed with myeloid tissue and fat, through which course the fine capillaries and sinusoids that support both marrow and bone cells. Unlike the arterial capillaries, the sinusoids have no adventitial layer and their patency is determined by the shape and volume of the surrounding structures (Branemark, 1959). The system functions essentially as a closed compartment within which one element can expand only at the expense of the others. On haemodynamic principles, bone ischaemia can be brought about in four different ways: (1) interruption of the arterial inflow; (2) occlusion of the venous

---

CAUSES OF BONE NECROSIS

Interruption of arterial supply
Fracture
Dislocation
Infection

Arteriolar occlusion
Sickle-cell disease
Vasculitis
Caisson disease

Capillary compression
Gaucher's disease
Fatty infiltration due to corticosteroids or alcohol abuse

---

outflow; (3) intravascular blockage of arterioles and capillaries; and (4) expansion of the marrow components, causing collapse of the sinusoids.

This is the basis of a pathogenetic classification of ischaemic necrosis. In practice, several mechanisms usually come into play simultaneously or as a cascade of events leading to increasingly severe bone cell anoxia.

ARTERIAL INSUFFICIENCY Post-traumatic osteonecrosis is assumed to be due to interruption of the arterial supply in areas with poor collateral circulation. However, even in such obvious examples as femoral neck fracture, slipped epiphysis or dislocation of the hip, there may be some element of venous tamponade due to intra-articular bleeding and stretching of the capsule.

VENOUS OCCLUSION Extraosseous venous occlusion must needs be very extensive to produce vascular stasis and bone ischaemia, because the communicating diaphyseal medullary veins provide such effective collateral drainage (Cuthbertson, Siris and Gilfillan, 1965). But what if the intraosseous veins are thrombosed (e.g. in osteomyelitis)? In children, diaphyseal venous drainage might be less effective because of the vascular isolation of the epiphysis; could this be why ischaemic necrosis occurs so readily after trauma to the proximal femoral epiphysis? Venous drainage of the femoral head is also reduced in Perthes' disease (Green and Griffin, 1982) and there is some evidence to suggest that this is due to venous tamponade associated with capsular distension following non-specific synovitis (Launder, Hungerford and Jones, 1981).

INTRAVASCULAR CAPILLARY OCCLUSION In sickle-cell disease clumping of abnormal red cells may lead to diminished capillary perfusion (Rickles and O'Leary, 1974). A similar mechanism was believed to apply in dysbaric ischaemia (caisson disease), where too rapid atmospheric decompression causes nitrogen bubbles to come out of solution in the blood; however, Pooley and Walder (1984) have shown that prolonged compression also causes swelling of the marrow fat cells and decreased intramedullary blood flow, effects that are attributed to oxygen toxicity.

Osteonecrosis due to alcohol abuse or corticosteroid administration has been attributed to intraosseous fat embolism, a consequence of the hyperlipidaemia and fatty infiltration of the liver which occurs in both conditions (Jones, 1985). Undoubtedly fat globules do appear in the subchondral capillaries of osteonecrotic femoral heads (Cruess, Ross and Crawshaw, 1975), but whether they cause the necrosis is unproven.

INTRAOSSEOUS CAPILLARY TAMPONADE Perhaps the commonest example of vascular tamponade causing osteonecrosis is in bone infection; it is the danger of bone death that dictates the urgency of treatment. In Gaucher's disease, osteonecrosis has been attributed to compression of the marrow capillaries and sinusoids by masses of large macrophages stuffed abnormally with glycocerebroside (Jaffe, 1972).

The mechanism of capillary tamponade offers an alternative explanation for corticosteroid- and alcohol-induced osteonecrosis. In both disorders marrow fat cell volume is significantly increased (Solomon, 1981), intramedullary pressure is markedly elevated and venous drainage is impaired (Ficat and Arlet, 1980). Similar changes probably occur in endogenous Cushing's disease and in familial hyperlipidaemia. Moreover, it has now been suggested that fat cell swelling may contribute to the ischaemic changes in dysbaric osteonecrosis (Pooley and Walder, 1984), and a similar

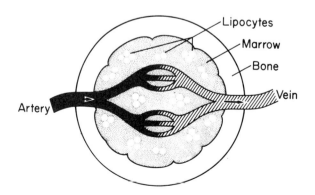

6.1 Avascular necrosis – pathogenesis The medullary cavity of bone is virtually a closed compartment containing myeloid tissue, marrow fat and capillary blood vessels. Any increase in fat cell volume will reduce capillary circulation and may result in bone ischaemia.

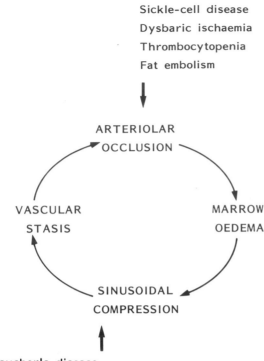

Sickle-cell disease
Dysbaric ischaemia
Thrombocytopenia
Fat embolism

ARTERIOLAR
OCCLUSION

VASCULAR
STASIS

MARROW
OEDEMA

SINUSOIDAL
COMPRESSION

Gaucher's disease
Tuberculosis
Cortisone/alcohol
Dysbaric ischaemia

6.2 Avascular necrosis Algorithm showing how various disorders may enter the vicious cycle of capillary stasis and marrow engorgement.

increase in fat cell density is seen in sickle-cell disease (Cabannes and Mambo-Sombo, 1984).

OSTEONECROSIS AS A COMPARTMENT SYNDROME
Except in traumatic osteonecrosis, where vessels are completely ruptured, vascular insufficiency in cancellous bone probably triggers a cascade of events resembling the familiar soft-tissue compartment syndrome of the forearm or leg. It matters little whether the initiating factor was capillary occlusion (as in sickle-cell disease), venous occlusion (as suggested for Perthes' disease) or intramedullary tamponade (in Gaucher's disease or, putatively, in hypercortisonism); the result is a diffuse ischaemia involving all these elements in greater or lesser degree.

Pathology

Dead bone is structurally indistinguishable from live bone; it is only when secondary features of mechanical failure and repair make their appearance that the radiographic abnormality is revealed. The changes begin within a week of the ischaemic episode and evolve over a period of 2–4 years; they are essentially the same for all types of osteonecrosis, though distinctive features of the underlying disorder may be present as well. The extent of the bone abnormality varies according to the degree of vascular insufficiency: if a large area is involved, fragmentation is the rule because new bone

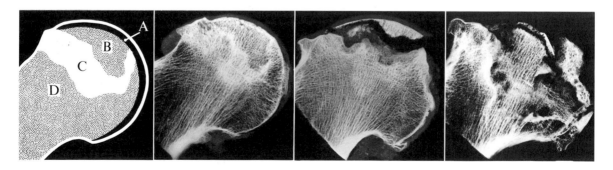

6.3 Avascular necrosis of bone – pathology These fine-detail x-rays of necrotic femoral heads show the progress of osteonecrosis. The articular cartilage (A) remains intact for a long time. The necrotic segment (B) has a texture similar to that of normal bone, but it may develop fine cracks. New bone surrounds the dead trabeculae and causes marked sclerosis (C). Beyond this the bone remains unchanged (D). In the later stages the necrotic bone breaks up and finally the joint surface is destroyed.

formation cannot keep pace with the cumulative loading stresses; if necrosis is limited to a small subchondral zone, repair may be complete and structural failure is by no means inevitable.

Bone cells die after 12–48 hours of anoxia, yet for days or even weeks the gross appearance of the affected segment remains unaltered. During this time the most striking histological changes are seen in the marrow: loss of fat cell outlines, infiltration by collections of round cells, the appearance of tissue histiocytes, and eventual replacement of necrotic marrow by undifferentiated mesenchymal tissue. Even at this very early stage one may see osteoblastic proliferation, the prelude to bone repair, on the trabecular surfaces. As the necrotic sector becomes demarcated, vascular granulation tissue grows in from the surviving tissues and new bone is laid down upon the dead; it is this increase in mineral mass that produces the radiographic appearance of sclerosis.

Even as reparative new bone formation proceeds, structural failure begins to appear in the necrotic bone. This takes three forms: (1) fine cracking of the subchondral bone, probably due to fatigue failure in dead bone; (2) a linear tangential fracture, close to the articular surface, which may be initiated by osteoclastic resorption at the periphery of the necrotic zone

(Glimscher and Kenzora, 1979a, b); and (3) a shearing fracture at the deep interface between dead bone and live bone.

Until very late the articular cartilage retains its thickness and viability. In the final stages, however, fragmentation of the necrotic bone leads to progressive deformity and eventual destruction of the joint surface.

Two questions arise: is avascular necrosis reversible? and does the fully established lesion ever go on to complete healing by new bone formation? The answer to both is, 'Yes, under certain conditions'. Doubtless there are numerous examples of bone cell death attributable to anoxia which never progress to full-blown segmental osteonecrosis; these lesions are seen in necropsy specimens from a variety of disorders and even in normal aged individuals. There is also evidence that in some cases the very early stage of bone ischaemia is reversible if the compartment syndrome is relieved by decompression (Ficat and Arlet, 1980; Solomon, 1981; Hungerford and Lennox, 1985). However, once segmental bone death has occurred the change is not reversible in any true sense. Nevertheless, new bone formation can effect repair without structural failure, provided (1) the necrotic lesion is not too large and (2) osteogenesis is vigorous. These conditions are most likely to be met in children with limited Perthes' disease, and least likely in the very old or in patients on corticosteroids in whom bone turnover is depressed.

Clinical features

The earliest stage of bone death is asymptomatic; by the time the patient presents, the lesion is usually well advanced.

Pain is the usual complaint. It is felt in or near a joint, and perhaps only with certain movements. Some patients complain of a 'click' in the joint, probably due to snapping or catching of a loose articular fragment. In the later stages the joint becomes stiff and deformed. Local tenderness may be present and, if a superficial bone (such as the carpal lunate) is affected, there may be some swelling. Movements – or perhaps one particular movement – may be restricted; in advanced cases there may be fixed deformities.

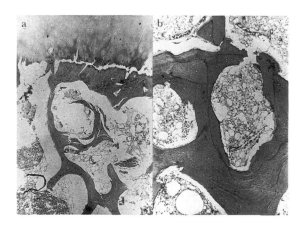

6.4 Avascular necrosis – histology (a) Section across the junction between articular cartilage and bone shows living cartilage cells but necrotic subchondral marrow and bone. (b) A high power view shows islands of dead bone with empty osteocytic lacunae enfolded by new, living bone.

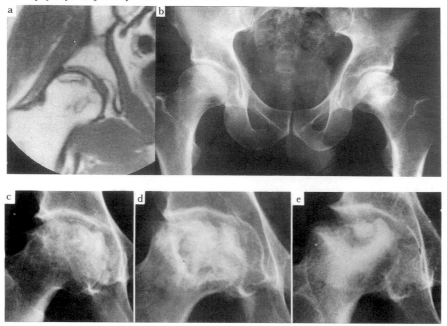

6.5 Avascular necrosis – x-rays   (a) The earliest changes are seen in the MRI: increased signal intensity from the abnormal marrow. (b) X-ray of the same patient shows only a hint of sclerosis in the right femoral head but well-marked changes on the left. (c–e) In long-standing cases the details may differ but the major features are constant: increased bone density and distortion of the bone architecture, but an intact joint space. Sometimes the necrotic segment separates ('dissects') as a discrete fragment (e).

X-RAY   The classic x-ray sign of avascular necrosis is increased bone density. This may be seen within weeks of the infarction and at that stage is due not to any change in the necrotic segment but to reactive new bone formation in the surrounding living tissue. It takes several forms: a subchondral flush of sclerosis, more diffuse density in a large segment of bone or patchy sclerosis further away from the articular surface. Suitable views may also show a thin tangential fracture line just below the articular surface – the 'crescent sign', which occurs in over 60% of cases. In the late stages there may be distortion of the articular surface and more intense sclerosis, now partly due to bone compression in a collapsed segment. Occasionally the necrotic portion separates from the parent bone as a discrete fragment. With all these changes (and this is the cardinal feature distinguishing primary avascular necrosis from the sclerotic forms of osteoarthritis) the articular 'space' retains its normal thickness.

OTHER DIAGNOSTIC IMAGING   X-ray changes are late; early signs of ischaemia may be found on radionuclide scintigraphy or MR imaging.

Radionuclide scanning   with ^{99m}TC-sulphur colloid, which is taken up in myeloid tissue, may reveal an avascular segment. This is most likely in traumatic avascular necrosis, where a large segment of bone is involved, or in sickle-cell disease where a 'cold' area contrasts significantly with the generally high nuclide uptake due to increased erythroblastic activity. ^{99m}Tc-HDP scans (in the bone phase) may also show a 'cold' area, particularly if a large segment of bone is avascular (e.g. after fracture of the femoral neck). More often, however, the picture is dominated by *increased* activity, reflecting hyperaemia and new bone formation in the area around the infarct.

Magnetic resonance imaging may show decreased signal intensity due to ischaemic changes in the marrow long before any abnormality

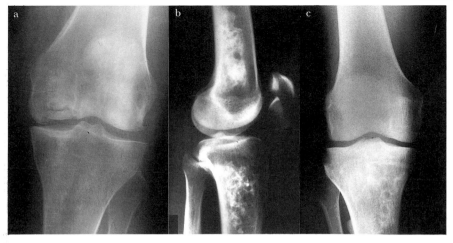

6.6 Avascular necrosis – x-rays (a) Osteonecrosis of the femoral condyle always affects the highest point of the articular surface, thus distinguishing it from osteochondritis dissecans which occurs adjacent to the intercondylar notch. (b) Medullary sclerosis, like puffs of smoke inside the bone away from the articular surface, is typical of asymptomatic bone infarction; this patient was x-rayed only because he fractured his patella. (c) A less common type of bone infarction appearing as rings of increased density in the metaphysis.

is obvious on plain x-rays. This is useful in diagnosing osteonecrosis in high-risk patients (i.e. those with conditions commonly associated with osteonecrosis) who have no overt symptoms or signs.

TESTS FOR HAEMODYNAMIC FUNCTION During the early stage of ischaemic necrosis the intramedullary pressure is often markedly raised. A cannula introduced into the metaphysis enables measurements to be taken (1) at rest and (2) after rapid injection of saline. The normal resting pressure is 10–20 mmHg, rising by about 15 mm after saline injection; in ischaemic bone the pressure may be increased three- or fourfold. Venous stasis can also be demonstrated by venography after injection of radio-opaque medium into the bone. While in no way diagnostic of osteonecrosis, these tests can warn of increasing ischaemia at a stage where further change may be prevented by drilling and decompression of the bone.

Staging the lesion

Ficat and Arlet (1980) have emphasized the importance of distinguishing between the very early and potentially reversible changes of bone ischaemia, the later abnormalities associated with bone death and progressive collapse, and the most advanced stage of articular destruction.

STAGE I This is the preclinical phase of ischaemia and early necrosis in which there is no radiographic abnormality. The diagnosis is suggested by demonstrating abnormally high intramedullary pressures and venous stasis in a patient known to be at risk. MRI may also show early changes in the marrow. The diagnosis can be confirmed by bone biopsy.

STAGE II This stage is painful and is characterized by early radiographic changes with a normal (or near normal) bone contour.

STAGE III This again shows clear-cut radiographic features of osteonecrosis, but now accompanied by definite structural damage and an abnormal bone outline. At this stage the intramedullary pressure may be normal, presumably because bone fracture has, in a sense, decompressed the area.

STAGE IV This is marked by collapse of the articular surface and secondary changes of degenerative arthritis.

Although based on a knowledge of the underlying morbid anatomy, this is a clinical rather than a pathological classification, with practical implications for treatment.

Diagnosis of the underlying disorder

In most cases of osteonecrosis the underlying disorder will be obvious from the history: a known episode of trauma, an occupation such as deep-sea diving or working under compressed air, a family background of Gaucher's disease or sickle-cell disease.

There may be a record of high-dosage corticosteroid administration; for example, after renal transplantation where the drug is used for immunosuppression. However, much smaller doses (e.g. for asthma or systemic lupus erythematosus) can also be dangerous; occasionally the drug has been given without the patient's knowledge. Combinations of drugs (e.g. corticosteroids and azathioprine, or corticosteroids after a period of alcohol abuse) are potent sources of osteonecrosis.

Alcohol abuse is often difficult to determine because patients tend to hide the information. There is no biochemical marker that is specific for high alcohol intake, but Whitehead, Clarke and Whitfield (1978) have shown that elevation of three or four of the following is highly suggestive: aspartate transaminase, γ-glutamyl transpeptidase, serum urate, serum triglyceride and mean red cell volume.

After careful clinical, haematological and biochemical investigation, very few cases of osteonecrosis remain unexplained. For these few the unsatisfactory term 'idiopathic necrosis' may still be used.

Treatment

In planning treatment, all the factors that influence the natural course of the condition must be taken into account: the type of ischaemic necrosis, the area affected, its stage of development, the patient's age and capacity for bone repair, the persistence or otherwise of the aetiological agent and its effect on bone turnover.

The results of non-operative management of established osteonecrosis have been disappointing. Steinberg, Hayken and Steinberg (1984) followed the progress of 48 hips treated conservatively and found that 44 of these eventually required arthroplasty; partial weightbearing and non-weightbearing appeared not to influence the outcome at all.

Such pessimism has fostered the attitude that the condition should be allowed to run its course (with nothing more than symptomatic treatment) until it eventually requires reconstructive surgery. This can take many years and, in some cases, the need for operation might never arise. Such an approach is more applicable to the shoulder than to the hip, to patients with a short life expectancy, to the very old (whose functional demands may be minimal) and to the very young (who have an enviable capacity for bone remodelling).

PREVENTION
The risk of developing osteonecrosis can be reduced by attention to well-established protective measures: prompt aspiration of hip effusions or haemarthrosis to prevent capsular tamponade; a policy of using corticosteroids only when essential and in minimal effective dosage; rigorous application of decompression procedures for divers and compressed-air workers; care in preventing anoxia in patients with haemoglobinopathies.

EARLY (STAGE I OR II) OSTEONECROSIS
While the bone contour is intact there is always the hope that structural failure can be prevented. Small lesions probably do heal spontaneously and with minimal deformity; this is seen especially in the femoral condyles and the talus, where one can afford to pursue a waiting policy. Osteonecrosis of the non-weightbearing joints also may interfere very little with function, so there is no need for early operative treatment. However, femoral head necrosis has a more ominous prognosis, which has prompted a swing towards operative treatment for early osteonecrosis. Two procedures are considered: medullary decompression and bone grafting.

MEDULLARY DECOMPRESSION Because decompression is meant to relieve the compartment syndrome in bone with an intact arterial supply, it is obviously not suitable for most cases of post-traumatic osteonecrosis.

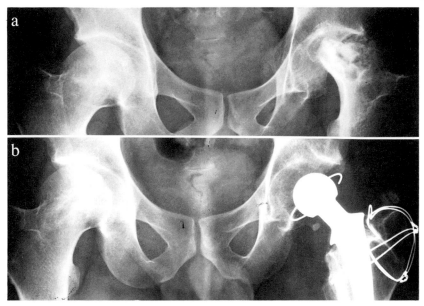

6.7 Osteonecrosis – treatment (a) Alcohol abuse has led to bilateral femoral head necrosis, advanced on the left but early on the right. (b) Drilling of the femoral neck to decompress the bone was in time to save the right hip; the left had to be replaced.

The ideal indication is non-traumatic stage I ischaemic necrosis. Unfortunately the condition is seldom diagnosed at this stage. Where there is a strong suspicion that it exists (e.g. in the contralateral asymptomatic hip) the patient is prepared for measurement of intraosseous pressure under general anaesthesia. If this shows a marked rise (normal = 10–25 mmHg), a 7 mm core of bone is removed from the femoral neck under image intensification fluoroscopy. Zizic and Hungerford (1985), in a follow-up of 211 patients treated in this way, found that further operation was required in only 4% of those with stage I and 23% of those with stage II osteonecrosis. The effect of decompression is maintained after the defect heals, possibly because of the improved venous drainage conferred by newly vascularized bone.

BONE GRAFTING   Free strut grafts placed up the femoral neck have been used in early cases of femoral head necrosis, with good results (Enneking, 1975). This provides both decompression and mechanical support. Vascularized grafts are even better in preventing collapse of the femoral head (Ganz and Buchler, 1983); however, this is mainly a mechanical effect and it is unlikely that a truly necrotic segment can be revascularized in any real sense.

LATE (STAGE III OR IV) OSTEONECROSIS
Once there is structural damage and distortion of the articular surface, conservative procedures (such as decompression) are wholly inappropriate. Operative treatment can usually be deferred until pain or loss of function make it necessary. Three procedures are employed: realignment osteotomy, arthroplasty and arthrodesis.

REALIGNMENT OSTEOTOMY   Provided that the damaged area is not too large, bone realignment can be planned to transfer load away from the necrotic segment to an undamaged part of the joint. This is certainly worth considering in younger patients (those under 45 years) with necrosis of the femoral head or one of the femoral condyles.

ARTHROPLASTY   For advanced osteonecrosis with severe joint dysfunction, partial or total joint replacement may be necessary. In older patients the decision is easy; indeed, there is a strong argument for treating all elderly patients with osteonecrosis in this way, rather than submit them to lesser procedures with less predictable results. However, for the younger patient with high functional demands joint replacement should be undertaken only after carefully weighing up all the alternatives.

Osteonecrosis of the head of the humerus poses special problems. Despite their disability, most patients manage at least as well as they would after any operation; provided pain can be controlled with analgesics and palliative physiotherapy, no specific treatment is required. About a third have severe pain, stiffness or deformity (Cruess, 1976); for these, shoulder arthroplasty may be justified.

ARTHRODESIS Patients who are too young to be considered for arthroplasty of a weightbearing joint may be offered the alternative of arthrodesis. Fusion of the ankle is certainly acceptable for necrosis of the talus. However, the question is less easily resolved where the hip or knee is involved. The publicity accorded to total joint replacement has made arthrodesis an unpopular option, the more so if the joint – though painful – still has a good range of movement.

Specific types of avascular necrosis (AVN)

Drug-induced necrosis

Alcohol, corticosteroids, immunosuppressives and cytotoxic drugs, either singly or in combination, are potent sources of avascular necrosis; their role in the pathogenesis of 'idiopathic' osteonecrosis has already been discussed.

Sickle-cell disease

Red cells containing the abnormal haemoglobin S (Hb-S) may become sickle shaped, leading to bone infarction. This is particularly likely in homozygous sickle-cell disease (where two Hb-S genes have been inherited), but may also occur in the heterozygous disorders, Hb-S/C haemoglobinopathy and Hb-S/thalassaemia. Inheritance of one Hb-S gene and one normal β-globin gene results in the *sickle-cell trait* in which sickling occurs only under conditions of hypoxia (e.g. under anaesthesia, in extreme cold or at high altitudes).

The abnormal Hb-S gene is limited to people of Central and West African Negro descent; it is fairly common in Nigeria, around the Mediterranean, in the West Indies and in the USA (about 10% of American Negroes have the sickle-cell trait). Below the equator it is virtually unknown.

In the established disorder there is increased aggregation of the haemoglobin molecules and subsequent distortion of red cell shape; this is most marked in deoxygenated blood. Clumping of the sickle-shaped cells causes diminished capillary flow and repeated episodes of pain ('bone crises') or, if more severe, ischaemic necrosis. Almost any bone may be involved and there is a tendency for the infarcts to become infected, sometimes with unusual organisms such as *Salmonella*.

Diagnosis

Patients with sickle-cell disease may present with acute osteomyelitis (sometimes multifocal), hyperuricaemia and gout (common in adults) with painful swollen joints, and sometimes with typical features of avascular necrosis.

On x-ray the tubular bones (including the phalanges) may show irregular endosteal destruction and medullary sclerosis, together with periosteal new bone formation. Not only does this resemble osteitis but also true infection is often superimposed on the infarct. Medullary calcification is common and may be very extensive. In children, femoral head necrosis could be mistaken for Perthes' disease were it not that the latter is known to be uncommon in Africans. Involvement of the spine may lead to vertebral collapse. Bone scanning with ^{99m}Tc-sulphur colloid may show localized areas of diminished uptake, many of which are asymptomatic. The definitive diagnosis of the underlying haemoglobinopathy is made by special haematological tests.

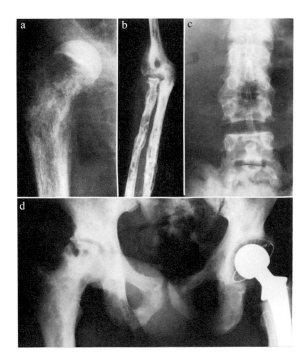

6.8 Sickle-cell disease   (a) Typical changes in the femur due to marrow hyperplasia, with bone infarction and necrosis of the femoral head. (b) In severe cases infarctions of tubular bones may resemble osteomyelitis, with sequestra and a marked periosteal reaction (sometimes a true salmonella infection supervenes). (c) The spine also may be involved. (d) In adults osteoporosis is followed by endosteal sclerosis, seen clearly in the right femur; the left hip has already been replaced following femoral head necrosis.

Treatment

Bone crises are treated by rest and analgesics, followed by physiotherapy to minimize stiffness. Established necrosis is treated according to the principles on p. 97, but with the emphasis on conservatism. Anaesthesia carries serious risks and may even precipitate vascular occlusion in the central nervous system, lungs or kidneys; moreover, the chances of postoperative infection are high.

Caisson disease and dysbaric osteonecrosis

Decompression sickness (caisson disease) and osteonecrosis are important causes of disability in deep-sea divers and compressed-air workers building tunnels or underwater structures. Under increased air pressure the blood and other tissues (especially fat) become supersaturated with nitrogen; if decompression is too rapid the gas is released as bubbles, which cause local tissue damage and generalized embolic phenomena. The symptoms of decompression sickness, which may develop within minutes, are pain near the joints ('the bends'), breathing difficulty and vertigo ('the staggers'). In the most acute cases there can be circulatory and respiratory collapse, severe neurological changes, coma and death. Only 10% of patients with bone necrosis give a history of decompression sickness.

Radiological bone lesions have been found in 17% of compressed-air workers in Britain; almost half the lesions are juxta-articular – mainly in the humeral head and femoral head – but microscopic bone death is much more widespread than x-rays suggest.

The bone infarction may be due to one or more of the following: (1) intravascular capillary obstruction by nitrogen bubbles; (2) extravascular capillary compression by gas released from the supersaturated marrow fat in the non-expandable bone; (3) intravascular fat embolism or thromboembolism resulting from tissue disruption when gas bubbles are released (Cryssanthou, 1978).

Clinical and x-ray features

The necrosis may cause pain and loss of joint movement, but many lesions remain 'silent' and are found only on routine x-ray examination. Medullary infarcts cause mottled calcification or areas of dense sclerosis. Juxta-articular changes are similar to those in other forms of osteonecrosis.

Management

The aim is prevention; the incidence of osteonecrosis is proportional to the working pressure, the length of exposure, the rate of decompression and the number of exposures. Strict enforcement of suitable working schedules has reduced the risks considerably. The treatment of established lesions follows the principles already outlined.

Gaucher's disease (see also p. 155)

This familial disease occurs predominantly in Ashkenazi Jews. Deficiency of the specific enzyme causes an abnormal accumulation of glucocerebroside in the macrophages of the reticuloendothelial system. The effects are seen chiefly in the liver, spleen and bone marrow, where the large polyhedral 'Gaucher cells' accumulate; their pressure on the bone sinusoids may be the cause of the bone necrosis.

Necrosis of the femoral head is not uncommon. It may occur at any age and presents with pain and limp; movements become gradually more restricted. Other areas may be similarly affected. There is a tendency for the Gaucher deposits to become infected and the patient may present with septicaemia. Blood tests reveal anaemia, leucopenia and thrombocytopenia. A diagnostic, though inconstant, finding is a raised serum acid phosphatase level.

X-RAY The appearances resemble those in other types of osteonecrosis, and 'silent' lesions may be found in a number of bones. A special feature (due to replacement of myeloid tissue by Gaucher cells) is expansion of the tubular bones, especially the distal femur, producing the Erlenmeyer flask appearance. Cortical thinning and osteoporosis may lead to pathological fracture.

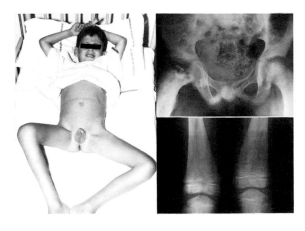

6.9 Gaucher's disease This young boy, whose sister also had Gaucher's disease, developed pain in the right hip; abduction was limited and painful. X-rays show necrosis of the right femoral head and widening of the femoral shafts (the Erlenmeyer flask appearance).

TREATMENT of the osteonecrosis follows the general principles outlined earlier. Femoral head replacement is often advisable – the prosthesis should be uncemented and antibiotics continued for 5 days.

Radiation necrosis

Ionizing radiation, if sufficiently intense or prolonged, may cause bone death. This is due to the combined effects of damage to small blood vessels, marrow cells and bone cells. Such changes, which are dose-related, often occurred in the past when low-energy radiation was in use. Nowadays, with megavoltage apparatus and more sophisticated planning techniques, long-term bone damage is much less likely; patients who present with osteonecrosis are usually those who were treated some years ago. Areas affected are mainly the shoulder and ribs (after external irradiation for breast cancer), the sacrum, pelvis and hip (after irradiation of pelvic lesions) and the jaws (after treatment of tumours around the head and neck).

Pathology

Unlike the common forms of ischaemic necrosis, which always involve subchondral bone, radiation necrosis is more diffuse and the effects more variable. Marrow and bone cells die, but for months or even years there may be no structural change in the bone. Gradually, however, stress fractures appear and may result in widespread bone destruction. A striking feature is the absence of repair and remodelling. The surrounding bone is usually osteoporotic; in the jaw, infection may follow tooth extraction.

Clinical features

The patient usually presents with pain around the shoulder, the hip, the sacrum or the pubic symphysis. There will always be a history of previous treatment by ionizing radiation, though this may not come to light unless appropriate questions are asked.

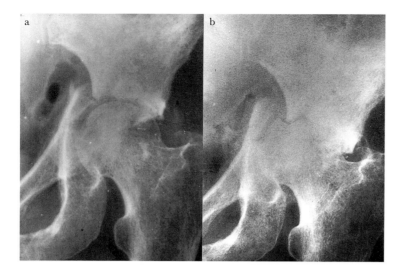

6.10 Radiation necrosis – x-rays This patient received radiation therapy for carcinoma of the bladder. One year later he developed pain in the left hip and x-ray showed (a) a fracture of the acetabulum. Diagnosis of radiation necrosis was confirmed when (b) the fracture failed to heal and the joint crumbled.

There may be local signs of irradiation, such as skin pigmentation, and the area is usually tender. Movements in the nearby joint are restricted. General examination may reveal scars or other evidence of the original lesion.

X-RAYS show areas of bone destruction and patchy sclerosis; in the hip there may be an unsuspected fracture of the acetabulum or femoral neck, or collapse of the femoral head.

Treatment

Treatment depends on the site of osteonecrosis, the quality of the surrounding bone and the life expectancy of the patient. If a large joint is involved (e.g. the hip), replacement arthroplasty may be considered; however, bone quality is often poor and there is a high risk of early implant loosening. Nevertheless, if pain cannot be adequately controlled, and if the patient has a reasonable life expectancy, joint replacement is justified.

Osteochondritis (osteochondrosis)

The term 'osteochondritis' is applied to a group of conditions in which there is compression, fragmentation or separation of a small segment of bone, usually at the bone end and involving the attached articular surface. The affected portion of bone shows many of the features of ischaemic necrosis, including loss of bone cells together with increased vascularity and reactive sclerosis in the surrounding bone. These conditions tend to occur in children and adolescents, often during phases of rapid growth and increased physical activity. Segmental ischaemia may be caused by trauma or repetitive stress to the epiphysis; indeed, this may simply be a stress fracture of a relatively isolated (unfused) epiphysis or small cuboidal bone, with damage to the segmental blood supply. Despite the name, there are no signs of inflammation.

Three types of osteochondritis are identified: 'crushing', 'splitting' and 'pulling'.

Table 6.1 The types of osteochondritis

Type	Bone	Eponym
Crushing	Metatarsal	Freiberg
	Navicular	Köhler
	Lunate	Kienböck
	Capitulum	Panner
Splitting	Femoral condyle	
	Elbow	
	Talus	
	Metatarsal	
Pulling	Tibial tuberosity	Osgood–Schlatter
	Calcaneum	Sever

Crushing osteochondritis

This is usually seen in late adolescence and is characterized by apparently spontaneous necrosis of the ossific nucleus in a long-bone epiphysis or one of the cuboidal bones of the wrist or foot. Local anatomical features (e.g. a metatarsal bone that is longer than usual, or disproportion in the lengths of radius and ulna) which could result in undue compressive stress being applied to the bone, can sometimes be identified and it is thought that this may compromise the local blood supply.

The pathological changes are the same as those in other forms of osteonecrosis: bone death, fragmentation or distortion of the necrotic segment, and new bone formation of the ischaemic trabeculae.

Pain and limitation of joint movement are the usual complaints. Tenderness is sharply localized to the affected bone. X-rays show the characteristic increased density, accompanied in the later stages by distortion and collapse of the necrotic segment.

The common examples of crushing osteochondritis have, by long tradition, acquired eponymous labels: Freiberg's disease of the metatarsal; Köhler's disease of the navicular; Keinböck's disease of the carpal lunate; and Panner's disease of the capitulum.

Vertebral osteochondritis (*Scheuermann's disease*) is similar in kind but without any evidence of bone death. Compression and fragmentation of the vertebral epiphyseal plates lead to wedging of the vertebral bodies. It occurs during adolescence and may cause back pain and dorsal kyphosis. Although x-rays show sclerosis and irregularity or fragmentation of the vertebral end-plates, this is not osteonecrosis.

Splitting osteochondritis (osteochondritis dissecans)

A small segment of articular cartilage and the subjacent bone may separate (dissect) as an avascular fragment. It occurs typically in young adults, usually men, and affects particular sites: the lateral surface of the medial femoral condyle in the knee, the anteromedial corner of the talus in the ankle, the superomedial part of the femoral head, the humeral capitulum and the first metatarsal head.

The cause is almost certainly repeated minor trauma resulting in osteochondral fracture of a convex surface; the fragment loses its blood supply. However, there must be other predisposing factors, for the condition is sometimes multifocal and sometimes runs in families.

The knee is much the commonest joint to be affected. The patient presents with intermittent pain, swelling and joint effusion. If the necrotic fragment becomes completely detached, it may cause locking of the joint or unexpected episodes of giving way. Less frequently, similar episodes occur in the hip or ankle.

X-rays must be taken with the joint in the appropriate position to show the affected part of the articular surface in tangential projection. The dissecting fragment is defined by a radio-

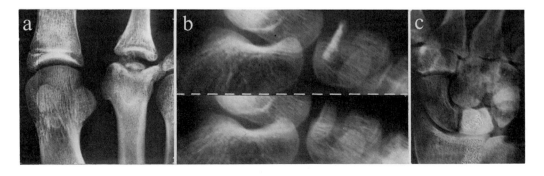

6.11 Crushing osteochondritis   (a) Freiberg's disease of the second metatarsal; (b) Köhler's disease of the navicular, compared with the normal side below; (c) Kienböck's disease of the lunate.

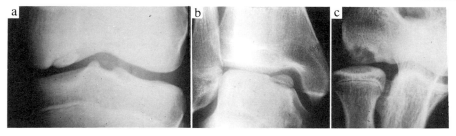

6.12 Splitting osteochondritis The osteochondral fragment usually remains in place at the articular surface. The most common sites are (a) the medial femoral condyle, (b) the talus and (c) the capitulum.

lucent line of demarcation. When it separates, the resulting 'crater' may be obvious.

The early changes (i.e. before demarcation of the dissecting fragment) are better shown by MRI: there is decreased signal intensity in the area around the affected osteochondral segment. Radionuclide scanning with ^{99m}Tc-HDP shows markedly increased activity in the same area. Treatment in the early stage consists of load reduction (crutches if necessary) and restriction of activity. In children, complete healing may occur, though it takes up to 2 years; in adults, it is doubtful whether the future

course of events can be significantly influenced. If the fragment becomes detached and causes symptoms, it should be fixed back in position or else completely removed.

Pulling osteochondritis (traction apophysitis)

Excessive pull by a large tendon may damage the unfused apophysis to which it is attached; this occurs typically at two sites – the tibial

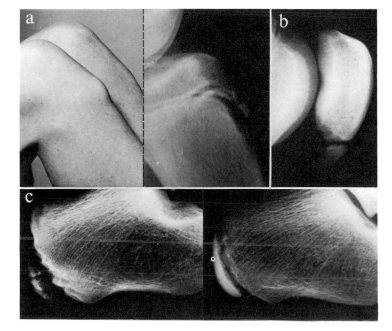

6.13 Pulling osteochondritis These are merely traction lesions, but dignified by eponyms: (a) Osgood–Schlatter's disease involves the apophysis into which the extensor mechanism is inserted; (b) in Johannson–Larsen's disease the calcification is a sequel to the patellar ligament partially pulling away from the bone; (c) Sever's disease, compared with the normal side.

tuberosity (Osgood–Schlatter's disease) and the calcaneal apophysis (Sever's disease). These lesions do not produce bone necrosis. The traumatized apophysis becomes painful and there may an associated tenosynovitis of the attached tendon.

References and further reading

Branemark, P.I. (1959) Vital microscopy of the bone marrow in the rabbit. *Scandinavian Journal of Clinical and Laboratory Investigation* **2**, suppl. 38, 5–82

Cabannes, R. and Mambo-Sombo, F. (1984) Anatomical and pathological aspects of bone changes in sickle cell disease. In *Bone Circulation* (eds. J. Arlet, R.P. Ficat and D.S. Hungerford), Williams & Wilkins, Baltimore, pp. 265–273

Cruess, R.L. (1976) Steroid-induced avascular necrosis of the head of the humerus. Natural history and management. *Journal of Bone and Joint Surgery* **58B**, 313–317

Cruess, R.L., Ross, D. and Crawshaw, E. (1975) The aetiology of steroid-induced avascular necrosis of bone. A laboratory and clinical study. *Clinical Orthopaedics and Related Research* **113**, 178–183

Cryssanthou, C.P. (1978) Dysbaric osteonecrosis. Etiological and pathogenetic concepts. *Clinical Orthopaedics and Related Research* **130**, 94–106

Cuthbertson, E., Siris, E. and Gilfillan, R.S. (1965) The femoral diaphyseal medullary venous system as a venous collateral channel in the dog. *Journal of Bone and Joint Surgery* **47A**, 965–974

Enneking, W.F. (1975) The choice of surgical procedures in idiopathic aseptic necrosis. In *The Hip*, Proceedings of the Seventh Open Scientific Meeting of the Hip Society, C.V. Mosby, St Louis MO, pp. 238–243

Ficat, R.P. and Arlet, J. (1980) *Ischemia and Necroses of Bone* (edited and adapted by D.S. Hungerford), Williams & Wilkins, Baltimore

Ganz, R. and Buchler, V. (1983) Overview of attempts to revitalize the dead head in aseptic necrosis of the femoral head – osteotomy and revascularization. In *The Hip*, Proceedings of the Eleventh Open Scientific Meeting of the Hip Society, C.V. Mosby, St Louis MO, pp. 296–305

Glimscher, M.J. and Kenzora, J.E. (1979a) The biology of osteonecrosis of the human femoral head and its clinical implications. I. Tissue biology. *Clinical Orthopaedics and Related Research* **138**, 284–309

Glimscher, M.J. and Kenzora, J.E. (1979b) The biology of osteonecrosis of the human femoral head and its clinical implications. II. The pathological changes in the femoral head as an organ and in the hip joint. *Clinical Orthopaedics and Related Research* **139**, 283–312

Green, N.E. and Griffin, P.P. (1982) Intra-osseous venous pressure in Legg–Perthes disease. *Journal of Bone and Joint Surgery* **64A**, 666–671

Hungerford, D.S. and Lennox, D.W. (1985) The importance of increased intra-osseous pressure in the development of osteonecrosis of the femoral head: implications for treatment. *Orthopedic Clinics of North America* **16**, 635–654

Jaffe, H.L. (1972) *Metabolic, Degenerative and Inflammatory Disease of Bones and Joints*, Lea and Febiger, Philadelphia

Jones, J.P. (1985) Fat embolism and osteonecrosis. *Orthopedic Clinics of North America* **16**, 595–634

Launder, W.J., Hungerford, D.S. and Jones, L.H. (1981) Hemodynamics of the femoral head. *Journal of Bone and Joint Surgery* **63A**, 442–448

Pooley, J. and Walder, D.N. (1984) The effect of compressed air on bone marrow blood flow and its relationship to caisson disease of bone. In *Bone Circulation* (eds. J. Arlet, R.P. Ficat and D.S. Hungerford), Williams & Wilkins, Baltimore, pp. 63–67

Rickles, F.R. and O'Leary, D.S. (1974) Role of coagulation system in pathophysiology of sickle cell disease. *Archives of Internal Medicine* **133**, 635–641

Sevitt, S. and Thompson, R.G. (1965) The distribution and anastomoses of arteries supplying the head and neck of the femur. *Journal of Bone and Joint Surgery* **47B**, 560–573

Solomon, L. (1981) Idiopathic necrosis of the femoral head: pathogenesis and treatment. *Canadian Journal of Surgery* **24**, 573–578

Steinberg, M.E., Hayken, G.D. and Steinberg, D.R. (1984) The 'conservative' management of avascular necrosis of the femoral head. In *Bone Circulation* (eds. J. Arlet, R.P. Ficat and D.S. Hungerford), Williams & Wilkins, Baltimore, pp. 338–342

Whitehead, T.P., Clarke, C.A. and Whitfield, A.G.W. (1978) Biochemical and haematological markers of alcohol intake. *Lancet* **1**, 978–981

Zizic, T.M. and Hungerford, D.S. (1985) Avascular necrosis of bone. In *Textbook of Rheumatology*, 2nd edn (eds. W.N. Kelley, E.D. Harris, S. Ruddy and C.B. Sledge), W.B. Saunders, Philadelphia, pp. 1689–1710

Metabolic and endocrine disorders 7

Bones have obvious biomechanical functions: they support and protect the soft tissues and transmit load and muscular force from one part of the body to another. Bone tissue has an equally important role as a mineral reservoir which helps to regulate the composition – and in particular the calcium ion concentration – of the extracellular fluid. For all its solidity, bone is in a continuous state of flux, its internal shape and structure changing from moment to moment in concert with the normal variations in mechanical function and mineral exchange. All modulations in bone structure and composition are brought about by cellular activity, which is regulated by hormones and local factors; these agents, in turn, are controlled by alterations in mineral ion concentrations. The metabolic bone disorders are conditions in which generalized skeletal abnormalities result from disruption of this complex interactive system.

Bone composition

Bone consists of a largely collagenous matrix which is impregnated with mineral salts and populated by cells.

THE MATRIX is composed of *type I collagen* lying in a *mucopolysaccharide* ground substance. There are also small amounts of non-collagenous protein, mainly in the form of *proteoglycans* and the bone-specific proteins *osteonectin*, which appears to be involved in bone mineralization, and *osteocalcin* – or Gla protein – whose function is unknown. Gla protein is produced only by osteoblasts and its concentration in the blood is, to some extent, a measure of osteoblastic activity. The unmineralized matrix is known as *osteoid*; normally it is seen only as a thin layer on surfaces where active new bone formation is taking place, but the proportion of osteoid to mineralized bone increases significantly in rickets and osteomalacia.

BONE MINERAL, which occupies almost half the bone volume, consists mainly of *calcium* and *phosphate* in the form of *crystalline hydroxyapatite*. It is laid down in osteoid at the calcification front; this interface between bone and osteoid can be labelled by administering tetracycline, which is taken up avidly in newly mineralized bone and shows as a fluorescent band on ultraviolet light microscopy. In mature bone the proportions of calcium and phosphate are constant and the molecule is firmly bound to collagen; 'demineralization' occurs only by resorption of the entire matrix.

BONE CELLS are of three kinds: osteoblasts, osteocytes and osteoclasts. *Osteoblasts* are concerned with bone formation; they are derived from local mesenchymal precursors and form rows of small (20 μm) cuboidal cells along the free surfaces of trabeculae and haversian systems where new bone is laid down. They are rich in alkaline phosphatase and are responsible for both the production and the mineralization of bone matrix (Peck and Woods, 1988). At the end of a bone remodelling cycle the osteoblast either remains on the newly formed surface as a quiescent lining cell or becomes enveloped in the matrix as a resting osteocyte.

Osteocytes can therefore be regarded as spent osteoblasts. Lying in their bony lacunae, they communicate with each other and with the surface lining cells by slender cytoplasmic processes. Their function is obscure: they may, under the influence of parathyroid hormone, participate in bone resorption ('osteocytic osteolysis') and calcium ion transport (Peck and Woods, 1988). It has also been suggested that they are sensitive to mechanical stimuli and communicate information and changes in stress and strain to the active osteoblasts (Sherry et al., 1989). *Osteoclasts* are the principal mediators of bone resorption. These large multinucleated cells are derived from monocytic precursors in the marrow and are attracted to free bone surfaces by chemotactic stimuli. With resorption of the organic matrix, the osteoclasts are left in shallow excavations along the surface – Howship's lacunae. These excavations help to distinguish 'resorption surfaces' from the smooth 'formation surfaces' or 'resting surfaces' in histological sections.

Bone structure

Bone in its immature state is called *woven bone*; the collagen fibres are arranged haphazardly and the cells have no specific orientation. Typically it is found in the early stages of fracture healing, where it acts as a temporary weld before being replaced by mature bone. The mature tissue is *lamellar bone*, in which the collagen fibres are arranged parallel to each other to form multiple layers (or laminae) with the osteocytes lying between the lamellae. Unlike woven bone, which is laid down in fibrous tissue, lamellar bone forms only on existing surfaces.

Lamellar bone exists in two structurally different forms. *Compact (cortical) bone* is dense to the naked eye. It is found where support matters most: the outer walls of all bones but especially the shafts of tubular bones, and the subchondral plates supporting articular cartilage. It is made up of compact units – haversian systems or osteons – each of which consists of a central canal containing blood vessels, lymphatics and nerves enclosed by whorled lamellae of bone. The haversian canal offers a free surface lined by bone cells; its size varies, depending on whether the osteon is in a phase of resorption or formation.

The vessels of the haversian canals communicate with those of the marrow and periosteum. Blood flow in this capillary network is normally centrifugal – from the medullary cavity outwards – but if the medullary vessels are blocked or destroyed the periosteal circulation can take over and the direction of flow is reversed.

Cancellous (trabecular) bone is spongy or porous in appearance; it makes up the interior meshwork of all bones and is particularly well developed in the ends of the tubular bones and the vertebral bodies. The structural units of trabecular bone are flattened sheets or spars that can be thought of as unfolded osteons. Three-dimensionally the trabecular sheets are interconnected (like a honeycomb) and arranged according to the mechanical needs of the structure, the thickest and strongest along the lines of compressive stress and the thinnest in the planes of tensile stress. The interconnectedness of this meshwork lends added strength to cancellous bone beyond the simple effect of tissue mass. The spaces between trabeculae – the 'opened out' vascular spaces – contain the marrow and the fine sinusoidal vessels that course through the tissue, nourishing both marrow and bone.

Trabecular bone is obviously more porous than cortical bone. Though it makes up only one-quarter of the total skeletal mass, it provides two-thirds of the total bone surface. Add to this the fact that it is covered with marrow and it is easy to understand why the effects of metabolic disorders are usually seen first in trabecular bone.

Bone remodelling

New bone growth occurs in two different ways: (1) by ossification of proliferating cartilage (*endochondral ossification*), typically at the epiphyseal growth plate (physis) or during bone repair; and (2) by direct ossification in connective tissue (*membranous ossification*), as seen in the formation of subperiosteal new bone.

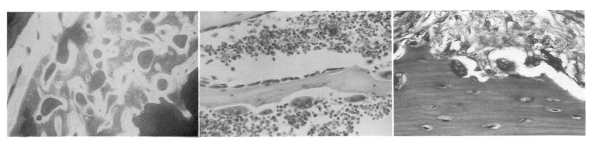

a   b   c

7.1 Bone turnover (a) Bone can be 'labelled' by administering tetracycline which appears in newly mineralized bone as a fluorescent band. Actively forming osteons are easily identified. (b) The cells that govern bone turnover are the osteoclasts (along the scalloped surface of this trabeculum) and the more populous osteoblasts (lining the opposite, bone-forming surface). (c) High-power view of osteoclasts in Howship's lacunae.

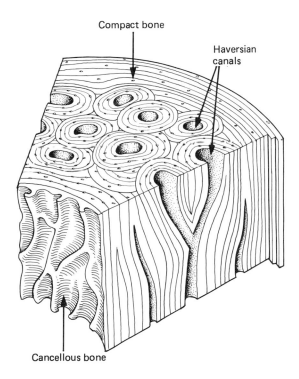

Compact bone

Haversian canals

Cancellous bone

7.2 Bone structure A slice of cortex shows the basic elements of compact bone: outer laminae of sub-periosteal bone, densely packed osteons each made up of concentric layers of bone and osteocytes around a central haversian canal which contains the vessels, and the inner surface (endosteum) which merges into a lattice of trabecular bone.

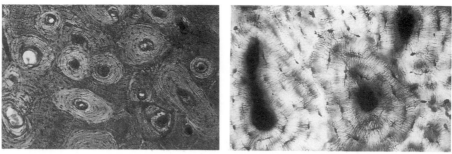

7.3 Histology (a) Low-power and (b) high-power views showing the osteons in various stages of formation and resorption.

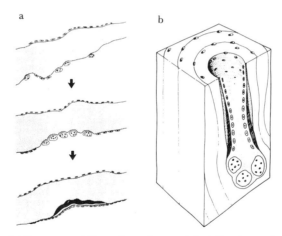

7.4 Bone remodelling Bone is remodelled like clay under the hands of a sculptor. (a) Open surfaces are first excavated by osteoclasts and then lined and filled in again by a following train of osteoblasts. (b) In compact bone the osteoclasts burrow deeply to produce a cutting cone, with the osteoblasts appearing behing them to reline the cavity with new bone.

Formed bone was once thought to be almost inert. This is far from the truth; it is in a constant state of resorption in one place and formation in another – a process known as *remodelling* or *turnover*. This is the means whereby bone is renewed and repaired throughout life. At each remodelling site work proceeds in an orderly sequence: osteoclasts gather on a free bone surface and excavate a cavity; they disappear and, after a period of quiescence, are replaced by osteoblasts which proceed to fill in the excavation with new bone. Each cycle of bone turnover – which takes from 4 to 6 months – is conducted by groups of cells that appear to work in concert; together they make a *bone remodelling unit*.

Resorption starts when osteoclasts are activated and attracted by chemotaxis to a mineralized surface. The organic matrix and mineral are removed together; on a trabecular plate this produces a simple excavation, but in cortical bone the cells burrow inwards as a *cutting cone* – like miners sinking a new shaft. After 2–3 weeks resorption ceases and the osteoclasts disappear. A week or two later the cavity surface is covered with osteoblasts and for the next 3 months bone *formation and mineralization* slowly restore the lost tissue.

During bone remodelling, resorption and formation are *coupled*, the one ineluctably following the other. This ensures that, at least over the short term, a balance is maintained, though at any moment and at any particular site one or other process may predominate.

Age-related changes in bone

Bone turnover or remodelling goes on throughout life. It varies in rate, extent and distribution according to the demands of growth, mechanical stress and biochemical exchange. During *growth* the entire bone increases in size and changes somewhat in shape. At the epiphyseal growth plate (physis), new bone is added by endochondral ossification; on the surface, bone is formed directly by subperiosteal appositional ossification; the medullary cavity is expanded by endosteal bone resorption; bulbous bone ends are re-formed and sculpted continuously by co-ordinated formation and resorption. Although during growth each bone gets longer and wider, the bone tissue of which it is made remains quite light and porous. *Between 20 and 40 years of age* the haversian canals and intertrabecular spaces are to some extent filled in, and the cortices increase in overall thickness; i.e. the bones become heavier and stronger. Somewhere in this period, each individual achieves a state of peak bone mass, which varies considerably from person to person. *From 40 years onwards* there is a slow but steady loss of bone; haversian spaces enlarge, trabeculae become thinner, the endosteal surface is resorbed and the medullary space expands – i.e. year by year the bones become more porous. In men, the diminution in bone mass proceeds at a rate of about 0.3% per year. In women it is quite different: at the menopause, and for 5–10 years afterwards, bone loss is markedly accelerated –

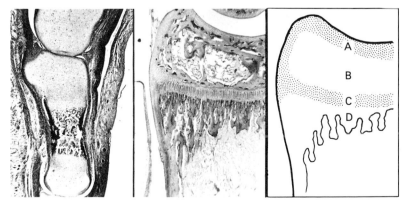

7.5 Bone growth On the left a fetal phalanx, with bone forming in its cartilage model. By the time the child is born, the bone (on the right) shows the familiar separation into (A) articular cartilage, (B) epiphysis, (C) cartilaginous growth plate (or physis), and (D) newly formed juxtaepiphyseal bone.

a state referred to rather loosely as *postmenopausal osteoporosis*. This is mainly due to the loss of gonadal hormone; thus it also occurs in younger women about 5 years after oöphorectomy. By 70 years of age the rapid postmenopausal depletion tails off and from then onwards men and women go on losing bone at about the same rate; this later phase of depletion is referred to as *senile* (or *involutional*) *osteoporosis*. It is important to recognize that although *bone mass* (i.e. the net quantity of bone per unit volume) decreases after middle age, *bone density* (i.e. the degree of mineralization) varies very little with age, or from one individual to another.

The progressive loss of bone tissue implies that remodelling is out of balance. Postmenopausal osteoporosis is due mainly to excessive resorption; osteoclastic activity has, in a sense, 'escaped' from the normal control of gonadal hormone. In senile osteoporosis, reduced osteoblastic activity may be more important (Parfitt, 1988).

The associated loss of bone strength – and the increased susceptibility to fracture – is explained in a number of ways. (1) The absolute diminution in bone mass is the most important, but not the only, factor. (2) With increased postmenopausal bone resorption there is perforation of the plates and spars in trabecular bone – defects that are never repaired; the loss of structural connectivity results in disproportionate loss of strength. (3) In old age the decrease in bone cell activity makes for a slow remodelling rate; old bone takes longer to be replaced and microtrauma to be repaired; stress failure is consequently more likely.

Regulation of bone turnover and calcium exchange

Over 98% of the body's calcium and 85% of its phosphorus are tightly packed in bone and capable of only very slow exchange. A small amount of mineral is in a rapidly exchangeable form, either in partially formed crystals or in the extracellular fluid where calcium and phosphate concentrations depend mainly on intestinal absorption and renal excretion; transient alterations in serum levels are accommodated quickly by changes in renal tubular absorption. The control of calcium is much more critical than that of phosphate; thus, in persistent calcium deficiency the extracellular calcium ion concentration is maintained by drawing on bone, whereas phosphate deficiency simply leads to lowered serum phosphate concentration. The regulation of calcium exchange is therefore linked inescapably to that of bone formation and bone resorption. The complex balance between calcium absorption, renal tubular excretion, extracellular circulation and calcium turnover in bone is controlled by an array of systemic and local factors.

Calcium and phosphorus

Calcium is essential for normal cell function and physiological processes such as nerve conduction and muscle contraction. The normal calcium concentration in plasma and extracellular fluid is 2.2–2.6 mmol/l (8.8–10.4 mg/dl). Much of this is bound to protein; about half is ionized and effective in cell metabolism and the regulation of calcium homoeostasis. The recommended daily intake of calcium is 10–20 mmol (400–800 mg), of which half enters the circulation; intestinal absorption is promoted by vitamin D metabolites. Urinary excretion varies between 2.5 and 10.0 mmol (100 and 400 mg) per 24 hours; if calcium intake is reduced, urinary excretion is adjusted by increasing tubular reabsorption. If calcium concentration is persistently reduced, calcium is drawn from the skeleton by increased bone resorption. These compensatory shifts in intestinal absorption, renal excretion and bone remodelling are regulated by parathyroid hormone and vitamin D metabolites.

Phosphorus is needed for many important metabolic processes. Plasma concentration – almost entirely in the form of ionized inorganic phosphates – is 0.9–1.3 mmol/l (2.8–4.0 mg/dl). It is abundantly available in the diet and is absorbed in the small intestine, more or less in proportion to the amount ingested; however, absorption is reduced in the presence of antacids such as aluminium hydroxide, which binds phosphorus in the gut. Phosphate excretion is extremely efficient, but 90% is reabsorbed in the proximal tubules. Tubular reabsorption is decreased (and overall excretion increased) by parathyroid hormones.

Parathyroid hormone

Parathyroid hormone (PTH) is the fine regulator of calcium exchange; its function is to maintain the extracellular calcium concentration between very narrow limits; production and release are stimulated by a fall and suppressed (up to a point) by a rise in plasma ionized calcium); target organs are the renal tubules, bone and (indirectly) the gut. The active terminal fragment of the PTH molecule can be readily estimated in blood samples.

In the *renal tubules* PTH increases phosphate excretion by restricting its reabsorption, and it conserves calcium by increasing its reabsorption. These responses rapidly compensate for any change in plasma ionized calcium.

In *bone* PTH promotes osteoclastic resorption and the release of calcium and phosphate into the blood. This it does, not by any direct action on osteoclasts but by stimulating the osteoblasts to prepare the bone surface for resorption and to initiate osteoclast chemotaxis; the net effect is a prolonged rise in plasma calcium. There may also be a rapid stimulation of osteocytic osteolysis.

In the *intestine* PTH indirectly stimulates calcium absorption by promoting the conversion of vitamin D to its active metabolite in the kidney.

Calcitonin

Calcitonin, which is secreted by the C cells of the thyroid, does the very opposite of PTH: it suppresses bone resorption and increases renal calcium excretion. This occurs especially when bone turnover is high, as in Paget's disease. Its secretion is stimulated by a rise in serum calcium concentration above 2.25 mmol/l (9 mg/dl).

Vitamin D

Vitamin D, through its active metabolites, is principally concerned with bone remodelling

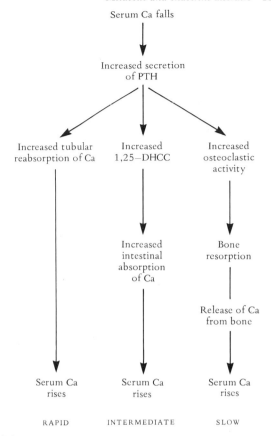

7.6 Homoeostatic loop Effect of a fall in serum calcium.

and the mass movement of calcium. Target organs are the small intestine and bone.

Naturally occurring vitamin D_3 (cholecalciferol) is derived from two sources: directly from the diet and indirectly by the action of ultraviolet light on precursors in the skin. The normal requirement is about 400 IU per day. In most countries this is obtained mainly from exposure to sunlight; those who lack such exposure are likely to suffer from vitamin D deficiency.

Vitamin D itself is inactive. Conversion to active metabolites (which function as hormones) takes place first in the liver by 25-hydroxylation to form 25-hydroxycholecalciferol (25-HCC), and then in the kidney by a further 1_α-hydroxylation to give 1,25-dihydroxycholecalciferol (1,25-DHCC). The concentration of these metabolites can be measured in serum samples.

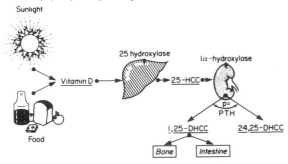

7.7 Vitamin D metabolism Cholecalciferol is derived either from the diet or by conversion of precursors when the skin is exposed to sunlight. This inactive 'vitamin' is hydroxylated, first in the liver and then in the kidney, to form the active metabolite 1,25-dihydroxycholecalciferol.

The terminal metabolite, 1,25-DHCC, is the most active form; it stimulates the uptake of calcium by the small intestine and promotes increased bone resorption. The 'liver' metabolite, 25-HCC, has similar though weaker effects. Other, less active, vitamin D metabolites are formed by the kidney. Indeed, 24,25-DHCC is normally present in far greater quantity than 1,25-DHCC, and it is only under conditions of need that the production of 1,25-HCC increases. This switch is controlled by parathyroid hormone (PTH) and by the serum phosphate concentration; a rise in PTH or a fall in phosphate increases 1,25-DHCC synthesis and decreases 24,25-DHCC production proportionately. A fall in serum calcium does the same indirectly, by stimulating PTH production; the increased 1,25-DHCC then promotes intestinal absorption of calcium and the serum level is restored.

In bone, 1,25-DHCC has a twofold action: stimulation of osteoclastic resorption and enhancement of calcium transport. There is also an indirect effect on bone formation, because increased intestinal absorption of calcium and phosphate promotes osteoid mineralization.

Other hormones

A number of hormones that influence epiphyseal growth, bone formation and bone resorption play a secondary role in calcium balance. *Oestrogen* is thought to stimulate calcium absorp-
tion and to protect bone from the unrestrained action of PTH. Its withdrawal leads to osteoporosis. *Adrenal corticosteroids* in excess cause osteoporosis due to a combination of increased bone resorption, diminished bone formation and decreased intestinal calcium absorption; collagen synthesis may also be defective. *Thyroxine* increases both formation and resorption, but more so the latter; hyperthyroidism is associated with high bone turnover and osteoporosis.

Local factors

Systemic hormones have a large-scale effect on bone turnover; they translate the shifts in calcium and phosphate balance to the workfront where bone remodelling takes place. But the intimate processes of signalling between osteoblasts and osteoclasts, cell recruitment and activation, spatial organization and mineral transport are mediated by local factors derived from bone cells, matrix components and cells of the immune system. Some serve as messengers between systemic and local agents; others behave as autocrines and paracrines. *Insulin-like growth factor I (somatomedin C)* is produced by osteoblasts and enhances osteoblast proliferation. *Transforming growth factors* produced during bone resorption can stimulate osteoblastic activity; this may account for the coupling of resorption and formation. *Interleukin-1* (IL-1) and *osteoclast-activating factor* (OAF), cytokines derived from monocytes and lymphocytes, are powerful activators of bone resorption; they are thought to be responsible for osteoporosis in inflammatory disorders, multiple myeloma and other malignant tumours. *Prostaglandins* are produced by bone cells and regulate both osteoclastic and osteoblastic activity. They are important in promoting bone resorption in inflammatory disorders and fractures (Dekel, Lenthall and Francis, 1981) and may also account for the bone destruction and hypercalcaemia in metastatic bone disease (Tashjian, 1975). *Bone morphogenetic protein* (BMP), which can be extracted from bone matrix, induces chondrogenesis and bone formation (Harakas, 1984). This process – known as bone induction – may be important in fracture healing and bone graft replacement.

Mechanical stress

It is well known that the direction and thickness of trabeculae in cancellous bone are related to regional stress trajectories. This is recognized in Wolff's law [1896], which says that the architecture and mass of the skeleton are adjusted to withstand the prevailing forces imposed by functional need or deformity. Physiological stress is supplied by gravity, loadbearing, muscle action and vascular pulsation. If a bending force is applied, more bone will form on the concave surfaces (where there is compression) and bone will thin down on the convex surfaces (which are under tension). Weightlessness, prolonged bed rest, lack of exercise, muscular weakness and limb immobilization are all associated with osteoporosis. How physical signals are transmitted to bone cells is not known, but they almost certainly operate through local growth factors.

Electrical stimulation

When bone is loaded or deformed, small electrical potentials are generated – negative on compressed surfaces and positive on surfaces under tension (Brighton and McCluskey, 1986). This observation led to the idea that stress-generated changes in bone mass may be mediated by electrical signals; from this it was a logical step to show that induced electrical potentials can affect bone formation and resorption. How, precisely, this is mediated remains unknown. Electromagnetic field potentials have been used for the treatment of delayed fracture union and regional osteoporosis, so far with inconclusive results.

Other environmental factors

It has been shown experimentally that bone formation is increased by a moderate rise in temperature or oxygen tension. Acid–base balance affects bone resorption, which is increased in chronic acidosis and decreased in alkalosis. Increased phosphate or pyrophosphate concentration can inhibit bone resorption. Pyrophosphate analogues (bisphosphonates)* are used therapeutically: they appear to inhibit both resorption and formation.

* The terms 'bisphonates', 'biphosphonates' and 'diphosphonates' are interchangeable.

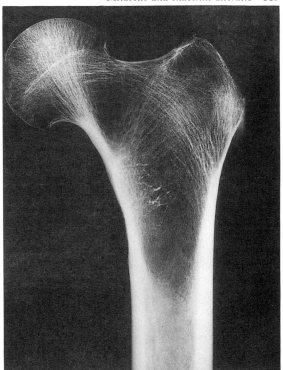

7.8 Wolff's law The elegant trabecular pattern of the upper femur shows how well the anatomical structure conforms to the imposed forces; the thickest trabeculae lie in the lines of the greatest stress.

Evaluation of bone metabolic disorders

Patients with metabolic bone disorders usually present with the symptoms and signs of *osteopenia*. This term, which means, literally, lack of bone, covers both *osteoporosis* (abnormal diminution of bone mass) and *osteomalacia* (defective mineralization of bone). In either case the clinical features are essentially those of *skeletal failure*: bone pain, fractures and deformity. In addition, there may be systemic features of *hypercalcaemia* (anorexia, abdominal pain, depression, renal stone or metastatic calcification), or of some *underlying hormone disorder*. X-rays may show *stress fractures, vertebral compression, cortical thinning, loss of trabecular structure* or merely an ill-defined *loss of bone density*. These appearances are so common in old people that they seldom lead on to detailed investigation. However, in patients under the age of 50, those with repeated fractures or bone deformities and those with associated systemic features, a full *clinical, radiological and biochemical evaluation* is essential.

History

The duration of symptoms and their relationship to previous disease, drug therapy or operations are important. Other causal associations are retarded growth, malnutrition, dietary fads, intestinal malabsorption, alcohol abuse and cigarette smoking.

Examination

The patient's appearance may be a giveaway: the moon face and cushingoid build of hypercortisonism; the smooth, hairless skin of testicular atrophy; physical underdevelopment in rickets. Thoracic kyphosis is a non-specific feature of spinal osteoporosis.

X-rays

Decreased skeletal radiodensity is a late and unreliable sign of osteopenia; it becomes apparent only after a 30% reduction in mineral or bone mass. There may be obvious fractures – new and old – especially in the spine, ribs, pubic rami or corticocancellous junctions of the long bones. Small stress fractures are more difficult to detect: they may be found in the superior cortex of the femoral shaft or the proximal end of the tibia. The vertebral bodies may show frank compression fractures, minor wedging at multiple levels, or biconcave distortion of the end-plates due to bulging of intact intervertebral discs. In addition to these general signs of osteopenia, there may be specific features of bone disorders such as rickets, hyperparathyroidism, metastatic bone disease or myelomatosis.

X-ray measurement of bone mass

There is no reliable method of measuring bone mass – or the degree of osteopenia – by x-rays. Various 'indices' have been devised and, while they are useful for epidemiological studies in large populations, they are too crude to record progress in an individual patient.

The *cortical index* is a measure of cortical thickness in relation to the diameter of the bone shaft. Measurements can be taken from x-rays of the metacarpals, the radius or the femoral shaft. The combined width of the cortices should be at least 50% of the total width of the bone at mid-diaphyseal level.

The *trabecular index* (Singh et al., 1970) is a semi-quantitative method of assessing bone mass from the radiographic pattern of trabecular distribution in the proximal femur; a similar index can be derived from the calcaneum. Their usefulness is limited by the fact that there is a large overlap of values in 'normal' and 'osteoporotic' individuals.

Photon absorption can be measured by directing a radioactive beam across the bone and recording the photon alteration on the far side. This can be applied in the radius, the lumbar spine and the femoral neck with a good level of reproducibility; losses of 5–10% of bone mass can be detected in sequential scans, thus permitting reliable evaluation of progressive bone loss or the response to treatment.

Quantitated computed tomography can be used in a similar manner to assess bone mass in the vertebral bodies.

NOTE   It is important to recognize that measurements at one site (e.g. the radius) do not accurately reflect changes at another site of interest (e.g. the femoral neck).

Biochemical tests

Serum calcium and phosphate concentrations should be measured in the fasting state, and it is the ionized calcium fraction that is important. The serum alkaline phosphatase level is an index of osteoblastic activity; it is raised in osteomalacia and in certain phases of Paget's disease.

Osteocalcin (Gla protein) is a more specific marker of bone formation; elevated serum levels suggest increased bone turnover.

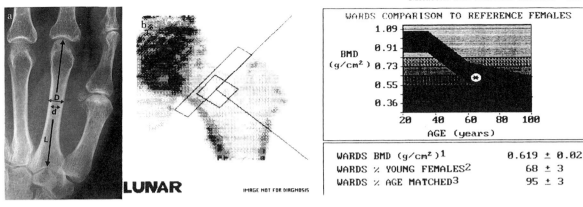

7.9 Bone mass   (a) Bone mass can be assessed very simply (but not very reliably) by measuring the thickness of cortex in relation to the overall thickness of the bone at a fixed point, e.g. the mid-shaft of the second metacarpal. $D^2 - d^2$ is an index of relative cortical area; $(D^2 - d^2)/D^2$ is a formula which corrects for variations in size of different individuals. (b) More accurate, more reproducible and specifically related to the particular area of interest is the photon scan. This printout from a DEXA (dual energy x-ray absorptionometry) scan showed that bone density in the femoral neck lay towards the lower limit of the band for normal individuals of different ages.

Parathyroid hormone activity can be estimated from serum assays of the COOH terminal fragment. However, in renal failure the test is unreliable because there is reduced clearance of the COOH fragment.

Vitamin D uptake is assessed by measuring the serum 25-HCC activity. Serum 1,25-DHCC levels do not necessarily reflect vitamin uptake but are reduced in advanced renal disease.

Urinary calcium and phosphate excretion can be measured. Significant alterations are found in malabsorption disorders, hyperparathyroidism and other conditions associated with hypercalcaemia.

Urinary hydroxyproline excretion is a measure of bone resorption. It may be increased in high-turnover conditions such as Paget's disease but it is not sensitive enough to reflect lesser increases in bone resorption.

Excretion of pyridinium compounds derived from bone collagen cross-links is a much more sensitive index of bone resorption (Seibel, Duncan and Robins, 1989; Uebelhart et al.,

1990). This may be useful in monitoring the progress of hyperparathyroidism and other types of osteoporosis. However, excretion is also increased in chronic arthritis associated with bone destruction.

Bone biopsy

Standardized bone samples are easily obtained from the iliac crest and can be examined (without prior decalcification) for histological bone volume, osteoid formation and the relative distribution of formation and resorption surfaces. The rate of bone remodelling can also be gauged by labelling the bone with tetracycline on two occasions (2 weeks apart) before obtaining the biopsy. Tetracycline is taken up in new bone and produces a fluorescent strip on ultraviolet light microscopy. By measuring the distance between the two labels, the rate of new bone formation can be calculated. Characteristically in osteomalacia there is a decrease in the rate of bone turnover and an increase in the amount of uncalcified osteoid.

Metabolic disorders

The common metabolic bone disorders are associated, in varying degree, with depletion of bone tissue or bone mineral. They fall into three groups: (1) osteoporosis, where the quantity of bone (bone mass) is abnormally low; (2) osteomalacia, where bone (osteoid) is present but insufficiently mineralized; and (3) osteitis fibrosa, in which parathyroid hormone (PTH) overproduction leads to bone resorption and replacement by fibrous tissue.

Osteoporosis

Osteoporosis, in the broadest sense, describes a state in which bone is fully mineralized but its structure is abnormally porous and its strength is less than normal for a person of that age. That there is an abnormal diminution of bone mass per unit volume is self-evident, but this alone is not enough to account for the increased fragility; bone resorption unbalanced by formation leads to perforation of trabecular plates and spars, thus further weakening the structure as a whole. It is the bone fragility – the increased tendency to fracture – rather than any absolute decrease in bone mass that defines osteoporosis as a clinical disorder.

Osteoporosis is conveniently classified as primary (which is related to ageing processes and decreased gonadal activity) and secondary (due to a variety of endocrine, metabolic and neoplastic disorders).

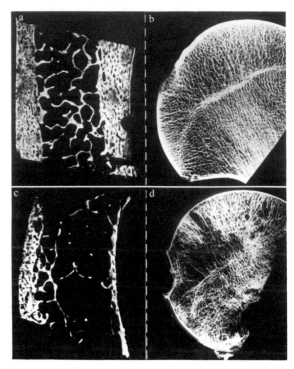

7.10 Osteoporosis   Fine-detail x-rays of iliac crest biopsies and femoral head slices, showing the contrast between trabecular density at the age of 40 (a, b) and aged 70 (c, d). No wonder old bones break easily.

Primary (postmenopausal, involutional) osteoporosis

The physiological, age-related, changes in bone mass and structure are described on p. 108. When these changes are exaggerated and associated with skeletal failure the condition becomes pathological.

POSTMENOPAUSAL OSTEOPOROSIS   Women at the menopause – and for the next 10 years – lose bone at an accelerated rate (about 3% per year compared with 0.3% during the preceding decade). This is due mainly to increased resorption, the withdrawal of oestrogen removing one of the normal restraints on osteoclastic activity. In some cases (perhaps they are a subgroup of 'fast losers') this leads to skeletal failure, with

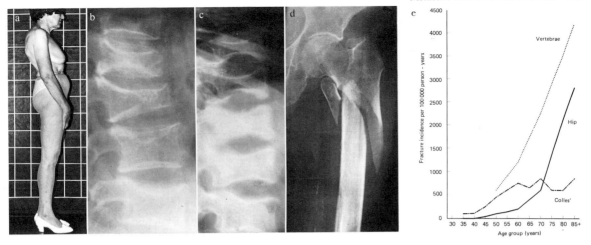

7.11 Osteoporosis (a) This woman noticed that she was becoming more and more 'round-shouldered'; she also had chronic backache and her x-rays (b) show compression of vertebral bodies. (c) The spine of a similar patient who, 6 years after this film was taken, fell in her kitchen and sustained the fracture shown in (d). The fracture incidence in women rises steeply after the menopause (e).

overt symptoms and signs. A number of *risk factors* for this group have been identified: race (Caucasians are more susceptible than Negroes); heredity (a family history of osteoporosis); asthenic build (body fat supplies oestradiol); premature menopause; early hysterectomy; cigarette smoking; and alcohol abuse. The question of low calcium intake as a risk factor is controversial, with conflicting evidence both for and against.

Clinical features A woman at or near the menopause develops back pain and increased thoracic kyphosis. X-rays show wedging or compression of one or more vertebral bodies. This is the typical picture, but sometimes the first clinical event is a fracture of the distal radius or one of the other bone ends. Photon absorptiometry may show markedly reduced bone content in the vertebral bodies. The rate of bone turnover is more or less normal (or slightly increased) and biochemical tests are usually negative.

Prevention and treatment Women with multiple risk factors, and even more so those with vertebral compression fractures, should be encouraged to take a normal diet with adequate calcium (at least 1500 mg per day), to keep up a

high level of physical activity, and to avoid smoking and excessive consumption of alcohol. In addition, those with oestrogen deficiency (premature or surgically induced menopause) and those with severe bone changes should receive oestrogen replacement therapy: this has

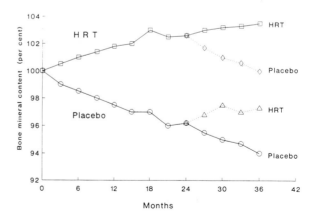

7.12 Postmenopausal osteoporosis – treatment Controlled trials have shown that hormone replacement therapy can prevent the otherwise inevitable bone loss that occurs after the menopause. When HRT is replaced by placebo (crossover trials), there is a significant drop in bone mineral content (after Lindsay, Hart and Clark, 1984).

been shown beyond any doubt to prevent the accelerated bone loss and to reduce the incidence of further fractures (Lindsay, Hart and Clark, 1984; Etlinger, Genant and Cann, 1985). However, there are drawbacks to hormone replacement therapy (HRT), notably the risk of recurrent bleeding after the menopause and slight increases in the incidence of breast and uterine cancer after long-term treatment. This has inhibited its more general acceptance. If practical and reliable screening tests (bone densitometry, biochemical investigations or a combination of both) could identify 'fast losers' in the perimenopausal period, preventive HRT would be more widely applied. If HRT is contraindicated, calcitonin or bisphosphonates can be given instead; both have been shown to prevent or slow down postmenopausal bone loss.

SENILE OSTEOPOROSIS Fifteen years after the menopause in women, and at the same age (the seventh or eight decade) in men, there is still a steady loss of bone mass – about 0.5% per year. This is so universal as to be regarded as a physiological manifestation of ageing. However, in some people (and much more often in women) bone loss reaches the point where fractures occur after comparatively minor trauma. This is most likely to happen in women who have already shown signs of poor bone mass around the menopause; significantly, the incidence of vertebral fracture rises steadily from the age of 50 onwards, and by 70 years almost a third of Caucasian women will have at least one vertebral fracture. Worse still, after 65 there is a rising incidence of femoral neck fracture – again more marked in women than in men, and much more marked in Caucasians than in Negroes. However, measurements of bone mass at that age show that there is considerable overlap between those who fracture and those who don't; the assumption is that qualitative changes contribute increasingly to bone fragility in old age. A new set of *risk factors* comes into play. Prolonged menopausal bone loss may be important; there is a high incidence of chronic illness, mild urinary insufficiency, muscular atrophy, dietary deficiency, lack of exposure to sunlight, and an increased tendency to fall. Moreover, many old people suffer from vitamin D deficiency and they have mild osteomalacia – which further weakens frail bones.

Clinical features are essentially an exaggeration of those seen in postmenopausal osteoporosis. There may be fractures of the ribs or the pubic rami. The classic 'event' is a fracture of the femoral neck, usually after minimal trauma. X-rays may reveal obvious loss of trabecular markings in the femoral neck and vertebral bodies. Serum and urinary biochemistry is normal – unless there is associated osteomalacia; if this is suspected, iliac crest biopsy will give the diagnosis.

Treatment is directed, initially, at management of the fracture. This will often require internal fixation; the sooner these patients are mobilized and rehabilitated the better. Thereafter the question of general treatment may be considered. Obvious factors such as concurrent illness, dietary deficiencies, lack of exposure to sunlight and lack of exercise will need attention. Beyond this, treatment is hampered by two factors: very few drugs have any positive effect on bone formation; and at that age bone turnover is so slow that metabolic manipulation takes a long time to produce any noticeable increase in bone mass. Sodium fluoride stimulates osteoblastic activity; it is given in doses of 60–80 mg per day, usually combined with calcium and vitamin D to promote mineralization of the newly formed bone. Although this produces a measurable increase in vertebral bone mass, there is some doubt about the strength of the new bone. If fluoride is used, bone status should be carefully monitored by x-rays, biochemical tests and serial iliac crest biopsy.

Secondary osteoporosis

There are numerous causes of secondary osteoporosis (Table 7.1). The most important are hypercortisonism, gonadal hormone deficiency, hyperthyroidism, multiple myeloma, chronic alcoholism and immobilization. It is impractical to screen all osteoporotic patients for these conditions, but those under 50 years – and older patients with rapidly increasing osteoporosis – should be fully investigated to exclude any potentially reversible disorder.

Table 7.1 Some causes of osteoporosis

Nutritional	*Malignant disease*
Scurvy	Carcinomatosis
Malnutrition	Multiple myeloma
Malabsorption	Leukaemia
Endocrine disorders	*Non-malignant disease*
Hyperparathyroidism	Rheumatoid arthritis
Gonadal insufficiency	Ankylosing spondylitis
Cushing's disease	Tuberculosis
Thyrotoxicosis	Chronic renal disease
Drug-induced	*Idiopathic*
Corticosteroids	Juvenile osteoporosis
Alcohol	Postclimacteric osteoporosis
Heparin	

HYPERCORTISONISM Corticosteroid overload occurs in endogenous Cushing's disease or after prolonged treatment with corticosteroids. This often results in severe osteoporosis, especially if the condition for which the drug is administered is itself associated with bone loss – for example, rheumatoid arthritis (Dykman et al., 1985). The deleterious effect on bone is mainly by suppression of osteoblast function, but there is also reduced calcium absorption, increased calcium excretion and stimulation of PTH secretion (Hahn, 1980). Bone resorption is markedly increased and formation is suppressed.

The clinical appearance in hypercortisonism is characteristic: there is obesity of the trunk and rounding of the face ('moon face'). X-rays show generalized osteoporosis; fractures of the vertebrae, pelvis and femoral neck are common. Biochemical tests are usually normal, but there may be a slight increase in calcium excretion.

Problems for the orthopaedic surgeon are manifold: fractures and wounds heal slowly, bones provide little purchase for internal fixation, wound breakdown and infection are more common than usual, and the patients are generally less fit.

Prevention means using systemic corticosteroids only when essential and in low dosage. If treatment is prolonged, calcium supplements (at least 1500 mg per day) should be given. Bisphosphonates may also be effective in slowing the rate of bone loss and preventing further fractures.

Treatment is essentially the management of fractures and general measures to control bone pain.

GONADAL HORMONE INSUFFICIENCY Oestrogen lack is an important factor in postmenopausal osteoporosis. It also accounts for osteoporosis in younger women who have undergone oöphorectomy, and in pubertal girls with ovarian agenesis and primary amenorrhoea (Turner's syndrome). Further bone loss can be prevented by long-term hormone replacement therapy. Amenorrhoeic female athletes, and adolescents with anorexia nervosa, may become osteoporotic; fortunately these conditions are usually self-limiting.

A decline in testicular function probably contributes to the continuing bone loss and rising fracture rate in men over 70 years of age. A more obvious relationship is found in young men with overt hypogonadism; this may require long-term treatment with testosterone.

HYPERTHYROIDISM Thyroxine speeds up the rate of bone turnover, but resorption exceeds formation. Osteoporosis is quite common in hyperthyroidism, but fractures usually occur

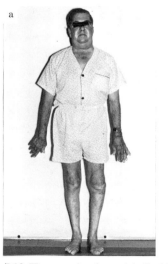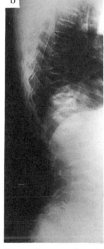

7.13 Hypercortisonism (a) Cushing's syndrome, due in this instance to prolonged corticosteroid treatment for rheumatoid disease. (b) On x-ray the bones look 'washed-out' and there may be spontaneous compression fractures.

only in older women who suffer the cumulative effects of the menopause and thyroid overload. Treatment is needed for both conditions.

MULTIPLE MYELOMA AND CARCINOMATOSIS Generalized osteoporosis, anaemia and a high ESR are characteristic features of myelomatosis and metastatic bone disease. Bone loss is due to overproduction of local osteoclast-activating factors (see p. 111).

ALCOHOL ABUSE This is a common (and often neglected) cause of osteoporosis at all ages, with the added factor of an increased tendency to falls and other injuries. Bone changes are due to a combination of decreased calcium absorption, liver failure and a toxic effect on osteoblast function.

IMMOBILIZATION The worst effects of stress reduction are seen in states of weightlessness; bone resorption, unbalanced by formation, leads to hypercalcaemia, hypercalciuria and severe osteoporosis. Lesser degrees of osteoporosis are seen in bedridden patients, and regional osteoporosis is common after immobilization of a limb. The effects can be mitigated by encouraging mobility, exercise and weightbearing.

OTHER CONDITIONS There are many other causes of secondary osteoporosis, including hyperparathyroidism (which is considered below), rheumatoid arthritis (p. 54), ankylosing spondylitis (p. 61) and even subclinical forms of osteogenesis imperfecta (p. 151). The associated clinical features usually point to the diagnosis.

Rickets and osteomalacia

Rickets and osteomalacia are different expressions of the same disease: inadequate mineralization of bone. In children (rickets) this chiefly affects areas of active endochondral growth; in adults new bone throughout the skeleton is incompletely calcified, and therefore 'softened' (osteomalacia). The inadequacy may be due to calcium deficiency, marked hypophosphataemia, or defects anywhere along the metabolic pathway for vitamin D: nutritional lack, underexposure to sunlight, intestinal malabsorption, decreased 25-hydroxylation (liver disease, anticonvulsants) and reduced 1_α-hydroxylation (renal disease, nephrectomy, 1_α-hydroxylase deficiency). The rate of bone formation is slowed

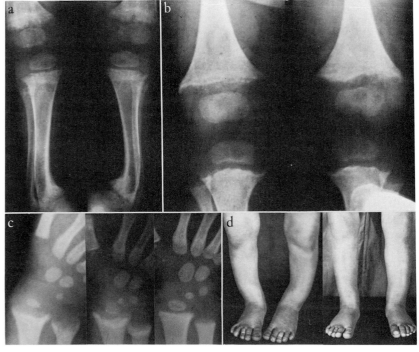

7.14 Rickets (a, b) Florid disease; (c) series showing the response to treatment; (d) before and after osteotomy for the neglected case.

down and unmineralized osteoid accumulates along the surfaces of the new bone.

Clinical features

The infant with *rickets* may present with tetany or convulsions. There is failure to thrive, listlessness and muscular flaccidity. Early bone changes are deformity of the skull (craniotabes) and thickening of the knees, ankles and wrists from epiphyseal overgrowth. Enlargement of the costochondral junctions ('rickety rosary') and lateral indentation of the chest (Harrison's sulcus) may also appear. Distal tibial bowing has been attributed to sitting or lying cross-legged. Once the child stands, lower limb deformities increase, and stunting of growth may be obvious. In severe rickets there may be spinal curvature, coxa vara and bending or fractures of the long bones.

Osteomalacia has a much more insidious course and patients may complain of bone pain, backache and muscle weakness for many years before the diagnosis is made. Vertebral collapse causes loss of height, and existing deformities such as mild kyphosis or knock knees – themselves perhaps due to adolescent rickets – may increase in later life. Unexplained pain in the hip or one of the long bones may presage a stress fracture.

X-RAYS In active rickets there is thickening and widening of the growth plate, cupping of the metaphysis and, sometimes, bowing of the diaphysis. The metaphysis may remain abnormally wide even after healing has occurred.

The stamp of osteomalacia is the Looser zone, a thin transverse band of rarefaction in an otherwise normal-looking bone. These zones, seen especially in the shafts of long bones and the axillary edge of the scapula, are due to incomplete stress fractures which heal with callus lacking in calcium. More often, however, there is simply a slow fading of skeletal structure, resulting in biconcave vertebrae (from disc pressure), lateral indentation of the acetabula ('trefoil' pelvis) and spontaneous fractures of the ribs, pubic rami, femoral neck or the metaphyses above and below the knee.

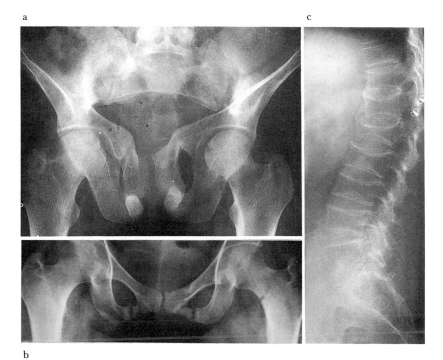

a

c

b

7.15 Osteomalacia Three characteristic features of osteomalacia: (a) indentation of the acetabula producing the trefoil or champagne-glass pelvis; (b) Looser's zones in the pubic rami and left femoral neck; (c) biconcave (codfish) vertebrae.

Secondary hyperparathyroidism occurs if the serum calcium is persistently low. In children the resulting subperiosteal erosions are at the sites of maximal remodelling (medial borders of the proximal humerus, femoral neck, distal femur and proximal tibia, lateral borders of the distal radius and ulna). In adults the middle phalanges of the fingers are more often affected, and in severe cases brown tumours ('cysts') are seen in the long bones.

Biochemistry

Changes common to almost all types of rickets and osteomalacia are diminished levels of serum calcium and phosphate, increased alkaline phosphatase and diminished urinary excretion of calcium. In vitamin D deficiency the 25-HCC levels also are low. The 'calcium phosphate product' (derived by multiplying calcium and phosphorus levels expressed in mmol/l), normally about 3, is diminished in rickets and osteomalacia, and values of less than 2.4 are diagnostic.

Bone biopsy

With clear-cut clinical and x-ray features the diagnosis is obvious. In less typical cases a bone biopsy will provide the answer. Osteoid seams are both wider and more extensive, and tetracycline labelling shows that mineralization is defective.

Table 7.2

Osteomalacia	Osteoporosis
Common in ageing women	
Prone to pathological fracture	
Decreased bone density	
Ill	Not ill
Generalized chronic ache	Pain only after fracture
Muscles weak	Muscles normal
Looser's zones	No Looser's zones
Alkaline phosphatase increased	Normal
Serum phosphorus decreased	Normal
Ca × P < 2.4 mmol/l	Ca × P > 2.4 mmol/l

Clinical varieties of rickets and osteomalacia

Vitamin D deficiency

Vitamin D deficiency may be due to dietary lack, underexposure to sunlight, malabsorption or a combination of these. Dietary lack of vitamin D (less than 100 IU per day) is common in strict vegetarians and in old people who often eat very little; if there is also reduced exposure to sunlight, osteomalacia may result. Even mild osteomalacia can be harmful if it is superimposed on postmenopausal or senile osteoporosis (Solomon, 1974). Treatment with vitamin D (400–1000 IU per day) and calcium supplements is usually effective; however, elderly people often require larger doses of vitamin D (up to 2000 IU per day).

Intestinal malabsorption – especially fat malabsorption – can cause vitamin D deficiency (fat and vitamin D absorption normally go hand in hand). If vitamin D supplements are administered they have to be given in large doses (50 000 IU per day). Gastrectomy is sometimes followed by osteomalacia; why this should be is unknown, as intestinal absorption is not affected.

Deficiency of vitamin D metabolites

Some patients with typical osteomalacia have no obvious vitamin lack and fail to respond to physiological doses of vitamin D. In some cases there is defective conversion to (or too-rapid breakdown of) the liver metabolite 25-HCC. This is seen in severe liver disease or after long-term administration of anticonvulsants or rifampicin; if these drugs are prescribed it is wise to give vitamin D at the same time. Established osteomalacia requires treatment with vitamin D in large doses.

Patients with early renal failure sometimes develop osteomalacia; this is thought to be due to reduced 1_α-hydroxylase activity resulting in deficiency of 1,25-DHCC. It can be treated with 1,25-DHCC (or else with very large doses of vitamin D).

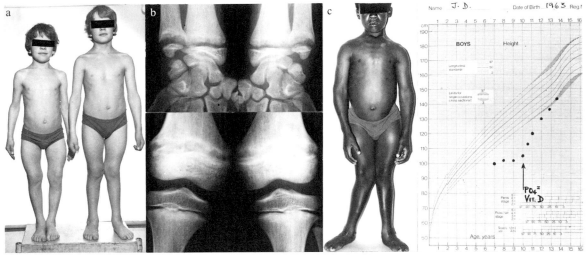

7.16 Renal tubular rickets – familial hypophosphataemia   (a) These brothers presented with knee deformities: their x-rays (b) show defective juxtaepiphyseal calcification. (c) Another example of hypophosphataemic rickets; his growth chart shows that he was well below the normal range in height, but improved dramatically on treatment with vitamin D and inorganic phosphate.

Patients with advanced renal disease treated by haemodialysis develop a more complex syndrome – renal osteodystrophy. This is considered below.

Hypophosphataemic rickets and osteomalacia

Chronic hypophosphataemia occurs in a number of disorders in which there is impaired renal tubular reabsorption of phosphate. Calcium levels are normal but bone mineralization is defective.

Familial hypophosphataemic rickets (vitamin D-resistant rickets) is probably the commonest form of rickets seen today. It is an X-linked genetic disorder with dominant inheritance, starting in infancy or soon after and causing severe bony deformity. The children are dwarfed, boys more so than girls. There is no myopathy. X-rays show marked epiphyseal changes but, because the serum calcium is normal, there is no secondary hyperparathyroidism. Treatment is by large doses of vitamin D (50 000 IU or more) and up to 4 g of inorganic phosphate per day (with careful monitoring to prevent overdosage), continued until growth ceases. Bony deformities may require bracing or osteotomy. If the child needs to be immobilized, vitamin D must be stopped temporarily to prevent hypercalcaemia from the combined effects of treatment and disuse bone resorption.

Table 7.3   Characteristics of different types of rickets

	Vitamin D deficiency	Renal tubular	Renal glomerular
Family history	−	+	−
Myopathy	+	−	+
Growth defect	±	++	++
Serum:			
Ca	↓	N	↓
P	↓	↓	↑
Alk. phos.	↑	↑	↑
Urine:			
Ca	↓	↓	↓
P	↓	↑	↓
Osteitis fibrosa	±	+	++
Other	Dietary deficiency or malabsorption	Amino-aciduria	Renal failure Anaemia

Adult-onset hypophosphataemia, though rare, must be remembered as a cause of unexplained bone loss and polyarthralgia. It responds dramatically to treatment with phosphate, vitamin D and calcium.

More severe *renal tubular defects* can produce a variety of biochemical abnormalities, including chronic phosphate depletion and osteomalacia. If there is acidosis, this must be corrected; in addition, patients may need phosphate replacement, together with calcium and vitamin D.

Hyperparathyroidism

Excessive secretion of PTH may be primary (usually due to an adenoma or hyperplasia), secondary (due to persistent hypocalcaemia) or tertiary (when secondary hyperplasia leads to autonomous overactivity).

Pathology

Overproduction of PTH enhances calcium conservation by stimulating tubular absorption, intestinal absorption and bone resorption. The resulting hypercalcaemia so increases glomerular filtration of calcium that there is hypercalciuria despite the augmented tubular reabsorption. Urinary phosphate also is increased, due to suppressed tubular reasbsorption. The main effects of these changes are seen in the kidney: calcinosis, stone formation, recurrent infection and impaired function. There may also be calcification of soft tissues.

There is a general loss of bone substance. In more severe cases, osteoclastic hyperactivity produces subperiosteal erosions, endosteal cavitation and replacement of the marrow spaces by vascular granulations and fibrous tissue (osteitis fibrosa cystica). Haemorrhage and giant-cell reaction within the fibrous stroma may give rise to brownish, tumour-like masses, whose liquefaction leads to fluid-filled cysts.

Primary hyperparathyroidism

Patients are usually middle-aged (40–65 years) and women are affected twice as often as men. Many remain asymptomatic and are diagnosed only because of their abnormal biochemistry.

Clinical features are mainly due to hypercalcaemia: anorexia, nausea, abdominal pain, depression, fatigue and muscle weakness. They

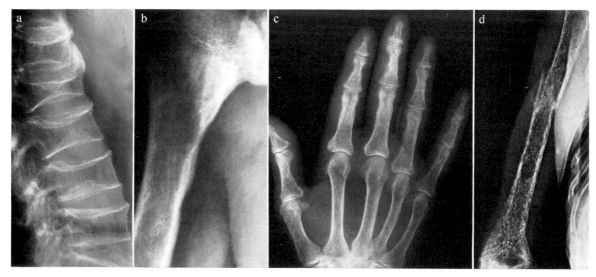

7.17 Hyperparathyroidism   (a) This hyperparathyroid patient with spinal osteoporosis later developed pain in the right arm; an x-ray (b) showed cortical erosion of the humerus; he also showed (c) typical erosions of the phalanges. (d) Another case, showing 'brown tumours' of the humerus and a pathological fracture.

may develop polyuria, kidney stones or nephrocalcinosis due to chronic hypercalciuria. Some complain of joint symptoms, due to chondrocalcinosis. Only a minority (probably less than 10%) present with bone disease – and this is usually generalized osteoporosis rather than the classic features of osteitis fibrosa, bone cysts and pathological fractures.

X-rays may show the characteristic subperiosteal bone resorption, particularly in the middle phalanges, the clavicles and proximal ends of the humeri.

Biochemical tests show hypercalcaemia, hypophosphataemia and a raised serum PTH concentration. Serum alkaline phosphatase is raised with osteitis fibrosa.

Diagnosis involves the exclusion of other causes of hypercalcaemia (multiple myeloma, metastatic disease, sarcoidosis) in which PTH levels are usually depressed.

Treatment is usually conservative and includes adequate hydration and decreased calcium intake. The indications for parathyroidectomy are marked and unremitting hypercalcaemia, recurrent renal calculi, progressive nephrocalcinosis and severe osteoporosis.

Postoperatively there is a danger of severe hypocalcaemia due to brisk formation of new bone (the 'hungry bone syndrome'). This must be treated promptly, with one of the vitamin D metabolites.

Secondary hyperparathyroidism

Parathyroid oversecretion is a predictable response to chronic hypocalcaemia. Secondary hyperparathyroidism is seen, therefore, in various types of rickets and osteomalacia, and accounts for some of the radiological features in these disorders. Treatment is directed at the primary condition.

Renal osteodystrophy

Patients with chronic renal failure are liable to develop diffuse bone changes which are a variable combination of rickets or osteomalacia, secondary hyperparathyroidism, osteoporosis and osteosclerosis. Uraemia and phosphate retention are accompanied by a fall in serum calcium which is due partly to the hyperphosphataemia and partly to 1,25-DHCC deficiency. It is now recognized that the bone changes are aggravated by aluminium retention or contamination of dialysing fluids.

Renal abnormalities precede the bone changes by several years. Children are clinically more severely affected than adults: they are stunted, pasty-faced and have marked rachitic deformities. Myopathy is common. *X-rays* show widened and irregular epiphyseal plates. In older children with long-standing disease there

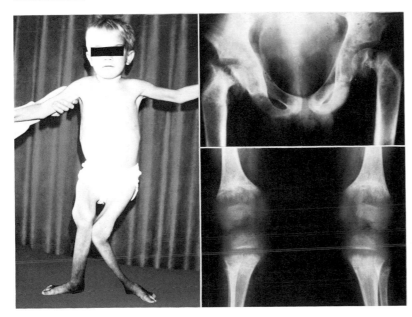

7.18 Renal glomerular osteodystrophy This young boy with chronic renal failure has severe abnormality of epiphyseal growth; the upper femoral epiphyses are grossly displaced.

may be displacement of the epiphyses (epiphyseolysis). Osteosclerosis is seen mainly in the axial skeleton and is more common in young patients: it may produce a 'rugger jersey' appearance in lateral x-rays of the spine, due to alternating bands of increased and decreased bone density. Signs of secondary hyperparathyroidism may be widespread and severe.

Biochemical features are low serum calcium, high serum phosphate and elevated alkaline phosphatase levels. Urinary excretion of calcium and phosphate is diminished. Plasma PTH levels may be raised.

The renal failure, if irreversible, may require haemodialysis or renal transplantation. The osteodystrophy should be treated, in the first instance, with large doses of vitamin D (up to 500 000 IU daily); in resistant cases, small doses of 1,25-DHCC may be effective. Epiphyseolysis may need internal fixation and residual deformities can be corrected once the disease is under control.

Scurvy

Vitamin C (ascorbic acid) deficiency causes failure of collagen synthesis and osteoid formation. The result is osteoporosis, which in infants is most marked in the juxtaepiphyseal bone. Spontaneous bleeding is common.

The infant is irritable and anaemic. The gums may be spongy and bleeding. Subperiosteal haemorrhage causes excruciating pain and tenderness near the large joints. Fractures or epiphyseal separations may occur.

X-rays show generalized bone rarefaction, most marked in the long bone metaphyses. The normal calcification in growing cartilage produces dense transverse bands at the juxtaepiphyseal zones and around the ossific centres of the epiphyses (the 'ring sign'). The metaphyses may be deformed or fractured. Subperiosteal haematomas show as soft-tissue swellings or periosseous calcification.

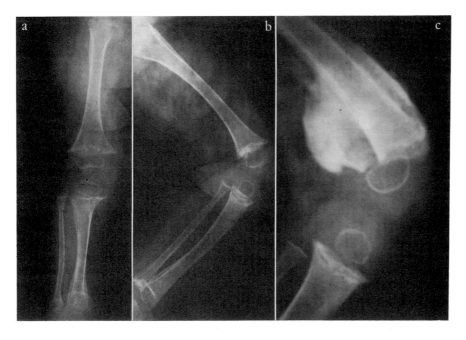

7.19 Scurvy   (a, b) The ring sign, the corner sign and small subperiosteal haemorrhages; (c) the femoral epiphysis has displaced and the subperiosteal haemorrhage has calcified.

Hypervitaminosis

Hypervitaminosis A occurs in children following excessive dosage; in adults it seldom occurs except in explorers who eat Polar bear livers. There may be bone pain, and headache and vomiting due to raised intracranial pressure. X-ray shows increased density in the metaphyseal region and subperiosteal calcification.

Hypervitaminosis D occurs if too much vitamin D is given. It exerts a PTH-like effect and so, as in the underlying rickets, calcium is withdrawn from bones; but metastatic calcification occurs. In treatment the dose of vitamin D must be properly regulated and the infant given a low-calcium diet but plentiful fluids.

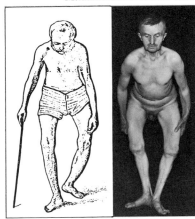

7.20 Paget's disease Paget's original case compared with a modern photograph.

Paget's disease (osteitis deformans)

Paget's disease is characterized by enlargement and thickening of the bone, but the internal architecture is abnormal and the bone is unusually brittle. The condition has a curious ethnic and geographic distribution, being relatively common in North America, Britain, Germany and Australia (more than 3% of people aged over 40) but rare in Asia, Africa and the Middle East. The cause is unknown, although the discovery of inclusion bodies in the osteoclasts has suggested a viral infection (Rebel et al., 1980).

Pathology

The disease may appear in one or several sites; in the tubular bones it starts at one end and progresses slowly towards the diaphysis, leaving a trail of altered architecture behind. The characteristic cellular change is a marked increase in osteoclastic and osteoblastic activity. Bone turnover is accelerated, plasma alkaline phosphatase is raised (a sign of osteoblastic activity) and there is increased excretion of hydroxyproline in the urine (due to osteoclastic activity).

In the osteolytic (or 'vascular') stage there is avid resorption of existing bone by large osteoclasts, the excavations being filled with vascular fibrous tissue. In adjacent areas osteoblastic activity produces new woven and lamellar bone, which in turn is attacked by osteoclasts. This alternating activity extends on both endosteal and periosteal surfaces, so the bone increases in thickness but is structually weak and easily deformed. Gradually, osteoclastic activity abates and the eroded areas fill with new lamellar bone, leaving an irregular pattern of cement lines that mark the limits of the old resorption cavities; these 'tidemarks' produce a marbled or mosaic appearance on microscopy. In the late, osteoblastic, stage the thickened bone becomes increasingly sclerotic and brittle.

Clinical features

Paget's disease affects men and women equally. Only occasionally does it present in patients under 50, but from that age onwards it becomes increasingly common. The disease may for many years remain localized to part or the whole of one bone – the pelvis and tibia being the commonest sites, and the femur, skull, spine and clavicle the next commonest.

Most people with Paget's disease are asymptomatic, the disorder being discovered when an x-ray is taken for some unrelated condition. When patients do present, it is usually because of pain or deformity, or some complication of the disease.

The pain is a dull constant ache, worse in bed when the patient warms up, but rarely severe unless a fracture occurs or sarcoma supervenes.

Deformities are seen mainly in the lower limbs. Long bones bend across the trajectories of mechanical stress; thus the tibia bows anteriorly and the femur anterolaterally. The limb looks bent and feels thick, and the skin is unduly warm – hence the term 'osteitis deformans'. If the skull is affected, it enlarges; the patient may complain that old hats no longer fit. The skull base may become flattened (platybasia), giving the appearance of a short neck. In generalized Paget's disease there may also be considerable kyphosis, so the patient becomes shorter and ape-like, with bent legs and arms hanging in front of him.

Cranial nerve compression may lead to impaired vision, facial palsy, trigeminal neuralgia or deafness. Another cause of deafness is otosclerosis. Vertebral thickening may cause spinal cord or nerve root compression.

Steal syndromes, in which blood is diverted from internal organs to the surrounding skeletal circulation, may cause cerebral impairment and spinal cord ischaemia. If there is also spinal stenosis the patient develops typical symptoms of 'spinal claudication' and lower limb weakness.

X-RAYS The appearances are so characteristic that the diagnosis is seldom in doubt. During the resorptive phase there may be localized areas of osteolysis; most typical is the flame-shaped lesion extending along the shaft of the bone, or a circumscribed patch of osteoporosis in the skull (osteoporosis circumscripta). Later the bone becomes thick and sclerotic, with coarse trabeculation. The femur or tibia sometimes develops fine cracks on the convex surface – stress fractures that heal with increasing deformity of the bone. Occasionally the diagnosis is made only when the patient presents with a pathological fracture. Silent lesions are revealed by increased activity in the radionuclide scan.

BIOCHEMICAL INVESTIGATIONS Disease activity is gauged by the increase in serum alkaline phosphatase and urinary hydroxyproline levels. Patients who are immobilized may develop hypercalcaemia.

Complications

NERVE COMPRESSION AND SPINAL STENOSIS are sometimes the first abnormalities to be detected, and may call for definitive surgical treatment.

FRACTURES are common, especially in the weightbearing long bones. In the femoral neck they are often vertical; elsewhere the fracture line is usually partly transverse and partly oblique, like the line of section of a felled tree. In the femur there is a high rate of non-union; for femoral neck fractures prosthetic replacement and for shaft fractures early internal fixation are recommended. Small stress fractures may be very painful; they resemble Looser's zones on x-ray, except that they occur on convex surfaces.

OSTEOARTHRITIS of the hip or knee is not merely a consequence of abnormal loading due to bone deformity; in the hip it seldom occurs unless the innominate bone is involved. The x-ray appearances suggest an atrophic arthritis with sparse remodelling, and at operation joint vascularity is increased.

BONE SARCOMA in the elderly is almost always due to Paget's disease. The frequency of malignant change is probably around 1%. It should always be suspected if a previously diseased bone becomes more painful, swollen and tender. Occasionally it presents as the first evidence of Paget's disease. The prognosis is extremely grave.

HIGH-OUTPUT CARDIAC FAILURE, though rare, is an important general complication. It is due to prolonged, increased bone blood flow.

HYPERCALCAEMIA may occur if the patient is immobilized for long.

In spite of all these complications, most patients with Paget's disease come to terms with the condition and live to a ripe old age.

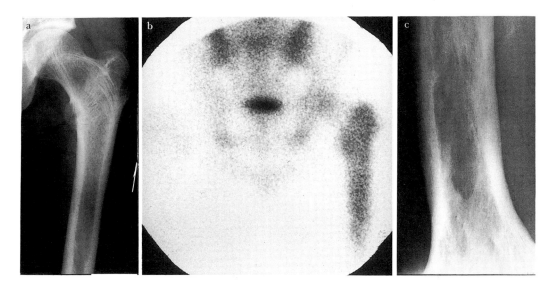

7.21 Paget's disease (a, b) In this early case the x-ray is almost normal, but the radionuclide scan of the same femur shows increased activity. (c) Flame-shaped area of osteopenia.

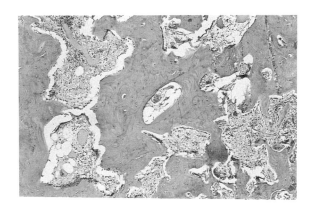

7.22 Paget's disease – histology Section from pagetic bone, showing the mosaic pattern due to overactive bone resorption and bone formation. The trabeculae are thick and patterned by cement lines. Some surfaces are excavated by osteoclastic activity whilst others are lined by rows of osteoblasts. The marrow spaces contain fibrovascular tissue.

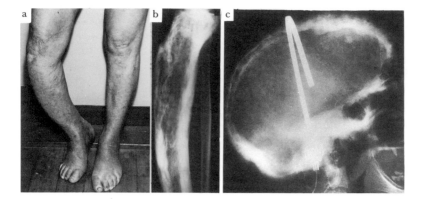

7.23 Paget's disease (a, b) The typical thick bent tibia. (c) The skull is enlarged, the vault thickened and the base flattened; x-ray or not, he clung to his hearing aid.

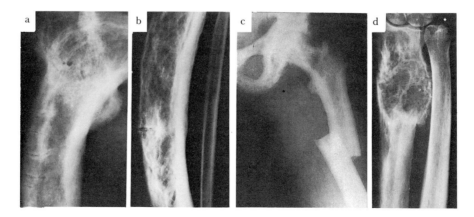

7.24 Paget complications (a) Fine cracks (microfractures) on the convex aspect, often associated with pain. (b) Incomplete fracture. (c) Complete fracture. This patient also has 'Paget's arthritis' of the hip. (d) Osteosarcoma.

Treatment

Most patients with Paget's disease never have any symptoms and require no treatment. Sometimes pain is due to an associated arthritis rather than bone disease, and this may respond to non-steroidal anti-inflammatory therapy.

The indications for specific treatment are: (1) persistent bone pain; (2) repeated fractures; (3) neurological complications; (4) high-output cardiac failure; (5) hypercalcaemia due to immobilization; and (6) for some months before and after major bone surgery where there is a risk of excessive haemorrhage.

Drugs that suppress bone turnover, notably calcitonin and diphosphonates, are most effective when the disease is active and bone turnover is high.

Calcitonin is the most widely used. It reduces bone resorption by decreasing both the activity and the number of osteoclasts; serum alkaline phosphatase and urinary hydroxyproline levels are lowered. Salmon calcitonin is more effective than the porcine variety; subcutaneous injections of 50–100 MRC units are given daily until pain is relieved and the alkaline phosphatase levels are reduced and stabilized. Maintenance injections once or twice weekly may have to be continued indefinitely, but some authorities advocate stopping the drug and resuming treatment if symptoms recur. Drug resistance due to antibody formation may occur, but this will be avoided when human calcitonin is more generally available.

Diphosphonates bind to hydroxyapatite crystals, inhibiting their rate of growth and dissolution. It is claimed that the reduction in bone turnover following their use is associated with the formation of lamellar rather than woven bone and that, even after treatment is stopped, there may be prolonged remission of disease (Bickerstaff et al., 1990). Etidronate can be given orally (always on an empty stomach) but dosage should be kept low (e.g. 5 mg/kg per day for up to 6 months) lest impaired bone mineralization results in osteomalacia. Diphosphonate derivates, such as pamidronate and clodronate, are more effective and produce remissions even with short courses of 1 or 2 weeks.

Surgery The main indication for operation is a pathological fracture, which (in a long bone) usually requires internal fixation. When the fracture is treated the opportunity should be taken to straighten the bone. Other indications for surgery are painful osteoarthritis (total joint replacement), nerve entrapment (decompression) and severe spinal stenosis (decompression). An osteosarcoma, if detected early, may be resectable, but generally the prognosis is grave.

Endocrine disorders

A number of endocrine disorders are associated with bone disease. Normally there is a fine balance between pituitary growth hormone (which stimulates epiphyseal growth) and gonadal hormone (which promotes growth-plate maturation and closure). Thus, at the end of puberty, as gonadal development evolves, growth slows down and the epiphyses fuse. If this balance is disturbed, abnormalities may occur.

Hypopituitarism

Growth hormone deficiency produces two distinct disorders: (1) *proportionate dwarfism (Lorain type)* due to epiphyseal growth retardation; and (2) delayed skeletal maturation associated with adiposity and hypogonadism (*Fröhlich's adiposogenital syndrome*). In both, the epiphyses remain unfused and, especially in the adiposo-

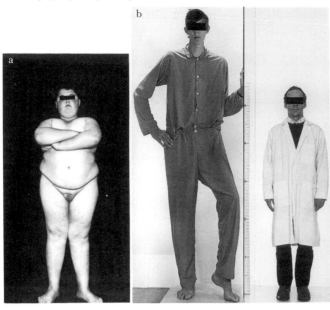

7.25 Endocrine disorders (a) A boy of 12 with the unmistakable build of Frölich's adiposogenital syndrome. (b) This young giant, only 16 years old, suffered from a pituitary adenoma; comparison with the photographer is quite startling. His peculiar stance is due to an undetected slipped upper femoral epiphysis on the left.

genital syndrome, there is danger of epiphyseal slipping at the hip or knee.

In the acquired types the disorder may be reversible; for example, by removing a craniopharyngioma. In others, growth hormone has been used.

Hyperpituitarism

Acidophil cell hypersecretion results in skeletal overgrowth, the effects of which vary according to the age at onset.

GIGANTISM An acidophil adenoma in childhood stimulates epiphyseal growth. Patients are excessively tall, often with sexual immaturity and mental retardation. Slipping of the upper femoral epiphysis may occur.

ACROMEGALY Hyperpituitarism starting in adulthood stimulates appositional bone growth and hypertrophy of articular cartilage. The jaw enlarges; together with thickening of the skull this produces a characteristic facies. The hands and feet are big and the long bone ends are markedly thickened; osteoarthritis is common.

Cushing's syndrome

Cushing's syndrome may be due to hypersecretion by the adrenal cortex, but is more often due to corticosteroid therapy. There is a characteristic obesity of the face and trunk, and generalized osteoporosis. With very large doses of steroids there is danger of bone necrosis (see p. 92).

Infantile hypothyroidism (cretinism)

With congenital thyroid deficiency the child is severely dwarfed and mentally retarded. Irregular epiphyseal ossification may be mistaken for avascular necrosis. These changes can be prevented by early treatment with thyroid hormone.

Myxoedema

Adult hypothyroidism may result from some primary disorder of thyroid function (including Hashimoto's disease) or iatrogenic suppression during the treatment of hyperthyroidism. These patients often develop *joint pain* (sometimes associated with CPPD crystal deposition), muscle weakness or *nerve compression* syndromes, all of which respond to treatment of the underlying disorders.

Hyperthyroidism

Hyperthyroidism in adults may give rise to osteoporosis. The investigation of unexplained bone loss should include tests for thyroid function. Treatment of the primary disorder results in improved bone mass.

Pregnancy

Women, during pregnancy, often develop musculoskeletal symptoms, some of which have been ascribed to the increased weight and unusual posture, others to hormonal changes.

Backache is common during the latter months. The lordotic posture may be to blame and postural exercises are a help. But there is also increased laxity of the pelvic joints due to secretion of relaxin, and this may play a part. Back pain may persist after childbirth and x-rays sometimes show increased sclerosis near the sacroiliac joint – *osteitis condensans ilii*. This is, in all probability, due to increased stress or minor trauma to the bone associated with sacroiliac laxity.

Carpal tunnel syndrome is common; it is probably due to fluid retention and soft-tissue swelling. Operation should be avoided; symptoms can be controlled with a wrist splint and the condition does not recur after the end of pregnancy.

Rheumatic disorders respond in unusual ways. Patients with rheumatoid arthritis often improve dramatically, while those with systemic lupus erythematosus sometimes develop a severe exacerbation of the disease.

References and further reading

Bickerstaff, D.R., Douglas, D.L., Burke, P.H. et al. (1990) Improvement in the deformity of the face in Paget's disease treated with diphosphonates. *Journal of Bone and Joint Surgery* **72B**, 132–136

Brighton, C.T. and McCluskey, W.P. (1986) Cellular response and mechanisms of action of electrically induced osteogenisis. In *Bone and Mineral Research/4* (ed. W.A. Peck), Elsevier, Amsterdam

Dekel, S., Lenthall, G. and Francis, M.J.O. (1981) Release of prostaglandins from bone and muscle after tibial fracture. An experimental study in rabbits. *Journal of Bone and Joint Surgery* **63B**, 185–189

Dykman, T.R., Gluck, O.S., Murphy, W.A. et al. (1985) Evaluation of factors associated with glucocorticoid-induced osteopenia in patients with rheumatic disease. *Arthritis and Rheumatism* **28**, 361–368

Etlinger, B., Genant, H.K. and Cann, C.E. (1985) Long-term estrogen therapy prevents bone loss and fracture. *Annals of Internal Medicine* **102**, 319–324

Hahn, T.J. (1980) Drug-induced disorders of vitamin D and mineral metabolism. *Clinics in Endocrinology and Metabolism* **9**, 107–129

Harakas, N.K. (1984) Demineralized bone-matrix-induced osteogenesis. *Clinical Orthopaedics and Related Research* **188**, 239–251

Lindsay, R., Hart, D.M. and Clark, D.M. (1984) The minimum effective dose of estrogen for prevention of postmenopausal bone loss. *Obstetrics and Gynecology* **63**, 759–763

Parfitt, A.M. (1988) Bone remodelling: relationship to the amount and structure of bone, and the pathogenesis and prevention of fractures. In *Osteoporosis* (eds. B.L. Riggs and L.J. Nelton III), Raven Press, New York, pp. 45–93.

Peck, W.A. and Woods, W.L. (1988) The cells of bone. In *Osteoporosis* (eds. B.L. Riggs and L.J. Melton III), Raven Press, New York, pp. 1–44

Rebel, A., Basle, M., Poulard, A. et al. (1980) Towards a viral aetiology for Paget's disease of bone. *Metabolic Bone Disorders and Related Research* **3**, 235–238

Seibel, M.J., Duncan, A. and Robins, S.P. (1989) Urinary hydroxypyridinium crosslinks provide indices of cartilage and bone involvement in arthritic disease. *Journal of Rheumatology* **16**, 964–970

Singh, M., Nagrath, A.R., Maini, P.S. and Haryana, R. (1970) Changes in trabecular pattern of the upper end of the femur as an index of osteoporosis. *Journal of Bone and Joint Surgery* **52A**, 457–467

Skerry, T.M., Bitensky, L., Chayen, J. and Lanyon, L.E. (1989) Early strain-related changes in enzyme activity in osteocytes following bone loading in vivo. *Journal of Bone and Mineral Research* **4**, 783–788

Solomon, L. (1974) Fracture of the femoral neck in the elderly. Bone ageing or disease? *South African Journal of Surgery* **11**, 269–279

Tashjian, A. (1975) Prostaglandins, hypercalcemia and cancer. *New England Journal of Medicine* **293**, 1317–1318

Uebelhart, D., Gineyts, E., Chapuy, M.-C. and Delmas, P.D. (1990) Urinary excretion of pyridium crosslinks: a new marker of bone resorption in metabolic bone disease. *Bone and Mineral* **8**, 87–96

Genetic disorders, dysplasias and malformations

8

There can be few diseases in which genetic factors do not play some role – if only in ensuring a background favourable to the operation of some more immediate pathogen. Sometimes, however, a genetic defect is the major – or the only – determinant of an abnormality that is either present at birth (i.e. congenital) or inevitably evolves in later years. Such conditions can be broadly classified into three categories: chromosome disorders, single gene disorders and polygenic or multifactorial disorders. Various anomalies may also result from injury to the formed embryo. Many of these conditions affect the musculoskeletal system, producing *bone dysplasia* (abnormal bone growth and/or modelling), *malformations* (e.g. absence or duplication of certain parts) or *structural defects of soft connective tissue*. In some a specific *metabolic abnormality* has been identified.

There are many different musculoskeletal dysplasias, but each individual one is rare, so the general orthopaedic surgeon is unlikely to see more than the very occasional case. Nevertheless their total number is not inconsiderable (probably more than double that of haemophilia) and in recent years their importance has increased because (1) prenatal diagnosis is often possible, (2) genetic counselling has become more precise and (3) even when the exact diagnosis is not known, modern surgical procedures such as joint replacement and limb lengthening are sometimes indicated.

Genetic order

The life-imparting material in the nucleus of every cell is *deoxyribonucleic acid* (DNA). Each of the 46 *chromosomes* in the human cell consists of a single molecule of DNA; unravelled it would be several centimetres long, a double-stranded chain along which thousands of segments are defined and demarcated as genes.

The *genes* are the basic units of inherited biological information, each one coding for the synthesis of a specific protein. Working as a set (or *genome*) they tell the cells how to develop, differentiate and function in specialized ways.

Chromosomes can be identified and numbered by microscopic examination of suitably prepared blood cells or tissue samples. Of the 46 chromosomes in human cells, 44 (the *autosomes*) are disposed in 22 homologous pairs: one of each pair, carrying the same type of genetic information, is derived from each parent. The remaining two are the *sex chromosomes*: females have two X chromosomes (one from each parent); males have one X chromosome (from the mother) and one Y chromosome (from the father).

Genetic studies are much more complicated and involve the mapping of molecular sequences by specialized techniques after fragmenting the chains of DNA by means of restriction enzymes. Each gene occurs at a specific point, or *locus*, on the chromosome. The chromosomes being paired, there will be two forms, or *alleles*, of each gene (one maternal, one paternal) at each locus; if the two alleles coding for a particular trait are identical, the person is said to be *homozygous* for that trait; if they are not identical, the individual is *heterozygous*.

The full genetic make-up of an individual is called the *genotype*. The finished person – a product of inherited traits and environmental forces – is the *phenotype*.

An important part of the unique human genotype is the *major histocompatibility complex* (MHC), also known as the *HLA system* (after human leucocyte antigen). This is a cluster of genes on chromosome 6 that is responsible for immunological specificity. The proteins for which they code are attached to cell surfaces and act as 'chaperones' for foreign antigens which have to be accompanied by HLA before they are recognized and engaged by the body's T-cells.

HLA proteins can be identified by serological tests and are registered according to their corresponding genetic loci on the short arm of chromosome 6. HLA typing is particularly important in tissue transplantation: acceptance or rejection of the transplant hinges on the degree of matching between the HLA genes of donor and recipient.

Genetic disorder

Any serious disturbance of either the quantity or the arrangement of genetic material may result in disease. Three broad categories of abnormality are recognized: chromosome disorders, single gene disorders and polygenic or multifactorial disorders.

Chromosome disorders

Additions, deletions and changes in chromosomal structure usually have serious effects, and affected fetuses are either still-born or give rise to infants with severe physical and mental abnormalities. In live-born children there are a few chromosome disorders with significant orthopaedic abnormalities: Down's syndrome, in which there is one extra chromosome 21 (trisomy 21), Turner's syndrome, in which one of the X chromosomes is lacking (monosomy X), and Klinefelter's syndrome, in which there is one Y but several X chromosomes.

Single gene disorders

Gene mutation may occur by insertion, deletion, substitution or fusion of amino-acids or nucleotides in the DNA chain – sometimes with profound consequences for cell metabolism. The abnormality is then passed on to future generations according to simple mendelian rules (see below). The clinical phenotype may show various kinds of growth disorder, structural abnormalities of connective tissue, or enzyme defects resulting in perturbed metabolism. There are literally thousands of single gene disorders, accounting for over 5% of child deaths, yet it is rare to see any one of them in an orthopaedic practice.

Polygenic and multifactorial disorders

Many normal traits (body build, for example) derive from the interaction of multiple genetic and environmental influences. Likewise, certain diseases have a polygenic background, and some occur only when a genetic predisposition combines with an appropriate environmental 'trigger'. Gout, for example, is more common than usual in families with hyperuricaemia: the uric acid level is a polygenic trait, reflecting the interplay of multiple genes; it is also influenced by diet and may be more than usually elevated after a period of overindulgence. Finally, a slight bump on the toe acts as the proximate trigger for an acute attack of pain and swelling.

Non-genetic disorders

Many developmental abnormalities occur sporadically and have no genetic background. Most of these are of unknown aetiology, but some have been linked to specific teratogenic agents which damage the embryo or the placenta during the first few months of gestation. Suspected or known teratogens include viral infections (e.g. rubella), certain drugs (e.g. thalidomide) and ionizing radiation. The clinical features are usually asymmetrical and localized, ranging from mild morphological defects to severe malformations such as spina bifida or phocomelia ('congenital amputations').

Patterns of inheritance

The single gene disorders have characteristic patterns of inheritance, which may be autosomal or X-linked, and dominant or recessive.

Autosomal dominant disorders are inherited even if only one of a pair of alleles on a non-sex chromosome is abnormal – i.e. the patient may be heterozygous. A typical example is hereditary multiple exostoses. Either parent may be affected and half the children of both sexes develop exostoses. The pedigree shows a 'vertical' pattern of inheritance, with several affected siblings in successive generations. Sometimes both parents appear to be normal: the patient may be the first member of the family to suffer the effects of a mutant gene; or (as often happens) the disease shows variable expressivity, some members of the family (in this example) developing many large exostoses and

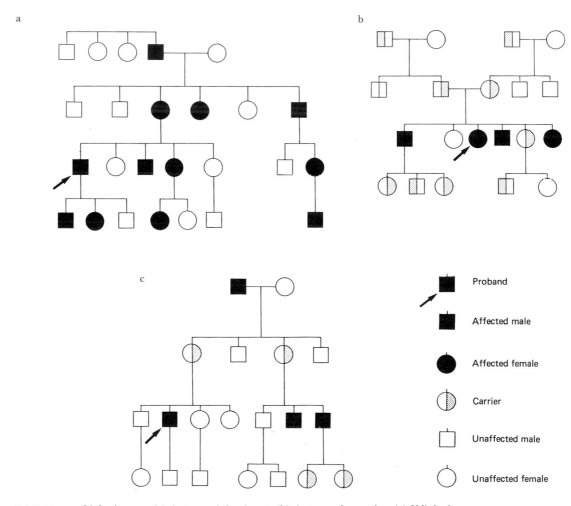

8.1 Patterns of inheritance (a) Autosomal dominant. (b) Autosomal recessive. (c) X-linked.

severe bone deformities, while others have only a few small and well-disguised nodules.

Autosomal recessive disorders appear only when both alleles of a pair are abnormal – i.e. the patient is always homozygous. Each parent contributes a faulty gene, though if both are heterozygous they will be clinically normal. Theoretically 1 in 4 of the children will be homozygous and will therefore develop the disease; 2 out of 4 will be heterozygous carriers of the faulty gene. The typical pedigree shows a 'horizontal' pattern of inheritance: several siblings in one generation are affected but neither their parents nor their children have the disease.

X-linked disorders are caused by a faulty gene in the X chromosome. Characteristically, therefore, they never pass directly from father to son because the father's X chromosome inevitably goes to the daughter, and the Y chromosome to the son. X-linked dominant disorders (e.g. hypophosphataemic rickets) pass from an affected mother to half of her daughters and half of her sons, or from an affected father to all of his daughters but none of his sons. Not surprisingly, they are twice as common in girls as in boys. X-linked recessive disorders – of which the most notorious is haemophilia – have a highly distinctive pattern of inheritance: an affected male will pass the gene only to his daughters, who will become unaffected heterozygous carriers; they, in turn, will transmit it to half of their daughters (who will likewise be carriers) and half of their sons (who will develop the disease). Thus a haemophilic man will have normal children but his daughters will be carriers and half his grandsons will be bleeders.

In-breeding

All types of genetic disease are more likely to occur in the children of consanguineous marriages or in closed communities where many people are related to each other. The rare recessive disorders, in particular, are seen in these circumstances, where there is an increased risk of a homozygous pairing between two mutant genes.

Genetic heterogenicity

The same phenotype (i.e. a patient with a set of clinical features) can result from widely different gene mutations. For example, there are four different types of osteogenesis imperfecta (brittle bone disease), some showing autosomal dominant and some autosomal recessive inheritance. Where this occurs, the recessive form is usually the more severe. Subtleties of this kind must be borne in mind when counselling parents.

Genetic markers

Many common disorders show an unusually close association with certain blood groups, tissue types or other serum proteins that occur with higher than expected frequency in the patients and their relatives. These are referred to as genetic markers; they arise from gene sequences that do not cause the disease but are either 'linked' to other (abnormal) loci or else express some factor that predisposes the individual to a harmful environmental agent. A good example is ankylosing spondylitis: over 90% of patients, and 60% of their first-degree relatives, are positive for HLA-B27. In this case (as in other autoimmune diseases) the HLA marker gene may provide the necessary conditions for invasion by a foreign viral fragment.

Gene mapping

With advancing recombinant DNA technology, the genetic disorders are gradually being mapped to specific loci. In some cases (e.g. Duchenne muscular dystrophy) the mutant gene itself has been cloned, holding out the possibility of effective treatment in the future.

Prenatal diagnosis

Many genetic disorders can be diagnosed before birth, thus giving the parents the choice of selective abortion. Ultrasound imaging is harmless and is now done almost routinely. On the other hand, tests that involve amniocentesis or chorionic villus sampling carry a risk of injury to the fetus and are therefore used only when there is reason to suspect some abnormality. Indications are: (1) maternal age over 35 years (increased risk of Down's syndrome) or an unduly high paternal age (increased risk of achondroplasia); (2) a previous history of chromosomal abnormalities (e.g. Down's syndrome) or genetic abnormalities amenable to biochemical diagnosis (neural tube defects, or inborn errors of metabolism); or (3) to confirm non-invasive tests suggesting an abnormality.

Maternal screening

Fetal neural tube defects are associated with increased levels of *alpha-fetoprotein* (AFP) in the amniotic fluid and, to a lesser extent, the maternal blood. Women with positive blood tests may be given the option of further investigation by amniocentesis. It has also been noted that abnormally low levels of AFP are associated with Down's syndrome.

Amniocentesis

Under local anaesthesia, a small amount (about 20 ml) of fluid is withdrawn from the amniotic sac with a needle and syringe. (It is best to determine the position of the fetus beforehand by ultrasonography.) The procedure is usually carried out between the 14th and 18th weeks of pregnancy. The fluid can be examined directly for *AFP* and desquamated fetal cells can be collected and cultured for *chromosomal studies* and *biochemical tests* for enzyme disorders.

Chorionic villus sampling

Under ultrasound screening, a fine catheter is passed through the cervix and a small sample of chorion is sucked out. This is usually done between the 8th and 10th weeks of pregnancy. Mesenchymal fibroblasts can be cultured and used for *chromosomal studies, biochemical tests* and *DNA analysis*. Rapid advances in DNA technology have made it possible to diagnose sickle-cell anaemia and haemophilia (among other disorders) during early pregnancy.

Fetal imaging

After the 20th week of pregnancy, *ultrasonography* may show anatomical abnormalities such as open neural tube defects and short limbs. In late pregnancy, *x-ray* examination will reveal any marked change in bone density (osteopetrosis) and multiple fractures (osteogenesis imperfecta).

Diagnosis in childhood

Physical abnormalities may be obvious *at birth*; for example, disproportionately short limbs, an abnormally shaped skull, localized malformations of the face, hands or feet, absence of a limb (or part of a limb), soft-tissue contractures, club foot or spina bifida.

During infancy the reasons for presentation are failure to grow normally, disproportionate shortness of the limbs, delay in walking, fractures or the discovery of exostoses.

The growing child should be measured at regular intervals and a record kept of height, length of lower segment (pubis to heel), upper segment (pubis to cranium), span, head circumference and chest circumference. Examination should include tests for hearing and visual acuity.

Radiologically most dysplasias can be diagnosed by three films: (1) an anteroposterior (AP) of the pelvis and hips; (2) an AP of the wrists and hands; and (3) a lateral of the spine. Sometimes a complete survey is needed and it is always important to note which portion of the long bones (epiphysis, metaphysis or diaphysis) is affected. With severe and varied changes in the metaphyses, periosteal new bone formation or epiphyseal separation *always consider the possibility of non-accidental fractures – the battered baby syndrome* (Horan and Beighton, 1980).

Biochemical tests may reveal increased production and excretion of abnormal metabolites in the storage disorders. Specific enzyme activity can be measured in serum, blood cells or cultured skin fibroblasts.

Bone biopsy is occasionally helpful in disorders of bone density.

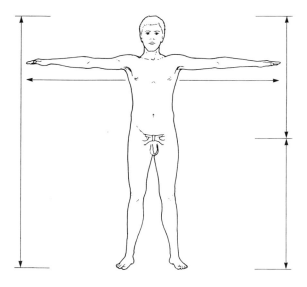

8.2 Normal arthropometry Upper segment = lower segment. Total height = span.

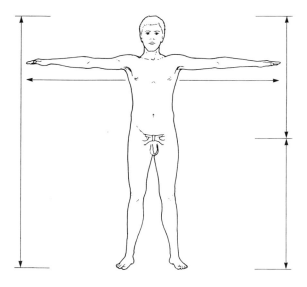

characteristic patterns of inheritance which may be helpful in diagnosis.

The family history should include information about similar disorders in close relatives, previous deaths in the family (and the cause of death), abortions and intermarriage.

Racial background is important: some diseases are almost confined to a racial group – for example, sickle-cell disease in Negroes and Gaucher's disease in Ashkenazi Jews.

Previous medical history

Always ask about exposure to teratogenic agents during the early months of pregnancy: x-rays, cytotoxic drugs or virus infections.

Adult presentation

In the worst of the genetic disorders the fetus is still-born or survives for only a short time. Those who reach adulthood, though recognizably abnormal, may lead active lives, marry and have children of their own. Nevertheless, they often seek medical advice for several reasons: (1) short stature – especially disproportionate shortness of the lower limbs; (2) local bone deformities or exostoses; (3) secondary osteoarthritis, due to epiphyseal dysplasia; (4) joint laxity or instability; (5) spinal stenosis; and (6) repeated fractures.

The milder grades of disorder are often missed and may be passed off as 'hip dysplasia' or 'double-jointedness'.

Management

Management of the individual patient depends on the diagnosis, the pattern of inheritance, the type and severity of deformity or disability, mental capacity and social aspirations. However, it is worth noting some general principles.

Communication

The first step, once the diagnosis has been made, is to explain as much as possible about the disorder to the patient (if old enough) and the parents. The rare developmental disorders are best treated in a centre that offers a 'special interest' team consisting of a paediatrician, medical geneticist, orthopaedic surgeon, psychologist, social worker, occupational therapist, orthotist and prosthetist.

The family history

A careful family history should be obtained. However, the fact that a parent or relative is said to be 'normal' does not exclude the possibility that they are either very mildly affected or have a biochemical defect without any physical abnormality. Many developmental disorders have

Counselling

Patients and families may need expert counselling about (1) the likely outcome of the disorders; (2) what will be required of the family; and (c) the risk of siblings or children being affected. Where there are severe deformities or mental retardation, the entire family may need psychological help.

Specific treatment

Genetic faults cannot (yet) be corrected, but in some cases their immediate effects can be counteracted; for example, haemophilia can be treated with factor VIII, and sickle-cell crises can often be prevented (see p. 100). One of the hopes for the future is that missing enzymes will be replaced.

Correction of deformities

Anomalies such as coxa vara, genu valgum, club foot, radial club hand or scoliosis (and many others outside the field of orthopaedics) are amenable to corrective surgery. In recent years, with advances in methods of limb lengthening, many short-limbed dwarfs have benefited from this operation; however, the risks should be carefully explained and the expected benefits should not be exaggerated.

Spinal surgery

Several developmental disorders are associated with potentially dangerous spinal anomalies: for example, spinal stenosis and cord compression in achondroplasia; atlantoaxial instability, due to odontoid aplasia, in any disorder causing vertebral dysplasia; or severe kyphoscoliosis, which occurs in a number of conditions. Cord decompression or occipitocervical fusion are perfectly feasible, but surgical correction of congenital kyphoscoliosis carries considerable risks and should be undertaken only in specialized units.

Joint reconstruction

Some of the generalized skeletal dysplasias cause joint incongruity – especially of the hip or knee. This may need corrective surgery at a later stage when secondary osteoarthritis supervenes.

Classification

There is no completely satisfactory classification of developmental disorders. The same genetic abnormality may be expressed in different ways, while a variety of gene defects may cause almost identical clinical syndromes. The grouping used here is no more than a convenient way of dividing the various clinical syndromes.

Skeletal dysplasias

All the skeletal dysplasias affect growth and may result in dwarfism, a term that defies precise definition, since racial differences are considerable; adults whose height is less than 1.25 metres are often labelled as 'dwarfs', a term that they resent, preferring to be known as 'individuals of retarded growth'. Diagnostically it is useful to know if the shortness of stature is *proportionate* (limbs and trunk related as in normal individuals) or *disproportionate* (in which usually the limbs are affected more than the trunk). In disproportionate limb shortening the fingertips do not reach the mid-thigh.

Diagnosis of the dysplasias is made less confusing by dividing the disorder into four categories: (1) those with predominantly *physeal and metaphyseal* changes; (2) those with predominantly *epiphyseal and/or vertebral body* changes; (3) those with mainly *diaphyseal* changes; and (4) those with a *mixture* of epiphyseal, metaphyseal, vertebral and cranial abnormalities.

Dysplasias with predominantly physeal and metaphyseal changes

In these disorders there is abnormal physeal growth, defective metaphyseal modelling and shortness of the tubular bones. The axial skeleton is affected too, but the limbs are disproportionately short compared to the spine.

Hereditary multiple exostosis (diaphyseal aclasis)

The most common, and least disfiguring, of the skeletal dysplasias is multiple exostosis.

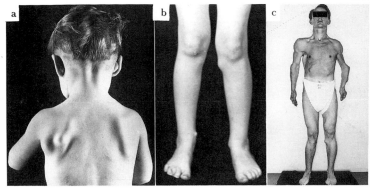

8.3 Hereditary multiple exostoses
Clinical presentation at (a) 3 years,
(b) 6 years, and (c) 28 years. In (c)
note the numerous small exostoses,
the one large tumour near the right
shoulder, bowing of the left radius,
shortening of the left forearm and
valgus deformity of the right knee.

CLINICAL FEATURES The condition is usually discovered in childhood; hard lumps appear at the ends of the long bones and along the apophyseal borders of the scapula and pelvis. As the child grows, these lumps enlarge and some may become hugely visible, especially around the knee. The more severely affected bones are abnormally short; this is seldom so marked as to cause dwarfism, but on measurement the lower body segment is shorter than the upper and span is less than height (Solomon, 1963). In the forearm and leg, the thinner of the two bones (the ulna or fibula) is usually the more defective, resulting in typical deformities: ulnar deviation of the wrist, bowing of the radius, subluxation of the radial head, valgus knees and valgus ankles. Bony lumps may cause pressure on nerves or vessels. Occasionally one of the cartilage-capped exostoses goes on growing into adult life and transforms to a chrondrosarcoma; this is said to occur in 1–2% of patients.

X-RAY Typically the long-bone metaphyses are broad and poorly modelled, with sessile or pedunculated exostoses arising from the cortices – almost as if longitudinal growth has been squandered in profligate lateral expansion. A stippled appearance around a bony excrescence indicates calcification in the cartilage cap. The distal end of the ulna is sometimes tapered or carrot-shaped.

PATHOLOGY Each exostosis has the typical appearance of an osteochondroma: the bony projection is surrounded by a cap of hyaline cartilage.

GENETICS The condition is inherited as an autosomal dominant trait; half the children are affected, both boys and girls. However, expression is variable and some people are so mildly affected as to be unaware of the disorder.

MANAGEMENT Exostoses may need removal because of pressure on a nerve or vessel, because of their unsightly appearance, or because they tend to get bumped during everyday activities. They should stop growing when the parent bone does; any subsequent enlargement suggests malignant change and calls for wide local resection (see p. 178). Deformities of the legs or forearms may be severe enough to warrant treatment by osteotomy; this is best postponed till late adolescence.

Achondroplasia

This is the commonest form of true dwarfism. Severe, disproportionate shortening of the limb bones may be diagnosed by x-ray before birth.

CLINICAL FEATURES The abnormality is obvious in childhood: growth is severely stunted; the limbs (particularly the proximal segments) are disproportionately short and the skull is quite large with prominent forehead and saddle-shaped nose. The fingers appear stubby and somewhat splayed (trident hands). The trunk seems too long by comparison with the limbs, and the posture when standing is typical: the back is excessively lordotic, the buttocks prominent, the hips flexed, the legs bowed and the elbows bent. In infancy there is often a thor-

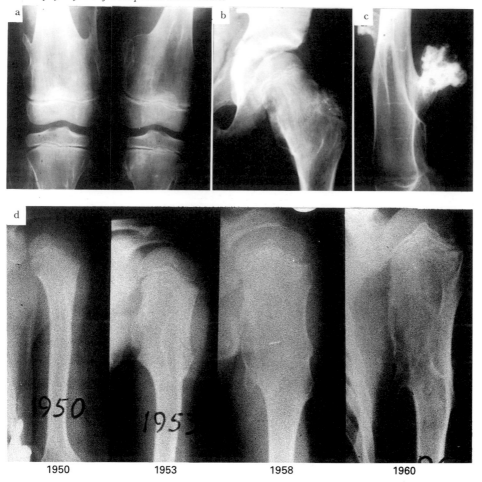

1950   1953   1958   1960

8.4 Hereditary multiple exostoses – x-rays (a) Typical x-ray appearances of the knees. (b) Sessile exostoses of the femoral neck. (c) A large pedunculated exostosis of the distal femur. (d) Evolution of the wide metaphysis during growth.

acolumbar gibbus, which disappears after a year or two. Shortening of the lumbar vertebral pedicles may lead to spinal stenosis, and disc prolapse (which is common in adult dwarfs) has exceptionally severe effects. Mental development is normal.

X-RAYS The tubular bones are short, the metaphyscs wide and the physeal lines somewhat irregular; the epiphyses are usually normal. The pelvic cavity is small (too small for normal delivery) and the iliac wings are flared, producing an almost horizontal acetabular roof. The skull vault is large but the base rather short and the foramen magnum smaller than usual.

GENETICS Achondroplasia occurs in about 1 in 25 000 births. There is autosomal dominant inheritance, but, because few achondroplastic people have children, over 80% of cases are sporadic.

DIAGNOSIS Achondroplasia should not be confused with other types of short-limbed dwarfism. In some (e.g. Morquio's disease) the shortening affects distal segments more than proximal and there may be widespread associated abnormalities. Others (e.g. the epiphyseal dysplasias) are distinguished by the fact that the epiphyses are abnormal whereas the head is not enlarged.

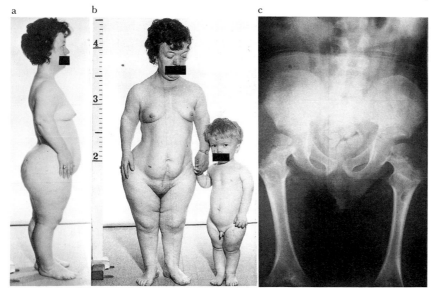

8.5 Achondroplasia (a) A typical achondroplastic patient with disproportionate shortening of the limbs. (b) Her son has clearly inherited the disorder. (c) The iliac wings have been likened to elephants' ears.

MANAGEMENT Achondroplastic dwarfs often develop neurological symptoms, and sometimes severe muscle weakness or paraplegia (Lutter and Langer, 1977). This may be due to spinal stenosis, intervertebral disc prolapse superimposed on a narrow spinal canal, or progressive spinal deformity. Any of these conditions may need operative treatment, which is rendered difficult by the fact that the posterior vertebral elements are abnormally short yet very thick.

Tibial blowing may need correction by osteotomy.

Advances in methods of external fixation have made leg lengthening a feasible option. However, there are drawbacks: complications, including bony non-union, infection and nerve palsy, may be disastrous; and the cosmetic effect of long legs and short arms may be less pleasing than anticipated.

8.6 Achondroplasia The smile reflects the patient's satisfaction with the increased height achieved by lengthening the lower limbs. (Courtesy of Mr M. Saleh.)

Hypochondroplasia

This has been described as a very mild form of achondroplasia. However, apart from shortness of stature (with the emphasis on proximal limb segments) and noticeable lumbar lordosis, there is little to suggest any abnormality; many of those affected pass for normal stocky individuals. X-rays may show slight pelvic flattening and thickening of the long bones. The condition is inherited as an autosomal dominant. Those affected sometimes ask for limb lengthening; after careful discussion, this may be done with a considerable chance of success.

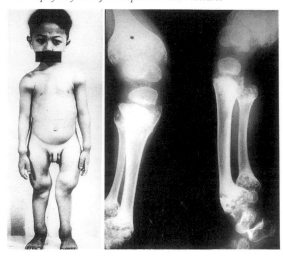

8.7 Metaphyseal chondrodysplasia This boy with the rare Jansen type shows the typical shortening of the lower limbs and metaphyseal swelling of the long bones. The x-rays show that the changes are confined to the metaphyses.

Metaphyseal chondrodysplasia

This term describes a type of short-limbed dwarfism in which the bony abnormality is virtually confined to the metaphyses. The epiphyses are unaffected but the metaphyseal segments adjacent to the growth plates are broadened and mildly scalloped, somewhat resembling rickets. Apart from a lordotic posture, the spine is normal. The main deformities are around the hips and knees.

There are several forms of metaphyseal chondrodysplasia. The best known (Schmid type) has the classic features described above, with autosomal dominant inheritance. Another group (McKusick type) is associated with sparse hair growth and is sometimes complicated by Hirschsprung's disease; inheritance shows an autosomal recessive pattern. The rarest of all (Jansen type) is usually sporadic and may be associated with deafness.

Operative correction (osteotomy) may be needed for coxa vara or tibia vara.

Dyschondroplasia (Ollier's disease)

This is a rare, but easily recognized, disorder in which there is defective transformation of physeal cartilage columns into bone.

CLINICAL FEATURES Typically the disorder is unilateral; indeed only one limb or even one bone may be involved. An affected limb is short and, if the growth plate is asymmetrically involved, the bone grows bent. Common deformities are valgus or varus at the knee and ankle, and relative shortening of the ulna such that the radius is curved and sometimes dislocated. The fingers or toes frequently contain multiple enchondromata, which are characteristic of the disease and may be so numerous that the hand is crippled. A rare variety of dyschondroplasia is associated with multiple haemangiomata (Maffucci's disease).

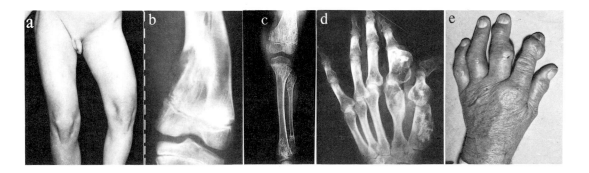

8.8 Dyschondroplasia (a, b) The bent femur in this boy is due to slow growth of half the lower femoral physis. (c) Incomplete ossification of the cartilage columns accounts for the curious metaphyseal appearance. (d, e) Two patients with multiple chondromas.

X-RAYS The characteristic change in the long bones is radiolucent streaking extending from the physis into the metaphysis – the appearance of persistent, incompletely ossified cartilage columns trapped in bone. If only half the physis is affected, growth is asymmetrically retarded and the bone becomes curved. With maturation the radiolucent columns eventually ossify. In the hands and feet the cartilage islands characteristically produce multiple enchondromata.

GENETICS The condition is not inherited; indeed, it is probably an embryonal rather than a genetic disorder.

MANAGEMENT Bone deformity may need correction, but this should be deferred until growth is complete; otherwise it is likely to recur.

MALIGNANCY A significant proportion of patients with Ollier's disease develop a low-grade chondrosarcoma or non-osseous malignancies; the risk with Maffucci's disease is still greater (Schwartz et al., 1987).

Dysplasias with predominantly epiphyseal changes

This group of disorders is characterized by abnormal development and ossification of the epiphyses, resulting in distortion of the bone ends. Limb length may be affected, though usually not as severely as in achondroplasia.

Multiple epiphyseal dysplasia

Multiple epiphyseal dysplasia (MED) varies in severity from a trouble-free disorder with mild anatomical abnormalities to a severe crippling condition.

CLINICAL FEATURES Children may present with stunted growth or, occasionally, with joint pain and progressive deformity. The face, skull and spine are normal. In adult life, residual bone defects may lead to joint incongruity and secondary osteoarthritis.

X-RAY Changes are apparent from early childhood. Epiphyseal ossification is delayed, and

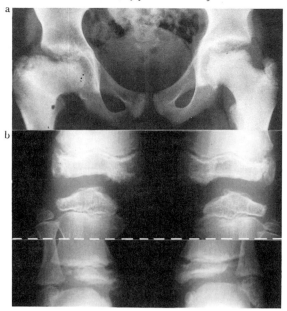

8.9 Multiple epiphyseal dysplasia (a) The grossly abnormal epiphyses led to a mistaken diagnosis of late Perthes' disease. (b) This girl had many epiphyses involved; her sister was similarly affected. Note the characteristic flattening of the femoral condyles.

when it appears it may be irregular or abnormal in outline. In the growing child the epiphyses are misshapen, and in the hips this may be mistaken for bilateral Perthes' disease. The vertebral ring epiphyses may be affected, but only mildly. At maturity the femoral heads and femoral condyles are flattened; secondary osteoarthritis may ensue and, if many joints are involved, the patient can be severely crippled.

VARIATIONS In some cases only one or two pairs of joints are involved, while in others the condition is widespread; sometimes there are striking changes in the hands or feet. Whether these are variations of one disorder or expressions of several different disorders is unknown.

GENETICS This appears to be a heterogeneous disorder but most cases have an autosomal dominant pattern of inheritance.

DIAGNOSIS MED is often confused with other childhood disorders.

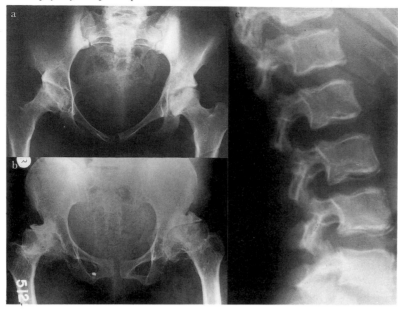

8.10 Multiple epiphyseal dysplasia (a) The typical irregular shape of the upper femoral epiphyses. This may lead to (b) severe osteoarthritis at a relatively young age. (c) The appearance of the vertebral ring epiphyses.

Perthes' disease is confined to the hips and shows a typical cycle of changes from epiphyseal irregularity to fragmentation, flattening and healing.

Cretinism, if untreated, causes progressive and widespread epiphyseal dysplasia. However, these children have other clinical and biochemical abnormalities and they are mentally retarded.

Pseudoachondroplasia is a rare disorder which resembles achondroplasia in causing disproportionate short-limbed dwarfism, but the head and face are normal and there is widespread involvement of the epiphyses. It differs from MED in showing more generalized skeletal abnormality (e.g. metaphyseal splaying, vertebral dysplasia, pelvic hypoplasia) and joint hypermobiity.

MANAGEMENT Children may complain of slight pain and limp, but little can (or need) be done about this. At maturity, bony deformities sometimes require corrective osteotomy. In later life, secondary osteoarthritis may call for reconstructive surgery.

Spondyloepiphyseal dysplasia

The term 'spondyloepiphyseal dysplasia' (SED) encompasses a heterogeneous group of disorders in which epiphyseal dysplasia is associated with well-marked vertebral changes – delayed ossification, flattening of the vertebral bodies (platyspondyly), irregular ossification of the ring epiphyses and indentations of the endplates (Schmorl's nodes). The mildest of these disorders is indistinguishable from MED; the more severe forms have characteristic appearances.

SED CONGENITA

An autosomal dominant disorder, SED congenita can be diagnosed in infancy: the limbs are short, but the trunk is even shorter and the neck hardly there. Older children develop a dorsal kyphosis and a typical barrel-shaped chest; they stand with the hips flexed and the lumbar spine in marked lordosis. By adolescence they often have scoliosis.

X-RAYS show widespread epiphyseal dysplasia and the characteristic vertebral changes. Odontoid hypoplasia is common and may lead to

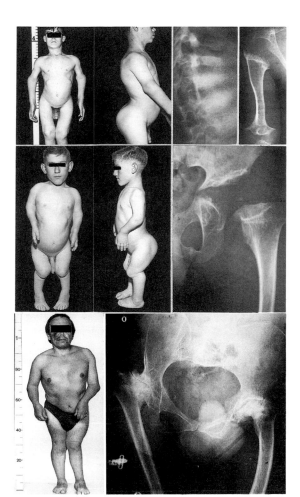

8.11 Spondyloepiphyseal dysplasia
Top: Usual variety.
Middle: Pseudoachondroplastic type.
Bottom: Pseudoachondroplastic type with severe secondary osteoarthritis.

anaesthesia; if there is evidence of subluxation atlantoaxial fusion may be advisable.

SED TARDA

An X-linked recessive disorder, SED tarda is much less severe and may become apparent only after the age of 5 years when the child fails to grow normally and develops a kyphoscoliosis. Adult men show disproportionate shortening of the trunk and a tendency to barrel chest. They may develop backache or secondary osteoarthritis of the hips.

X-RAYS show the characteristic platyspondyly and abnormal ossification of the ring epiphyses, together with more widespread dysplasia.

TREATMENT may be needed for backache or (in older adults) for secondary osteoarthritis of the hips.

Dysplasia epiphysealis hemimelica (Trevor's disease)

This is a curious 'hemidysplasia' affecting only one limb and only one-half (the medial or lateral half) of each epiphysis. Usually it appears at the ankle or knee. The child (usually a boy) presents with a bony swelling on one side of the joint; several sites may be affected – all on the same side in the same limb, but rarely in the upper limb (Kettelkamp, Cambell and Bonfiglio, 1966). X-ray shows an irregular, asymmetrical enlargement of the bony epiphysis and distortion of the adjacent joint. If this interferes with joint function, the excess bone is best removed, taking care not to damage the articular cartilage or ligaments. The condition is always sporadic.

atlantoaxial subluxation and cord compression.

DIAGNOSIS is not always easy; there are obvious similarities to Morquio's disease but, in the latter, shortening is in the distal limb segments and urinalysis shows increased excretion of keratan sulphate.

MANAGEMENT may involve corrective osteotomies for severe coxa vara or knee deformities. Odontoid hypoplasia increases the risks of

Chondrodyplasia punctata (stippled epiphyses)

Patchy epiphyseal ossification may be seen in children with MED, Down's syndrome or cretinism. Chrondrodysplasia punctata (or Conradi's disease) is a generalized, multisystem disorder producing facial abnormalities, vertebral anomalies, asymmetrical epiphyseal changes and bone shortening. In severe cases there may also be cardiac anomalies, congenital

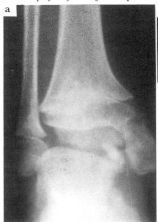

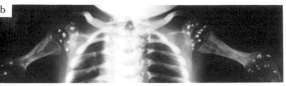

8.12 Epiphyseal dysplasia (a) Trevor's disease. (b) Conradi's disease – the spots disappeared later.

cataracts and mental retardation; some of these children die during infancy. The characteristic x-ray feature is a punctate stippling of the cartilaginous epiphyses and apophyses. This disappears by the age of 4 years but is often followed by epiphyseal irregularities and dysplasia. Orthopaedic management is directed at the deformities that develop in older children: joint contractures, limb length inequality or scoliosis.

Dysplasias with predominantly metaphyseal and diaphyseal changes

Most of the 'metaphyseal' and 'diaphyseal dysplasias' appear to be the result of defective bone modelling. Unlike the physeal and epiphyseal disorders, dwarfing is not a feature. There may be associated thickening of the skull bones, with the risk of foraminal occlusion and cranial nerve entrapment.

Fibrous dysplasia is dealt with on p. 169.

Metaphyseal dysplasia (Pyle's disease)

The only significant clinical feature in this disorder is genu valgum – or rather valgus angulation of the bones on either side of the knee. X-rays show a typical 'bottle shape' of the distal femur or proximal tibia – the so-called Erlenmeyer flask deformity – suggesting a

failure of bone modelling. Inheritance pattern is autosomal recessive. Treatment is seldom needed.

Craniometaphyseal dysplasia

This condition, of autosomal dominant inheritance, is similar to Pyle's disease, but here the tubular defect is associated with progressive thickening of the skull and mandible resulting in a curiously prominent forehead, a large jaw and a squashed-looking nose. Foraminal occlusion may cause cranial nerve compression – sometimes severe enough to require operative treatment.

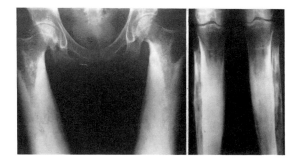

8.13 Engelmann's disease This patient had considerable discomfort from her long bones – all of which were wide and looked dense on x-ray.

Diaphyseal dysplasia (Engelmann's or Camurati's disease)

This rare, autosomal dominant disorder of tubular modelling is notable because of its association with muscle pain and weakness. Children complain of 'tired legs' and have a typical wide-based or waddling gait. There may be muscle wasting and failure to thrive. X-rays show fusiform widening and sclerosis of the shafts of the long bones, and sometimes thickening of the skull. Muscle pain may need symptomatic treatment. Milder cases usually clear up spontaneously by the age of 25.

Craniodiaphyseal dysplasia

This rare autosomal recessive disorder is characterized by cylindrical expansion of the long bones and gross thickening of the skull and facial bones. Prominent facial contours may appear in early childhood and are the most striking feature of the condition – giving rise to the name 'leontiasis'. Foraminal occlusion may cause deafness or visual impairment.

Osteopetrosis (marble bones, Albers–Schönberg disease)

The common form of osteopetrosis is a fairly benign, autosomal dominant disorder that seldom causes symptoms and may only be discovered in adolescence or adulthood after a pathological fracture or when an x-ray is taken for other reasons – hence the designation *tarda*.

Appearance and function are unimpaired, unless there are complications: pathological fracture or cranial nerve compression due to bone encroachment on foramina. Sufferers are also prone to bone infection, particularly of the mandible after tooth extraction. X-rays show increased density of all the bones: cortices are widened, leaving narrow medullary canals; sclerotic vertebral end-plates produce a striped appearance ('rugger-jersey spine'); the skull is thickened and the base densely sclerotic. Treatment is required only if complications occur.

A rare, autosomal recessive form – *osteopetrosis congenita* – is present at birth and causes severe disability. Bone encroachment on marrow results in pancytopenia, haemolysis, anaemia and hepatosplenomegaly. Foraminal occlusion may cause optic or facial nerve palsy. Repeated haemorrhage or infection usually leads to death in early childhood. Treatment, in recent years, has focused on methods of enhancing bone resorption. This has been achieved by transplanting marrow from normal donors (Marks, 1984), suggesting that the condition is due to lack of marrow cells that control osteoclastic activity.

Pyknodysostosis

Interest in this rare disorder owes something to the suggestion that the French impressionist, Toulouse-Lautrec, was a victim (Maroteaux and Lamy, 1965). Clinical features are shortness of stature, frontal bossing, underdevelopment of

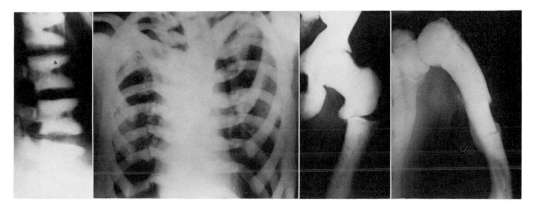

8.14 Marble bones Despite the remarkable density, the bones break easily; but, as in this humerus, union occurs although rather slowly.

the mandible and abnormal dentition. The presence of blue sclerae and proneness to fracture may cause confusion with osteogenesis imperfecta. On x-ray the bones are dense; the skull is enlarged, with wide suture lines and open fontanelles, but the facial bones and mandible are hypoplastic, thus accounting for the typical 'triangular' facies. The condition is inherited as an autosomal recessive trait. Despite appearances, it causes little trouble (apart from the odd pathological fracture) and needs no treatment.

Candle bones, spotted bones and striped bones

Candle bones (melorheostosis, Leri's disease) is not familial. The patient presents with pain and stiffness, usually confined to one limb. X-rays show irregular patches of sclerosis, usually distributed in linear fashion through the limb; the appearance is reminiscent of the wax that congeals on the side of a burning candle. Scleroderma and joint contractures may be associated.

In *spotted bones* (osteopoikilosis) numerous white spots are seen in the x-rays of many bones; there may also be whitish spots in the skin (disseminated lenticular dermatofibrosis). The condition is inherited as an autosomal dominant trait.

In *striped bones* (osteopathia striata) x-rays show lines of increased density parallel to the shafts of long bones, but radiating like a fan in the pelvis. The condition is symptomless. Some cases show autosomal dominant inheritance.

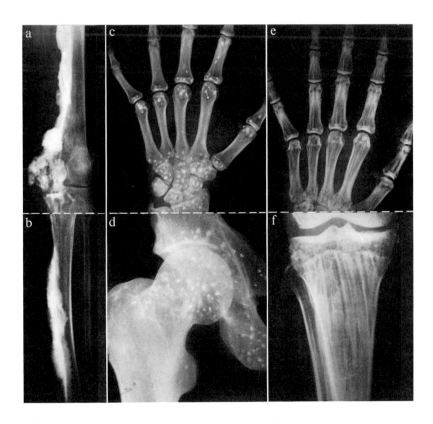

8.15 Radiological curiosities

(a) (b)
Candle
bones

(c) (d)
Spotted
bones

(e) (f)
Striped
bones

Combined and mixed dysplasias

A number of disorders show a mixture of physeal, metaphyseal and vertebral defects – i.e. dwarfism combined with epiphyseal maldevelopment, abnormal modelling of the metaphyses and platyspondyly.

Spondylometaphyseal dysplasia

This is the commonest of the 'mixed' dysplasias. There may be severe vertebral flattening and kyphoscoliosis. Epiphyseal changes are usually mild but the metaphyses are broad and ill-formed. Patients may need treatment for spinal deformity or malalignment of the hip or knee.

Pseudoachondroplasia

There is short-limbed dwarfism (as in achondroplasia), hypermobility of the joints and valgus or varus knees. However, unlike achondroplasia, there is also epiphyseal dysplasia and the skull is normal.

Diastrophic dysplasia

This autosomal recessive disorder affects all types of cartilage. Infants are severely dwarfed and distorted, with deformities of the hands ('hitch-hiker's thumb'), club feet, joint contractures, dislocations, 'cauliflower' ears and cleft palate. Softening of the laryngeal cartilage may produce respiratory distress. In older children the main problems are scoliosis and joint contractures. *X-rays* show epiphyseal hypo-

plasia and maldevelopment, metaphyseal thickening, flattening of the pelvis and kyphoscoliosis. Odontoid hypoplasia is usual.

Management involves early correction of joint contractures and treatment of club foot and hand deformities. Scoliosis may require correction and spinal fusion.

Cleidocranial dysplasia

This disorder, of autosomal dominant inheritance, is characterized by hypoplasia of the clavicles and flat bones. In a typical case the patient is somewhat short, with a large head, frontal prominence, a flat-looking face and drooping shoulders. The teeth appear late and develop poorly. Because the clavicles are hypoplastic or absent, the chest seems narrow and the patient can bring his shoulders together anteriorly. The pelvis is narrow but the symphysis pubis may be unduly wide and there may be some disproportion of the forearm or finger bones.

X-rays show a brachycephalic skull and persistence of wormian bones. Characteristically there is underdevelopment of the clavicles, scapulae and pelvis. Much of the clavicle may be missing, leaving a nubbin of bone at the medial or lateral end. Scoliosis and coxa vara are common.

Treatment is unnecessary unless the patient develops severe coxa vara or scoliosis; dental anomalies may need attention.

Nail–patella syndrome

This curious condition is relatively common and is inherited as an autosomal dominant trait.

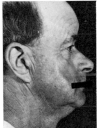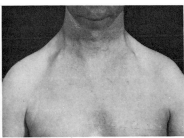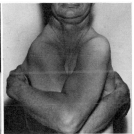

8.16 Cleidocranial dysplasia The squashed face and sloping shoulders which can be brought together anteriorly are pathognomonic.

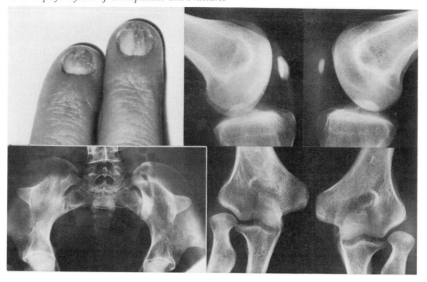

8.17 The nail–patella syndrome   The dystrophic nails, minute patellae, pelvic 'horns' and subluxed radii combine to make an unmistakable picture.

The nails are hypoplastic and the patellae unusually small or absent. The radial head is subluxed laterally and the elbows may lack full extension. Congenital nephropathy may be associated. The characteristic x-ray features are hypoplastic or absent patellae and the presence of bony protuberances ('horns') on the lateral aspect of the iliac blades.

Craniofacial dysplasia

Many disorders – some inherited, some not – are distinguished primarily by the abnormal appearance of the face and skull. Other bones may be affected as well, but it is the odd facial appearance that is most striking. Premature fusion of the cranial sutures may lead to exophthalmos and mental retardation. Orthopaedic problems arise from the associated anomalies of the hands and feet.

The best-known of these conditions is *Apert's syndrome* (acrocephalosyndactyly). The head is somewhat egg-shaped: flat at the back, narrow anteroposteriorly, with a broad, towering forehead, depressed face, bulging eyes and prominent jaw. The hands and feet are misshapen, with syndactyly or synostosis of the medial rays.

The condition sometimes shows autosomal dominant inheritance, but most cases are sporadic.

Cerebral compression can be prevented by early craniotomy and the facial appearance may be improved by maxillofacial reconstruction. Syndactyly may need operative treatment.

Connective tissue disorders

Collagen is the commonest form of body protein, making up 90% of the non-mineral bony matrix and 70% of the structural tissue in ligaments and tendons. Over ten types of collagen have been identified; those distributed most abundantly in the musculoskeletal system are *type I* (in bone, ligament, tendon and skin), *type II* (in cartilage) and *type III* (in blood vessels, muscle and skin).

Heritable defects of collagen synthesis give rise to a number of disorders involving either

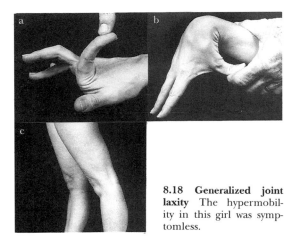

8.18 Generalized joint laxity The hypermobility in this girl was symptomless.

Marfan's syndrome

This is a generalized disorder affecting the skeleton, joint ligaments, eyes and cardiovascular structures. It is thought to be due to a cross-linkage defect in collagen and elastin.

CLINICAL FEATURES Patients are tall, with disproportionately long legs and arms, and often with flattening or hollowing of the chest (pectus excavatum). Typically, lower segment length is greater than upper segment, and arm span exceeds height. The digits are unusually long, giving rise to the term 'arachnodactyly' or 'spider fingers'. Spinal abnormalities include spondylolisthesis and scoliosis. There is an increased incidence of slipped upper femoral epiphysis. Generalized joint laxity is usual and patients may develop flat feet or dislocation of the patella or shoulder. Associated abnormalities include a high arched palate, hernias, lens dislocation, retinal detachment, aortic aneurysm and mitral or aortic incompetence.

X-RAYS Bone structure appears normal (apart from excessive length), but x-rays may reveal complications such as spondylolisthesis or slipped epiphysis.

GENETICS The condition is inherited as an autosomal dominant trait.

DIAGNOSIS 'Marfanoid' features are quite common and it is now thought that there are several *variants* of the underlying condition; in some, arachnodactyly is complicated by joint contractures. *Homocystinuria*, an inborn error of

the soft connective tissues or bone, or both. In some cases the specific collagen defect can be identified by special investigations.

Generalized (familial) joint laxity

About 5% of normal people have joint hypermobility. This trait runs in families and is inherited as a mendelian dominant. The condition is not in itself disabling but it may predispose to congenital dislocation of the hip in the newborn or recurrent dislocation of the patella or shoulder in later life. Transient joint pains are common and there is an increased risk of ankle sprains.

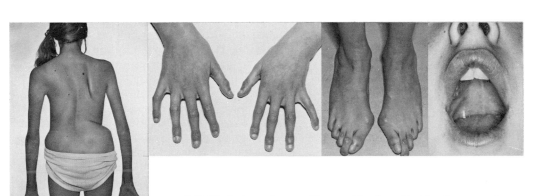

8.19 Marfan's syndrome The combination of spider fingers and toes with scoliosis is characteristic; the high-arched palate is sometimes associated.

methionine metabolism, has in the past been confused with Marfan's syndrome.

MANAGEMENT Patients occasionally need treatment for progressive scoliosis or flat feet. The heart should be carefully checked before operation.

Ehlers–Danlos syndrome

Ehlers–Danlos syndrome (EDS) is a heterogeneous condition characterized by unusual skin laxity, joint hypermobility and vascular fragility.

CLINICAL FEATURES Babies may show marked hypotonia and joint laxity. Hypermobility persists and older patients are often capable of bizarre feats of contortion. The skin is soft and hyperextensible; it is easily damaged and vascular fragility may give rise to 'spontaneous' bleeding. Joint instability, recurrent dislocations and scoliosis are common.

GENETICS Of the nine or ten types of EDS so far described, over 90% show autosomal dominant inheritance.

MANAGEMENT Complications (e.g. recurrent dislocation or scoliosis) may need treatment. However, if joint laxity is marked, soft-tissue reconstruction usually fails to cure the tendency to dislocation. Blood vessel fragility may cause severe bleeding at operation.

Larsen's syndrome

This is a heterogeneous condition, the more severe (recessive) forms presenting in infancy

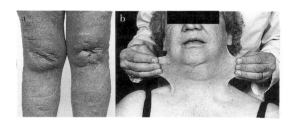

8.20 Ehlers–Danlos syndrome (a) This woman presented with these unpleasant but characteristic scars. (b) She also shows the usual remarkable skin hyperextensibility.

with marked joint laxity and dislocation of the hips, instability of the knees, subluxation of the radial head, equinovarus deformities of the feet and 'dish-face' appearance. Spinal deformities are common in older children. Mild forms of the same condition show autosomal dominant inheritance.

Operative treatment may be needed for joint instability and dislocation.

Osteogenesis imperfecta (brittle bones)

Osteogenesis imperfecta (OI) is one of the commonest of the heritable bone disorders, with an estimated incidence of 1 in 20 000. Because of the marked skeletal abnormalities it is often included among the bone dysplasias. However, it is basically a connective tissue disorder (defective synthesis of type I collagen) with generalized involvement of the bones, teeth, ligaments, sclerae and skin. It is a heterogeneous condition and there are at least four subgroups showing variations in phenotype and pattern of inheritance (Sillence, 1981). What they have in common are (1) osteopenia, (2) proneness to fracture and (3) laxity of ligaments. About two-thirds of patients have (4) blue sclerae and about half have (5) 'crumbling teeth', or dentinogenesis imperfecta.

CLINICAL FEATURES Following Sillence (1981), OI is separated into four clinical types.

OI type I (mild) This, the commonest variety, is a comparatively mild autosomal dominant disorder. Some children have broken bones at birth, but the majority develop fractures a year or two later – generally after minor trauma and often without local bruising or swelling. Fractures heal without difficulty and, provided alignment is maintained, deformities of the long bones are not severe. There may be delayed closure of the anterior fontanelle and head circumference is usually increased.

A characteristic and striking feature is the deep blue colour of the sclerae (due to defective scleral collagen tissue). In some families the teeth are affected as well; dentin is thin and breaks down easily. Generalized joint laxity is usual.

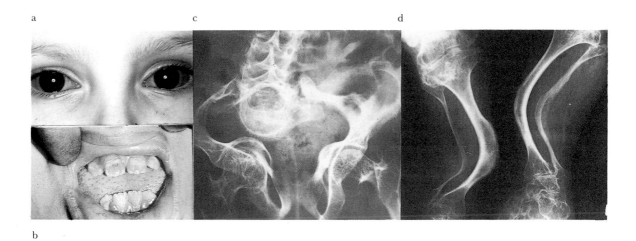

a

c

d

b

8.21 Osteogenesis imperfecta   (a) The typical blue sclerae and (b) faulty dentine in type I disease. (c, d) The deformities in a patient with type III disease.

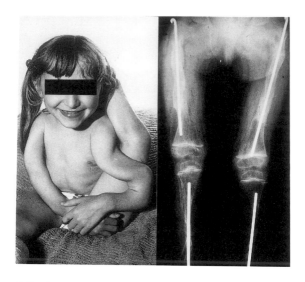

8.22 Osteogenesis imperfecta This patient had severe deformities of both legs; these were corrected by multiple osteotomies and 'rodding'.

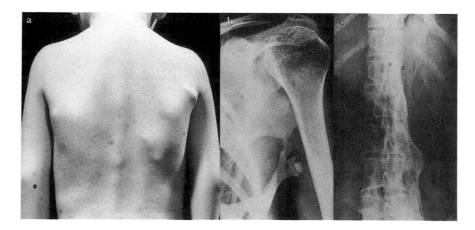

8.23 Fibrodysplasia ossificans progressiva (a) The lumps in this boy's back were hard and his back movements were limited. (b, c) This adult shows the extensive soft-tissue ossification.

After adolescence fractures become less frequent, but early deformities persist and mild kyphoscoliosis is common. There is usually only moderate shortness of stature. Adults often develop impaired hearing.

X-rays show osteopenia and thinning of the cortices. Old fractures are usually evident and there may be some bowing of the long bones. Adults may present with early-onset vertebral osteoporosis. In very mild cases the diagnosis may be missed altogether.

OI type II (lethal)   This severe, lethal disorder may be diagnosed before birth by x-ray or ultrasound imaging. Some infants are still-born, and those who survive have multiple fractures and deformities of the long bones, giving the extremities a crumpled appearance. The skull is large but poorly ossified, with wormian bones. Surprisingly the sclerae look normal. Respiratory difficulties are common and the infant seldom survives more than a few weeks. Most cases are sporadic but some show autosomal recessive inheritance.

OI type III (severe, deforming)   This is the classic, though not the commonest, form of OI. It is sometimes diagnosed at birth and by the age of 6 years the child has had numerous fractures and has usually developed severe deformities of the limbs and kyphoscoliosis. Joint laxity is marked. There is delayed closure of the fontanelles and enlargement of the skull with a pinched, somewhat triangular, face. The sclerae may be blue–grey at first but gradually become lighter. X-rays reveal severe osteopenia and multiple fractures in various stages of healing. Hyperplastic callus may develop after a femoral fracture and is occasionally mistaken for sarcoma! There are wormian bones in the skull. This autosomal recessive disorder is not as severe as type II, but few of the children survive into adulthood; those who do are markedly dwarfed and disabled.

OI type IV (moderately severe)   This autosomal dominant disorder is similar to type I. Fractures may be present at birth or later in childhood, but they become less frequent after adolescence. Deformities, including scoliosis and short stature, are usual. However, unlike type I, the sclerae are only a pale blue and they become normal in colour in adult life; hearing is seldom affected.

MANAGEMENT   The most severe forms of OI (type II) defy treatment and none is indicated apart from sympathetic nursing care. For other types of OI, treatment is aimed at: (1) gentle nursing of infants to prevent fractures as far as possible; (2) prompt splinting when fractures do occur, to prevent unnecessary deformity; (3) mobilization, to prevent further osteoporosis; and (4) correction of deformities, if necessary by multiple osteotomies, bone realignment and intramedullary fixation (Sofield and Millar, 1959). To allow for growth, elongating rods may be used (Marafioti and Westin, 1977; Lang-Stevenson and Sharrard, 1984).

Scoliosis is particularly difficult to treat. Bracing is ineffectual and progressive curves require operative stabilization and spinal fusion (Benson, Donaldson and Millar, 1978).

After adolescence, fractures are much less common and patients may pursue a reasonably comfortable and useful life.

Fibrodysplasia ossificans progressiva

This rare condition, formerly known as myositis ossificans progressiva, is characterized by widespread ossification of the connective tissue of muscle, mainly in the trunk. It starts in early childhood with episodes of fever and soft-tissue inflammation around the shoulders and trunk. As this subsides the tissues harden and plaques of ossification extend throughout the affected areas. In the worst cases movements are restricted and the patient is severely disabled. Associated anomalies are shortening of the big toe and thumb. The condition is probably transmitted as an autosomal dominant but, since affected individuals seldom have children, most cases result from new mutations. Treatment with diphosphonates may prevent progression.

Storage disorders and other metabolic defects

Many single gene disorders are expressed as undersecretion of an enzyme that controls a specific stage in the metabolic chain; the undegraded substrate accumulates and may be stored, with harmful effects, in various tissues or be excreted in the urine. Conditions involving the musculoskeletal system are the mucopolysaccharidoses (MPS), Gaucher's disease, homocystinuria, alkaptonuria and congenital hyperuricaemia. All these inborn errors of metabolism are inherited as recessive traits.

Mucopolysaccharidoses

The polysaccharide glycosaminoglycans (GAGs) form the side-chains of macromolecular proteoglycans, a major component of the matrix in bone, cartilage, intervertebral discs, synovium and other connective tissues. Defunct proteoglycans are degraded by lysosomal enzymes. Deficiency of any of these enzymes causes a hold-up on the degradative pathway. Partially degraded GAGs accumulate in the lysosomes in the liver, spleen, bones and other tissues, and spill over in the blood and urine where they can be detected by suitable biochemical tests. Confirmation of the enzyme lack can be obtained by tests on cultured fibroblasts.

CLINICAL FEATURES Depending on the specific enzyme deficiency and the type of GAG storage, at least six clinical syndromes have been defined. As a group they have certain recognizable features: dwarfism with vertebral deformity, coarse facies, hepatosplenomegaly and (in some cases) mental retardation. X-rays show bone dysplasia affecting the vertebral bodies, epiphyses and metaphyses; typically the bones have a spatulate appearance.

There is a superficial similarity to spondyloepiphyseal and spondylometaphyseal dysplasia. However, careful observation reveals several points of difference, and the diagnosis can be confirmed by testing for abnormal GAG excretion or demonstrating the enzyme deficiency in blood cells or cultured skin fibroblasts.

Hurler's syndrome (MPS I) Infants look normal at birth but over the next 2–3 years they gradually develop a typical appearance: they are undersized, with increasing kyphosis, hepatosplenomegaly, coarse facies, protruding tongue and mental retardation. Joints are stiff and

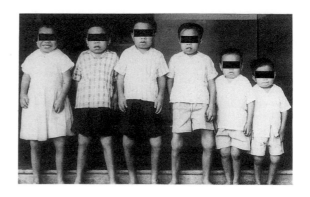

8.24 Mucopolysaccharidoses The appearance of a group of children with Hurler's syndrome. (Courtesy of Prof. K. Bose of Singapore.)

there may be corneal opacities, respiratory difficulty and cardiac anomalies. X-rays usually show unmistakable features such as hypoplastic epiphyses and vertebral bodies, poorly modelled metaphyses, short but wide metacarpals, underdeveloped mandible, spatulate ribs and clavicles, flared iliac blades and shallow acetabuli. Cardiac or respiratory complications usually cause death in later childhood.

Hunter's syndrome (MPS II) This is also a recessive disorder, but X-linked – so all patients are male. Clinical features are similar to those of Hurler's syndrome, but less severe.

Morquio–Brailsford syndrome (MPS IV) Development seems normal for the first year or two. Thereafter the child beings to look dwarfed, with a moderate kyphosis, short neck and protuberant sternum. There is joint laxity and progressive genu valgum. However, the face is unaffected and intelligence is normal. X-rays of the spine show the typical ovoid, hypoplastic vertebral bodies, which end up abnormally flat (platyspondyly) and peculiarly pointed anteriorly. Odontoid hypoplasia is usual. A marked manubriosternal angle (almost 90 degrees) is pathognomonic. By the age of 5 years the femoral head epiphyses are underdeveloped and flat, and the acetabuli abnormally shallow. The long bones are of normal width but the metacarpals may be short and broad, and pointed at their proximal ends.

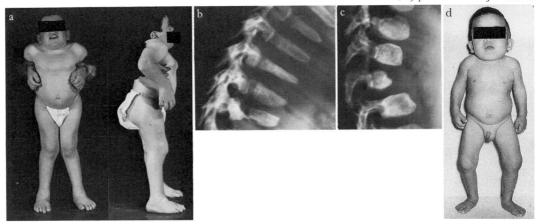

8.25 Mucopolysaccharidoses (a) Morquio–Brailsford syndrome – note the manubriosternal angle. (b) Platyspondyly in a similar patient, contrasted with (c) the sabot appearance in Hurler's syndrome. (d) A boy with Hunter's syndrome; his appearance is similar to that in Hurler's syndrome.

MANAGEMENT There is no specific treatment for the mucopolysaccharide disorder. Hurler's syndrome has a very poor prognosis but the complications (e.g. respiratory infection) may need treatment. Morquio's syndrome presents several orthopaedic problems. Genu valgum may need correction by femoral osteotomy, though this should be delayed till growth has ceased. Coxa valga and subluxation of the hips, if symmetrical, may cause little disability; unilateral subluxation may need femoral or acetabular osteotomy. Atlantoaxial instability may threaten the cord and require occipitocervical fusion. All the 'spondylodysplasias' carry a risk of atlantoaxial subluxation during anaesthesia and intubation, and special precautions are needed during operation (Kopits et al., 1972).

Table 8.1 Enzyme defect and GAG excretion in the commoner mucopolysaccharidoses

Syndrome	Enzyme defect	GAG excretion
Hurler (MPS I)	Iduronidase	Dermatan sulphate Heparan sulphate
Hunter (MPS II)	Iduronate sulphatase	Dermatan sulphate Heparan sulphate
Morquio (MPS IV)	N-Acetylgalactosamine-4-sulphatase.	Keratan sulphate

Gaucher's disease

Lack of the enzyme β-glycosidase results in macromolecular cerebrosides accumulating in the reticuloendothelial cells of the marrow, spleen and other tissues. A rare lethal form causes infiltration of the brain. A chronic form of the disorder, most common in Jews of the Ashkenazi sect, causes marked bone changes and splenomegaly. Like other storage disorders, it is inherited as an autosomal recessive trait.

CLINICAL FEATURES Patients present in childhood or adult life, with bone pain and loss of movement in one of the larger joints. There may be acute crises, closely resembling osteomyelitis or septic arthritis. Indeed, Gaucher's disease predisposes to infection and this may be a source of confusion. Pathological fracture is rare. The spleen may be enlarged – or it may have been removed.

X-RAYS show a variable pattern of radiolucency or patchy density, more marked in cancellous bone. The distal end of the femur may be expanded – the Erlenmeyer flask appearance. Avascular necrosis of the femoral head is a frequent complication. Gaucher crises can be distinguished from infection by an early bone scan: a 'cold' scan strongly suggests a crisis.

MANAGEMENT Bone pain may need symptomatic treatment. For the acute crisis, hyperbaric oxygen is recommended. Avascular necrosis

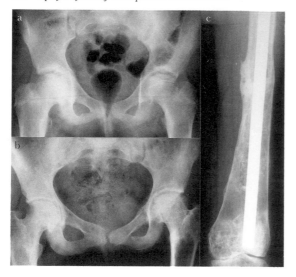

8.26 Gaucher's disease X-rays taken (a) at the age of 12 and (b) at 25 show avascular necrosis of the femoral head and an area of increased radiolucency in the proximal femur on the left side. (c) Two years later this patient was treated for a pathological fracture of the left femur. The distal end of the bone shows the typical modelling defect; there are also sclerotic patches in the metaphysis suggesting medullary infarcts.

may call for operation (see p. 102). Recently, replacement therapy with macrophage targeted glucocerebrosidase has shown promising results (Barton et al., 1991).

Homocystinuria

This rare disorder is due to deficiency of the enzyme cystathionine β-synthetase and accumulation of homocysteine and methionine. Patients are tall and thin and may have joint laxity and dislocation of the lens – features reminiscent of Marfan's disease (p. 151). However, unlike Marfan's disease, homocystinuria is of autosomal recessive inheritance and is associated with marked osteoporosis and mental retardation. Thromboembolic disease is common and may be fatal. Homocysteine levels are raised in the blood and urine. The enzyme deficiency may be detected in fibroblast cultures. Though rare, the condition should be diagnosed because it can be treated: about half

the patients are 'cured' by pyridoxine administered from early childhood (Rowe and Shapiro, 1989). Others may be helped by a low methionine, cysteine-supplemented diet.

Alkaptonuria

Deficiency of the enzyme homogentisic acid oxidase leads to accumulation of homogentisic acid, which is deposited in connective tissue and excreted in the urine. On standing the urine turns dark (hence the name, alkaptonuria); cartilage and other connective tissues are stained grey – a condition referred to as ochronosis. Clinical problems arise from degenerative changes in articular cartilage with the development of osteoarthritis, and from calcification of the intervertebral discs.

Congenital hyperuricaemia

The Lesch–Nyhan syndrome is a rare, X-linked recessive disorder causing absence of the enzyme hypoxanthine-guanine phosphoribosyltransferase (HGPRT). This enzyme controls a 'salvage pathway' in the complex purine metabolic chain; absence of HGPRT results in excessive uric acid formation and gout. The young boys are mentally retarded and prone to self-mutilation (gnawing the ends of their fingers). Milder cases present simply as early-onset severe gout. Diagnosis can be confirmed by measuring HGPRT in red cell preparations.

Chromosome disorders

Chromosome disorders are common but usually result in fetal abortion. Of the nonlethal conditions, several produce bone or joint abnormalities.

Down's syndrome (trisomy 21)

This condition results from having an extra copy of chromosome 21. It is much more common than any of the skeletal dysplasias, with an overall incidence of 1 per 800 live births – and 1 in 250 if the mother is over 37 years of age. Affected infants can be recognized at birth: the head is foreshortened and the eyes slant upwards, with prominent epicanthic folds; the nose is flattened, the lips are parted and the tongue protrudes. There may be abnormal palmar creases, clinodactyly and spreading of the first and second toes. The babies are unusually floppy (hypotonic) and skeletal development is delayed. Children are short and, because of their characteristic facial appearance, they tend to resemble each other. They show varying degrees of metal retardation.

Adults have a significant incidence of atlantoaxial instability, though fortunately this seldom causes neurological complications (Roy, Baxter and Roy, 1990). Associated anomalies, particularly cardiac defects, are common, and there is diminished resistance to infection. Life expectancy is about 35 years.

There is no specific treatment but surgery can offer considerable cosmetic improvement, and attentive care will allow many of these individuals to pursue a pleasant and productive life.

Turner's syndrome

Congenital female hypogonadism is a rare abnormality caused by a defect in one of the X chromosomes. Those affected are phenotypically female, with a normal vagina and uterus, but the ovaries are markedly hypoplastic or absent. Patients are short, with webbing of the neck, barrel chest and increased carrying angle of the elbows. Cardiovascular and renal abnormalities are common. They have primary amenorrhoea, and hypogonadism leads to early-onset osteoporosis. Treatment consists of oestrogen replacement from puberty onwards.

Klinefelter's syndrome

The Klinefelter syndrome, a form of male hypogonadism, occurs in about 1 per 1000 males. Those affected have more than one X chromosome (as well as the usual Y chromosome). They are recognizably male, but they have eunuchoid proportions, with gynaecomastia and underdeveloped testicles. The condition should be borne in mind as a cause of osteoporosis in men (see p. 119). Treatment with androgens may improve bone mass.

Localized malformations

Localized malformations of the vertebrae or limbs are common. The majority cause no disability and may be discovered incidentally during investigation of some other disorder. Some have a genetic background and similar malformations are seen in association with generalized skeletal dysplasia. Most are sporadic and probably non-genetic – i.e. caused by injury to the developing embryo, especially during the first 3 months of pregnancy. In some cases there is a known teratogenic agent; for example, maternal infection or drug administration. Usually, however, the exact cause is unknown.

Vertebral anomalies

These are of three main kinds: (1) agenesis, with total absence of vertebrae; (2) dysgenesis, with hemivertebrae, or with vertebrae fused together (sometimes called errors of segmentation); and (3) dyraphism, with deficiencies of the neural arch. These are considered in the sections on spinal deformity and spina bifida. Corresponding sacral anomalies are also encountered; associated visceral anomalies are common in sacral dysgenesis but not in agenesis, and dysraphism may be complicated by urogenital problems.

Klippel–Feil syndrome

In this segmentation defect there is fusion of two or more cervical vertebrae. The patient has an unusually short neck, sometimes with webbing, and neck movements are restricted. Associated anomalies are common and include hemivertebra, posterior arch defects, cervical

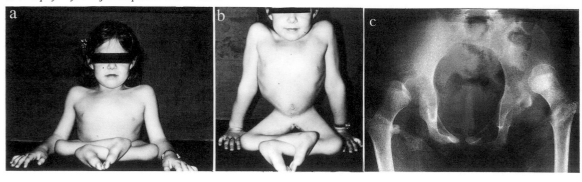

8.27 Sacral agenesis This girl shows (a) the characteristic sitting posture and (b) the spinal hump. (c) The sacrum is absent and the hips are dislocated.

meningomyelocele, thoracic defects, scapular elevation and visceral abnormalities. X-rays may show various combinations of these disorders, together with scoliosis or kyphosis. Treatment is usually not necessary, but scoliosis may require correction and fusion; occasionally, operative relief is needed for threatened cord compression.

Thoracospinal anomalies

Segmentation defects in the thoracic regions usually involve the ribs as well; for example, hemivertebrae may be associated with fusion of adjacent ribs or other types of dysplasia. Some of these disorders are of autosomal dominant inheritance. Clinically, patients present in childhood with scoliosis or kyphoscoliosis, sometimes leading to paraplegia. X-rays may show various combinations of thoracic vertebral fusion or dysgenesis and rib anomalies, together with scoliosis and marked distortion of the thorax. Operative treatment may be needed for threatened cord compression.

Elevation of the scapula (Sprengel deformity)

Mild degrees of congenital elevation of the scapula are common. In the full-blown Sprengel deformity the child has obvious asymmetry

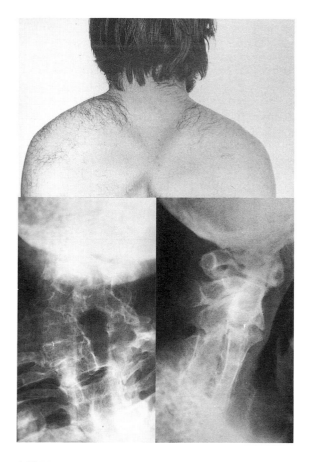

8.28 Klippel–Feil syndrome The short neck and vertebral anomalies in a typical patient.

of the shoulders, with elevation and under-development of the affected side. The scapula is abnormally small and too high. Sometimes the clavicle is affected as well. Shoulder movements, especially abduction, may be restricted. Occasionally both sides are involved.

This condition, which usually occurs sporadically, represents a failure of scapular descent from the cervical spine. Associated vertebral or rib anomalies are quite common.

Treatment is required only if shoulder movements are severely limited or if the deformity is particularly unsightly. The vertebroscapular muscles are released from the spine, the supraspinous part of the scapula is excised together with the omovertebral bar and the scapula is repositioned by tightening the lower muscles. The operation is best performed before the age of 6 years.

Limb anomalies

These include extra bones, absent bones, hypoplastic bones and fusions. Complete absence of a limb is called amelia, almost complete absence (a mere stub remaining) phocomelia and partial absence ectromelia; defects may be transverse or axial. In the hands and feet brachydactyly, syndactyly, polydactyly and symphalangism are among the many possibilities.

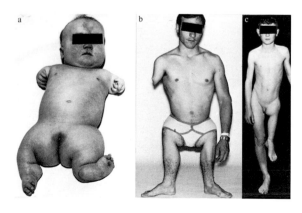

8.29 Congenital limb anomalies (a) A thalidomide baby, with all four limbs severely affected. (b) This man, with three limbs affected, had almost complete absence of his femora. (c) Severe dysplasia of one femur – leg length inequality was the major problem here.

Most of these defects are non-genetic but some are of autosomal dominant inheritance. Detailed elaboration of terminology interests the philologist more than the surgeon.

Radial deficiency

Absence or hypoplasia of the radius may occur alone or in association with visceral anomalies or – more rarely – certain blood dyscrasias. Sometimes the thumb is missing too, and the elbow is often abnormal. The clinical deformity (radial club hand) may look bizarre but children often acquire excellent function. If this seems unlikely, operative reconstruction may be advisable (usually after the age of 3 years).

Ulnar deficiency

Hypoplasia of the distal end of the ulna is usually seen as part of a generalized dysplasia, but occasionally it occurs alone. The radius is bowed (as if growth is tethered on the ulnar side) and the radial head may dislocate; the wrist is deviated medially. Only if function is severely disturbed should wrist stabilization be advised.

Femoral deficiency

In its most benign form shortening is less than 7 cm and treatment no different from that for other types of leg length inequality. But if the dysplasia is combined with coxa vara, shortening may be too severe for practicable leg lengthening; artificial extension may be feasible but amputation often permits greater prosthetic elegance. If the entire upper third of the femur is missing the situation is still worse; but the 'absent' part may in fact be cartilaginous, in which case bone grafting can provide hip stability and therefore more satisfactory limb-fitting. Good prognostic features are: a good acetabulum; a large gap between the acetabulum and the radiologically visible part of the upper femur; and a bulbous end to the upper femur. If the upper third (or even more) is truly absent the only prospect for even mediocre prosthetic fitting is to perform one of several heroic operations described by van Nes; for example, femoral rotation osteotomies to make the foot point backwards so that its muscles activate the 'knee' of a prosthesis.

Tibial and fibular deficiencies

Absence of the tibia is extremely rare and usually demands amputation.

Absence of part or all of the fibula – and sometimes the fourth and fifth rays of the foot as well – results in tibial bowing, shortening of the leg and valgus deformity of the foot. Leg lengthening is difficult and, if tibial osteotomy seems inappropriate, amputation is needed.

Synostosis

The various types of interosseous fusion (radio-ulnar, tibiofibular, carpal or tarsal) are discussed in the relevant chapters. They rarely cause significant disability, excepting tarsal synostosis (which may be associated with spastic flat foot) or radioulnar fusion which limits forearm supination (a considerable disability if both forearms are affected). In spastic flat foot, division or removal of the bony bridge may improve symptoms. Radioulnar fusion resists any form of operative mobilization, because of the associated soft-tissue involvement. However, the bones can be osteotomized and rotated to leave the hand in a more functional position.

Digital anomalies

There are numerous digital anomalies – missing digits, extra digits, fused digits, short digits or split deformities of the hand or foot – which may occur in isolation, in combination with each other or as part of a generalized dysplasia. Short digits seldom require any form of treatment. Extra digits, if simply hanging by a neck of skin, can be amputated at any time. The more complex anomalies, which involve not only bone but also the associated muscle and neurovascular structures, may be treated by operative reconstruction when the child is 3–4 years old – but only after painstaking assessment and by someone experienced in this branch of surgery.

'Congenital pseudarthrosis'

Fracture followed by intractable non-union is sometimes seen in the tibia or clavicle – but not necessarily at birth.

Tibial pseudarthrosis usually presents with anterior bowing of the tibia during the first 2 years of life. X-ray may show a gap, or marked thinning of the midshaft. Sometimes the fibula is affected too. Biopsy of the abnormal segment may show histological features of neurofibromatosis or fibrous dysplasia. The condition resists all attempts at promoting union by immobilization or internal fixation. Bone grafting and rigid immobilization in an external fixator may

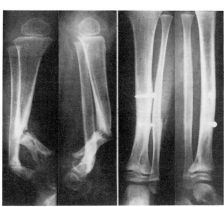
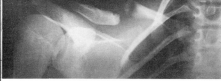

8.30 Congenital pseudarthrosis The tibia is the commonest site; in this case bone-grafting was successful. This clavicular pseudarthrosis (from a different patient) is of course on the right.

succeed, and transferring the unaffected fibula as a vascularized graft is nearly always successful (Weiland et al., 1990).

Pseudarthrosis of the clavicle is probably due to pressure by the subclavian artery on the developing bone. In every reported unilateral case the right side has been affected – except in the presence of dextrocardia. The child is brought up with a painless lump. Treatment, if required, is by excision or grafting.

References and further reading

Barton, N.W., Brady, R.O., Dambrosia, J.M. et al. (1991) Replacement therapy for inherited enzyme deficiency – macrophage targeted glucocerebrosidase for Gaucher's disease. *New England Journal of Medicine* **324**, 1464–1470

Benson, D.R., Donaldson, D.H. and Millar, E.A. (1978) The spine in osteogenesis imperfecta. *Journal of Bone and Joint Surgery* **60A**, 925–929

Goldblatt, J., Sachs, S. and Beighton, P. (1978) The orthopaedic aspects of Gaucher's disease. *Clinical Orthopaedics and Related Research* **137**, 208–214

Horan, F.T. and Beighton, P.H. (1980) Infantile metaphyseal dysplasias or 'battered babies'. *Journal of Bone and Joint Surgery* **62B**, 243–247

Kettelkamp, D.B., Campbell, C.J. and Bonfiglio, M. (1966) Dysplasia epiphysialis hemimelica. *Journal of Bone and Joint Surgery* **48A**, 746–766

Kopits, S.E. (1976) Orthopaedic complications of dwarfism. *Clinical Orthopaedics and Related Research* **114**, 153–179

Kopits, S.E., Perovic, M.N., McKusick, V.A., Robinson, R.A. and Bailey, J.A. (1972) Congenital atlantoaxial dislocations in various forms of dwarfism. *Journal of Bone and Joint Surgery* **54A**, 1349–1350

Lang-Stevenson, A.I. and Sharrard, W.J.W. (1984) Intramedullary rodding with Bailey–Dubow extensible rods in osteogenesis imperfecta. *Journal of Bone and Joint Surgery* **66B**, 227–232

Lutter, L.D. and Langer, L.O. (1977) Neurological complications in achondroplastic dwarfs – surgical treatment. *Journal of Bone and Joint Surgery* **59A**, 87–92

Marafioti, R.L. and Westin, G.W. (1977) Elongating intramedullary rods in the treatment of osteogenesis imperfecta. *Journal of Bone and Joint Surgery* **59A**, 467–472

Marks, S.C. Jr (1984) Congenital osteopetrotic mutations as probes of the origin, structure and function of osteoclasts. *Clinical Orthopaedics and Related Research* **189**, 239–263

Maroteaux, P. and Lamy, M. (1965) The malady of Toulouse-Lautrec. *Journal of the American Medical Association* **191**, 715–717

Rowe, D.W. and Shapiro, J.R. (1989) Heritable disorders of structural proteins. In *Textbook of Rheumatology* (eds. W.N. Kelley, E.D. Harris, S. Ruddy and C.B. Sledge), W.B. Saunders, Philadelphia, pp. 1691–1703

Roy, M., Baxter, M. and Roy, A. (1990) Atlantoaxial instability in Down's syndrome – guidelines for screening and detection. *Journal of the Royal Society of Medicine* **83**, 433–435

Schwartz, H.S., Zimmerman, N.B., Simon, M.A. et al. (1987) The malignant potential of enchondromatosis. *Journal of Bone and Joint Surgery* **69A**, 269–274

Sillence, D. (1981) Osteogenesis imperfecta: an expanding panorama of variants. *Clinical Orthopaedics and Related Research* **159**, 11–25

Sofield, H.A. and Millar, E.A. (1959) Fragmentation, realignment and intramedullary rod fixation of deformities of the long bones in children. *Journal of Bone and Joint Surgery* **41A**, 1371–1391

Solomon, L. (1963) Hereditary multiple exostosis. *Journal of Bone and Joint Surgery* **45B**, 292–304

Weiland, A.J., Weiss, A.-P.C., Moore, J.R. and Tolo, V.T. (1990) Vascularized fibular grafts in the treatment of congenital pseudarthrosis of the tibia. *Journal of Bone and Joint Surgery* **72A**, 654–662

Tumours

9

Tumours, tumour-like lesions and cysts are considered together, partly because their clinical presentation and management are similar and partly because the definitive classification of bone tumours is still evolving and some disorders may yet move from one category to another. Benign lesions are quite common, primary malignant ones rare; yet so often do they mimic each other, and so critical are the decisions on treatment, that a working knowledge of all the important conditions is necessary.

Classification

Most classifications of bone tumours are based on the recognition of the dominant tissue in the various lesions (Table 9.1). This has several drawbacks: (1) the most pervasive tissue is not necessarily the tissue of origin; (2) there is no pathological or clinical connection between the conditions in any particular category; (3) there is often no relationship between benign and malignant lesions with similar tissue elements (e.g. osteoma and osteosarcoma); and (4) some tumours named as simple entities (e.g. osteosarcoma) comprise several lesions with different behaviour patterns.

Clinical presentation

Age may be a useful clue. Many benign lesions present during childhood and adolescence –

162

Table 9.1 A classification of the less rare primary bone tumours

Cell type	Benign	Malignant
Bone	Osteoid osteoma	Osteosarcoma
Cartilage	Chondroma Osteochondroma	Chondrosarcoma
Fibrous tissue	Fibroma	Fibrosarcoma
Marrow	Eosinophilic granuloma	Ewing's sarcoma Myeloma
Vascular	Haemangioma	Angiosarcoma
Uncertain	Giant-cell tumour	Malignant giant-cell tumour

but so do some primary malignant tumours, notably Ewing's tumour and osteosarcoma. Chondrosarcoma and fibrosarcoma typically occur in older people (4th to 6th decades); and myeloma, the commonest of all primary malignant bone tumours, is seldom seen before the 6th decade. In patients over 70 years of age, metastasis is more common than all primary tumours together.

Patients may be completely *asymptomatic* until the abnormality is discovered on x-ray. This is much more likely with benign lesions; and, since some of these (e.g. non-ossifying fibroma) are common in children but rare after the age of 30, they must be capable of spontaneous resolution. Malignant tumours, too, may remain silent if they are slow-growing and situated where there is room for inconspicuous expansion (e.g. the cavity of the pelvis).

Pain is a common complaint and gives no indication of the nature of the lesion. It may be caused by rapid expansion with stretching of surrounding tissues, central haemorrhage or degeneration in the tumour, or a small fatigue fracture. However, even a tiny lesion may be very painful if it is encapsulated in dense bone (e.g. an osteoid osteoma).

Swelling, or the appearance of *a lump*, may be alarming. Often, though, patients seek advice only when a mass becomes painful or continues to grow.

A *history of trauma* is offered so frequently that it cannot be dismissed (Monkman, Orwoll and Ivins, 1974). Yet, whether the injury initiates a pathological change or merely draws attention to what is already there remains unanswered.

Neurological symptoms (paraesthesiae or numbness) may be caused by pressure upon or stretching of a peripheral nerve. Progressive dysfunction is more ominous and suggests invasion by an aggressive tumour.

Pathological fracture may be the first (and only) clinical signal. Suspicion is aroused if the injury was slight; in elderly people, whose bones usually fracture at the corticocancellous junctions, any break in the mid-shaft should be regarded as pathological until proved otherwise.

Examination focuses on the symptomatic part, but it should include also the area of lymphatic drainage and, often, the abdomen, chest and spine. If there is a *lump*, where does it arise? Is it discrete or ill-defined? Is it soft or hard? And is it tender? *Swelling* may be more diffuse, and the overlying skin warm and inflamed; it can be difficult to distinguish a tumour from haematoma or infection. With a tumour near the joint there may be an *effusion* and *limitation of movement*. Spinal lesions, whether benign or malignant, often cause painful *muscle spasm* and *back stiffness*.

Imaging

Plain x-rays are the most useful of all imaging techniques. General characteristics such as the site of the 'tumour', its size, outline and internal architecture, and the presence or

---

Questions to ask when looking at an x-ray (Watt, 1985)

Is the lesion solitary or multiple?
What type of bone is involved?
Where is the lesion in the bone?
Are the margins of the lesion well- or ill-defined?
Is there a bony reaction?
Does the lesion contain calcification?

---

absence of periosteal new bone, usually suggest – at the very least – a differential diagnosis. With benign lesions, the changes tend to be well defined: a bony outgrowth, or a circumscribed 'vacant area' with the appearance of a cyst; however, 'cystic' lesions are not necessarily hollow cavities: any radiolucent material (e.g. a fibroma) may look like a cyst. The boundary of the cyst may be well defined and even sclerotic (a 'hard' endosteal margin), suggesting a very slow-growing and probably benign lesion; or it may be more hazy and diffuse (a 'soft' endosteal margin), characteristic of osteoclastic bone resorption; most ominous is diffuse invasion of the bone with extensive areas of destruction. Diffuse periosteal new-bone formation and extension of the tumour into the soft tissues are likewise suggestive of malignant change. Serial x-rays are the best way of showing progressive (i.e. aggressive!) enlargement of a bone tumour. With suspected malignant tumours, a chest x-ray is essential.

For all its informative detail, the x-ray alone can seldom be relied on for a definitive diagnosis. With some notable exceptions, in which the appearances are pathognomonic (e.g. osteochondroma, non-ossifying fibroma, osteoid osteoma), further investigations are essential. *If further imaging is planned, this should be done before the biopsy*, which itself may distort the scintigraphic, CT or MR appearances.

Radionuclide scanning with ^{99m}Tc-HDP shows non-specific reactive changes in bone; this can be most helpful in revealing the site of a small tumour (e.g. an osteoid osteoma) that does not show up clearly on x-ray. Skeletal scintigraphy is also the best method of detecting skip lesions or 'silent' secondary deposits.

Computed tomography (CT) extends the range of x-ray diagnosis; it shows more accurately both intraosseous and extraosseous extension of the tumour and the relationship to surrounding structures. It may also reveal suspected lesions in inaccessible sites, like the vertebra or pelvis; and it is the most reliable method of detecting pulmonary metastases.

Magnetic resonance imaging (MRI) provides further refinement of diagnostic information. Its greatest value is in the assessment of tumour spread – (1) within the bone, (2) into a nearby joint and (3) into the soft tissues (Pettersson et al., 1987). Blood vessels and the relationship of the tumour to the perivascular space are well defined.

Laboratory investigations

Blood tests are often necessary to exclude other conditions (e.g. infection or metabolic bone disorders). *Anaemia*, increased *ESR* and elevated *serum alkaline phosphatase* levels are non-specific findings, but if other causes are excluded they may help in differentiating between benign and malignant bone lesions. *Serum protein electrophoresis* may reveal an abnormal globulin fraction and the urine may contain *Bence-Jones protein* in patients with myeloma. A raised *serum acid phosphatase* suggests prostatic carcinoma.

Biopsy

With few exceptions, biopsy is essential for accurate diagnosis and planning of treatment. If sufficient expertise is available, this can be done with a *large-bore needle*. However, this does not always yield sufficient material, and when it does the tissue may not be representative or suitable for accurate diagnosis; its greatest value is in sampling inaccessible tumours (e.g. in a vertebral body). *Open biopsy* is much more

reliable: the site is selected without exposing much of the tumour and a block of tissue is removed – ideally in the boundary zone so as to include normal tissue, pseudocapsule and abnormal tissue. If necessary, several samples can be obtained. If bone is removed the raw area is covered with bone wax or methylmethacrylate cement. The wound should be closed without drainage, so as to minimize the risk of tumour contamination. The biopsy is best performed in the centre where the patient will be treated; planning the site and the route of access is part of the definitive surgical management, because the biopsy scar may have to be included in the subsequent excision and it should be placed so as not to compromise any subsequent ablative operation.

For benign tumours an *excisional biopsy* is permissible (the entire lesion is removed); with cysts that need operations, representative tissue can be obtained by careful curettage. In either case, histological confirmation of the diagnosis is essential.

When dealing with tumours that could be malignant, there is a strong temptation to perform the biopsy as soon as possible; as this may alter the CT and MRI appearances, it is important to delay the biopsy until all the imaging studies have been completed.

Differential diagnosis

A number of conditions may mimic a tumour, either clinically or radiologically. It is vital to exclude these common dissemblers before making the final diagnosis.

Haematoma

A large, clotted subperiosteal or soft-tissue haematoma may present as a painful lump in the arm or lower limb. Sometimes the x-ray shows an irregular surface on the underlying bone. Important clues are the history and the rapid onset of symptoms.

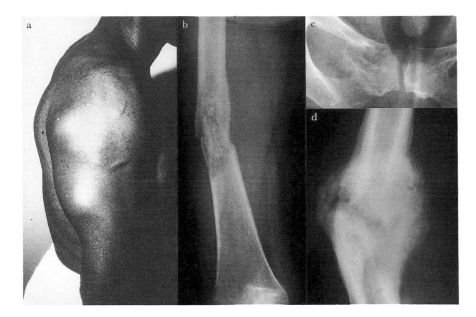

9.1 Tumours – differential diagnosis (1) (a) This huge swelling was simply a clotted haematoma. (b) Fracture through an area of osteomyelitis. (c) Stress fracture in an old woman. (d) Florid callus.

Infection

Osteomyelitis typically causes pain and swelling near one of the larger joints; as with primary bone tumours, the patients are usually children or young adults. X-rays may show an area of destruction with periosteal new bone in the metaphysis. Systemic features, especially if the patient has been treated with antibiotics, may be mild. If the area is explored, tissue should be submitted for both bacteriological and histological examination.

Stress fracture

Some of the worst mistakes have been made in misdiagnosing a stress fracture. The patient is often a young adult with localized pain near a large joint; x-rays show a dubious area of cortical 'destruction' and overlying periosteal new bone; if a biopsy is performed the healing callus may show histological features resembling those of osteosarcoma. If the pitfall is recognized, and there is adequate consultation between surgeon, radiologist and pathologist, a serious error can be prevented.

Myositis ossificans

Though rare, this may be a source of confusion. Following an injury the patient develops a tender swelling in the vicinity of a joint; the

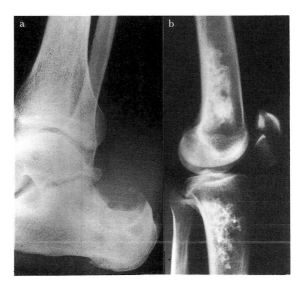

9.2 Tumours – differential diagnosis (2) (a) Tophaceous gout. (b) Bone infarcts.

x-ray shows fluffy density in the soft tissue adjacent to bone. Unlike a malignant tumour, however, the condition soon becomes less painful and the new bone better defined and well demarcated.

Gout

Occasionally a large gouty tophus causes a painful swelling at one of the bone ends, and x-ray shows a large, poorly defined excavation. If it is kept in mind the diagnosis will be easily confirmed – if necessary by obtaining a biopsy from the lump.

Staging

In treating tumours we strive to reconcile two conflicting principles: the lesion must be removed as widely as is necessary; but damage must be kept to a minimum. Choosing the boundary between these objectives depends on knowing (1) how the tumour usually behaves (i.e. how aggressive it is) and (2) how far it has spread. The answers to these two questions are embodied in the staging system developed by Enneking (1986).

Aggressiveness

Tumours are graded not only on their cytological characteristics but also on their clinical behaviour; i.e. the likelihood of recurrence and spread after surgical removal. Benign lesions, by definition, occupy the lowest grade: the meekest of them either remain quiescent or disappear spontaneously (e.g. non-osteogenic fibroma); the worst of them are difficult to distinguish from a low-grade sarcoma and sometimes undergo malignant change (e.g. aggressive osteoblastoma). They are usually amenable to local (marginal) excision with little risk of recurrence. Sarcomas are divided into 'low-grade' and 'high-grade'; the former are

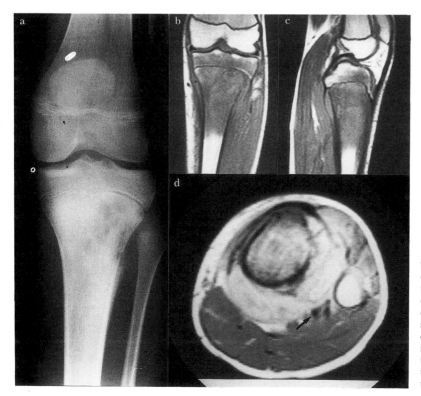

9.3 Staging (a) Plain x-ray shows a destructive lesion of the proximal tibia, almost certainly an osteosarcoma; but is it locally resectable? (b, c) Coronal and sagittal MR images show the tumour extending medially and laterally and posteriorly into the soft tissue. (d) Transectional MRI shows that the abnormal tissue extends posteriorly right up to the vascular compartment (arrow).

only moderately aggressive and take a long time to metastasize (e.g. secondary chondrosarcoma or parosteal osteosarcoma), while the latter are usually very aggressive and metastasize early (e.g. osteosarcoma or fibrosarcoma).

Spread

Assuming that there are no metastases, the local extent of the tumour is the most important factor in deciding how much tissue has to be removed. Lesions that are confined to an enclosed tissue space (e.g. a bone, a joint cavity or a muscle group within its fascial envelope) are called 'intracompartmental'. Those that extend into interfascial or extrafascial planes with no natural barrier to proximal or distal spread (e.g. perivascular sheaths, pelvis, axilla) are designated 'extracompartmental'. The extent of the tumour and adjacent 'contaminated' tissue is shown by advanced imaging (scintigraphy, CT and MRI).

Surgical stage

All low-grade sarcomas are designated stage I; high-grade lesions are stage II; and those with metastases are stage III. Each category is further subdivided into A (intracompartmental) and B (extracompartmental). Thus, a localized chondrosarcoma arising in a cartilage-capped exostosis is designated IA; it could be treated by wide excision without exposing the tumour. An osteosarcoma confined to bone would be IIA – operable by wide excision or amputation with a low risk of local recurrence; if it has spread into the soft tissues it would be IIB – less suitable for wide excision and preferably treated by radical resection or disarticulation through the proximal joint. If there are pulmonary metastases it becomes stage III.

The point of the staging exercise is to select the operation best suited to that particular patient, and carrying a low risk of recurrence. Locally recurrent sarcomas tend to be (1) more aggressive, (2) more often extracompartmental and (3) more likely to metastasize than the original tumour (Enneking, 1983).

Principles of management

For all but the simplest and most obvious of benign tumours, management calls for close co-operation and consultation between the orthopaedic surgeon, radiologist, pathologist and (certainly in the case of malignant tumours) the oncologist, prosthetic designer and rehabilitation therapist as well. Clinical and x-ray examination having suggested the most likely diagnosis, further management proceeds as follows.

Benign, asymptomatic lesions

If the diagnosis is beyond doubt (e.g. a non-ossifying fibroma or a small osteochondroma) one can afford to temporize; treatment may never be needed. However, if the appearances are not pathognomonic, a biopsy is advisable and this may take the form of an excisional biopsy (or curettage).

Benign, symptomatic or enlarging tumours

Painful lesions, or tumours that continue to enlarge after the end of normal bone growth, require biopsy and confirmation of the diagnosis. Unless they are unusually aggressive, they can generally be removed by local (marginal) excision or (in the case of benign cysts) curettage.

Suspected malignant tumours

If the lesion is thought to be a primary malignant tumour, the patient is admitted for more detailed examination, blood tests, chest x-ray, further imaging (including pulmonary CT) and biopsy. This should allow a firm diagnosis and staging. The various treatment options can then be discussed with the patient (or the parents, in the case of a young child). There are choices between amputation, limb-sparing operations and different types of adjuvant therapy, and the patient must be fully informed about the pros and cons of each.

Methods of treatment

Tumour excision

Operative removal, either alone or combined with some form of adjuvant therapy, is the most effective way of treating most tumours. In Enneking's (1983) terminology, *intracapsular excision* or *curettage* provides subtotal removal, while *marginal excision* goes beyond the capsule; both are suitable for different types of benign lesion. *Wide local excision* means removal of the tumour together with a wide margin of normal tissue; this is appropriate for low-grade intra-compartmental lesions (IA), and somewhat less so for high-grade intracompartmental tumours (IIA). *Radical resection* implies removal of the entire bone (or muscle compartment) in which

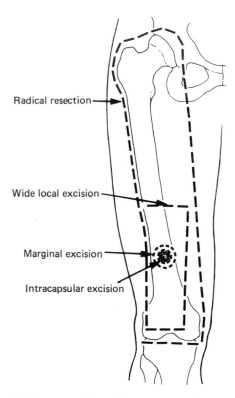

Radical resection —►

Wide local excision —►

Marginal excision —►

Intracapsular excision —►

9.4 Tumour excision The more aggressive a tumour is, and the wider it has spread, the more widely does it need to be excised. Local excision is suitable only for low-grade tu-mours that are confined to a single compart-ment. Radical resection may be needed for high-grade tumours and this often means amputation at a level above the compart-ment involved.

the tumour lies; this provides more effective treatment for high-grade lesions (IIA or IIB). The same principles apply to the different levels of amputation.

MARGINAL EXCISION Benign bone lesions are excised with a minimum of normal tissue. Even so this sometimes leaves a gap which may have to be filled with graft. Curettage, no matter how meticulous, cannot remove every shred of abnormal tissue and should be reserved for benign lesions with a low risk of local recur-rence. Here, again, the cavity is packed with graft bone, autogenous if possible or freeze-dried allograft if the space is very large.

LIMB-SPARING SURGERY With more accurate stag-ing procedures and advances in chemotherapy (to control tumour spread), amputation is no longer the automatic choice for tumour abla-tion (Mankin and Gebhardt, 1985; Enneking, 1987). For an intracompartmental tumour, wide excision and replacement by bone grafts or a custom-made prosthesis may be preferred provided that certain conditions are fulfilled: (1) there must be no skip lesions further up the bone; (2) for a high-grade tumour the entire compartment containing the tumour must be removed – this may mean excision of a muscle or group of muscles from origin to insertion; (3) the resulting loss of function should not be so great as to make the limb useless; and (4) replacement must be technically feasible. Cus-tom-made prostheses have to be specially de-signed for each situation; they are difficult to fix to bone and the operation carries a higher-than-usual risk of complications such as wound breakdown and pathological fracture. More-over, in children, allowance must be made for length inequality due to growth of the normal limb; an 'expandable' prosthesis may be used, or further operations will be needed. If large bone grafts are used, they take many months to join with the host bone and they are never completely revitalized. In some situations vascu-larized grafts are feasible.

AMPUTATION Considering the difficulties of limb-sparing surgery – particularly for high-grade tumours or if there is doubt about whether the lesion is intracompartmental – amputation and early rehabilitation may be more sensible. For stage IA lesions, the amputation can go through the proximal part of the involved bone; for more aggressive tumours, proximal disarticulation is wiser.

Radiotherapy

High-energy irradiation has long been used to destroy radiosensitive tumours or as adjuvant therapy before operation. Nowadays the indications are more restricted. For highly sensitive tumours (such as Ewing's sarcoma) it offers an alternative to amputation; it is then combined with adjuvant chemotherapy. The same combination can be used for tumours in inaccessible sites, lesions that are inoperable because of size or local spread, metastatic deposits and marrow-cell tumours such as myeloma and malignant lymphoma. It is usually given in divided doses over 4 weeks up to a total of 6000 cGy.

Chemotherapy

This is now the preferred adjuvant treatment for malignant bone and soft-tissue tumours. For some years following its introduction in the 1970s there was doubt as to whether it really improved the chances of long-term survival. Evidence is now available to show that, for sensitive tumours, chemotherapy effectively reduces the size of the primary lesion and prevents metastatic seeding (Rosen, 1987). Drugs currently in use are methotrexate, doxorubicin (adriamycin), cyclophosphamide, vincristine and cis-platinum. Treatment is started preoperatively and the effect is assessed by examining the resected tumour; if there is little or no necrosis, a different drug is selected for postoperative treatment.

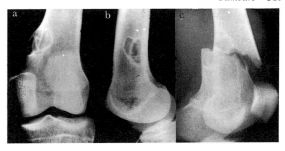

9.5 Non-ossifying fibroma (a) The x-ray always shows a cortical defect although, in some projection planes, this looks deceptively like a medullary lesion (b). The bone may fracture through the weakened area (c).

some years before ossifying. It is asymptomatic and is almost always encountered in children as an incidental finding on x-ray. The commonest sites are the metaphyses of long bones; occasionally there are multiple lesions.

The x-ray appearance is unmistakable. There is a more or less oval radiolucent area surrounded by a thin margin of dense bone; views in different planes may show that a lesion that appears to be 'central' is actually adjacent to or within the cortex, hence the alternative name 'fibrous cortical defect'.

PATHOLOGY Although it looks cystic on x-ray, it is a solid lesion consisting of unremarkable fibrous tissue with a few scattered giant cells.

As the bone grows the defect becomes less obvious and it eventually heals spontaneously. However, it sometimes enlarges to several centimetres in diameter and there may be a pathological fracture. There is no risk of malignant change.

TREATMENT is usually unnecessary. If the defect is very large or has led to repeated fractures, it can be treated by curettage and bone grafting.

Benign bone lesions

Non-ossifying fibroma (fibrous cortical defect)

This, the commonest benign lesion of bone, is a developmental defect in which a nest of fibrous tissue appears within the bone and persists for

Fibrous dysplasia

Fibrous dysplasia is a developmental disorder in which areas of trabecular bone are replaced by cellular fibrous tissue containing flecks of osteoid and woven bone. It may affect one bone (monostotic), one limb (monomelic) or many bones (polyostotic). If the lesions are large, the bone is considerably weakened and pathological fractures or progressive deformity may occur.

Small, single lesions are asymptomatic. Large, monostotic lesions may cause pain or may be discovered only when the patient develops a pathological fracture. Patients with polyostotic disease present in childhood or adolescence with pain, limp, bony enlargment, deformity or pathological fracture. Untreated, the characteristic deformities persist through adult life. Occasionally the bone disorder is associated with café-au-lait patches on the skin and (in girls) precocious sexual development (Albright's syndrome).

X-rays show radiolucent 'cystic' areas in the metaphysis or shaft; because they contain fibrous tissue with diffuse spots of immature bone, the lucent patches typically have a slightly hazy or 'ground-glass' appearance. The weight-bearing bones may be bent, and one of the classic features is the 'shepherd's crook' deformity of the proximal femur. Radioscintigraphy shows marked isotope uptake in the lesion.

PATHOLOGY   At operation the lesional tissue has a coarse, gritty feel (due to the specks of immature bone). The histological picture is of loose, cellular fibrous tissue with widespread patches of woven bone and scattered giant cells.

Both clinically and histologically the monostotic condition may resemble either a bone-forming tumour or hyperparathyroidism. However, detailed x-ray and laboratory studies will exclude these disorders.

Malignant transformation to fibrosarcoma occurs in 5–10% of patients with polyostotic lesions, but only rarely in monostotic lesions.

TREATMENT   depends on the extent of the defect and the presence or absence of deformities. Small lesions need no treatment. Those that are large and painful or threatening to fracture (or have fractured) can be curetted and grafted, but there is a strong tendency for the abnormality to recur. A mixture of cortical and cancellous bone grafts may provide added strength even if the lesion is not eradicated. For very large lesions, the grafts can be supplemented by methylmethacrylate cement. De-

formities may need correction by suitably designed osteotomies.

With large cysts, the bone often bleeds profusely at operation: forewarned is forearmed.

Compact osteoma (ivory exostosis)

This rare benign 'tumour' appears as a localized thickening on the outer or inner surface of compact bone. An adolescent or young adult presents with a painless, ivory-hard lump, usually on the outer surface of the skull, occasionally on the subcutaneous surface of the tibia. If it occurs on the inner table of the skull, it may cause focal epilepsy; sometimes it protrudes into the paranasal sinuses. On x-ray a sessile plaque of exceedingly dense bone with a well-circumscribed edge is seen. This might suggest a parosteal osteosarcoma, but the long history, the absence of pain and the smooth outline will dispel this suspicion.

TREATMENT   Unless the tumour impinges on important structures, it need not be removed. However, the patient may want to be rid of it; excision is easier if a margin of normal bone is taken with it.

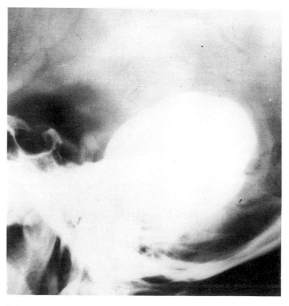

9.6 Compact osteoma   This was as hard as ivory, but quite painless.

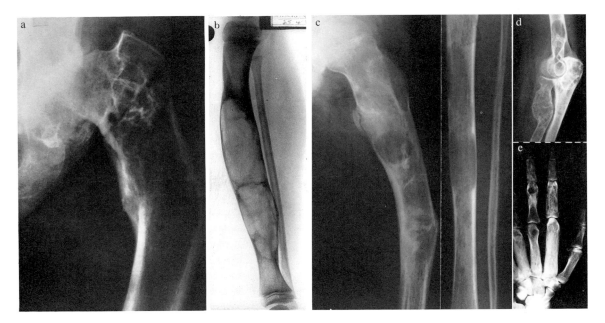

9.7 Fibrous dysplasia (a) Monostotic fibrous dysplasia of the upper femur (with the so-called 'shepherd's crook' appearance) and (b) of the tibia. (c, d, e) From three patients with polyostotic fibrous dysplasia.

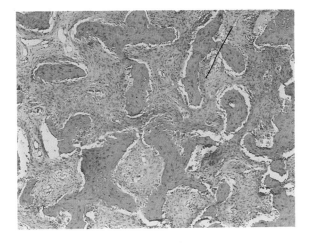

9.8 Fibrous dysplasia – histology Microscopic islands of woven bone lie scattered in a bed of cellular fibrous tissue. Occasional giant cells are seen. (× 120)

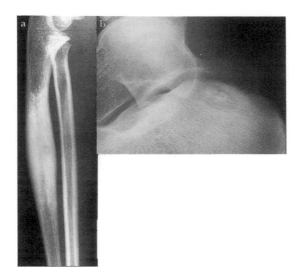

9.9 Osteoid osteoma The x-ray appearance depends on the site of the lesion. (a) With cortical tumours there is marked reactive bone thickening leaving a small lucent nidus, which may itself have a central speck of ossification. (b) Lesions in cancellous bone produce far less periosteal reaction and are easily mistaken for a Brodie's abscess.

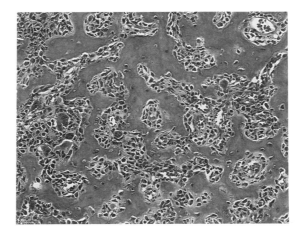

9.10 Osteoid osteoma – histology The histological features are characteristic: the nidus consists of sheets of pink-staining osteoid in a fibrovascular stroma. Giant cells and osteoblasts are prominent. (× 300)

Osteoid osteoma

This tiny bone tumour causes symptoms out of all proportion to its size. Patients are usually under 30 years of age and males predominate. Any bone except the skull may be affected, but over half the cases occur in the femur or tibia. The patient complains of persistent pain, sometimes well localized but sometimes referred over a wide area. Typically the pain is relieved by salicylates. If the diagnosis is delayed, other features appear: a limp or muscle wasting and weakness; spinal lesions may cause intense pain, muscle spasm and scoliosis.

The important x-ray feature is a small radiolucent area, the so-called 'nidus'. Lesions in the diaphysis are surrounded by dense sclerosis and cortical thickening; this may be so marked that the nidus can be seen only in tomograms. Lesions in the metaphysis show less cortical thickening. Further away the bone may be osteoporotic. ^{99m}Tc-HDP scintigraphy reveals intense, localized activity.

It is sometimes difficult to distinguish an osteoid osteoma from a small Brodie's abscess without biopsy. Ewing's sarcoma and chronic periostitis must also be excluded.

PATHOLOGY The excised lesion appears as a dark-brown or reddish 'nucleus' surrounded by dense bone; the central area consists of unorganized sheets of osteoid and bone cells.

There is no risk of malignant transformation.

TREATMENT The only effective treatment is complete removal of the nidus. The lesion is carefully localized by multiple x-ray and excised in a small block of bone; the specimen should be x-rayed to confirm that it does contain the little tumour. If the tumour is difficult to locate, a sterilizable radiation probe is helpful (Colton and Hardy, 1983). If the excision is likely to weaken the host bone (especially in the vulnerable medial cortex of the femoral neck), prophylactic internal fixation may be needed.

Osteoblastoma (giant osteoid osteoma)

This tumour is in some ways similar to an osteoid osteoma, but it is larger, more cellular and sometimes more ominous in appearance. It is usually seen in young adults, more often in men than in women. It tends to occur in the spine and the flat bones, and patients present with pain (much less than in osteoid osteoma) and local muscle spasm.

X-ray shows a well-demarcated osteolytic lesion which may contain small flecks of ossification. There is surrounding sclerosis but this is not always easy to see – especially with lesions in the flat bones or the vertebral pedicle. A radioisotope scan will reveal the 'hot' area. Larger lesions may appear 'cystic', and sometimes a typical aneurysmal bone cyst appears to have arisen in an osteoblastoma.

PATHOLOGY When the tumour is exposed it has a somewhat 'fleshy' appearance. Histologically it resembles an osteoid osteoma, but the cellularity is more striking. Occasionally the picture may suggest a low-grade osteosarcoma.

TREATMENT consists of excision and bone grafting. With lesions in the vertebral pedicle, or the floor of the acetabulum, this is not always easy and removal may be incomplete; local recurrence is common and malignant transformation has been reported (McLeod, Dahlin and Beabout, 1976).

Chondroma (enchondroma)

Islands of cartilage may persist in the metaphyses of bones formed by endochondral ossification; sometimes they grow and take on the characteristics of a benign tumour. Chondromas are usually asymptomatic and are discovered incidentally on x-ray or after a pathological fracture. They are seen at any age (but mostly in young people) and in any bone preformed in cartilage (most commonly the tubular bones of the hands and feet). Lesions may be solitary or multiple and part of a generalized dysplasia (see p. 142).

X-ray shows a well-defined, centrally placed radiolucent area at the junction of metaphysis and diaphysis; sometimes the bone is slightly expanded. In mature lesions there are flecks or wisps of calcification within the lucent area;

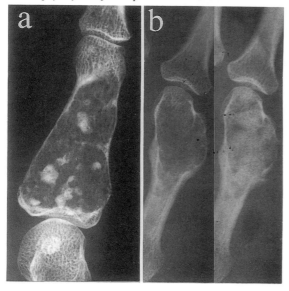

9.11 Chondroma (a) The hand is a common site. (b) Another chondroma before and after curettage and bone grafting.

when present, this is a pathognomonic feature.

PATHOLOGY When it is exposed the lesion is seen to consist of pearly-white cartilaginous tissue, often with a central area of degeneration and calcification. Histologically the appearances are those of simple hyaline cartilage.

TREATMENT is not always necessary, but if the tumour appears to be enlarging, or if it presents as a pathological fracture, it should be removed as thoroughly as possible by curettage; the defect is filled with bone graft. There is a fairly high recurrence rate and the tissue may be seeded in adjacent bone or soft tissues. Chondromas in expendable sites are better removed en bloc. There is a small but significant risk of malignant change (probably less than 2% and hardly ever in a child). Signs of malignant transformation in patients over 30 years are (1) the onset of pain; (2) enlargement of the lesion; (3) cortical erosion. Unfortunately, biopsy is of little help in this regard as the cartilage usually looks benign during the early stages of malignant transformation. If the other features are present, and especially in older patients, the lesion should be treated as a stage

IA malignancy; the biopsy then serves chiefly to confirm the fact that it is a cartilage tumour.

Periosteal chondroma

These are rare developmental lesions arising in the deep layer of the periosteum. A cartilaginous lump bulges from the bone into the soft tissues and causes some alarm when it is discovered by the patient. Because the cartilage remains uncalcified, the lesion itself does not show on x-ray, but the surface of the bone may be irregular or scalloped. MRI may reveal the full extent of the tumour. Histologically the lesion is composed of highly cellular cartilage.

TREATMENT Because of its propensity to recur, it is best removed by marginal excision (taking a rim of normal bone). Recurrent lesions may look more aggressive but the lesion probably does not undergo malignant change.

Chondroblastoma

This benign tumour of immature cartilage cells is one of the few lesions to appear primarily in the epiphysis, usually of the proximal humerus, femur or tibia. Patients are affected around the end of the growth period or in early adult life; there is a predilection for males. The presenting symptom is a constant ache 'in the joints'; the tender spot is actually in the adjacent bone.

X-ray shows a rounded, well-demarcated radiolucent area in the epiphysis; the site is so unusual that the diagnosis springs readily to mind. However, sometimes the lesion extends across the physeal line. Occasionally the articular surface is breached. Like osteoblastoma, the lesion sometimes expands and acquires the features of an aneurysmal bone cyst.

PATHOLOGY The histological appearances are fairly typical – there are large collections of chondroblasts set off by the surrounding matrix of immature fibrous tissue. Within the stroma are scattered giant cells. In expansile lesions, the edge may resemble that of an aneurysmal bone cyst.

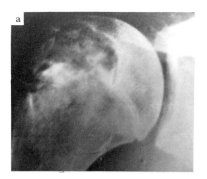

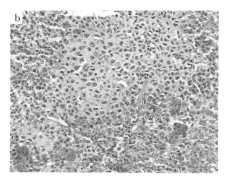

9.12 Chondroblastoma (a) X-ray shows a cyst-like lesion occupying the epiphysis, and sometimes extending across the physis into the adjacent bone. (b) The characteristic features in this photomicrograph are the more faintly staining islands of chondroid tissue composed of round cells ('chondroblasts') and scattered multinucleated giant cells. (×300)

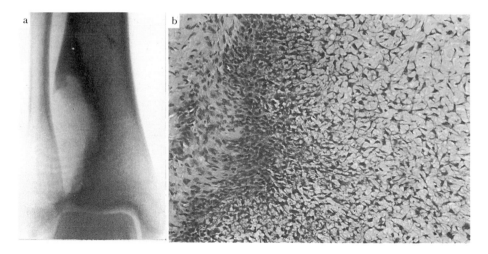

9.13 Chondromyxoid fibroma (a) The x-ray is quite typical: there is an eccentric cyst-like lesion with a densely sclerotic endosteal margin often extending like a tongue towards the diaphysis. (b) The section shows predominantly myxomatous cells and fibrous tissue; elsewhere chondroid tissue and giant cells were more obvious. (×300)

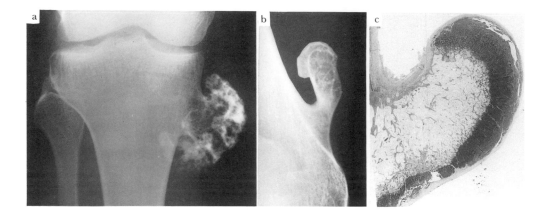

9.14 Osteochondroma (a, b) The lesion is a cartilage-capped exostosis but the cartilage does not show on x-ray unless it is calcified. The bony part may be pedunculated, sessile or cauliflower-like. (c) A section through the exostosis shows that it is always covered by hyaline cartilage from which the bony excrescence grows.

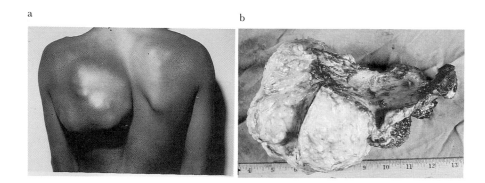

9.15 Osteochondroma – treatment (a) This 20-year-old man had known about the lump on his left scapula for many years. He stopped growing at the age of 18 but the tumour continued to enlarge. (b) Despite the benign histology in the biopsy, the tumour together with most of the scapula was removed; sections taken from the depths of the lesion showed atypical cells suggestive of malignant change.

These tumours do not undergo malignant change but they may be locally aggressive and extend into the joint.

TREATMENT In children the risk of damage to the physis makes one hesitate to remove the lesion. After the end of the growth period the lesion can be removed – by marginal excision wherever possible or (less satisfactory) by curettage – and replaced with autogenous bone grafts. There is a high risk of recurrence after incomplete removal, and if this happens repeatedly there may be serious damage to the nearby joint. Occasionally one is forced to excise the recurrent lesion with an adequate margin of bone and accept the inevitable need for major joint reconstruction.

Chondromyxoid fibroma

Like other benign cartilaginous lesions, this is seen mainly in adolescents and young adults. It may occur in any bone but is more common in those of the lower limb.

Patients seldom complain and the lesion is usually discovered by accident or after a pathological fracture.

X-rays are very characteristic: there is a rounded or ovoid radiolucent area placed eccentrically in the metaphysis; in children it may extend up to or even slightly across the physis. The endosteal margin may be scalloped, but is almost always bounded by a dense zone of reactive bone extending tongue-like towards the diaphysis. The cortex may be asymmetrically expanded. Sometimes there is calcification in the vacant area.

PATHOLOGY Although the lesion looks 'cystic' on x-ray, it contains mucinous material and bits of cartilage. Histologically the three types of tissue can usually be identified: patches of myxomatous tissue with delicate, stellate cells; islands of hyaline cartilage; and areas of fibrous tissue with cells of varying degrees of maturity.

Malignant change has been recorded but this must be extremely rare.

TREATMENT Where feasible, the lesion should be excised but often one can do no more than a thorough curettage – followed by autogenous bone grafting. There is considerable risk of recurrence; if repeated operations are needed, care should be taken to prevent damage to the physis (in children) or the nearby joint surface.

Osteochondroma (cartilage-capped exostosis)

This, one of the commonest 'tumours' of bone, is a developmental lesion which starts as a small overgrowth of cartilage at the edge of the physeal plate and develops by endochondral ossification into a bony protuberance still covered by the cap of cartilage. Any bone that develops in cartilage may be involved; the commonest sites are the fast-growing ends of long bones and the crest of the ilium. In long bones, growth leaves the bump stranded further down the metaphysis. Here it may go on growing but at the end of the normal growth period for that bone it stops enlarging. Any further enlargement after that is suggestive of malignant transformation.

The patient is usually a teenager or young adult when the lump is first discovered. Occasionally there is pain due to an overlying bursa or impingement on soft tissues, or, rarely, paraesthesia due to stretching of an adjacent nerve.

The x-ray appearance is pathognomonic. There is a well-defined exostosis emerging from the metaphysis, its base co-extensive with the parent bone. It looks smaller than it feels because the cartilage cap is usually invisible; however, large lesions undergo cartilage degeneration and calcification and then the x-ray shows the bony exostosis surrounded by clouds of calcified material.

Multiple lesions may develop as part of a heritable disorder – hereditary multiple exostosis – in which there is abnormal bone growth resulting in characteristic deformities (p. 138).

PATHOLOGY At operation the cartilage cap is seen surmounting a narrow base or pedicle of bone. The cap consists of simple hyaline cartilage; in a growing exostosis the deeper cartilage cells are arranged in columns, giving rise to the formation of endochondral new bone. Large lesions may have a 'cauliflower' appearance, with degeneration and calcification in the centre of the transected specimen. The incidence of malignant transformation is difficult to assess because 'troublesome' lesions are so often removed before they are histologically malignant. Figures usually quoted are 1% for solitary lesions and 6% for multiple.

TREATMENT   If the tumour causes symptoms it should be excised; if, in an adult, it has recently become bigger or painful then operation is urgent, for these features suggest malignancy. This is seen most often with pelvic exostoses – not because they are inherently different but because considerable enlargement may, for long periods, pass unnoticed. If there are suspicious features, further imaging and staging should be carried out before doing a biopsy. If the histology is that of 'benign' cartilage but the tumour is known for certain to be enlarging after the end of the growth period, it should be treated as a chondrosarcoma.

Simple bone cyst

This lesion (also known as a solitary cyst or unicameral bone cyst) appears during childhood, typically in the metaphysis of one of the long bones and most commonly in the proximal humerus or femur. It is not a tumour, tends to heal spontaneously and is seldom seen in adults. The condition is usually discovered after a pathological fracture or as an incidental finding on x-ray.

X-rays show a well-demarcated radiolucent area in the metaphysis, often extending up to the physeal plate; the cortex may be thinned and the bone expanded.

Diagnosis is usually not difficult but other cyst-like lesions may need to be excluded. Non-osteogenic fibroma, fibrous dysplasia and the benign cartilage tumours are solid and merely look cystic on x-ray. In doubtful cases a needle can be inserted into the lesion under x-ray control: with a simple cyst, straw-coloured fluid will be withdrawn. Very seldom will there be any need for biopsy. However, if curettage is thought to be necessary, material from the cyst should be submitted for examination.

PATHOLOGY   The lining membrane consists of flimsy fibrous tissue, often containing giant cells. In an actively growing cyst, there is osteoclastic resorption of the adjacent bone.

TREATMENT   depends on whether the cyst is symptomatic, actively growing or involved in a fracture. Asymptomatic lesions in older children can be left alone but the patient should be cautioned to avoid injury which might cause a fracture. 'Active' cysts (those in young children, usually abutting against the physeal plate and obviously enlarging in sequential x-rays) should be treated, in the first instance, by aspiration of fluid and injection of 80–160 mg of methylprednisolone. This often stops further enlargement and leads to healing of the cyst (Scaglietti, Marchetti and Bartolozzi, 1979). If the cyst goes on enlarging, or if there is a pathological fracture, the cavity should be thoroughly cleaned by curettage and packed with bone chips. There is a considerable risk of recurrence and more than one operation may be needed. Care should be taken not to damage the nearby physeal plate.

Aneurysmal bone cyst

Aneurysmal bone cyst may be encountered at any age and in almost any bone – though more often in young adults and in the long-bone metaphyses. Usually it arises spontaneously but it may appear after degeneration or haemorrhage in some other lesion (Levy et al., 1975).

With expanding lesions, patients may complain of pain. Occasionally, a large cyst may cause a visible or palpable swelling of the bone.

X-rays show a well-defined radiolucent cyst, often trabeculated and eccentrically placed. In a growing tubular bone it is always situated in the metaphysis and therefore may resemble a simple cyst or one of the other cyst-like lesions. Occasional sites include vertebrae and the flat bones. In an adult an aneurysmal bone cyst may be mistaken for a giant-cell tumour but, unlike the latter, it usually does not extend right up to the articular margin. Occasionally it causes marked ballooning of the bone end.

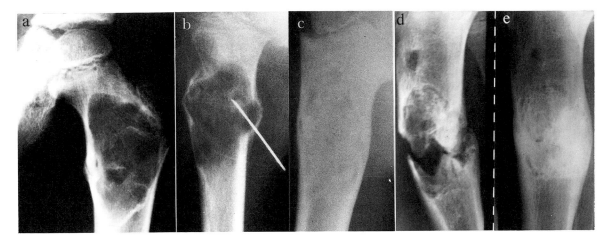

9.16 Simple bone cysts (a) A typical solitary (or unicameral) cyst – on the shaft side of the physis and expanding the cortex. (b) Injection with methylprednisolone, and (c) healing. (d) Fracture through a cyst, leading to (e) healing.

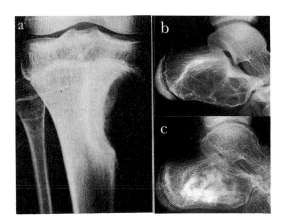

9.17 Aneurysmal bone cyst (a) The outer wall of this cyst is so thin that it barely shows on the x-ray. (b) The soap-bubble appearance in this lesion is produced by ridges on the walls of the cyst. (c) After curettage and packing with bone chips the lesion healed.

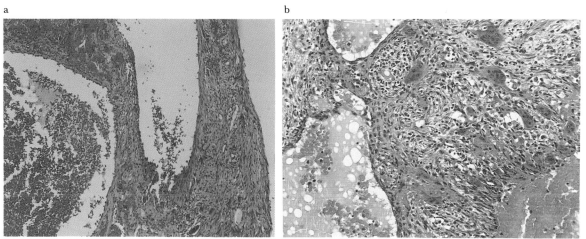

9.18 Aneurysmal bone cyst – histology (a) The cyst contained blood and was lined by loose fibrous tissue containing numerous giant cells. ($\times$120) (b) A high-power view of the same. ($\times$300)

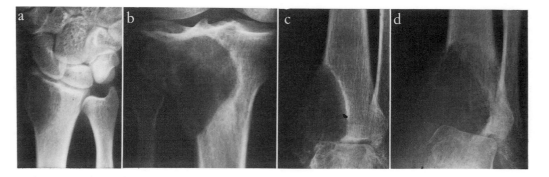

9.19 Giant-cell tumours   (a, b, c) In each of these the tumour abuts against the joint margin, and is asymmetrically placed – these are characteristic features; in (d) malignant change has supervened and the junction of the tumour with the rest of the bone is no longer well defined.

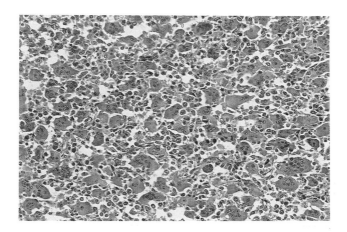

9.20 Giant-cell tumour – histology   A low-power view of the biopsy shows the abundant multinucleated giant cells lying in a stroma composed of round and polyhedral tumour cells. There are numerous mitotic figures.

PATHOLOGY When the cyst is opened it is found to contain clotted blood, and during curettage there may be considerable bleeding from the fleshy lining membrane. Histologically the lining consists of fibrous tissue with vascular spaces, deposits of haemosiderin and multinucleated giant cells. Occasionally the appearances so closely resemble those of giant-cell tumour that only the most experienced pathologists can confidently make the diagnosis. Malignant transformation does not occur.

TREATMENT calls for thorough curettage and packing with bone grafts. Even then the graft may be resorbed with recurrence of the lesion, necessitating a second or third operation. In these cases, packing with methylmethacrylate cement may be more effective. However, if the cyst is in a 'safe' area (with no risk of fracture) there is no hurry to reoperate; the lesion occasionally heals spontaneously (Malghem et al., 1989).

Giant-cell tumour

Giant-cell tumour is a lesion of uncertain origin that appears in mature bone, most commonly in the distal femur, proximal tibia, proximal humerus and distal radius, but other bones may be affected. It is hardly ever seen before closure of the physis in that region and characteristically it extends up to the subarticular bone plate. Rarely, there are multiple lesions.

The patient is usually a young adult who complains of pain at the end of a long bone; sometimes there is slight swelling. A history of trauma is not uncommon and pathological fracture occurs in 10–15% of cases. On examination there may be a palpable mass with warmth of the overlying tissues.

X-rays show a radiolucent area situated eccentrically at the end of a long bone and bounded by the subchondral bone plate. The endosteal margin may be quite obvious, but in aggressive lesions it is ill-defined. The centre sometimes has a soap-bubble appearance due to ridging of the surrounding bone. The cortex is thin and sometimes ballooned; aggressive lesions extend into the soft tissue. The appearance of a 'cystic' lesion in mature bone, extending right up to the subchondral plate, is so characteristic that the diagnosis is seldom in doubt.

Because of the tumour's potential for aggressive behaviour, detailed staging procedures are essential. CT scans and MRI will reveal the extent of the tumour, both within the bone and beyond. It is important to establish whether the articular surface has been broached; arthroscopy may be helpful.

Biopsy is essential. This can be done either as a frozen section before proceding with operative treatment or (especially if more extensive operation is contemplated) as a separate procedure.

PATHOLOGY The tumour has a reddish, fleshy appearance; it comes away in pieces quite easily when curetted but is difficult to remove completely from the surrounding bone. Aggressive lesions have a poorly defined edge and extend well into the surrounding bone. Histologically the striking feature is an abundance of multinucleated giant cells scattered on a background of stromal cells with little or no visible inter-

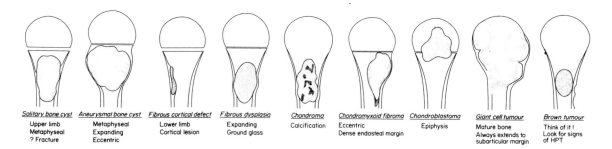

Solitary bone cyst — Upper limb / Metaphyseal / ? Fracture *Aneurysmal bone cyst* — Metaphyseal / Expanding / Eccentric *Fibrous cortical defect* — Lower limb / Cortical lesion *Fibrous dysplasia* — Expanding / Ground glass *Chondroma* — Calcification *Chondromyxoid fibroma* — Eccentric / Dense endosteal margin *Chondroblastoma* — Epiphysis *Giant cell tumour* — Mature bone / Always extends to subarticular margin *Brown tumour* — Think of it! / Look for signs of HPT

9.21 Cysts and cyst-like lesions of bone.

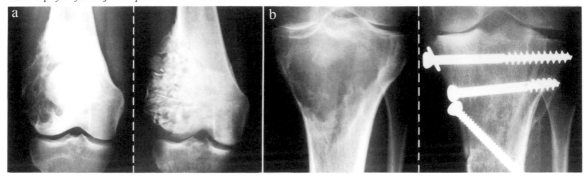

9.22 Giant-cell tumour – treatment   (a) Excision and bone grafts. (b) Block resection and replacement with a large osteocartilaginous graft from another individual (who had died after a road accident).

cellular tissue. Aggressive lesions tend to show more cellular atypia and mitotic figures, but histological grading is unreliable as a predictor of tumour behaviour.

TREATMENT   is planned on the basis of surgical staging. Well-confined, slow-growing lesions with 'benign' histology can safely be treated by thorough curettage and 'stripping' of the cavity wall with burrs and gouges, followed by packing with bone chips or methylmethacrylate cement. More aggressive tumours, and recurrent lesions, should be treated by excision followed, if necessary, by bone grafting or prosthetic replacement. Tumours in awkward sites (e.g. the spine) may be difficult to eradicate and surgery may have to be supplemented by radiotherapy.

GIANT-CELL SARCOMA

Giant-cell sarcoma is an unequivocally malignant lesion with x-ray features like those of a highly aggressive benign giant-cell tumour. There is a high risk of metastasis and treatment requires radical resection or amputation.

Eosinophilic granuloma and histiocytosis

The lipid storage disorders which Lichtenstein (1964) grouped as 'histiocytosis-X' may cause osteolytic lesions resembling bone tumours. The commonest of these – and the one present-

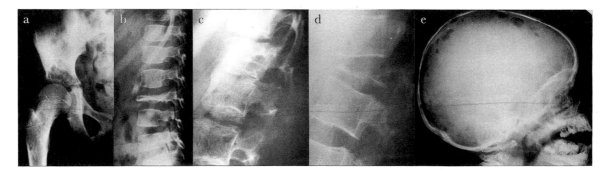

9.23 Lipid storage disorders   (a) An eosinophilic granuloma which went on to spontaneous healing. (b) Calvé's disease with a flattened vertebral body but discs of normal height. (c, d) The development of Calvé's disease from an eosinophilic granuloma. (e) Hand–Schüller–Christian disease.

ing as a pure bone lesion – is *eosinophilic granuloma*. Cells of the reticuloendothelial system (histiocytes and eosinophils) form granulomatous collections. Marrow-containing bone is resorbed and one or more lytic lesions may appear – usually in the flat bones or the metaphyses of long bones. The patient is usually a child; there is seldom any complaint of pain and the condition is discovered incidentally or after a pathological fracture. X-ray shows a well-demarcated oval area of radiolucency within the bone; sometimes this is associated with marked reactive sclerosis. There may be multiple lesions and in the skull they have a characteristic punched-out appearance. Vertebral collapse may result in a flat wedge (vertebra plana) which is pathognomonic.

The condition usually heals spontaneously and is therefore rarely seen in adults. Occasionally, however, a solitary lesion may herald the onset of one of the generalized disorders (see below). Operation is usually done to obtain a biopsy; if the lesion is easily accessible it may be completely excised.

Hand–Schüller–Christian disease is a disseminated form of the same condition. The patient is a child, usually with widespread lesions involving the skull, vertebral bodies, liver and spleen. There may be anaemia and a marked tendency to recurrent infection. In severely affected children there is a considerable mortality rate. There is no effective treatment.

Letterer–Siwe disease is an extremely rare (and severe) form of histiocytosis. It is seen in infants and usually progresses rapidly to a fatal outcome.

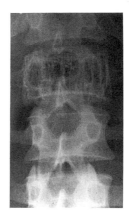

9.24   Haemangioma
This haemangioma was symptomless; it was discovered accidentally.

pelvis where the appearance may suggest malignancy, but there is no associated cortical or medullary destruction. In the trabecular bones the presenting feature may be a pathological fracture. If operation is needed there is a risk of profuse bleeding, and embolization may be a useful preliminary.

Haemangioma

Osseous haemangiomas consist of vascular channels (capillary, venous or cavernous) and are usually seen in middle-aged patients, the spine being the commonest site. They may cause backache but are often symptomless and discovered accidentally when the back is x-rayed for some other reason. Radiologically there is coarse vertical trabeculation (the 'corduroy appearance'). Other sites include the skull and

Osteolysis ('disappearing bones')

In massive osteolysis (Gorham's disease) there is progressive disappearance of bone, associated with haemangiomatosis or multiple lymphangiectases. Usually the progression involves contiguous bones, but occasionally multiple sites are affected. Patients may present with mild pain or with a pathological fracture. No effective treatment is known, but spontaneous arrest has been described. Occasionally, however, the process spreads to vital structures and the outcome is fatal (Cannon, 1986).

Primary malignant bone tumours

Chondrosarcoma

Chondrosarcoma can occur either as a primary tumour or as secondary change in a pre-existing cartilaginous lesion. Both types have their highest incidence in the fourth and fifth decades, and men are affected more often than women. The tumours are slow growing and are usually present for many months before being discovered. Patients may complain of a dull ache or a gradually enlarging lump. Medullary lesions may present as a pathological fracture.

Primary chondrosarcoma   may occur in any bone that develops in cartilage but is usually seen in the metaphysis of one of the tubular bones. X-rays show a radiolucent area with central flecks of calcification. Rarely, the tumour appears as a globular mass on the surface of the bone; this distinguishes the so-called 'peripheral chondrosarcoma' from the more common 'central chondrosarcoma'.

Secondary chondrosarcoma   usually arises in the cartilage cap of an exostosis (osteochondroma) that has been present since childhood. Exostoses of the pelvis and scapula seem to be more susceptible than others to malignant change, but perhaps this is simply because the site allows a tumour to grow without being detected and removed at an early stage. X-rays show the bony exostosis, often surmounted by clouds of patchy calcification in the otherwise unseen lobulated cartilage cap. A tumour that is very large and calcification that is very fluffy and poorly outlined are suspicious features, but the clearest sign of malignant change is a demonstrable progressive enlargement of an osteochondroma after the end of normal bone growth.

A medullary chondroma (enchondroma) may also undergo malignant transformation, but it is difficult to be sure that the lesion was not a slowly evolving sarcoma from the outset.

If a chondrosarcoma is suspected, CT scans and MRI should be carried out to show the extent of the tumour.

PATHOLOGY   A biopsy is essential to confirm the diagnosis. However, low-grade chondrosarcoma may show histological features no different from those of an aggressive benign cartilaginous lesion. High-grade tumours are more cellular, and there may be obvious abnormal features of the cells, such as plumpness, hyperchromasia and mitoses. The term 'dedifferentiated' chondrosarcoma is used when the usual appearances are associated with areas that look more malignant.

TREATMENT   depends on the results of the staging procedures. These tumours are slow-growing and metastasize late. They present the ideal case for wide excision and prosthetic replacement, provided it is certain that the lesion can be completely removed without exposing the tumour and without causing an unacceptable loss of function. In that case amputation may be preferable.

Chondrosarcomas do not respond to either radiotherapy or chemotherapy.

Osteosarcoma

In its classic form, osteosarcoma is a highly malignant tumour arising within the bone and spreading rapidly outwards to the periosteum and surrounding soft tissues. It is said to occur predominantly in children and adolescents, but a recent epidemiological study suggests that between 1972 and 1981 the age of presentation rose significantly (Stark et al., 1990). It may affect any bone but most commonly involves the long-bone metaphyses, especially around the knee and at the proximal end of the humerus.

Pain is usually the first symptom; it is constant, worse at night and gradually increases in severity. Sometimes the patient presents with a lump. Pathological fracture is rare. On examination there may be little to find except local tenderness. In later cases there is a palpable mass and the overlying tissues may appear swollen and inflamed. The ESR is usually raised and there may be an increase in serum alkaline phosphatase.

X-ray appearances are variable: hazy osteolytic areas may alternate with unusually dense osteoblastic areas. The endosteal margin is poorly defined. Often the cortex is breached and the tumour extends into the adjacent tissues; when this happens, streaks of new bone

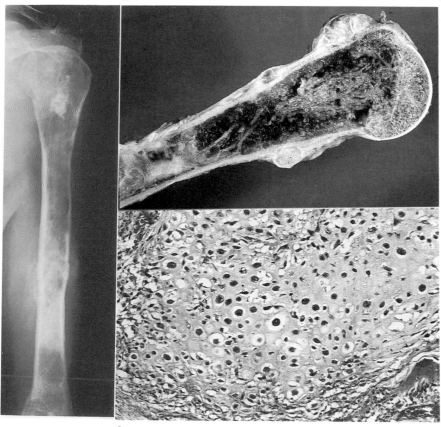

9.25 Chondrosarcoma   (a) This patient presented with a suspected pathological fracture of the humerus. X-rays showed rarefaction of the bone with central flecks of calcification. At the fracture site the lesion extends into the soft tissues. (b) Radical resection was carried out. Pale, glistening cartilage tissue was found in the medullary cavity and, in several places, spreading beyond the cortex. Much of the bone is occupied by haemorrhagic tissue. (c) The histological sections show lobules of highly atypical cartilage cells, including binucleate cells.

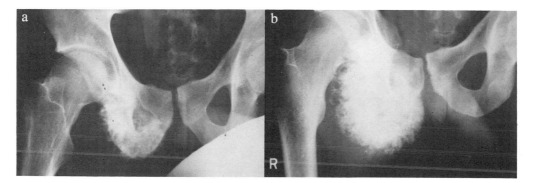

9.26 Chondrosarcoma   At the age of 20 this young man complained of pain in the right groin; x-ray showed an osteochondroma of the right inferior pubic ramus (a). A biopsy showed 'benign cartilage' but a year later the tumour had doubled its size (b), a clear sign that it was a chondrosarcoma.

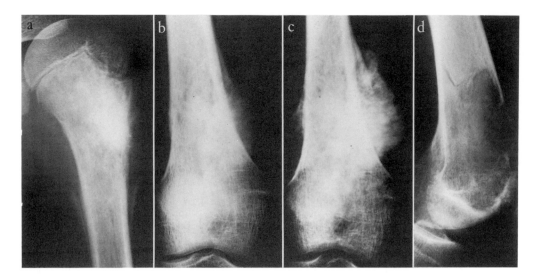

9.27 Osteosarcoma (a) The metaphyseal site: increased density, cortical erosion and periosteal reaction are characteristic. (b) Sunray spicules and Codman's triangle; (c) the same patient after radiotherapy. (d) A predominantly osteolytic tumour.

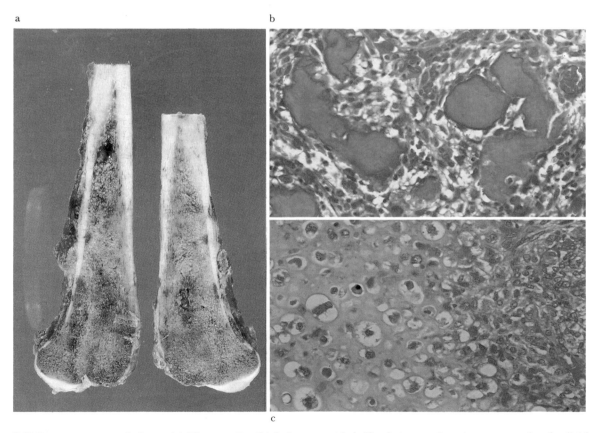

9.28 Osteosarcoma – pathology (a) After resection this lesion was cut in half; pale tumour tissue is seen occupying the distal third of the femur and extending through the cortex. (b) The dominant features in the histological sections were malignant stromal tissue showing osteoid formation (pink masses). ($\times$ 480) (c) The same tumour showed areas of chondroblastic differentiation. ($\times$ 480)

appear, radiating outwards from the cortex – the so-called 'sunburst' effect. Where the tumour emerges from the cortex, reactive new bone forms at the angles of periosteal elevation (Codman's triangle). While both the sunburst appearances and Codman's triangle are typical of osteosarcoma, they may occasionally be seen in other rapidly growing tumours.

In most cases the diagnosis can be made with confidence on the x-ray appearances, but other imaging studies are essential for staging purposes. Radioisotope scans may show up skip lesions, but a negative scan does not exclude them. CT and MRI reliably show the extent of the tumour. Chest x-rays are done routinely, but pulmonary CT is a much more sensitive detector of lung metastases.

Conditions to be excluded in the differential diagnosis are post-traumatic swellings, infection, stress fracture and the more aggressive 'cystic' lesions. A biopsy should always be carried out before commencing treatment; it must be carefully planned to allow for complete removal of the track when the tumour is excised.

PATHOLOGY The tumour is usually situated in the metaphysis of a long bone, where it destroys and replaces normal bone. Areas of bone loss and cavitation alternate with dense patches of abnormal new bone. The tumour extends within the medulla and across the physeal plate. There may be obvious spread into the soft tissues with ossification at the periosteal margins and streaks of new bone extending into the extraosseous mass.

The histological appearances show considerable variation: some areas may have the characteristic spindle cells with a pink-staining osteoid matrix; others may contain cartilage cells or fibroblastic tissue with little or no osteoid. Several samples may have to be examined; pathologists are reluctant to commit themselves to the diagnosis unless they see evidence of osteoid formation.

TREATMENT The appalling prognosis that formerly attended this tumour has markedly improved, partly as a result of better diagnostic and staging procedures, and possibly because the average age of the patients has increased,

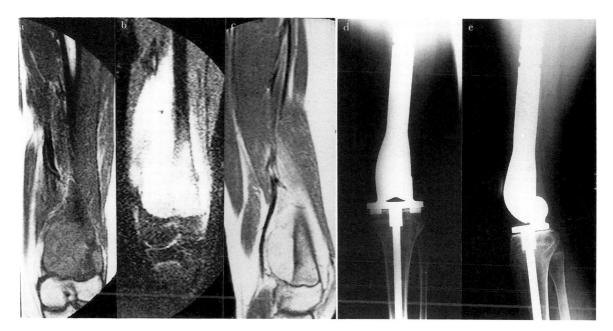

9.29 Staging and treatment (a) MRI T_1 sequence showing the tumour (an osteosarcoma) in the distal femur but not penetrating the joint. (b) STIR sequence (fat suppression) gives a more realistic picture of spread into the soft tissues. (c) Proton density sequence showing posterior extension of the tumour up to (but not into) the vascular compartment. (d, e) Wide excision and replacement with large 'extending' prosthesis. (Courtesy of Mr John Dixon.)

but mainly because of advances in chemotherapy to control metastatic spread. However, it is still important to eradicate the primary lesion completely; the mortality rate after local recurrence is far worse than following effective ablation at the first encounter. Most osteosarcomas are high-grade lesions with extracompartmental spread (stage IIB). The fundamentals of treatment are straightforward: radical surgery combined with adjuvant chemotherapy; and radiotherapy in reserve.

Radical surgery offers the best chance of preventing recurrence. This means amputation through or even above the joint proximal to the tumour, and also above the origin of any affected muscle. Lesser procedures (e.g. amputation through the affected bone or wide excision with limb salvaging) may be contemplated provided the patient is informed that (1) this carries a somewhat higher risk of recurrence and (2) limb-sparing operations are attended by serious complications in about one-third of cases (see p. 168).

Chemotherapy – usually high dosage methotrexate – is started preoperatively. When the tumour is removed the response to treatment is assessed. If tumour destruction is marked, methotrexate is continued postoperatively; if the response is poor, a different chemotherapeutic agent may be substituted. This regimen has produced relatively long-term survival in over 80% of patients (Rosen et al., 1982).

Radiotherapy is used to control tumours at inoperable sites such as the pelvis and jaw, or for patients who refuse operation.

Pulmonary metastases, especially if they are small and peripherally situated, may be completely resected with a wedge of lung tissue; the prognosis for survival is still reasonable.

Variants of osteosarcoma

Parosteal osteosarcoma

This is a low-grade sarcoma situated on the surface of one of the tubular bones, usually at the distal femoral or proximal tibial metaphysis. The patient is a young adult who presents with a slowly enlarging mass near the bone end.

X-ray shows a dense bony mass on the surface of the bone or encircling it; the cortex is not eroded and usually a fine gap remains between cortex and tumour. The picture is easily mistaken for that of a benign bone lesion and the diagnosis is often missed until the tumour recurs after local excision. CT and MRI will show the boundary between tumour and surrounding soft tissues. Although the lesion is outside the bone, it does not spread into the adjacent muscle compartment until fairly late. Staging, therefore, often defines it as a low-grade intracompartmental tumour (stage IA).

PATHOLOGY At biopsy the tumour appears as a hard mass. On microscopic examination the lesion consists of well-formed bone but without any regular trabecular arrangement. The spaces between trabeculae are filled with cellular fibroblastic tissue; a few atypical cells and mitotic figures can usually be found.

TREATMENT Despite its apparently non-aggressive behaviour, the tumour must be treated by wide excision. Amputation through the affected bone well proximal to the lesion gives a high cure rate (over 90%). For localized lesions in accessible sites, limb-sparing resection with prosthetic replacement is usually more acceptable. If wide excision cannot be assured, the operation should be followed by radiotherapy.

Periosteal osteosarcoma

This rare tumour is quite distinct from parosteal sarcoma; unlike the latter, it is a highly malignant osteosarcoma, but situated on the surface of the bone. It occurs in young adults and causes local pain and swelling. X-ray shows a superficial defect of the cortex and CT scan may reveal a larger soft-tissue mass. The appearances may suggest a periosteal chondroma (see p. 172). Histologically this is a true osteosarcoma, but characteristically the sections show a prominent cartilaginous element.

TREATMENT is the same as that of classic osteosarcoma.

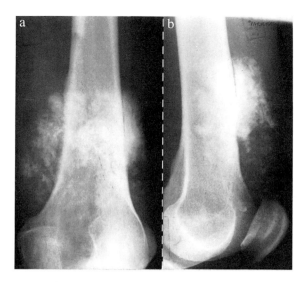

9.30 Parosteal osteosarcoma (a, b) X-rays show an ill-defined extraosseous tumour – note the linear gap between cortex and tumour.

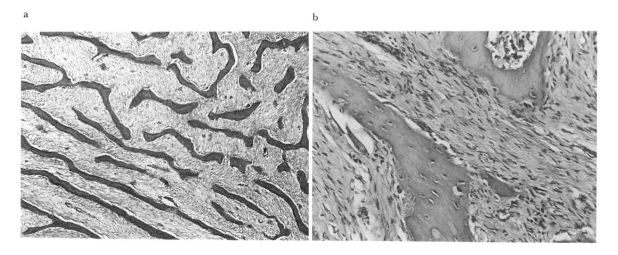

9.31 Parosteal osteosarcoma – histology (a) Histologically there were bony trabeculae and spindle-shaped, well-differentiated fibrous tissue with occasional mitotic figures. (× 120) (b) High-power view of the same. (× 300)

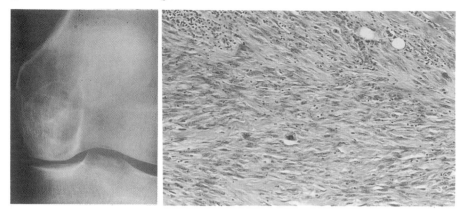

9.32 Fibrosarcoma (a) The area of bone destruction in the femoral condyle has no special distinguishing features. (b) The biopsy showed highly atypical fibroblastic tissue.

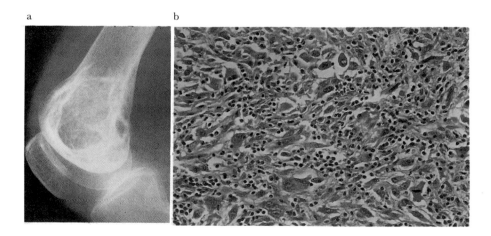

9.33 Malignant fibrous histiocytoma (a) X-ray showing a large 'cystic' lesion in the distal femur. The lesion may occur in an area of old 'bone infarct', which may account for the flecks of increased density in this x-ray. (b) Histology shows abnormal fibrohistiocytic cells, many of which are unusually large and some of which are binucleate or multinucleate. ($\times$ 480)

Paget's sarcoma

Although malignant transformation is a rare complication of Paget's disease, most osteosarcomas appearing after the age of 50 years fall into this category. Warning signs are the appearance of pain or swelling in a patient with long-standing Paget's disease. In late cases, pathological fracture may occur. X-ray shows the usual features of Paget's disease, but with areas of bone destruction and soft-tissue invasion.

This is a high-grade tumour – if anything, even more malignant than classic osteosarcoma. Staging usually shows that extracompartmental spread has occurred; most patients have pulmonary metastases by the time the tumour is diagnosed.

TREATMENT is disappointing. Even with radical resection or amputation and chemotherapy the 5-year survival rate is low. If the lesion is definitely extracompartmental, palliative treatment by radiotherapy and chemotherapy may be preferable.

Fibrosarcoma of bone

Fibrosarcoma is rare in bone, and is more likely to arise in previously abnormal tissue (a bone infarct, fibrous dysplasia or after irradiation). The patient – usually an adult – complains of pain or swelling; there may be a pathological fracture. X-ray shows an undistinctive area of bone destruction. CT or MRI will reveal the soft-tissue extension.

PATHOLOGY Histologically the lesion consists of masses of fibroblastic tissue with scattered atypical and mitotic cells. Appearances vary from well-differentiated to highly undifferentiated, and the tumours are sometimes graded accordingly.

TREATMENT Low-grade, well-confined tumours (stage IA) can be treated by wide excision with local prosthetic replacement. High-grade lesions (IIA or IIB) require radical resection or amputation; if this cannot be achieved, local excision must be combined with radiation therapy.

Malignant fibrous histiocytoma

Like fibrosarcoma, this tumour tends to occur in previously abnormal bone (old infarcts or Paget's disease). Patients are usually middle-aged adults and x-rays may reveal a destructive lesion adjacent to an old area of medullary infarction. Staging studies almost invariably show that the tumour has spread beyond the bone. Histologically it is a fibrous tumour, but the arrangement of the tissue is interweaving bundles, and the presence of histiocytes and of giant cells distinguishes it from the more uniform fibrosarcoma.

TREATMENT calls for radical resection or amputation and adjunctive chemotherapy. For inaccessible lesions, local radiotherapy may be needed.

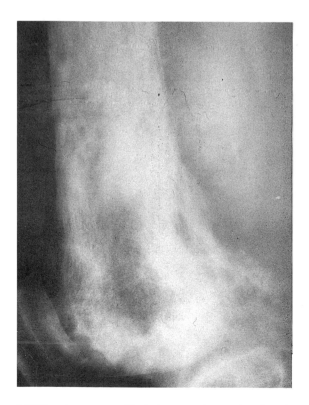

9.34 Paget's sarcoma The lesion, superimposed on Paget's disease, looks malignant – and it was.

Ewing's sarcoma

Ewing's sarcoma is believed to arise from endothelial cells in the bone marrow. It occurs most commonly between the ages of 10 and 20 years, usually in a tubular bone and especially in the tibia, fibula or clavicle.

The patient presents with pain – often throbbing in character – and swelling. Generalized illness, pyrexia, a warm, tender swelling and a raised ESR may suggest a diagnosis of osteomyelitis. X-rays usually show an area of bone destruction which, unlike that in osteosarcoma, is predominantly diaphyseal; formation of new bone may occur along the shaft and sometimes there is a fusiform layering of bone around the lesion – the so-called onion-peel effect. More often the tumour extends into the surrounding soft tissues, with radiating streaks of ossification and reactive periosteal bone at the proximal and distal margins. These features (the 'sunray' appearance and Codman's triangles) are usually associated with osteosarcoma, but they are just as common in Ewing's sarcoma. CT and MRI reveal the large extraosseous component. Radioisotope scans may show multiple areas of activity in the skeleton.

PATHOLOGY Macroscopically the tumour is lobulated and often fairly large. It may look grey (like brain) or red (like redcurrant jelly) if

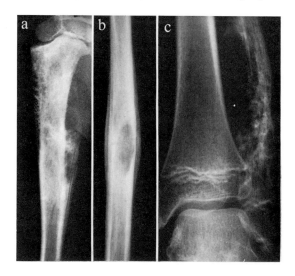

9.35 Ewing's tumour Examples of Ewing's tumour in (a) the humerus, (b) the mid-shaft of the fibula and (c) the lower end of the fibula.

haemorrhage has occurred into it. Microscopically, sheets of small dark polyhedral cells with no regular arrangement and no ground substance are seen.

DIAGNOSIS can be problematic. Clinically it is important rapidly to exclude bone infection. On biopsy the essential step is to recognize this as a malignant round-cell tumour, distinct from osteosarcoma. Other round-cell tumours that may resemble Ewing's are reticulum-cell sarcoma (see below) and metastatic neuroblastoma.

TREATMENT is somewhat controversial. The prognosis is always poor and surgery alone does little to improve it. Radiotherapy has a dramatic effect on the tumour but overall survival is not much enhanced. Chemotherapy is much more effective, offering a 5-year survival rate of about 50% (Souhami and Craft, 1988). The best results are achieved by a combination of all three methods: a course of preoperative chemotherapy; then wide excision or amputation if the tumour is in a favourable site, or radiotherapy followed by local excision if it is less accessible; and then a further course of chemotherapy for 1 year.

Reticulum-cell sarcoma (non-Hodgkin's lymphoma)

Like Ewing's sarcoma, this is a round-cell tumour of the reticuloendothelial system. It is usually seen in sites with abundant red marrow: the flat bones, the spine and the long-bone metaphyses. The patient, usually an adult of 30–40 years, presents with pain – or a pathological fracture. X-ray shows a mottled area of bone destruction in areas that normally contain red marrow; the radioisotope scan may reveal multiple lesions.

PATHOLOGY Histologically this is a marrow-cell tumour with collections of abnormal lymphocytes. Special reticulin stains are needed to show the fine fibrillar network that helps to distinguish the picture from that of Ewing's sarcoma. In recent years reticulum-cell sarcoma has come to be regarded as a variety of non-Hodgkin's lymphoma.

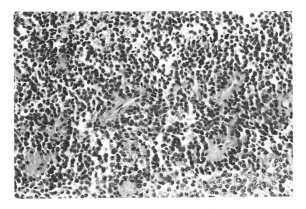

9.36 Ewing's sarcoma – histology There is a monotonous pattern of small round cells clustered around blood vessels. (× 480)

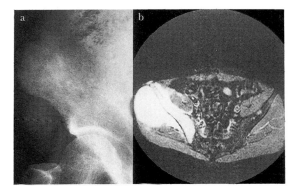

9.37 Reticulum-cell saroma (a) X-ray showing a rather nondescript mottled appearance of the ilium. (b) MRI reveals the extent of the soft-tissue lesion.

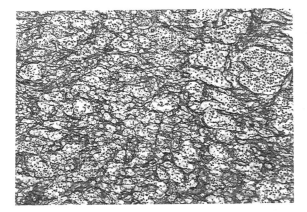

9.38 Reticulum-cell sarcoma – histology There is dense infiltration of abnormal lymphocytes (a typical 'round-cell tumour'), which is distinguished from Ewing's by the characteristic distribution of reticulin around collections of cells and between individual cells. (× 200; special reticulin stain)

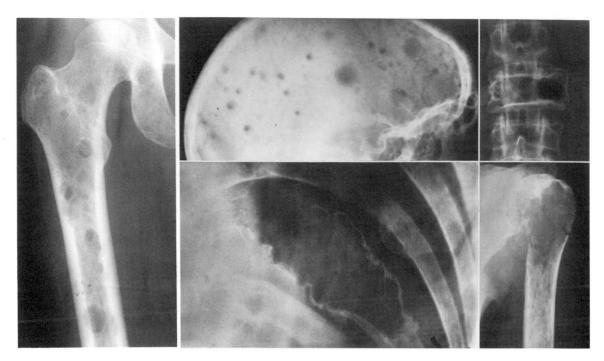

9.39 Myeloma The characteristic x-ray features are bone rarefaction, expanding lesions (typically in the ribs and pelvis) and punched-out areas in the skull and the long bones.

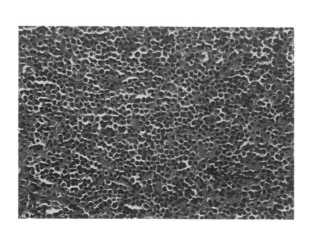

9.40 Myeloma – histology There are dense sheets of plasma cells with eccentric nuclei. (×480)

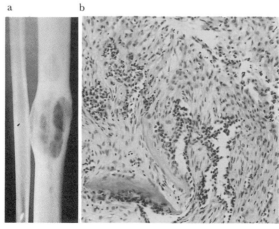

a b

9.41 Adamantinoma (a) The bubble-like appearance in the mid-shaft of the tibia is typical. (b) Histology typically shows epithelial-like cells, sometimes with an acinar arrangement. (×300)

TREATMENT is by chemotherapy and radical resection; radiotherapy is reserved for less accessible lesions.

Myeloma

Myeloma is believed to arise from plasma cells of the bone marrow. The tumours are found wherever red marrow occurs; that is, in the trunk bones, the skull and the proximal ends of femur and humerus. Sometimes it appears as a solitary tumour; usually the lesions are multiple from the start.

The patient, aged 45–65, presents with weakness, bone pain or a pathological fracture. The bone pain is constant and backache in particular is common; sometimes this is associated with root pain and, occasionally, lower limb weakness. Anaemia, cachexia and chronic nephritis all contribute to the general ill-health. There is almost invariably a high ESR. The usual cause of death is renal failure.

X-rays may show nothing more than overall reduction in density; myeloma is one of the commonest causes of secondary osteoporosis and vertebral compression fracture after the age of 45 years. Sometimes there are multiple punched-out defects with no marginal new bone around them. Thus, the x-ray features can be very similar to those of metastatic bone disease.

Investigations of importance in establishing a diagnosis are: urinalysis, which in over half the cases shows Bence-Jones protein; electrophoretic analysis of plasma and urine proteins, which shows a characteristic pattern; and sternal marrow puncture, which reveals the typical myeloma cells. Often an unusually high ESR (over 100) arouses suspicion and prompts the surgeon to undertake these investigations.

PATHOLOGY At operation the affected bone is often soft and crumbly. The typical microscopic picture is of sheets of plasmacytes with a large eccentric nucleus containing a spoke-like arrangement of chromatin.

TREATMENT Radiotherapy and chemotherapy relieve pain and pressure effects for a time, and may prolong survival. Pathological fractures in the limbs are best treated by internal fixation and packing of cavities with methylmethacrylate cement (which also helps to staunch the profuse bleeding that sometimes occurs). Perioperative antibiotic prophylaxis is important as there is a higher than usual risk of infection and wound breakdown. Spinal fractures are treated with a brace; unrelieved cord pressure may need decompression.

Plasmacytoma

This is the name often applied to a solitary myeloma. The patient presents with pain, a lump or a pathological fracture. X-ray shows a multilocular expanding osteolytic lesion in a red marrow area. Years may elapse before multiplicity becomes apparent. Treatment is by radiotherapy, combined when necessary with internal fixation and methylmethacrylate packing.

Chordoma

This rare malignant tumour arises from notochordal remnants. It affects young adults and usually presents as a slow-growing mass in the sacrum; however, it may occur elsewhere along the spine. The patient complains of longstanding backache. The tumour expands anteriorly and, if it involves the sacrum, may eventually (after months or even years) cause rectal or urethral obstruction. In late cases there may also be neurological signs. X-ray shows a radiolucent lesion in the sacrum. CT and MRI reveal the extent of intrapelvic enlargement.

TREATMENT This is a low-grade tumour, though often with extracompartmental spread. After wide excision there is little risk of recurrence. However, attempts to prevent damage to the pelvic viscera usually result in inadequate surgery. If there are doubts in this regard, operation should be combined with local radiotherapy.

Adamantinoma

This rare tumour has a predilection for the anterior cortex of the tibia but is occasionally found in other long bones. The patient is usually a young adult who complains of aching and mild swelling in the front of the leg. On examination there is thickening and tenderness along the subcutaneous border of the tibia. X-ray shows a typical bubble-like defect in the anterior tibial cortex; sometimes there is thickening of the surrounding bone.

Adamantinoma is a low-grade tumour which metastasizes late – and usually only after repeated and inadequate attempts at removal. Early on it is confined to bone; later, CT may show that the tumour has extended inwards to the medullary canal or outwards beyond the periosteum.

PATHOLOGY   The histological picture varies considerably but the most typical features are islands of epithelial-like cells on a densely populated stroma of spindle cells; the 'epithelial' nests may have an acinar arrangement.

TREATMENT   calls for wide local excision and a substantial margin of normal bone. Preoperative CT is essential to determine how deep the tumour penetrates; if it is confined to the anterior cortex, the posterior cortex can be preserved and this makes reconstruction much easier. If the lesion extends to the endosteal surface, a full segment of bone must be excised; the gap is filled with a vascularized graft. If there has been more than one recurrence, or if the tumour extends into the surrounding soft tissues, amputation is advisable.

Metastatic bone disease

The skeleton is one of the commonest sites of secondary cancer; in patients over 50 years bone metastases are seen more frequently than all primary malignant bone tumours together. The commonest source is carcinoma of the breast; next in frequency are carcinomas of the prostate, kidney, lung, thyroid, bladder and gastrointestinal tract. In about 10% of cases no primary tumour is found.

The commonest sites for bone metastases are the vertebrae, pelvis, the proximal half of the femur and the humerus. Spread is usually via the blood stream; occasionally, visceral tumours spread directly to adjacent bones (e.g. the pelvis or ribs).

Metastases are usually osteolytic, and pathological fractures are common. Bone resorption is due either to the direct action of tumour cells or to tumour-derived factors that stimulate osteoclastic activity. Osteoblastic lesions are uncommon; they usually occur in prostatic carcinoma.

Clinical features

The patient is usually aged 50–70 years; with any destructive bone lesion in this age group, the differential diagnosis must include metastasis.

Pain is the commonest – and often the only – clinical feature. The sudden appearance of backache or thigh pain in an elderly person – and especially someone known to have been treated for carcinoma in the past – is always suspicious. If x-rays do not show anything, a radionuclide scan might.

Some deposits remain clinically silent and are discovered incidentally on x-ray, or after a pathological fracture. Sudden collapse of a vertebral body or a fracture of the mid-shaft of a long bone in an elderly person are ominous signs; if there is no history and no clinical clue pointing to a primary carcinoma, a biopsy of the fracture area is essential.

In children under 6 years of age, metastatic lesions are most commonly from adrenal neuroblastoma. The child presents with bone pain and fever; examination reveals the abdominal mass.

Symptoms of hypercalcaemia may occur (and are often missed) in patients with skeletal metastases. These include anorexia, nausea, abdominal pain, general weakness, depression and polyuria.

X-RAYS   Most skeletal deposits are osteolytic and appear as rare areas in the medulla or produce a moth-eaten appearance in the cortex; sometimes there is marked bone destruction, with or without a pathological fracture. Osteoblastic deposits usually signify prostatic carcinoma; the pelvis may show a mottled increase in density which has to be distinguished from Paget's disease or lymphoma.

Radioscintigraphy with ^{99m}Tc-HDP is the most sensitive method of detecting 'silent' metastatic deposits in bone; areas of increased activity are selected for x-ray examination.

SPECIAL INVESTIGATIONS The ESR may be increased and the haemoglobin concentration is usually low. The serum alkaline phosphatase level is often increased, and in prostatic carcinoma the acid phosphatase also is elevated.

Patients with breast cancer can be screened by measuring blood levels of CA15–3, a breast tumour-associated antigen that serves as a reliable marker of bone metastases (O'Brien et al., 1992).

Treatment

By the time a patient has developed secondary deposits the prognosis, as far as life is concerned, is almost hopeless. Occasionally, radical treatment (by combined surgery and radiotherapy) of a solitary secondary deposit and of its parent primary may be rewarding and even apparently curative. This applies particularly to hypernephroma and thyroid tumours; but in the great majority of cases, and certainly in those with multiple secondaries, treatment is entirely symptomatic. For that reason, elaborate witch-hunts to discover the source of an occult primary tumour are to be deprecated; the search may be diagnostically satisfying but is therapeutically valueless and psychologically harmful.

Despite the ultimately hopeless prognosis, patients deserve to be made comfortable, to enjoy (as far as possible) their remaining months or years, and to die in a peaceful and dignified way. The active treatment of skeletal metastases contributes to this in no small measure. In addition, patients need sympathetic counselling and practical assistance with their material affairs.

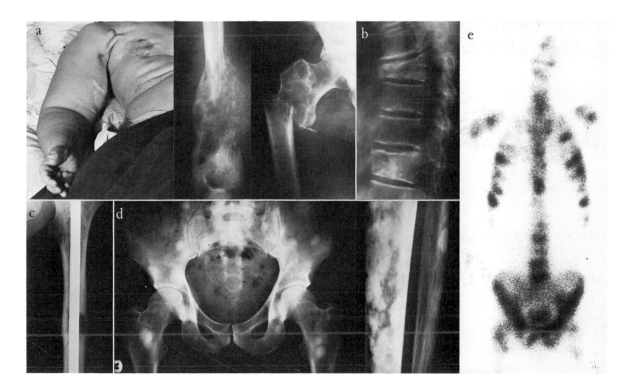

9.42 Metastatic deposits (a) This patient presents an all-too-familiar picture. (b) Spinal secondary deposits. (c) Osteolytic deposits are liable to fracture and invite prophylatic fixation. (d) Osteoblastic deposits in the pelvis and tibia, from prostatic carcinoma. (e) Radioscintigraphy revealed some silent deposits in this patient.

CONTROL OF PAIN AND METASTATIC ACTIVITY Most patients require analgesics, but the more powerful narcotics should be reserved for the terminally ill.

Unless specifically contraindicated, radiotherapy is used both to control pain and to reduce metastatic growth. This is often combined with other forms of treatment (e.g. internal fixation).

Secondary deposits from breast or prostate can often be controlled by hormone therapy: stilboestrol for prostatic secondaries and androgenic drugs or oestrogens for breast carcinoma. Disseminated secondaries from breast carcinoma are sometimes treated by oöphorectomy combined with adrenalectomy or by hypophyseal ablation.

Intractable pain occasionally requires nerve or spinal tract ablation.

Hypercalcaemia may have serious consequences, including renal acidosis, nephrocalcinosis, unconsciousness and coma. It should be treated by ensuring adequate hydration, reducing the calcium intake and, if necessary, administering diphosphonates.

TREATMENT OF FRACTURES Surgical timidity may condemn the patient to a painful lingering death, so shaft fractures should almost invariably be treated by internal fixation and (if necessary) packing with methylmethacrylate cement. If there are multiple fractures, several bones may be fixed at one sitting. Pain is immediately relieved, nursing is made easier and the patient can get up and about or attend for other types of treatment without unnecessary discomfort. Shaft fractures usually unite satisfactorily.

In most cases intramedullary nailing is the most effective method; fractures near joints (e.g. the distal femur or proximal tibia) may need fixation with plates or blade-plates.

Fractures of the femoral neck rarely, if ever, unite. They are best treated by prosthetic replacement: a hemiarthroplasty if the pelvis is intact, or total joint replacement if the acetabulum is involved. If the pelvic wall is destroyed, it can be reconstructed by large bone grafts or a custom-made prosthesis; however, if such extensive surgery is contraindicated, one may have to settle for a simple excisional arthroplasty.

Postoperative irradiation is essential to prevent further extension of the metastatic lesion.

PROPHYLACTIC FIXATION Large deposits that threaten to result in fracture should be treated by internal fixation while the bone is still intact. The principles are the same as for the management of fractures. A preoperative radionuclide scan will show whether other lesions are present in that bone, thus calling for more extensive fixation and postoperative radiotherapy.

SPINAL STABILIZATION Vertebral fractures usually require some form of support. If the spine is stable, a well-fitting brace may be sufficient. However, spinal instability may cause severe pain, making it almost impossible for the patient to sit or stand – with or without a brace. For these patients, operative stabilization is indicated – usually a posterior spinal fusion – followed by radiotherapy.

Preoperative assessment should include CT or MRI, and sometimes myelography, to establish whether the cord is threatened; if it is, spinal decompression should be carried out at the same time.

If there are overt symptoms and signs of cord compression, treatment is urgent. If the patient is expected to live for some time, surgical decompression and fusion are indicated; if not, it may be wiser (and more humane) to give radiotherapy, alone or together with corticosteroids and narcotics to control oedema and pain.

Soft-tissue tumours

Benign soft-tissue tumours are common, malignant ones rare. The distinction between these two groups is not always easy, and some lesions, treated confidently as 'benign', recur in more aggressive form after inadequate removal. Features suggestive of malignancy are: pain in a previously painless lump; a rapid increase in size; poor demarcation; and attachment to the surrounding structures. Sonograms of malignant lesions are said to show a discrete echo pattern, whereas with benign lesions the pattern may be ill-defined (Lange et al., 1987). When doubt exists, a biopsy is essential. Wherever possible this should take the form of an excisional biopsy, including a wide margin of normal tissue around the tumour. As with bone tumours, special imaging and staging should be carried out before the field is disturbed by operation. Chest x-rays and blood investigations may be necessary as well.

The account that follows is intended as a summary of those soft-tissue tumours likely to be encountered in orthopaedics.

Fatty tumours

Lipoma

A lipoma, one of the commonest of all tumours, may occur almost anywhere; sometimes there are multiple lesions. The tumour usually arises in the subcutaneous layer. It consists of lobules of fat with a surrounding capsule which may become tethered to neighbouring structures. The patient, usually aged over 50, complains of a painless swelling. The lump is soft and almost fluctuant; the well-defined edge and lobulated surface distinguish it from a chronic abscess. Fat is notably radiotranslucent, a feature that betrays the occasional subperiosteal lipoma.

If the lump is troublesome it may be removed by marginal excision. Prior biopsy is usually unnecessary. There is no risk of malignant transformation.

Liposarcoma

Liposarcoma is rare but should be suspected if a fatty tumour (especially in the buttock or thigh) goes on growing and becomes painful. The lump may feel quite firm and is usually not translucent. CT is essential to determine the extent of the tumour.

Treatment depends on the degree of malignancy. Low-grade lesions can be removed by wide excision; high-grade tumours need radical resection or amputation. For liposarcomas in inaccessible sites, radiation therapy is often effective.

Fibrous tumours

Fibroma

The common fibroma is a solitary, benign tumour of fibrous tissue. It is usually discovered as a small asymptomatic nodule or lump. Treatment is not essential; if it is removed, a marginal excision is adequate.

Palmar fibroma (Dupuytren's contracture)

A palmar fibroma may be the first evidence of Dupuytren's contracture (see p. 320).

Fibromatosis

This term is applied to lesions that are more aggressive than simple fibromas and have a

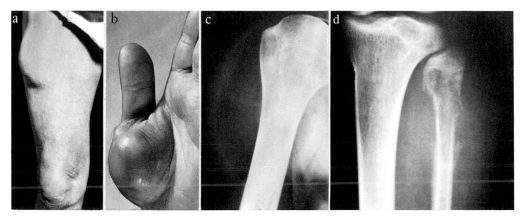

9.43 Fatty tumours   (a) Subcutaneous lipoma – like so many lipomas, this one felt almost fluctuant; (b) intramuscular lipoma; (c) subperiosteal lipoma; (d) liposarcoma – the cortex of the fibula has been eroded.

strong tendency to recur after excision. They appear, usually in young adults, as thick cords or plaques in the subcutaneous tissues of the limbs or trunk. If left, they grow into featureless masses with ill-defined margins, sometimes extending proximally up the limb or along the trunk. After local excision they tend to recur, and new lesions appear more and more proximally. Pressure on nerves may cause paraesthesiae. CT is useful to show the extent of this invasive tumour.

Although not malignant in the true sense of the term, the lesion can be highly aggressive. Local excision is often performed too timidly, and the recurrences are more and more invasive and difficult to eradicate without damage to nerves or blood vessels. Wide excision is essential, especially if the lesion threatens to involve the pelvis or axilla; once this has occurred, complete removal may be impossible. Occasionally, amputation is the only solution.

Microscopically these lesions vary from those with clearly benign cells to some whose appearance suggests malignancy (multinucleated cells with many mitoses). The differentiation from fribrosarcoma is difficult and demands considerable histological expertise; but it is important because fibromatosis does not metastasize and can be eradicated if surgery is sufficiently thorough.

Fibrosarcoma

Fibrosarcoma may occur in any area of connective tissue but is more common in the extremities. It presents as an ill-defined mass and may grow to a considerable size. The diagnosis is usually made only after biopsy and histological examination. Local extension can be shown on CT. There may be metastases in the lungs.

High-grade lesions showing atypical spindle cells are usually easy to diagnose. Low-grade lesions may be difficult to distinguish from fibromatosis.

For low-grade lesions, wide excision (sometimes combined with radiation therapy) is sufficient. For high-grade lesions, amputation may be the wisest choice.

Synovial tumours

Pigmented villonodular synovitis and giant-cell tumour of tendon sheath

These are two forms of the same condition – a benign disorder that occurs wherever synovial membrane is found: in joints, tendon sheaths or bursae.

Pigmented villonodular synovitis (PVNS) presents as a long-standing boggy swelling of the joint – usually the hip, knee or ankle – in an adolescent or young adult. X-ray may show excavations in the juxta-articular bone on either side of the joint. When the joint is opened, the synovium is swollen and hyperplastic, often covered with villi and golden-brown in colour – the effect of haemosiderin deposition. The juxta-articular excavations contain clumps of friable synovial material.

Tendon sheath lesions are seen mainly in the hands and feet, where they cause nodular thickening of the affected sheath. X-ray may show pressure erosion of an adjacent bone surface – for example, on one of the phalanges. At operation the boggy synovial tissue is often yellow; this type of lesion is sometimes called *xanthoma of tendon sheath.*

Histologically, joint and tendon sheath lesions are identical. There is proliferation and hypertrophy of the synovium, which contains fibroblastic tissue with foamy histiocytes and multinucleated giant cells. These features have engendered yet another name for the same condition: *giant-cell tumour of tendon sheath.*

Treatment is by synovectomy. Although the tumour does not undergo malignant change, the local recurrence rate is high unless excision is complete. In the knees (especially) this may be impossible and incomplete synovectomy is sometimes combined with local radiotherapy. If, despite such aggressive treatment, there are repeated recurrences, it may be necessary to sacrifice the joint and carry out arthroplasty or arthrodesis.

Synovial sarcoma (malignant synovioma)

This rare malignant tumour of synovium causes rapid enlargement of the joint, usually around the knee, hip or shoulder. Occasionally it presents as a small swelling in the hand or foot

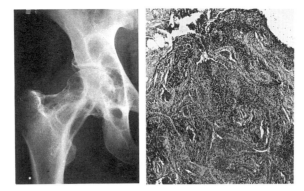

9.44 Pigmented villonodular synovitis (a) This farmer presented with pain in the hip. The x-rays showing cystic excavations on both sides of the joint at first suggested tuberculosis. However, there were no signs of infection. At operation the synovium was thick and golden in colour. (b) The biopsy showed dense proliferation of the synovium with scattered multinucleated giant cells. (× 120)

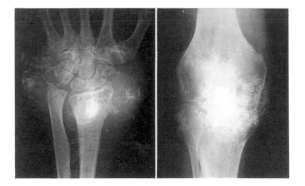

9.45 Malignant synoviomas They show the typical snow-storm appearance.

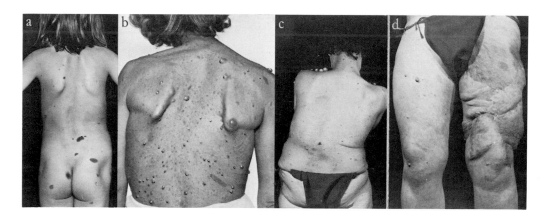

9.46 Neurofibromatosis   (a) Café-au-lait spots, (b) molluscum fibrosum with slight scoliosis; (c, d) a patient with scoliosis and elephantiasis.

and the histological diagnosis comes as a complete surprise. X-ray shows a soft-tissue mass, sometimes with extensive calcification. CT and MRI will help to outline the tumour. Biopsy reveals a fleshy tumour composed of proliferative synovial cells and fibroblastic tissue; characteristically the cellular areas are punctured by vacant slits that give the tissue an acinar appearance. Cellular abnormality and mitoses reflect the degree of malignancy.

Small, well-defined lesions can be treated by wide excision. High-grade lesions, which usually have ill-defined margins, require radical resection – and this usually means radical amputation – combined with radiotherapy and chemotherapy.

Blood vessel tumours

Haemangioma

This benign lesion, probably a hamartoma, is usually seen during childhood but may be present at birth. It occurs in two forms. The *capillary haemangioma* is more common; it usually appears as a reddish patch on the skin, and the congenital naevus or 'birthmark' is a familiar example. A *cavernous haemangioma* consists of a sponge-like collection of blood spaces; superficial lesions appear as blue or purple skin patches, sometimes overlying a soft subcutaneous mass; deep lesions may extend into the fascia or muscles, and occasionally an entire limb is involved. X-rays may show calcified phleboliths in the cavernous lesions.

There is no risk of malignant change and treatment is needed only if there is significant discomfort or disability. Local excision carries a high risk of recurrence, but more radical procedures seem unnecessarily destructive.

Glomus tumour

This rare tumour usually occurs around fine peripheral neurovascular structures, and especially in the nail beds of fingers or toes. A young adult presents with recurrent episodes of intense pain in the fingertip. A small bluish nodule may be seen under the nail; the area is sensitive to cold and exquisitely tender. X-rays sometimes show erosion of the underlying phalanx. Treatment is excision; the tumour, never larger than a pea, is easily shelled out of its fibrous capsule.

Nerve tumours

Neuroma

A neuroma is not a tumour but an overgrowth of fibrous tissue and randomly sprouting nerve fibrils following injury to nerve. It is often tender and local percussion may induce paraesthesiae distal to the lesion (Tinel's sign). Treatment can be frustrating, but a promising method of prophylaxis during amputations is to free the epineural sleeve from the nerve fascicles and to seal this sleeve with a synthetic tissue adhesive (Martini and Fromm, 1989).

Neurilemmoma

Neurilemmoma is a benign tumour of the nerve sheath. It is seen in the peripheral nerves and in the spinal nerve roots. The patient complains of pain or paraesthesiae; sometimes there is a small palpable swelling along the course of the nerve. Root lesions are a rare cause of 'sciatica', and x-rays of the spine may show erosion of an intervertebral foramen.

With careful dissection the tumour can be removed from its capsule without damage to the nerve.

Neurofibroma

This is a benign tumour of fibrous and neural elements; its origin in a peripheral nerve may be obvious, but it is also seen as a nodule in the skin or subcutaneous tissues where it presumably originates in fine nerve fibrils. Occasionally it arises directly in bone; more often it causes pressure erosion of an adjacent surface. Lesions may be solitary or multiple. Curiously, they are sometimes associated with skeletal abnormalities (scoliosis, pseudarthrosis of the tibia) or overgrowth of a digit or an entire limb, in which there is no obvious neural pathology.

The patient may present with a lump overlying one of the peripheral nerves, or with neurological symptoms such as paraesthesiae or muscle weakness. If a nerve root is involved, symptoms can mimic those of a disc prolapse; x-rays may show erosion of a vertebral pedicle or enlargement of the intervertebral foramen.

Multiple neurofibromatosis (von Recklinghausen's disease) is transmitted by autosomal dominant inheritance. Patients (usually children) develop numerous skin nodules and café-au-lait patches; there may be associated skeletal abnormalities. Malignant transformation is said to occur in 5–10% of cases.

The pathological appearances are characteristic: on cross-section the tumour consists of pale fibrous tissue with nerve elements running into and through the substance of the tumour. Microscopically, the fibrillar and cellular elements are arranged in a wavy pattern.

Treatment is needed only if pain or paraesthesiae become troublesome, or if a tumour becomes very large. The tumour cannot be separated from intact nerve fibres; if it involves an unimportant nerve, it can be excised en bloc; if nerve damage is not acceptable, intracapsular shelling out is preferable, notwithstanding the risk of recurrence.

Neurosarcoma (malignant schwannoma)

Malignant tumours may arise from the cells of the nerve sheath or from a pre-existing neurofibroma. Symptoms are due to local pressure; there may be a visible or palpable swelling, and percussion causes distal paraesthesiae.

Histologically this is a cellular fibrous lesion, similar to a fibrosarcoma. However, if it arises in the neurovascular bundle, spread is inevitable and local excision is not feasible without severe damage to important structures. For this reason, treatment usually involves radical amputation.

Muscle tumours

Tumours of muscle are rare; only those that occur in the striped muscle of the extremities are considered here.

Rhabdomyoma

A rhabdomyoma (tumour of a striped muscle) is rare and should not be confused with the lump that follows muscle rupture. Both are in the line of a muscle, can be moved across but not along it, and harden with muscle action; the muscle rupture, however, has a depression distal to the lump and the lump is not getting bigger. If a tumour is suspected, early exploration is advisable because malignant change is not uncommon; not infrequently the swelling proves to be normal muscle fibres in an anomalous situation.

Rhabdomyosarcoma

Malignant tumours are occasionally seen in the bulky muscles around the shoulder or hip. The patient – usually a young adult – presents with ache and an enlarging, ill-defined lump attached to and moving with the affected muscle. CT and MRI show that the mass is in the muscle, but the edge may be poorly demarcated because the tumour tends to spread along the fascial planes. At biopsy the tissue looks and feels different from normal muscle and microscopic examination shows clusters of highly abnormal muscle cells.

This is a high-grade lesion which requires radical resection of the affected muscle – i.e. from origin to insertion. If this cannot be assured or if the tumour has spread beyond the fascial sheath, amputation is advisable. Recurrent lesions are also treated by amputation. If complete removal is impossible, adjunctive radiotherapy may lessen the risk of recurrence.

References and further reading

Cannon, S.R. (1986) Massive osteolysis. *Journal of Bone and Joint Surgery* **68B**, 24–28

Colton, C.L. and Hardy, J.G. (1983) Evaluation of a sterilizable radiation probe as an aid to the surgical treatment of osteoid osteoma. *Journal of Bone and Joint Surgery* **65A**, 1019–1022

Enneking, W.F. (1983) *Musculoskeletal Tumour Surgery*, Churchill Livingstone, New York, Edinburgh, London, Melbourne

Enneking, W.F. (1986) A system of staging musculoskeletal neoplasms. *Clinical Orthopaedics and Related Research* **204**, 9–24

Enneking, W.F. (Ed.) (1987) *Limb Surgery in Musculoskeletal Oncology*, Churchill Livingstone, New York

Lange, T.A., Austin, C.W., Siebert, J.J., Angtuaco, T.L. and Yandow, D.R. (1987) Ultrasound imaging as a screening study for malignant soft tissue tumours. *Journal of Bone and Joint Surgery* **69A**, 100–105

Levy, W.M., Miller, A.S., Bonakdarpour, A. et al. (1975) Aneurysmal bone cyst secondary to other osseous lesions. A report of 57 cases. *American Journal of Clinical Pathology* **63**, 1–8

Lichtenstein, L. (1964) Histiocytosis X: further observations of pathologic and clinical importance. *Journal of Bone and Joint Surgery* **46A**, 76–90

McLeod, R.A., Dahlin, D.C. and Beabout, J.W. (1976) The spectrum of ostcoblastoma. *American Journal of Roentgenology* **126**, 321–335

Malghem, J., Maldague, B., Esselinckx, W., Noel, H., DeNayer, P. and Vincent, A. (1989) Spontaneous healing of aneurysmal bone cysts. *Journal of Bone and Joint Surgery* **71B**, 645–650

Mankin, H.J. and Gebhardt, M.C. (1985) Advances in the management of bone tumours. *Clinical Orthopaedics and Related Research* **200**, 73–84

Martini, A. and Fromm, B. (1989) A new operation for the prevention and treatment of amputation neuromas. *Journal of Bone and Joint Surgery* **71B**, 379–382

Monkman, G.R., Orwoll, G. and Ivins, J.C. (1974) Trauma and oncogenesis. *Mayo Clinic Proceedings* **49**, 157–163

O'Brien, D.P., Horgan, P.G., Gough, D.B. et al. (1992) CA15–3: a reliable indicator of metastatic bone disease in breast cancer patients. *Annals of the Royal College of Surgeons of England* **74**, 9–12

Pettersson, H., Gillespy, T., Hamlin, D.J. et al. (1987) Primary musculoskeletal tumors: examination with MR imaging compared with conventional modalities. *Radiology* **164**, 237–241

Rosen, G. (1987) Neoadjuvant chemotherapy for osteogenic sarcoma. In *Limb Salvage in Musculoskeletal Oncology* (ed. W.F. Enneking), Churchill Livingstone, New York, p. 260

Rosen, G., Caparrow, B., Huvos, A.G. et al. (1982) Pre-operative chemotherapy for osteogenic sarcoma: selection of post-operative chemotherapy based on the response of the primary tumor to pre-operative chemotherapy. *Cancer* **49**, 1221–1230

Scaglietti, O., Marchetti, P.G. and Bartolozzi, P. (1979) The effects of methylprednisolone acetate in the treatment of bone cysts. *Journal of Bone and Joint Surgery* **61B**, 200–208

Souhami, R.L. and Craft, A.W. (1988) Annotation. Progress in management of malignant bone tumours. *Journal of Bone and Joint Surgery* **70B**, 345–347

Stark, A., Kreicbergs, A., Nilsonne, U. and Sillvensward, L. (1990) The age of osteosarcoma patients is increasing. *Journal of Bone and Joint Surgery* **72**, 89–93

Watt, I. (1985) Radiology in the diagnosis and management of bone tumours. *Journal of Bone and Joint Surgery* **67B**, 520–529

Neuromuscular disorders 10

The neuron

The neuron is the specialized cell of the nervous system, capable of electrical excitation and conduction of impulses (action potentials) along one of its thread-like extensions – the axon. Motor axons carry efferent impulses to the periphery; sensory axons carry afferent impulses to the spinal cord or brain.

Peripheral nerves carry motor, sensory and autonomic fibres. *Motor axons* run from cells in the anterior horn of the spinal cord to striated muscle throughout the body. *Sensory neurons* have their cells in the dorsal root (or cranial nerve) ganglia; they carry impulses from receptors in the skin and deep structures. *Autonomic sympathetic axons* arise from cells in the thoracolumbar cord; preganglionic fibres leave with the ventral roots to enter the sympathetic chain and synapse with postganglionic fibres that supply blood vessels and sweat glands in the periphery. Parasympathetic fibres pass from the cord and synapse in ganglia close to their target organs.

Peripheral nerve structure is described in Chapter 11. Here it should merely be noted that they carry a mixture of myelinated and unmyelinated axons; the former include all motor axons and the larger sensory axons serving touch, pain and proprioception, while the latter (much the more numerous) are small-diameter sensory fibres serving crude touch, pain and warmth and sympathetic vaso-motor and sudomotor fibres. Damage to the myelin sheath – by either disease or injury – will cause slowing of conduction and, eventually, loss of sensory and motor functions.

Axons carry the impulse along the nerve pathway by a series of relays, or *synapses*, where the message is passed on by chemical neuro-transmitters – chiefly acetylcholine. For a motor neuron the cell body is in the anterior horn of the spinal cord and the terminal synapse is at the neuromuscular junction. Sensory neurons have their cell bodies in the dorsal root ganglia and their synapses in the spinal cord.

Each motor neuron innervates hundreds of muscle fibres. Normal resting muscle tone is maintained by a reflex arc consisting of fast-conducting sensory fibres from the muscle spindles (stretch receptors) and alpha motor neurons. Sudden stretching of the muscle (e.g. by tapping the tendon sharply) induces an involuntary muscle contraction – the stretch reflex. This reflex is normally monitored or controlled by impulses passing from the brain down the spinal cord. Interruption of the central nervous pathways (the upper motor neurons) results in undamped reflex contraction and *spastic paralysis*. Damage to the anterior horn cells or peripheral motor nerves causes *flaccid paralysis*.

Muscle

Skeletal muscle is *striated muscle*. Each muscle belly consists of thousands of *muscle fibres*, each of which is made up of many tiny (1 μm diameter) *myofibrils*. The motor neuron and the group of muscle fibres supplied by it make up a *motor unit*.

Muscle fibres are of different types, which can be distinguished by histochemical staining. *Type I fibres* contract slowly and are not easily fatigued; their prime function is postural control. *Type II fibres* are fast contracting and are rapidly fatigued; they are ideally suited to intense activities of short duration. The muscles of the body comprise a mixture of fibre types, the proportions varying from person to person. The average individual has 50% type I and 50% type II fibres, and long-distance runners have more of type I fibres.

Muscle wasting follows either disuse or denervation: in the former, the fibres are intact but thinner; in the latter, they degenerate and are replaced by fibrous tissue or fat.

Neurological disorders

Of the vast range of neurological disorders, there are several that produce characteristic – and often remediable – defects in musculoskeletal function. The following conditions are dealt with here: (1) cerebral palsy and other upper motor neuron (spastic) disorders, (2) spinocerebellar degeneration (Friedreich's ataxia, (3) compressive lesions of the spinal cord, (4) neural tube defects (spina bifida), (5) anterior poliomyelitis, (6) motor neuron disorders and (7) peripheral neuropathies. (Peripheral nerve injuries are considered in Chapter 11.)

Clinical assessment

Age   Cerebral palsy and spina bifida present during infancy. Poliomyelitis usually occurs in childhood, but may be seen at any age. Spinal cord lesions and peripheral neuropathies are more common in adults. However, the orthopaedic surgeon deals mainly with the residual effects of neurological disease, and these may require diagnosis and treatment throughout life.

Muscle weakness   may be due to upper motor neuron lesions (spastic paresis), lower motor neuron lesions (flaccid paresis) or muscle disorders. The type of weakness, its distribution and rate of onset are important clues to diagnosis.

Numbness and paraesthesiae   may be the main complaints. It is important to establish their exact distribution as this will often localize the lesion accurately. The rate of onset and the relationship to posture may, likewise, suggest the cause.

Other features,   such as headache, dizziness, loss of balance, change in visual acuity or hearing, disorder of speech and loss of bladder or bowel control may be significant.

Deformity   is a common complaint in long-standing disorders. It arises from muscle imbalance (see below) and therefore usually goes hand in hand with other symptoms. However, minor degrees of weakness in one muscle group may go unnoticed and the deformity appears so insidiously that its cause may escape detection (e.g. claw toes or scoliosis).

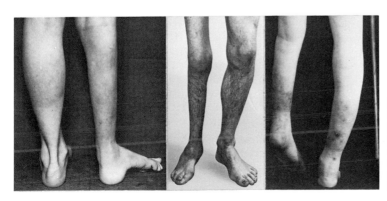

10.1 Some effects of neurological lesions These patients, all of whom had polio, illustrate some of the effects of paralysis – deformity, wasting and shortening; the trophic changes in the patient on the right suggest that, in her, the anterolateral horn cells also may have been damaged.

Examination should include a *complete neurological assessment* (see Chapter 1). Particular attention should be paid to the patient's *mental state*, natural *posture, gait, sense of balance, involuntary movements, muscle wasting, muscle tone* and *power, reflexes, skin changes*, the various *modes of sensibility* and autonomic functions such as *sphincter control, peripheral blood flow* and *sweating*.

The back should be examined for skin changes, local deformities (e.g. a kyphos) and mobility.

Grading muscle power

In assessment it is important to examine not only individual muscles but also functional groups. Grading muscle power is most valuable in the floppy type of paralysis associated with spina bifida and poliomyelitis; in cerebral palsy, grading is useful but difficult because spasticity obscures the undoubted weakness. Muscle charting pinpoints the site and severity of paralysis; repetition enables progress to be recorded. The following grades are standard:

0 total paralysis
1 barely detectable contracture
2 not enough power to act against gravity
3 strong enough to act against gravity
4 still stronger but less than normal
5 full power

Deformity

In long-standing disorders, deformity may become a major problem. It arises when one group of muscles is too weak to balance the pull of antagonists (*unbalanced paralysis*). At first it can be corrected passively but with time the joint structures contract and the deformity becomes fixed.

When all muscle groups are equally weak (*balanced paralysis*) the joint simply assumes the position imposed on it by gravity. The joint is unstable and, on examination, the limb feels floppy or flail.

Paralysis arising in childhood seriously affects *bone growth*. The bone is both thinner and shorter than normal and, in the absence of the mechanical stresses normally imposed by muscle pull, modelling is defective. The bone

ends may appear dysplastic and there may be loss of joint congruity. A good example is the common valgus deformity of the femoral neck, with acetabular dysplasia and hip subluxation, resulting from childhood weakness of the hip abductors.

Gait and posture

Watching the patient walk is most valuable. With experience, certain typical patterns will be recognized.

A *spastic gait* is stiff and jerky, often with the feet in equinus, the knees somewhat flexed and the hips adducted ('scissoring'). The term *dystonia* refers to abnormal posturing of any part of the body, often aggravated when the patient concentrates on movement (see box).

A *high-stepping gait*, where the legs are lifted unnecessarily high off the ground, signifies either a problem with proprioception and balance or bilateral foot drop.

A *drop-foot gait* is due to peripheral neuropathy or injury of the nerves supplying the dorsiflexors of the ankle. During the swing phase the foot falls into equinus ('drops') and if it were not lifted higher than usual the toes would drag along the ground.

A *waddling gait*, in which the trunk is thrown from side to side with each step, may be due to dislocation of the hips or to weakness of the abductor muscles.

Ataxia produces a more obvious and irregular loss of balance, which is compensated for by a broad-based gait, or sometimes uncontrollable staggering.

CAUSES OF DYSTONIA

Generalized
1. Cerebral disorders, most commonly cerebral palsy, stroke and Huntington's disease
2. Drug-induced

Focal dystonia
1. Stroke (hemiplegia or monoplegia)
2. Spasmodic torticollis
3. Writer's cramp

Imaging studies

Plain x-rays of the skull and/or spine are routine for all disorders of the central nervous system. If the diagnosis is not obvious, further studies by myelography, CT or MRI may be necessary.

Intraspinal compression

Imaging of the spine is essentially aimed at demonstrating compression of the spinal cord or nerve roots.

Fractures and dislocations usually show on the plain x-rays, but a CT scan will reveal the exact relationship of bone fragments to nerve structures.

Prolapsed intervertebral disc is usually diagnosed on clinical examination, but myelography or CT will help to establish the extent of the lesion and its exact site.

Narrowing of the spinal canal is best demonstrated by CT. The commonest cause is osteophytic overgrowth following disc degeneration and osteoarthritis of the facet joints. This is even worse when the spinal canal is congenitally narrow or trefoil-shaped (spinal stenosis).

Destructive lesions of the bones may be due to *infection* or *tumour* (usually metastatic lesions).

These may show on plain x-rays, but CT, MRI or myelography is usually helpful.

Electrodiagnosis

Neurophysiological studies, though hardly part of the routine examination, can be extremely helpful in elucidating less obvious syndromes.

Electromyography (EMG) records the motor response to nerve stimuli. It is of greatest use (1) in deciding whether the muscle weakness is due to nerve or muscle disorder, and (2) in establishing the site of compression in peripheral nerve entrapment.

Other special investigations

Depending on the type of disorder, diagnostic investigations may include *blood tests* (cell counts, ESR, serology, blood sugar, muscle enzymes), *cerebrospinal fluid examination* and specialized tests for *vision, hearing, speech* and *mental capacity.*

MUSCLE BIOPSY A biopsy may yield valuable information in diagnosing muscle disorders.

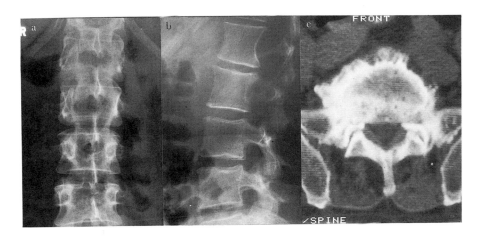

10.2 Imaging   (a) In the lower two vertebrae the pedicles are seen end on and look like eyes; the upper two vertebrae are 'blind' because the pedicles have been destroyed by tumour. (b) The scalloping at the back of the upper two vertebrae is typical of a neurofibroma. (c) This CT scan shows degeneration of the facet joints with encroachment on the intervertebral foramina and spinal canal.

However, for the findings to be reliable, certain precautions are necessary. The sample should be taken from an affected muscle, but one that is still working; the muscle itself must not be injected with local anaesthetic; the specimen, about 2 cm long and 1 cm wide, should be handled gently and kept at the natural fibre length by laying it on a wooden spatula and securing the two ends with stitches before placing it in fixative.

Specimens for light microscopy are fixed in 10% formalin; those for electron microscopy in glutaraldehyde; and those for histochemical staining are frozen at −160°C.

damage during early development. The incidence is about 2 per 1000 live births. Known causal factors are maternal toxaemia, prematurity, perinatal anoxia, kernicterus and postnatal brain infections or injury; birth injury, though often blamed, is a distinctly unusual cause. The main consequence is the development of neuromuscular incoordination, dystonia, weakness and spasticity; in addition there may be convulsions, perceptual problems, speech disorder and mental retardation or behavioral problems.

There are four main varieties of cerebral palsy: spastic (over 60% of all cases), athetotic, ataxic and rigid. In about 10% of cases there is a mixture of features.

Cerebral palsy

The term 'cerebral palsy' includes a group of disorders that result from non-progressive brain

Early diagnosis

The full-blown clinical picture may take months or even years to develop. Diagnosis in infancy calls for painstaking examination. A history of

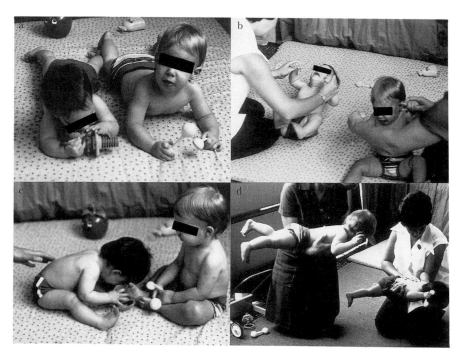

10.3 Cerebral palsy – early diagnosis By 6 months these twin brothers had developed quite differently, the one being smaller and showing (a) lack of head and arm control, (b) lack of body control when helped to the sitting position, (c) inability to sit unaided, and (d) lack of the normal extension response when turned face downwards.

prenatal toxaemia, haemorrhage, premature birth, difficult labour, fetal distress or kernicterus should arouse suspicion. Early symptoms include difficulty in sucking and swallowing, with dribbling at the mouth. The mother may notice that the baby feels stiff or wriggles awkwardly.

Gradually it becomes apparent that the milestones are delayed (the normal child holds up its head at 3 months, sits up at 6 months and begins walking at about 1 year). Neonatal reflexes (e.g. the grasp reflex, withdrawal reflexes and sucking reflexes) may be delayed.

Bleck (1987) has described seven tests for children over 1 year; these give an idea of severity and of the prognosis for walking. The primitive neck-righting reflex, asymmetrical and symmetrical tonic neck reflexes, the Moro reflex and the extensor thrust response should all have disappeared at 1 year. The 'parachute reflex' and the stepping reflex should be present. If several of these are abnormal, the prognosis for walking is poor.

Clinical features in children over 1 year

Since cerebral palsy is essentially a disorder of posture and movement, the child should be carefully observed sitting, standing, walking and lying. This is followed by a detailed examination of the limbs. It is important also to assess speech, hearing, visual acuity, intelligence, psychological attitude and social adjustment. Optimal management is provided by a multidisciplinary team consisting of a paediatrician, orthopaedic surgeon, neurologist, psychologist, speech therapist, physiotherapist, occupational therapist, remedial teacher and social worker.

Dystonia Some part of the body is held in an abnormal posture, which is aggravated when the child concentrates on movement.

SITTING POSTURE The child may find it difficult to sit unsupported; hypotonic children will slump forward. The lower limbs may be thrust into extension. Note also whether there is scoliosis or a skew pelvis.

STANDING POSTURE Scoliosis and pelvic obliquity are common; it is important to establish whether these deformities are fixed or correctible when the spine is flexed. In the typical spastic posture the child stands with the hips flexed, adducted and internally rotated, the knees bent and the feet in equinus. If the hamstrings are tight there may be flattening of the normal lumbar lordosis and the child may have difficulty standing unsupported. Indeed, any attempt to correct one spastic deformity may aggravate another and it is important to establish whether the deformity is primary or compensatory.

Equilibrium reactions are tested by gently pushing the child forwards, backwards or sideways; normal children take a step to maintain balance, spastic children may simply topple over.

GAIT If the child can walk unsupported, the elements of gait are analysed; it is important to observe limb movement in the swing phase as

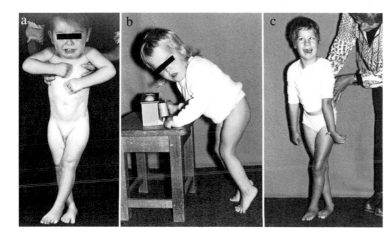

10.4 Cerebral palsy (a) Scissors stance; (b) flexion deformity of hips and knees with equinus of the feet; (c) characteristic facial expression and limb deformities.

well as limb posture in the stance phase. Ataxia or athetoid movement may now be obvious. The most common spastic abnormalities are a tendency to walk with the hips flexed and adducted (scissors gait); the trunk leans forward, the knees are flexed and the equinus may become exaggerated. The lack of free rotation at the hip makes it necessary to swivel the trunk from side to side as each leg swings through. The narrow walking base (due to hip adduction) and the tendency to fall forward (due to hip and knee flexion and equinus) are often dealt with by using crutches. Correction of these deformities is therefore an important objective.

Laboratory gait analysis, including video sequences, provides more detailed information than single observation, and energy expenditure can be measured at the same time.

NEUROMUSCULAR EXAMINATION Examination of the limbs shows the typical features of upper motor neuron or spastic paresis. Passive movements are resisted, the reflexes are exaggerated and there is a positive Babinski response. However, spasticity may obscure the fact that muscle power is actually weak.

DEFORMITIES should be carefully analysed. Contracture at one level may be markedly influenced by the position of the joints above or below. Equinus is often correctible if the knee is flexed; and knee flexion deformity (due to tight hamstrings) is made worse by flexing and abducting the hips. Flexion deformity of the hip may be unmasked by Thomas' test.

In the upper limb, fingers may be tightly flexed with the wrist in extension, but uncurl quite easily when the wrist is flexed. The child uses these fixed-length reactions to manipulate the hands and fingers in a variety of ways (so-called trick movements).

SENSATION Skin sensibility is usually present, if not completely normal. However, stereognosis may be impaired – an important factor which contributes to upper limb disability.

Overall assessment

For a more detailed description of the clinical features the reader is referred to the monograph by Bleck (1987). A full appreciation of the complex alterations in function is achieved only by repeated examination as the child develops.

SPASTIC PALSY The majority of patients will have a spastic palsy. The commonest features have been alluded to above; depending on their distribution, the condition is further classified as:

Monoplegia – about 5% of patients
Hemiplegia – about 40%
Diplegia – about 30% (usually lower limb palsy but sometimes together with mild features in the upper limbs)
Tetraplegia or triplegia – about 25%

ATHETOSIS is seldom seen nowadays. The writhing movements seem quite irregular and uncontrollable, but the patient is usually capable of a surprising degree of function. Tongue and speech muscles may be involved and this can give a mistaken impression of mental retardation. On the contrary, intelligence in this group is often far above average.

ATAXIA is rare. There is an irregular intention tremor and incoordination.

RIGIDITY is not to be confused with spasticity. The muscles are in a constant state of increased tone and, on examination, they do not 'give' like spastic muscles.

Secondary defects

MUSCLE 'CONTRACTURE' Long-standing spasticity leads to apparent fixed contraction or shortening of the muscle. Whether this is true shortening or a failure of muscle to grow along with skeletal growth remains unanswered. Unopposed, it will eventually lead to fixed deformities and alterations in joint congruity.

BONY DEFORMITY Persistent adduction of the hip leads to valgus of the femoral neck, acetabular dysplasia and subluxation of the hip. At the knee, flexion deformity is associated with upward displacement of the patella and patellofemoral pain. External tibial torsion may result in planovalgus deformity of the foot. Fixed deformities of the toes and foot may become painful.

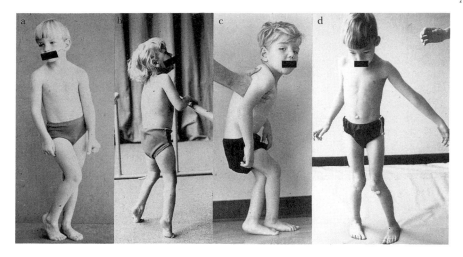

10.5 Spastic palsy   Common types of spastic palsy: (a) hemiplegic, (b) diplegic, (c) tetraplegic and (d) ataxic.

SCOLIOSIS This is most likely to occur in children with whole body involvement and adds greatly to the problems of rehabilitation.

Management

Any serious approach to treatment demands multidisciplinary skills; the team of therapists should meet as often as necessary to work out realistic objectives, discuss progress and plan further management. The objective is not merely to improve physical performance but to increase overall functional ability as well (Rang and Wright, 1989).

SETTING GOALS Based on the extent and severity of the neuromuscular disorder, realistic goals should be defined as early as possible. Even if the child is unlikely ever to walk, active treatment may enable him to sit and get about in a wheelchair – an infinitely better prospect than spending a lifetime lying flat. Children with cerebral diplegia and adequate trunk control can be treated as potential walkers, and the objectives then are to overcome or prevent progressive deformity and to provide stability and balance.

PHYSICAL THERAPY Although it is usually impossible to assess prognosis in children under a year old, physical treatment is begun early (1) to provide a setting for repeated observation and assessment, (2) to establish contact between patient and therapist, and (3) to provide a source of counselling and support for the parents.

Special Methods – with a capital M – abound (Bleck, 1987), but there is a paucity of objective comparative studies; any controlled trial is, for ethical reasons, impossible. What is agreed is that treatment should be concerned with broad functional patterns of movement and postural reactions. The most widely practised methods have been reviewed by Bleck (1987). Whatever line is followed, the physiotherapist must be skilled in neurophysiological assessment, in modern methods of movement therapy and in the conduct of interpersonal relationships.

Physiotherapy continues throughout childhood and early adolescence. Walking patterns are normally established by the age of 7 years, and children with spastic diplegia show a levelling off of motor development after that (Beals, 1966). However, physiotherapy goes hand in hand with other methods of treatment at all stages of development. Every decision on surgery is a combined decision by both surgeon and therapist.

SPLINTAGE Splints are used to prevent fixed deformity, to facilitate improved patterns of movement and to hold position after corrective surgery. For example, a spastic equinus that is passively correctible can be held corrected (or even overcorrected) in a splint; this prevents shortening of the calf muscles and may actually lessen dynamic spastic contraction in the proximal part of the limb. The splint is removed intermittently for physiotherapy. It may be abandoned altogether (1) because it cannot control the deformity or (2) because a permanent correction is achievable by operation.

Splintage can be applied by a plaster cast if it is only for a short period, or immediately after an operation. Long-term splintage is provided by plastic or more robust orthoses.

OPERATIONS   The indications for surgery are: (1) inability to control a spastic deformity by conservative measures; (2) fixed deformity that interferes with function; (3) secondary complications such as bony deformities or dislocation of the hip; and (4) joint instability.

Timing is crucial. That is why it is important for patients to be seen and reassessed repeatedly. As long as the dynamic spastic deformity is controlled by lesser measures, there is no urgency about operations; indeed, one approach is to deliberately put off all operations until the condition plateaus off after the age of 6 or 7 years and then do all the necessary corrective surgery at one sitting. However, if it becomes increasingly difficult to regain or maintain position, it may be better to operate before function deteriorates and certainly before fixed deformity supervenes. The physiotherapist's advice is often the most valuable.

Operative strategies are limited. (1) Tight muscles can be released or their tendons lengthened; but remember that this will also diminish muscle power and may therefore affect overall function. (2) Weak muscles can be augmented by tendon transfers; but beware the combined effect of enhancing power on one side of a joint and taking away the spastic antagonist – the patient may end up with severe overcorrection! (3) Fixed deformities can be corrected by osteotomy, by reshaping the bone ends and performing an arthrodesis, or by arthroplasty; but always consider what effect this will have on the position of other joints and on overall function.

Low intelligence is no bar to surgery; but whole body involvement, lack of trunk control or athetosis may be (Craig, 1967).

Regional survey

LOWER LIMB

In most patients (those with spastic diplegia) treatment is concentrated on the lower limbs. In the very young child, treatment consists of physiotherapy and splintage to prevent fixed contractures. Surgery is indicated either to correct structural defects (e.g. a fixed contracture or hip subluxation) or to improve gait. By 3–4 years of age the walking pattern can be observed and the functional needs assessed. Bleck (1987) advises that operative treatment be completed, if possible, between 4 and 8 years of age.

Although it is customary to consider each deformity individually, Evans (1971) emphasized the interrelationship between the various posture problems, especially lumbar lordosis, hip flexion, knee flexion and ankle equinus; this must be constantly borne in mind when surgery is being planned.

Hip adduction deformity   The child walks with the thighs together and sometimes even with the knees crossing ('scissoring'). This may be combined with spastic internal rotation. Adductor release is indicated if passive abduction is less than 30 degrees on each side (Hoffer, 1986). For most patients open tenotomy of adductor longus and division of gracilis will suffice. Only if this fails to restore passive abduction (a rare occurrence) should the other adductors be released. Anterior branch obturator neurectomy is hardly ever indicated.

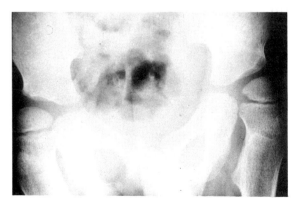

10.6 Spastic hips   X-ray of a boy with spastic adducted hips showing acetabular dysplasia and coxa valga on the left side.

Hip flexion deformity This is usually associated with compensatory knee flexion (the child walks with a 'sitting' posture) or else hyperextension of the lumbar spine. Operative correction is indicated if the hip deformity is more than 20 degrees. This consists of psoas tendon lengthening (complete division is avoided as this weakens hip flexion unduly).

Hip internal rotation deformity is usually combined with flexion and adduction. If so, adductor release and psoas lengthening are combined with division of the anterior half of gluteus medius. If, after a few years, rotation is still excessive, a derotation osteotomy of the femur (subtrochanteric or supracondylar) is advisable.

Hip subluxation A persistent flexion–adduction deformity leads to femoral neck anteversion. If the abductors are weak and the child is not fully weightbearing, there is a risk of subluxation and acetabular dysplasia; in non-walkers there may be complete dislocation (Scrutton, 1989). Correction of flexion and adduction deformities (see above) before the age of 6 years is the surest way of preventing subluxation. Older children may need varus-derotation osteotomy of the femur, perhaps combined with acetabular reconstruction (e.g. a Chiari pelvic osteotomy). Long-standing dislocation in a non-walker may be irreducible; if discomfort makes operation imperative, the proximal end of the femur can be excised.

Knee flexion deformity is usually due to hamstring spasticity or contracture, but is aggravated by any associated hip flexion deformity or weakness of ankle plantarflexion. All three factors must be considered in planning treatment. Flexion deformity with the patient lying flat (hip extended) must be due to capsular contracture. Spastic flexion deformity may be revealed only when the hip is flexed to 90 degrees so that the hamstrings are tightened. Hamstring lengthening is indicated if there is spastic flexion of more than 20 degrees during the stance phase of walking – *but only after carefully assessing the hip and foot.* (1) The hip extensors must be working, otherwise the weakened hamstrings will cause anterior tilting of the pelvis and excessive lumbar lordosis. (2) If there is any marked hip flexion deformity this must be corrected at the same time. (3) Knee extension is aided by plantarflexion of the foot in walking, so it is important not to weaken the triceps surae by overzealous lengthening of the Achilles tendon.

Sometimes hamstring contracture is associated with rectus femoris spasticity (co-spasticity) which prevents knee flexion during the swing phase; this may be corrected by combined hamstring lengthening and rectus femoris release at its distal end.

Spastic knee extension deformity can usually be corrected by simple tenotomy of the proximal end of rectus femoris.

External tibial torsion is easily corrected by supramalleolar osteotomy.

Equinus of the foot Spastic equinus in the young child can be treated by physiotherapy and intermittent splintage. Active plantarflexion is needed to assist knee extension in the stance phase of walking (see above), so Achilles tendon lengthening should be considered only if there is severe spastic deformity or fixed contracture, and should never be overdone.

Pes varus is associated with tightness of tibialis posterior and tibialis anterior. This can be corrected by tibialis posterior lengthening and tibialis anterior tendon transfer to the outer side of the foot. But only half the tendon is transferred, so as to avoid the risk of overcorrection into valgus. Older children with fixed deformity may need bone operations – calcaneal osteotomy or triple arthrodesis.

Pes valgus (pronated foot) may require subtalar arthrodesis.

UPPER LIMB

Upper limb deformities are seen most typically in the child with spastic hemiplegia and consist of flexion of the elbow, pronation of the forearm, flexion of the wrist, clenched fingers and adduction of the thumb. In the mildest cases, spastic postures emerge only when the child exerts himself (e.g. when running). Proprioception is often disturbed and this may preclude any marked improvement of function, whatever the kind of treatment. Operative treatment is usually delayed till after the age of 8 years; it is aimed at improving the resting position of the limb and restoring grasp.

Elbow flexion deformity   Provided the elbow can extend to a right angle, no treatment is needed.

Forearm pronation deformity   This is fairly common and may give rise to subluxation or dislocation of the radial head. Simple release of pronator teres may improve the position, or the tendon can be rerouted round the back of the forearm in the hope that it may act as a supinator. If the wrist is flexed, pronator release may be combined with flexor carpi ulnaris lengthening.

Wrist flexion deformity   may be improved by lengthening or releasing flexor carpi ulnaris; if extension is weak, the tendon is transferred into one of the wrist extensors.

Flexion deformity of the fingers   is due to spasticity of the flexor muscles. The flexor tendons can be lengthened individually, but if the deformity is severe a forearm muscle slide may be more appropriate. If the fingers can be unclenched only by simultaneously flexing the wrist, it is obviously important not to immobilize the wrist.

Thumb-in-palm deformity   This is due to spasticity of the thumb adductors, but later there is also contracture of flexor pollicis longus. In mild cases, function can be improved by splinting the thumb away from the palm, or by operative release of the adductor pollicis and first dorsal interosseous muscles. Resistant deformity is best treated by Matev's (1963) procedure: first the flexor pollicis longus is lengthened; then, through a palmar incision, all the thenar muscles are released; finally abduction and extension are reinforced by shortening the appropriate tendons or by tendon transfers.

SPINE AND PELVIS

Scoliosis is common in children with cerebral palsy and is evidently due to involvement of the trunk muscles. The curve is usually thoracolumbar; sometimes (especially in patients unable to walk) it incorporates the pelvis, which is tilted obliquely so that one hip is in abduction and one in adduction and threatening to dislocate. Deformity is usually progressive and treatment is more difficult than with idiopathic scoliosis. If the child can walk, treatment is the same as that of idiopathic scoliosis (see p. 355). Even in those with severe whole body involvement, if the child is alert and intelligent, corrective surgery may make it easier to sit upright, use a wheelchair and attend to hygiene and dressing (Louis et al., 1989). For those who need a wheelchair permanently, the Matrix seating system is useful (Trail and Galasko, 1990).

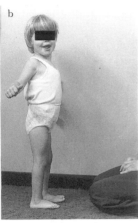
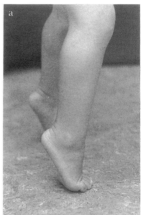
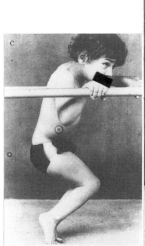
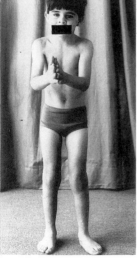

10.7 Spastic knee and foot   (a) This young girl had true spastic equinus deformities. (b) Tendo Achillis lengthening resulted in complete correction and a balanced posture. (c) This boy is also standing on his toes but he has a much more complex problem. He has spastic flexion of the knees due to tight hamstrings; close observation shows that the hindfeet are not really in equinus, and lengthening of the tendo Achillis would be disastrous. (d) Here he is after simple hamstring release.

Stroke – adult spastic paresis

Cerebral damage following a stroke may cause persistent spastic paresis in the adult; disturbance of proprioception and stereognosis may coexist.

In the early recuperative stage, physiotherapy and splintage are important in preventing fixed contractures; all affected joints should be put through a full range of movement every day, and deformities should be corrected and splinted until controlled muscle power returns. Proprioception and co-ordination can be improved by occupational therapy. Once maximal motor recovery has been achieved – usually by 9 months – residual deformity or joint instability may need surgical correction or permanent splinting.

In the lower limbs the principal deformities requiring correction are equinus or equinovarus of the foot, flexion of the knee and adduction of the hip. In the upper limb (where the chances of regaining controlled movement are less) the common residual deformities are adduction and internal rotation of the shoulder (often accompanied by shoulder pain), and flexion of the elbow, wrist and metacarpophalangeal joints. Treatment is similar to that of spastic deformity in the child, and is summarized in Table 10.1.

Table 10.1 Treatment of the principal deformities of the limbs

	Deformity	*Splintage*	*Surgery*
Foot	Equinus	Spring-loaded dorsiflexion	Lengthen tendo Achillis
	Equinovarus	Bracing in eversion and dorsiflexion	Lengthen tendo Achillis and transfer lateral half of tibialis anterior to cuboid
Knee	Flexion	Long caliper	Hamstring release
Hip	Adduction	–	Obturator neurectomy Adductor muscle release
Shoulder	Adduction	–	Subscapularis release
Elbow	Flexion	–	Release elbow flexors
Wrist	Flexion	Wrist splint	Lengthen or release wrist flexors

In severe cases there is progressive disability and cardiac involvement; patients eventually take to a wheelchair and may die before they are 30, usually from cardiac failure. In milder cases operative correction of the foot and spine deformities is well worth while (Makin, 1953).

Friedreich's ataxia

Friedreich's ataxia, though itself rare, is the commonest of the hereditary ataxias. It is an autosomal recessive disorder in which there is degeneration of the spinocerebellar tracts, the corticospinal tracts, the posterior columns of the cord and part of the cerebellum. It usually presents at the age of 5–6 years, with an awkward unsteady gait, a tendency to fall and clumsiness. Typical deformities are pes cavovarus with claw toes, and scoliosis, sometimes very mild. Neurological examination reveals ataxia and loss of vibration sense and two-point discrimination. There is marked slowing of sensory conduction.

Lesions of the spinal cord

The three major pathways in the spinal cord are the *corticospinal tracts* (in the anterior columns) carrying motor neurons, the *spinothalamic tracts* carrying sensory neurons for pain, touch and temperature, and the *posterior column tracts* serving deep sensibility (joint position and vibration).

Clinical features

With lesions of the spinal cord, patients complain of muscle weakness, numbness or loss of balance; bladder and bowel control may be impaired and men may complain of impotence. Examination reveals a spastic (upper motor neuron) paresis, with exaggerated reflexes and a Babinski response; there may be a fairly precise boundary of sensory change, suggesting the level of cord involvement. However, it should be remembered that extradural compressive lesions often involve the nerve roots as well, so there may be a combination of upper motor neuron (UMN) and lower motor neuron (LMN) signs. Several typical patterns are recognized.

Cervical cord compression causes LMN weakness and paraesthesiae or numbness in the arms, with UMN signs in the lower limbs. Bladder symptoms are usually frequency and incontinence but acute lesions may cause retention.

Thoracic cord lesions cause UMN paresis in the lower limbs and variable types of sensory impairment, depending on whether there is involvement of the spinothalamic tracts or posterior columns.

Lumbar lesions may involve the conus medullaris (L1) or the cauda equina (below L1) or both. Thus there may be a combination of UMN paresis and LMN signs. The typical *cauda equina syndrome* consists of lower limb weakness, depressed reflexes, impaired sensation and urinary retention with overflow.

The Brown-Séquard syndrome occurs with asymmetrical (hemisectional) lesions: below the lesion there is ipsilateral UMN weakness and posterior column dysfunction, with contralateral loss of skin sensibility; at the level of the lesion there is ipsilateral loss of sensibility.

Acute cord lesions at any level may present with flaccid paralysis which only later changes to the more typical UMN picture.

Diagnosis and management

The more common causes of spinal cord dysfunction are listed in Table 10.2. Traumatic and compressive lesions are the ones most likely to be seen by orthopaedic surgeons. Plain x-rays will show structural abnormalities of the spine; cord compression can be visualized by myelography, alone or combined with CT. Intrinsic

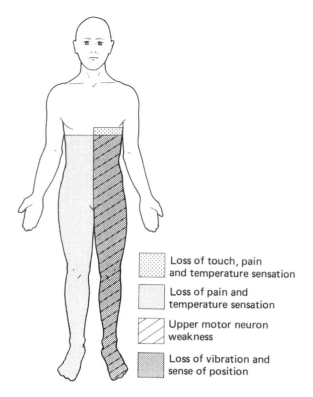

Loss of touch, pain and temperature sensation

Loss of pain and temperature sensation

Upper motor neuron weakness

Loss of vibration and sense of position

10.8 The Brown-Séquard syndrome

lesions of the cord require further investigation by blood tests, CSF examination and MRI.

Acute compressive lesions require urgent diagnosis and treatment if permanent damage is to be prevented. Bladder dysfunction is ominous: whereas motor and sensory signs may improve after decompression, *loss of bladder control, if present for more than 24 hours, is usually irreversible.*

Spinal injury is dealt with in Chapter 25. It is important to remember that (1) any spinal injury may be associated with cord damage, and great care is needed in transporting and examining the patient; (2) in the early period of 'spinal shock', the usual picture is one of flaccid paralysis; and (3) plain x-rays seldom show the full extent of bone displacement, which is much better displayed on CT. Unstable injuries usually need operative treatment; stable injuries can be treated conservatively. Corticosteroids are sometimes used to treat acute cord injuries, and there is some evidence that this can reduce

Table 10.2 Causes of spinal cord dysfunction

Acute injury
Vertebral fractures
Fracture-dislocation

Infection
Epidural abscess
Poliomyelitis

Intervertebral disc prolapse
Sequestrated disc
Disc prolapse in spinal stenosis

Vertebral canal stenosis
Congenital stenosis
Acquired stenosis

Vertebral bone disease
Tuberculous spondylitis
Metastatic disease

Spinal cord tumours
Neurofibroma
Meningioma

Intrinsic cord lesions
Tabes dorsalis
Syringomyelia
Other degenerative disorders

Miscellaneous
Spina bifida
Vascular lesions
Multiple sclerosis
Haemorrhagic disorders

the degree of permanent damage. However, the matter is highly controversial and patients should be informed that high-dosage corticosteroids may have serious side effects, including widespread avascular necrosis.

Epidural abscess is a surgical emergency. The patient rapidly develops acute pain and muscle spasm, with fever, leucocytosis and elevation of the ESR. X-rays may show disc space narrowing and bone erosion. Treatment is by immediate decompression and antibiotics.

Acute disc prolapse usually causes unilateral symptoms and signs. However, complete lumbar disc prolapse may present as a cauda equina syndrome with urinary retention and overflow; spinal canal obstruction is demonstrated by myelography or CT; operative discectomy is urgent.

Chronic discogenic disease is often associated with narrowing of the intervertebral foramina

and compression of nerve roots (radiculopathy), and occasionally with bony hypertrophy and pressure on the spinal cord (myelopathy). Diagnosis is usually obvious on x-ray and transectional imaging.

Spinal stenosis produces a typical clinical syndrome – due partly to direct pressure on the cord or nerve roots and partly to vascular obstruction and ischaemic neuropathy during hyperextension of the lumbar spine. The patient complains of 'tiredness', weakness and sometimes aching or paraesthesia in the lower limbs after standing or walking for a few minutes, symptoms that are completely relieved by bending forward, sitting or crouching so as to flex the lumbar spine. Congenital narrowing of the spinal canal is rare, except in developmental disorders such as achondroplasia. But a moderately narrow canal may be further constricted by osteophytes, thus compromising the cord and nerve roots. Treatment calls for laminectomy and bony decompression of the nerve structures.

Vertebral bone disease, such as tuberculosis or metastatic disease, may cause cord compression and paraparesis. The diagnosis is usually obvious on x-ray, but a needle biopsy may be necessary for confirmation. Management is usually by anterior decompression and, if necessary, internal stabilization. However, in metastatic disease, if the prognosis is poor it may be wiser to use radiotherapy and corticosteroids, plus narcotics for pain.

Spinal cord tumours are a comparatively rare cause of progressive paraparesis. X-rays may show bony erosion, widening of the spinal canal or flattening of the vertebral pedicles. Widening of the intervertebral foramina is typical of *neurofibromatosis*. Treatment usually involves operative removal of the tumour.

Intrinsic lesions of the cord produce slowly progressive neurological signs. Two conditions in particular – tabes dorsalis and syringomyelia – may present with orthopaedic problems because of neuropathic joint destruction.

Tabes dorsalis is a late manifestation of syphilis causing degeneration ('tabes' means wasting) of the posterior columns of the spinal cord. A pathognomonic feature is 'lightning pains' in the lower limbs. Much later other neurological features appear: sensory ataxia, which causes a stamping gait; loss of position sense and sometimes of pain sensibility; trophic lesions in the lower limbs; progressive joint instability; and almost painless destruction of joints (Charcot joints). There is no treatment for the cord disorder.

Syringomyelia In syringomyelia a long cavity (the syrinx) filled with CSF develops within the spinal cord, most commonly in the cervical region. Usually the cause is unknown but the condition is sometimes associated with prolapse of the cerebellar tonsils and hydrocephalus or, in later life, with spinal cord injury or tumour. Symptoms and signs are most evident in the upper limbs. The expanding cyst presses on the anterior horn cells, producing weakness and wasting of the hand muscles. And destruction of the decussating spinothalamic fibres in the centre of the cord produces a characteristic dissociated sensory loss in the upper limbs – impaired response to pain and temperature but preservation of touch. There may be trophic lesions in the fingers and neuropathic arthropathy ('Charcot joints') in the upper limbs. CT may reveal an expanded cord and the syrinx can be defined on MRI. Deterioration may be slowed down by decompression of the foramen magnum.

Spina bifida

Spina bifida is a congenital disorder in which the two halves of the posterior vertebral arch (or several arches) have failed to fuse. This is an embryonic defect, often associated with maldevelopment of the neural tube and the overlying skin; the combination of faults is called *dysraphism*. It usually occurs in the lumbar or lumbosacral region. If neural elements are involved there may be paralysis and loss of sensation and sphincter control.

Pathology

SPINA BIFIDA CYSTICA In severe forms of dysraphism the vertebral laminae are missing and the contents of the vertebral canal prolapse

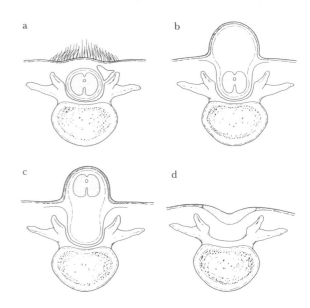

10.9 Dysraphism (a) Spina bifida occulta. (b) Meningocele. (c) Myelomeningocele. (d) Open myelomeningocele.

through the defect – either as a CSF-filled meningeal sac or *meningocele* or as a sac containing part of the spinal cord and nerve roots, a *myelomeningocele*. The cord may be in its primitive state, the unfolded neural plate forming part of the roof of the sac; this is an '*open*' *myelomeningocele* or *rachischisis*. In a '*closed*' *myelomeningocele* the neural tube is fully formed and covered by membrane and skin, though still outwith the bony canal.

SPINA BIFIDA OCCULTA In the mildest forms of dysraphism there is a midline defect between the laminae and nothing more; hence the term 'occulta' (meaning 'secret'). However, in some cases – and especially if several vertebrae are affected – there are telltale defects in the overlying skin; for example, a dimple, a pit or a tuft of hair. Occasionally there are associated intraspinal anomalies, such as tethering of the conus medullaris below L1, splitting of the spinal cord (diastematomyelia) and cysts or lipomas of the cauda equina.

HYDROCEPHALUS Distal tethering of the cord may cause herniation of the cerebellum and brainstem through the foramen magnum, resulting in obstruction to CSF circulation and hydrocephalus. The ventricles dilate and the skull enlarges by separation of the cranial sutures. Persistently raised intracranial pressure may cause cerebral atrophy and mental retardation.

NEUROLOGICAL DYSFUNCTION Myelomeningocele is always associated with neurological deficit below the level of the lesion. This may also occur – though less frequently and much less severely – in spina bifida occulta.

Incidence and screening

Isolated laminar defects are seen in over 5% of lumbar spine x-rays. By comparison, cystic spina bifida is rare at 2–3 per 1000 live births, but if one child is affected the risk for the next child is ten times greater.

Neural-type defects are associated with high levels of alpha-fetoprotein in the amniotic fluid and serum. This offers an effective method of antenatal screening.

Clinical features

SPINA BIFIDA OCCULTA Isolated laminar defects are often seen in normal people, and usually they can be ignored. However, a posterior midline dimple, a tuft of hair or a pigmented naevus signifies something more serious. Patients may present at any age with neurological symptoms – usually a partial cauda equina syndrome with enuresis, urinary frequency or incontinence; neurological examination may reveal weakness and some loss of sensibility in the lower limbs. X-rays will show the laminar defect and any associated vertebral anomalies. A midline ridge of bone suggests bifurcation of the cord (diastematomyelia). Intraspinal anomalies are best shown by myelography, CT and MRI.

SPINAL BIFIDA CYSTICA The saccular lesion over the lumbosacral spine is obvious at birth. It may be covered only with membrane, or with membrane and skin. In open myelomeningoceles the neural elements form the roof of the cyst, which merges into plum-coloured skin at its base. Meningoceles are covered by normal looking skin.

Hydrocephalus may be present at birth; with a communicating hyrocephalus the intracranial pressure may not be elevated until leakage from the spinal lesion is arrested by surgical closure.

The baby's posture may suggest the type of paralysis and sometimes indicates its neurological level. Deformities are common, especially hip dislocation, genu recurvatum, talipes and claw toes. Such deformities may be due to muscle imbalance, to abnormal positioning of

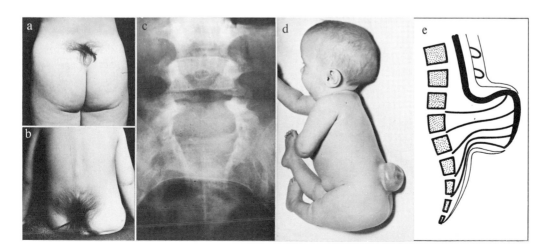

10.10 Dysraphism (a, b) Examples of the hairy patches which suggest a bony defect such as that in (c). (d) Spina bifida cystica. (e) Why traction lesions of the nerve roots develop with growth.

the limbs *in utero* or after birth, or to associated anomalies that are independent of the paralysis.

Muscle charting (p. 194) should be performed within 24 hours of birth in order to establish both the type and the level of neurological deficit. Sharrard has shown convincingly that this is perfectly practicable; he suggests that the untreated child may, within a few days, become increasingly paralysed as enlargement of the meningeal sac exerts traction on adherent nerve roots. In about one-third of infants with myelomeningocele there is complete lower motor neuron paralysis and loss of sensation and sphincter control below the affected level. In one-third there is a complete lesion at some level but a distal segment of cord is preserved, giving a mixed neurological picture with intact segmental reflexes and spastic muscle groups. In one-third the cord lesion is incomplete and some movement and sensation are preserved.

X-rays will show the extent of the bony lesion as well as other vertebral anomalies.

Treatment

Selection of patients for operative closure of the spinal lesion is ethically controversial. Most centres avoid urgent operation if the neurological level is high (above L1), if spinal deformities are severe or if there is marked hydrocephalus. In the remainder (about half) the skin lesion is closed early.

For subsequent management, teamwork is essential. The ideal is a combined clinic at which neurosurgery, orthopaedics, urology, paediatrics, physiotherapy and occupational therapy are all represented. As the child grows, help is likely to be needed from the splint maker, the social worker and possibly the psychotherapist. But above all, the child will need parental understanding and ceaseless devotion.

EARLY MANAGEMENT

SKIN CLOSURE should, in those patients with good prognostic signs, be performed within 48 hours. The neural plaque is carefully preserved and the skin widely undercut to facilitate closure. Only in this way can drying and ulceration be prevented.

HYDROCEPHALUS is the next priority. Usually it develops within a few days; treatment must not be delayed or brain damage follows. A ventriculocaval shunt containing a valve (e.g. Spitz–Holter) is inserted. As the baby grows, the shunt may need to be replaced.

DEFORMITIES must be kept under control. The orthopaedic surgeon is usually not called upon for 3 weeks, and then only if the child is thriving, the back healed and a shunt (if

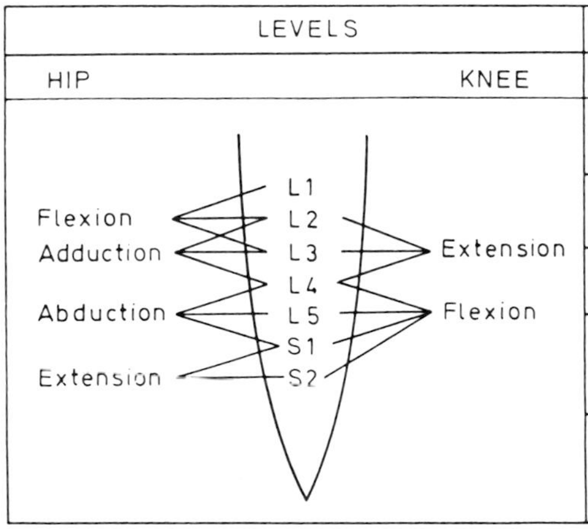

LEVELS			EARLY MANAGEMENT – TIMING	
HIP		KNEE	AGE	PROCEDURE
Flexion Adduction Abduction Extension	L1 L2 L3 L4 L5 S1 S2	Extension Flexion	1 DAY	Close skin defect
			1 WEEK	Ventriculo-caval shunt
			1 MONTH	Stretch and strap
			6 MONTHS TO 3 YEARS	Orthopaedic operations
			WHENEVER NEEDED	Urogenital operations

10.11 Spina bifida   The diagram shows the root levels concerned with hip and knee movements. The table is a simple guide to the timing of operations.

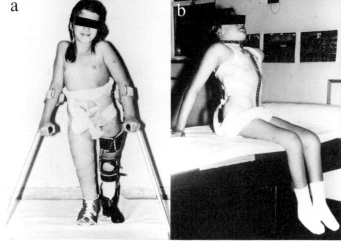

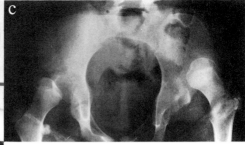

10.12 Spina bifida (a) Paralysis may require permanent splintage in a caliper, and crutch-walking for life. (b) Scoliosis is common and is treated in a brace until the child is old enough for fusion. (c) Muscle imbalance may lead to bilateral hip dislocation.

needed) working. At this stage muscle charting is repeated and a programme of stretching and strapping begun: stretching to keep deformity at a minimum; elastic strapping (or simple splints) to hold correction.

Two features dominate orthopaedic management: the bones are somewhat fragile (spontaneous fractures are common and frequently unite with excessive callus); and the skin is anaesthetic. Consequently manipulations must not be too forcible, and splintage should be intermittent. The skin must be protected from localized pressure and watched with extravagant vigilance.*

URINARY PROBLEMS develop in 90% of cases. Intravenous pyelography is used to detect any upper urinary tract dilatation, and is repeated at intervals. Males can usually be fitted with a penile appliance but in females urinary diversion is needed.

SUBSEQUENT MANAGEMENT OF PARALYSIS AND
DEFORMITY
The guiding principles are:

1. For the first 6–12 months deformities are treated by stretching and strapping (see above). Forcible overcorrection followed by plaster is forbidden: this combination, useful in other varieties of paralysis, is disastrous

*A sore which takes a day to form may take a month to heal.

with spina bifida; the bones may break and the skin will ulcerate.
2. Open methods of correcting deformity are best, but should be delayed until the child is several months old.
3. Proximal deformities are corrected before distal deformities. Short tendons should be divided and, where appropriate, transferred. Only when balance has been restored should any residual deformity be corrected by osteotomy.
4. Splints alone are never used to obtain correction; they may be used to maintain it but even then only intermittently; their action is reinforced by frequently repeated stretching.

Regional survey

SPINE
Apart from the posterior defect which constitutes spina bifida, many other vertebral anomalies can occur, such as unsegmented bars, hemivertebrae and fused ribs resulting in scoliosis, lordosis or kyphosis. Neonatal kyphosis may be so severe that spinal osteotomy is needed if the skin defect is to be closed.

Even moderate kyphosis or kyphos may later cause persistent skin ulceration; treatment consists in excising the kyphotic vertebrae and fixing the two halves of the spine together – a procedure less alarming than it sounds because the cord is already non-functioning. Many patients with high neurological lesions develop progressive lordoscoliosis aged 5 or 6 years. Bracing at best slows deterioration. When the child is old enough (aged about 10) operative correction and stabilization is often needed using a combination of Dwyer and Harrington instrumentation.

HIP

The aim is to secure hips straight enough to enable the child to stand in calipers, and flexible enough for him to sit. If the neurological level of the lesion is above L1, all muscle groups are equally paralysed (balanced); the hips are flail and no treatment other than splintage is needed. With a lesion from S1 downwards there may be pure flexion deformity; this can be corrected by elongation of the psoas tendon combined with detachment of the flexors from the ilium (Soutter).

Usually the lesion is between these levels and the commonest hip problem is dislocation: 50% of spina bifida children have subluxed or dislocated hips by the age of 2 years. Some may be coincidental congenital dislocations but most result from unbalanced paralysis; if the flexors and adductors can overpower the extensors and abductors, dislocation is almost inevitable. In infancy, reduction (closed or open) is usually possible, perhaps aided by adductor tenotomy; but, because postoperative splintage must be minimized, it is important to improve muscle balance. This is achieved by transferring the psoas tendon from the lesser to the greater trochanter; flexor power is reduced and extensor–abductor power may be increased. Sharrard advocates threading the detached psoas through a large hole in the ilium, while Mustard prefers moving the tendon across the front of the bone.

In older children it may be difficult or impossible to reduce a dislocation. The possibilities then are varus osteotomy of the upper femur or innominate osteotomy; often it is best not to intervene.

KNEE

Unlike the hip, the knee usually presents no problem, because the aim is simple – a straight knee suitable for straight calipers. Occasionally, recurvatum develops and cautious elongation of the quadriceps may be called for. In older children fixed flexion may follow prolonged sitting. If stretching and splintage fail, one or more of the hamstrings may be lengthened, divided or reinserted into the femur or patella. Not uncommonly the knees are straight and will not bend, making sitting difficult; extensive soft-tissue release may be needed if subcutaneous tenotomy proves inadequate.

FOOT

The aim is a plantigrade foot with plantar skin strong enough not to break down easily. The floppy foot of balanced paralysis needs no surgery; accurately fitting footwear with strong external bracing is adequate. The same is true of any deformity that can be corrected passively, though in every case the patient and parents must be taught an elaborate ritual of skin care; pressure sores must, at all costs, be prevented.

Fixed deformities are common and varied. Tendon operations are often helpful and are best performed at or before the age of 6 months: preoperative electrical testing may help in deciding if the short tendon is paralysed but contracted (in which case simple division is satisfactory) or is active but unopposed (in which case transfer is better). The common equinovarus deformity often requires extensive posteromedial release, also at the age of 6 months.

Vertical talus is not uncommon, with a rigid boat-shaped foot and possibly skin ulceration. Operative reduction is important and prefer-

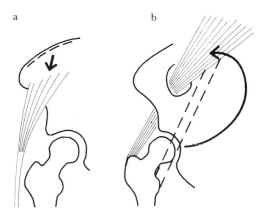

10.13 Spina bifida Two procedures for hip deformity: (a) Soutter's muscle slide; (b) Sharrard's iliopsoas transfer.

able to talectomy; it is performed at the age of 3 years or over. Still older children may need bone operations to restore a plantigrade foot. Should claw toes prove troublesome, flexor-to-extensor transfer is suitable for the outer four toes, and tenodesis of the long flexor (anchoring it to the proximal phalanx) for the hallux.

Long-term function

Despite the best of care and surgical skills, only one-third of all patients achieve independent walking. The remaining two-thirds use a wheelchair, and for them there are additional problems due to inacitivity: obesity, osteoporosis, pressure sores and urinary infection.

Many patients – especially among those with lesions below L5 – attain a good degree of social integration and they should be encouraged to extend their education and training so as to lead lives as near normal as possible.

Anterior poliomyelitis

Poliomyelitis is a viral infection of the anterior horn cells of the spinal cord and brainstem, which may lead to lower motor neuron paralysis of the affected muscle groups. In countries where vaccination is encouraged, it has become a rare disease, though the victims of earlier epidemics continue to pose challenging problems.

Pathology

The virus gains entry through the gut and usually produces no more than a mild influenza-like illness. Sometimes, however, it attacks the anterior horn cells, causing varying degrees of paralysis in isolated muscles or muscle groups. Some motor neuron cells, merely damaged by inflammation or oedema, survive, and the muscles they supply can regain their lost power. Residual paralysis 6 months after the infection will be permanent.

Clinical features

The disease strikes at any age. Following a trivial and often unrecognized minor illness (a sore throat or diarrhoea) a small proportion of patients develop acute meningitis, with fever, headache, neck stiffness and vomiting. The patient lies curled up with the joints flexed; the muscles are painful and tender, and passive stretching provokes painful spasms. Paralysis soon follows and reaches its maximum in 2–3 days. The limbs are weak and there may also be difficulty with breathing and swallowing. If the patient does not succumb from respiratory paralysis, pain and pyrexia subside after 7–10 days and the patient enters the convalescent stage. However, he should be considered to be infective for at least 4 weeks from onset.

Early treatment

During the acute phase the patient is isolated and kept at complete rest, with symptomatic treatment for pain and muscle spasm. Active movement is avoided but gentle passive stretching helps to prevent contractures. Respiratory paralysis calls for artificial respiration.

Once the acute illness settles, physiotherapy is stepped up; active movements are encouraged and every effort is made to regain maximum power. Between exercise periods, splintage may be necessary to prevent fixed deformities.

Muscle charting is carried out at monthly intervals. At first there may be some return of function, but after 6 months there will be no further recovery.

Residual paralysis

During the stage of residual paralysis there are five types of problem that may require treatment.

ISOLATED MUSCLE WEAKNESS WITHOUT DEFORMITY Quadriceps paralysis may make walking impossible; it is best managed with a splint (or caliper) which holds the knee straight. Elsewhere, isolated weakness (e.g. of thumb opposition) may be treated by tendon transfer.

DEFORMITY   Unbalanced paralysis may lead to deformity. At first this is passively correctible and can be counteracted by a splint (e.g. a caliper with corrective strap to control valgus or varus of the foot). However, an appropriate tendon transfer may solve the problem permanently.

Fixed deformity cannot be corrected by either splintage or tendon transfer alone; it is also necessary to restore alignment operatively, and to stabilize the joint (if necessary, by arthrodesis). This is especially applicable to fixed deformities of the ankle and foot, but the same principle applies in treating paralytic scoliosis.

Occasionally, fixed deformity is an advantage.

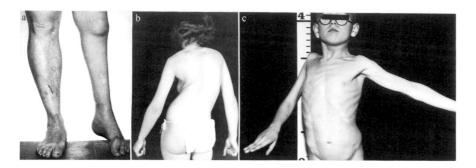

10.14 Polio   (a) Shortening and wasting of the left leg, with equinus of the ankle. (b) This long curve is typical of a paralytic scoliosis. (c) This boy is trying to abduct both arms, but the right deltoid and supraspinatus are paralysed.

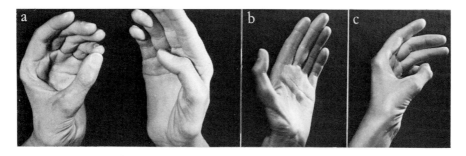

10.15 Tendon transfer   (a) In both hands the opponens pollicis was paralysed; in the left hand a superficialis transfer has restored opposition. (b, c) The transferred tendon in action.

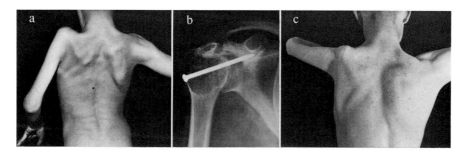

10.16 Arthrodesis   (a) This patient had paralysis of the left deltoid; after arthrodesis (b) he could lift his arm (c) by using his scapular muscles.

Thus, an equinus foot may help to compensate mechanically for quadriceps weakness; if so, it should not be corrected.

FLAIL JOINT   Balanced paralysis, because it causes no deformity, may need no treatment. However, if the joint is unstable or flail it must be stabilized, either by permanent splintage or by arthrodesis.

SHORTENING   Lack of muscle activity undermines normal bone growth. Leg length inequality of up to 3 cm can be compensated for by building up the shoe. Anything more is unsightly, and operative lengthening of the limb (or shortening of the opposite limb) may be preferable (see p. 245).

VASCULAR DYSFUNCTION   Sensation is intact but the paralysed limb is often cold and blue. Large chilblains sometimes develop and sympathectomy may be needed.

Regional survey

UPPER LIMB

Provided the scapular muscles are strong, abduction at the *shoulder* can be restored by arthrodesing the glenohumeral joint (50 degrees abducted and 25 degrees flexed). Contracted adductors may need division.

At the *elbow*, flexion can be provided by rerouting an intact pectoralis major; its tendon is detached from its insertion and sutured to the biceps tendon. Proximal advancement of the forearm flexors is a less effective way of restoring elbow flexion.

Wrist deformity or instability can be markedly improved by arthrodesis. Any active muscles can then be used to restore finger movement.

In the *thumb*, weakness of opposition can be overcome by a superficialis transfer; the tendon (usually of the ring finger) is wound round that of flexor carpi ulnaris (which acts as a pulley), threaded across the palm and fixed to the distal end of the first metacarpal.

TRUNK

Unbalanced paralysis causes *scoliosis*, frequently a long thoracolumbar curve which may involve the lumbosacral junction, causing pelvic obliquity. Operative treatment is often needed,

the most effective being a combination of Dwyer's anterior fusion with posterior Harrington rod instrumentation.

LOWER LIMB

At the hip balanced paralysis causes instability; the resulting Trendelenburg gait cannot be prevented except by arthrodesis, which is rarely advisable. Unbalanced paralysis causes deformities similar to those in spina bifida and cerebral palsy. Fixed flexion can be treated by Soutter's muscle slide operation or by transferring psoas to the greater trochanter. For fixed abduction with pelvic obliquity the fascia lata and iliotibial band may need division; occasionally, for severe deformity, proximal femoral osteotomy may be required as well. With this type of obliquity the 'higher' hip tends to be unstable and the 'lower' hip to have fixed abduction; if the abducted hip is corrected first the pelvis may level and the other hip become normal.

At the knee instability is dangerous. Unaided walking may still be possible provided the hip has good extensor power and the foot good plantarflexion power (or fixed equinus); with this combination the knee is stabilized by being thrust into hyperextension as body weight comes onto the leg. In the absence of such passive stabilization a full-length caliper is needed. Fixed flexion with flexors stronger than extensors is more common and must be corrected; the possibilities are hamstring division or hamstring to quadriceps transfer, but if fixed flexion remains, supracondylar extension osteotomy is needed. Marked hyperextension sometimes occurs, either as a primary deformity or secondary to fixed equinus. It can be improved by supracondylar flexion osteotomy; an alternative is to excise the patella and slot it into the upper tibia where it acts as a bone block (Hong-Xue Men et al., 1991).

In the foot instability can be controlled by a below-knee caliper, and foot drop by a toe-raising spring. Often there is imbalance causing varus, valgus or calcaneocavus deformity; fusion alone is unsatisfactory and should be combined with tendon rerouting to restore balance.

For varus or valgus the simplest procedure (Grice) is to slot bone grafts into vertical grooves on each side of the sinus tarsi; alternatively, a triple arthrodesis (Dunn) of subtalar and mid-tarsal joints is performed, relying on bone carpentry to correct deformity. With associated foot drop, Lambrinudi's modification is valuable: triple arthrodesis is performed but the fully plantarflexed talus is slotted into the navicular with the forefoot in only slight equinus: foot drop is corrected because the talus cannot plantarflex further, and slight equinus helps to stabilize the knee. With calcaneocavus deformity, Elmslie's operation is useful: triple arthrodesis is performed in the calcaneus position, but corrected at a second stage by posterior wedge excision combined with tenodesis using half of the tendo Achillis. Claw toes, if the deformity is mobile, are corrected by transferring the toe flexors to the extensors; if the deformity is fixed, the interphalangeal joints should be arthrodesed in the straight position and the long extensor tendons reinserted into the metatarsal necks.

Motor neuron disorders

Rare degenerative disorders of the large motor neurons may cause progressive and sometimes fatal paralysis.

Motor neuron disease (amyotrophic lateral sclerosis)

This is a degenerative disease of unknown aetiology. It affects both cortical (upper) motor neurons and the anterior horn cells of the cord, causing widespread UMN and LMN symptoms and signs. Patients usually present in middle age with dysarthria and difficulty in swallowing or, if the limbs are affected, with muscle weakness (e.g. clumsy hands or unexplained foot drop) and wasting in the presence of exaggerated reflexes. Sensation and bladder control are normal. Some of the features are also seen in spinal cord compression, which may have to be excluded by myelography. The disease is progressive and incurable. Patients usually end up in a wheelchair and have increasing difficulty with speech and eating.

Most of them die within 5 years from a combination of respiratory weakness and aspiration pneumonia.

Spinal muscular atrophy

In this rare group of heritable disorders there is widespread degeneration of the anterior horn cells in the cord, leading to progressive LMN weakness. The commonest form (*Werdnig–Hoffman disease*) is inherited as an autosomal recessive and is diagnosed at birth or soon afterwards. The baby is floppy and weak, feeding is difficult and breathing is shallow. Death occurs, usually within a year.

A less severe form (*Kugelberg–Welander disease*), of either dominant or recessive inheritance, is usually seen in adolescents or young adults who present with limb weakness, proximal muscle wasting and spinal deformity. However, it sometimes appears in early childhood as a cause of delayed walking. Patients may live to 30–40 years of age but are usually confined to a wheelchair.

Arthrogryposis multiplex congenita

Arthrogryposis is included in the neuromuscular disorders for want of certainty about its pathogenesis. It is a non-specific term applied to congenital disorders in which there is nonprogressive restriction of movement due to soft-tissue contractures. Neuropathic and myopathic varieties are described. In addition to the contractures there is stiffness of several joints, shapeless, cylindrical limbs and absence of skin creases. Typically the wrists and ankles are stiff in flexion, while elbows and knees may be either flexed or hyperextended. Equinovarus is common and difficult to treat. In the rarer myopathic form of the disease, children may develop spinal deformities. Brown, Robson and Sharrard (1980) have pointed out that the deformities are associated with unbalanced

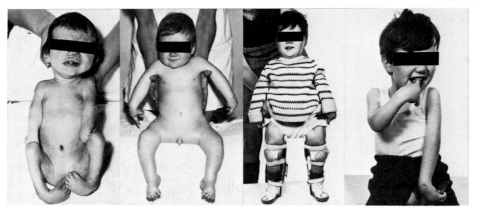

10.17 Arthrogryposis multiplex congenita Severe deformities are present at birth but surgery is possible and, as this bright lad shows, worth while. The lower limbs are tackled first (aiming at straight legs with plantigrade feet), then the upper limbs (where the minimum aim is getting a hand to the mouth).

muscle weakness which follows a neurosegmental distribution, and necropsy specimens show sparseness of anterior horn cells in the cervical and lumbar cord. Deformities and contractures develop *in utero* and remain largely unchanged throughout life.

Treatment begins soon after birth and initially consists of manipulation and splintage of deformed joints. Later, if progress is slow, tendon release, tendon transfers and osteotomies may become necessary. The contractures are notoriously resistant to all forms of treatment and recurrences of deformity are the rule rather than the exception.

Peripheral neuropathy

Disorders of the peripheral nerves may affect motor, sensory or autonomic functions, may be localized to a short segment or may involve the full length of the nerve fibres including their cell bodies in the anterior horn (motor neurons), posterior root ganglia (sensory neurons) and autonomic ganglia. In some cases spinal cord tracts are involved as well.

Pathology

There are essentially three types of nerve pathology: (1) acute interruption of axonal continuity; (2) axonal degeneration; and (3) demyelination. In all three, conduction is disturbed or completely blocked, with consequent loss of motor and/or sensory function.

Axonal degeneration occurs most typically after nerve division and is described in Chapter 11. Recovery, when it occurs, is slow (a new axon grows by 1–2 mm per day) and is often incomplete. Demyelination is less damaging and may be localized to a short segment of nerve; recovery usually takes less than 6 weeks.

Most of the chronic neuropathies show a mixture of degeneration and demyelination.

Classification

The clinical disorders are divided into:

1. *Mononeuropathy* – involvement of a single nerve (e.g. nerve entrapment)
2. *Multiple mononeuropathy* – involvement of several isolated nerves (e.g. leprosy)
3. *Polyneuropathy* – widespread symmetrical dysfunction (e.g. diabetic neuropathy, alcoholic

Table 10.3 Causes of polyneuropathy

Hereditary
Hereditary motor and sensory neuropathy
Friedreich's ataxia
Hereditary sensory neuropathy

Infections
Viral infections
Herpes zoster
Neuralgic amyotrophy
Leprosy

Inflammatory
Acute inflammatory polyneuropathy
Guillain–Barré syndrome
Systemic lupus erythematosus
Sarcoidosis

Nutritional and metabolic
Vitamin deficiencies
Diabetes
Myxoedema
Amyloidosis

Neoplastic
Primary carcinoma
Myeloma

Toxic
Alcohol
Lead

Drugs
Various

myopathy, vitamin deficiency or – perhaps the most common – idiopathic neuropathy (Table 10.3)

Disorders may be predominantly sensory (e.g. diabetic polyneuropathy), predominantly motor (e.g. peroneal muscular atrophy) or mixed. *Chronic motor loss with no sensory component is usually due to anterior horn cell disease rather than polyneuropathy.*

Clinical features

Patients usually complain of sensory symptoms: 'pins and needles', numbness, a limb 'going to sleep', 'burning', shooting pains or restless legs. They may also notice weakness or clumsiness, or loss of balance in walking. Occasionally (in the predominantly motor neuropathies) the main complaint is of progressive deformity; for example, claw hand or cavus foot.

The onset may be rapid (over a few days) or very gradual (over weeks or months). Sometimes there is a history of injury, infection, a known disease such as diabetes or malignancy, alcohol abuse or nutritional deficiency.

Examination may reveal motor weakness in a particular muscle group. In the polyneuropathies the limbs are involved symmetrically, usually legs before arms and distal before proximal parts. Reflexes are usually depressed, though in small-fibre neuropathies (e.g. diabetes) this occurs very late. In mononeuropathy, sensory loss follows the 'map' of the affected nerve. In polyneuropathy, there is a symmetrical 'glove' or 'stocking' distribution. Trophic skin changes may be present. Deep sensation is also affected and some patients develop ataxia. If pain sensibility and proprioception are depressed there may be joint instability or breakdown of the articular surfaces (Charcot joints).

Clinical examination alone may establish the diagnosis. Further help is provided by electromyography (which may suggest the type of abnormality) and nerve conduction studies (which may show exactly where the lesion is).

The *mononeuropathies* – mainly nerve injuries and entrapment syndromes – are dealt with in Chapter 11. The more common polyneuropathies are listed in Table 10.3 and some are described below. In over 50% of cases no specific cause is found.

Hereditary neuropathies

These rare disorders present in childhood and adolescence, usually with muscle weakness and deformity.

HEREDITARY MOTOR AND SENSORY NEUROPATHY (HMSN)
This group of conditions includes *peroneal muscular atrophy* and *Charcot–Marie–Tooth* disease, the commonest of the inherited neuropathies, which are usually passed on as autosomal dominant disorders. HMSN type I is seen in young children who have difficulty walking and develop claw toes and pes cavus or cavovarus. There may be severe wasting of the

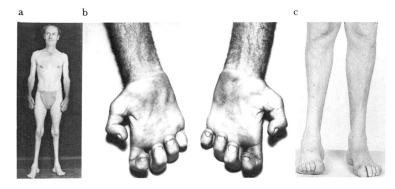

a　b　c

10.18 Hereditary neuropathies (a, b) The most severely affected muscles in this man with peroneal muscular atrophy are those which are most peripheral, producing cavus feet, claw toes and claw hands. He could ride a bicycle, but could scarcely walk until his foot deformities were corrected surgically. His hands were left untreated – it seems incredible but he made beautiful model ships as a hobby. (c) A much milder version, similar to that in his teenage daughter.

legs and (later) the upper limbs. Spinal deformity is common. This is a demyelinating disorder and nerve conduction velocity is markedly slowed. Type II HMSN occurs in adolescents and young adults, and is much less disabling than type I; it affects only the lower limbs, causing mild pes cavus and wasting of the peronei. Nerve conduction velocity is only slightly reduced, indicating primary axonal degeneration. If foot deformities are progressive or disabling, operative correction may bring marked improvement. Claw toes (due to intrinsic muscle weakness) can be corrected by transferring the toe flexors to the extensors, with or without fusion of the interphalangeal joints. Clawing of the big toe is best corrected by the Robert Jones procedure – transfer of the extensor hallucis longus to the metatarsal neck and fusion of the interphalangeal joint. The cavus deformity often needs no treatment, but if it causes pain it can be improved by calcaneal or dorsal mid-tarsal osteotomy.

FRIEDREICH'S ATAXIA

This is predominantly a spinocerebellar disorder, but there may also be degeneration of the posterior root ganglia and peripheral nerves. Patients present at around the age of 6 years with gait ataxia, lower limb weakness and deformities similar to those of severe Charcot–Marie–Tooth disease. Despite the poor prognosis, surgical correction of deformities is well worth while.

HEREDITARY SENSORY NEUROPATHY

Congenital insensitivity to pain and temperature is inherited as either a dominant or a recessive trait. Patients develop Charcot joints and ulceration of the feet.

Diabetic neuropathy

Diabetes is one of the commonest causes of peripheral neuropathy. Hyperglycaemia interferes with Schwann cell function, leading to demyelination and axonal degeneration. Microvascular occlusion may also play a part. Patients complain of numbness and paraesthesiae in the feet and hands. The onset is insidious and the condition often goes undiagnosed until complications arise – neuropathic ulcers of the feet, regional osteoporosis and fractures of the foot bones, or Charcot joints in the ankles and feet. There may be muscular weakness and loss of reflexes. A late feature is loss of balance. Treatment consists of skin care, management of fractures and splintage or arthrodesis of grossly unstable or deformed joints. The underlying disorder should, of course, be controlled. The diabetic foot is discussed on p. 489.

Leprosy

Although uncommon in Europe and North America, this is still a frequent cause of peripheral neuropathy in Africa and Asia.

Mycobacterium leprae, an acid-fast organism, causes a diffuse inflammatory disorder of the skin, mucous membranes and peripheral nerves. Depending on the host response, several forms of disease may evolve. The most severe neurological lesions are seen in *tuberculoid leprosy.* Anaesthetic skin patches develop over the extensor surfaces of the limbs; loss of motor function leads to weakness and deformities of the hands and feet. Thickened nerves

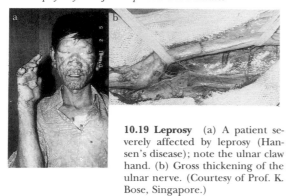

10.19 Leprosy (a) A patient severely affected by leprosy (Hansen's disease); note the ulnar claw hand. (b) Gross thickening of the ulnar nerve. (Courtesy of Prof. K. Bose, Singapore.)

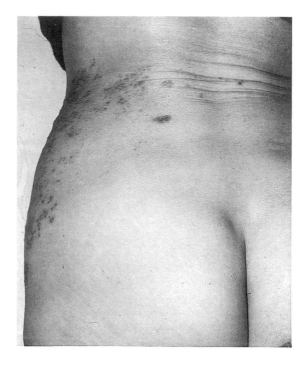

10.20 Herpes zoster This patient was treated for several weeks for 'sciatica' – then the typical rash of shingles appeared.

may be felt as cords under the skin or where they cross the bones (e.g. the ulnar nerve behind the medial epicondyle of the elbow). Trophic ulcers are common and may predispose to osteomyelitis. *Lepromatous leprosy* is associated with a symmetrical polyneuropathy, which occurs late in the disease.

Treatment by combined chemotherapy (mainly rifampicin and dapsone) is continued for 6 months to 2 years, depending on the response. Muscle weakness – particularly the intrinsic muscle paralysis due to ulnar nerve involvement – may require multiple tendon transfers.

Herpes zoster (shingles)

This common disorder is caused by varicella (chickenpox) virus infection of the dorsal root ganglia. Elderly or immunosuppressed patients are particularly susceptible. Following an injury or intercurrent illness, the patient develops severe unilateral pain in the distribution of several adjacent nerve roots. Involvement of the lumbar roots may closely mimic sciatica. Days or weeks later an irritating vesicular rash appears; characteristically it trails out along the dermatomes corresponding to affected nerves. The condition usually subsides spontaneously but neuralgia may persist for months or years. Treatment is symptomatic, though in severe cases systemic antiviral therapy may be justified.

Neuralgic amyotrophy (brachial neuritis)

This acute condition usually follows a flu-like illness or immunization. It causes intense pain in the shoulder followed by weakness, and sometimes sensory symptoms, in the distribution of the brachial plexus. It is, fortunately, self-limiting, but at the onset it is easily mistaken for an acute cervical disc prolapse.

Muscular dystrophies

The muscular dystrophies are rare hereditary disorders causing progressive muscle weakness and wasting.

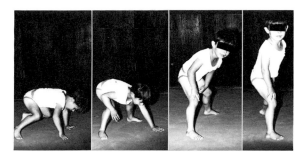

10.21 Muscle dystrophy This boy, with a Duchenne type of dystrophy, has to climb up his legs in order to achieve the upright position.

Duchenne muscular dystrophy

This is a progressive disease of X-linked inheritance. It is therefore seen only in boys (or in girls with sex chromosome disorders). It is usually unsuspected until the child starts to walk; he has difficulty standing and falls frequently. The muscles look bulky, but much of this is due to fat and the pseudohypertrophy belies the weakness, which is progressive and generalized. Compensatory postural deformities produce a typical stance and gait, with the feet in equinus, the pelvis tilted forward, the back arched in lordosis and the neck extended. A characteristic feature is the method of rising from the floor by climbing up his legs (Gowers' sign). By 10 years of age the child is unable to walk, and by 20 he may be dying of cardiac or respiratory failure.

Diagnostic tests are a raised level of serum creatinine phosphokinase,* characteristic EMG signs and histochemical findings on muscle biopsy.

While the child can still walk, physiotherapy and splintage or even tendon operations may help to prevent and correct joint deformities and so prolong the period of mobility. When he is wheelchair-bound, spinal deformity must be prevented and physiotherapy is directed at retaining muscle power for as long as possible. A method of treatment being tried is to inject cultured myoblasts from normal donors into affected muscles.

*This should be tested in any boy with a clumsy gait.

Limb girdle dystrophy

This disorder, of autosomal recessive inheritance, is even rarer than the Duchenne type and much less disabling. Symptoms usually start in late adolescence. Pelvic girdle weakness causes a waddling gait and difficulty in rising from a low chair; pectoral girdle weakness makes it difficult to raise the arms above the head. The disease is slowly progressive and by the 5th decade disability is usually marked. Treatment consists of physiotherapy and splintage to prevent contractures, and operative correction when necessary. Because the deltoid muscles are spared, shoulder movements can be improved by fixing the scapula to the ribs posteriorly, so improving deltoid leverage (Copeland and Howard, 1978).

Facioscapulohumeral dystrophy

This condition, of autosomal dominant inheritance, presents in early adult life with facial muscle weakness, winging of the scapulae and slight pelvic girdle weakness. Deterioration is slow and the life span normal. Treatment is the same as for limb girdle dystrophy.

Myotonic disorders

Myotonia is persistent muscle contraction after cessation of voluntary effort. It is a prominent feature in certain autosomal dominant genetic disorders.

Dystrophia myotonica

Patients present in adult life with distal muscle weakness and myotonia. Later there is more widespread involvement and the face and tongue may be affected as well. Patients usually have low intelligence. Complications are dysphagia, respiratory difficulty and cardiomyopathy. Foot deformities may need manipulation and splintage.

Myotonia congenita

Myotonia is present at birth and may cause feeding problems. Children have 'stiff joints' and muscle cramps, which are usually worse after rest. Limb muscles are quite bulky and in mild cases function is not severely disturbed.

References and further reading

Beals, R.K. (1966) Spastic paraplegia and diplegia: an evaluation of non-surgical and surgical factors influencing prognosis for ambulation. *Journal of Bone and Joint Surgery* **48A**, 827–846

Bleck, E.E. (1987) *Orthopaedic Management in Cerebral Palsy*, Blackwell Scientific, Oxford; Lippincott, Philadelphia

Brown, L.M., Robson, M.J. and Sharrard, W.J.W. (1980) The pathophysiology of arthrogryposis multiplex congenita neurologica. *Journal of Bone and Joint Surgery* **62B**, 291–296

Copeland, S.A. and Howard, R.C. (1978) Thoracoscapular fusion for facioscapulohumeral dystrophy. *Journal of Bone and Joint Surgery* **60B**, 547–551

Craig, J.J. (1967) Cerebral palsy. In *Modern Trends in Orthopaedics* (ed. W.D. Graham), Butterworths, London

Evans, E.B. (1971) Editorial. Hip flexion deformity in spastic cerebral palsy. *Journal of Bone and Joint Surgery* **53A**, 1465–1467

Hoffer, M.M. (1986) Management of the hip in cerebral palsy. *Journal of Bone and Joint Surgery* **68A**, 629–631

Hong-Xue Men, Chan-Hua Bian, Chan-Dou Yang, Zen-Long Zhang, Chi-Chang Wu and Bo-You Pang (1991) Surgical treatment of the flail knee after poliomyelitis. *Journal of Bone and Joint Surgery* **73B**, 195–199

Louis, D.S., Hensinger, R.M., Fraser, B.A., Phelps, J.A. and Jacques, K. (1989) Surgical management of the severely multiply handicapped individual. *Journal of Pediatric Orthopedics* **9**, 15–18

Makin, M. (1953) The surgical management of Friedreich's ataxia. *Journal of Bone and Joint Surgery* **35A**, 425–436

Matev, I. (1963) Surgical treatment of the spastic thumb in palm deformity. *Journal of Bone and Joint Surgery* **45B**, 703–708

Menelaus, M.B. (1980) *The Orthopaedic Management of Spina Bifida Cystica*, 2nd edn, Churchill Livingstone, Edinburgh

Rang, M. and Wright, J. (1989) What have 30 years of medical progress done for cerebral palsy? *Clinical Orthopaedics and Related Research* **247**, 55–60

Scrutton, D. (1989) The early management of hips in cerebral palsy. *Developmental Medicine and Child Neurology* **31**, 108–116

Sharrard, W.J.W. (1979) *Paediatric Orthopaedics and Fractures*, 2nd edn, Blackwell Scientific, Oxford

Sutherland, D.H., Ohlson, R., Cooper, L. and Woo, S.K. (1980) The development of mature gait. *Journal of Bone and Joint Surgery* **62A**, 336–353

Trail, I.A. and Galasko, C.S.B. (1990) The matrix seating system. *Journal of Bone and Joint Surgery* **72B**, 666–669

Peripheral nerve injuries 11

Nerve structure and function

Peripheral nerves are bundles of axons conducting efferent (motor) impulses from cells in the anterior horn of the spinal cord to the muscles, and afferent (sensory) impulses from peripheral receptors via cells in the posterior root ganglia to the cord. They also convey sudomotor and vasomotor fibres from ganglion cells in the sympathetic chain. Some nerves are predominantly motor, some predominantly sensory; the larger trunks are mixed, with motor and sensory axons running in separate bundles.

All motor axons and the large sensory axons serving touch, pain and proprioception are coated with *myelin*, a lipoprotein membrane derived from the accompanying *Schwann cells*. Depletion of this myelin sheath causes slowing – and eventually complete blocking – of axonal conduction.

Most axons – in particular the small-diameter fibres carrying crude sensation and the efferent sympathetic fibres – are unmyelinated but wrapped in Schwann cell cytoplasm. Damage to these axons causes unpleasant or bizarre sensations and various sudomotor and vasomotor effects.

Outside the Schwann cell membrane the axon is covered by a connective tissue stocking, the *endoneurium*. The axons that make up a nerve are separated into bundles – or fascicles – by fairly dense membranous tissue, the *perineurium*. In a transected nerve, these fascicles are seen pouting from the cut surface, their perineurial sheaths well defined and strong enough to be grasped by fine instruments. The nerve trunk itself is enclosed in an even thicker connective tissue coat, the *epineurium*.

The nerve is richly supplied by *blood vessels* that run on the surface of the nerve trunk in a layer of loose areolar tissue, before penetrating the various layers to become the *endoneurial capillaries*. These fine vessels may be damaged by stretching or rough handling of the nerve; however, they can withstand extensive mobilization of the nerve (Lundborg, 1988), making it feasible to repair or replace damaged segments by operative transposition or neurotization. The tiny blood vessels have their own *sympathetic nerve supply* coming from the parent nerve, and stimulation of these fibres (causing intraneural vasoconstriction) may be important in conditions such as reflex sympathetic dystrophy and other unusual pain syndromes.

Pathology

Nerve damage varies markedly in severity from transient and quickly recoverable loss of function to complete interruption and degeneration.

ISCHAEMIA Acute nerve compression causes numbness and tingling within 15 minutes, loss of pain sensibility after 30 minutes and muscle weakness after 45 minutes. Relief of compression is followed by intense paraethesiae lasting up to 5 minutes (the familiar 'pins and needles' after a limb 'goes to sleep'); feeling is restored within 30 seconds and full muscle power after about 10 minutes. These changes are due to transient endoneurial anoxia and they leave no trace of nerve damage.

NEURAPRAXIA Seddon (1942) coined the term 'neurapraxia' to describe a reversible physiological nerve conduction block in which there is loss of some types of sensation and muscle power followed by spontaneous recovery after a few days or weeks. It is due to mechanical pressure causing segmental demyelination and is seen typically in 'crutch palsy' and 'Saturday night paralysis'. It also accounts for tourniquet paralysis, in which the sites of nerve damage correspond to the edges of the cuff (Ochoa, Fowler and Gilliat, 1972).

AXONOTMESIS This is a more severe form of nerve injury, seen typically after closed fractures and dislocations. The term means, literally, axonal interruption. There is loss of conduction but the nerve is in continuity and the endoneurial tubes are intact. Distal to the lesion, and for a few millimetres retrograde, axons disintegrate and are resorbed by phagocytes. This *wallerian degeneration* takes only a few days and is accompanied by marked proliferation of Schwann cells and fibroblasts lining the endoneurial tubes. The denervated target organs (motor end-plates and sensory receptors) gradually atrophy, and if they are not re-innervated within 2 years they will never recover.

Axonal *regeneration* starts within hours of nerve damage. From the proximal stumps grow numerous fine unmyelinated tendrils, many of which find their way into the intact endoneurial tubes. These axonal processes grow at a speed of 1–3 mm per day, the larger fibres slowly acquiring a new myelin coat. Eventually they join to end-organs, which enlarge and start functioning again.

NEUROTMESIS In Seddon's original classification, neurotmesis meant division of the nerve trunk, such as may occur in an open wound. More accurately, it applies also to severe traction injuries, crushing injuries and damage due to intraneural injections where the nerve is in continuity. As in axonotmesis, there is rapid wallerian degeneration, but here the endoneurial tubes are destroyed over a variable segment and scarring thwarts any hope of regenerating axons entering the distal segment and regaining their target organs. Instead, regenerating fibres mingle with proliferating Schwann cells and fibroblasts in a jumbled knot, or 'neuroma', at the site of injury. Even after surgical repair, many new axons fail to reach the distal segment, and those that do may not find suitable Schwann tubes, or may not reach the correct end-organs in time, or may remain incompletely myelinated. Function may be adequate but is never normal.

Clinical features

Nerve injuries are easily missed. Following any kind of trauma, patients should be questioned about numbness, any change of feeling or weakness without waiting for them to complain. Partial lesions sometimes cause pain or paraesthesia. Late cases may present as joint stiffness, deformity or wasting. Examination requires painstaking observation. There may be a scar of the causal wound. Anaesthetic skin looks smooth and shiny, the affected fingers are thin and tapering and their nails abnormal. Trophic ulcers may be present, especially in the foot. Muscle wasting is apparent and the attitude of a paralysed limb is often characteristic.

The anaesthetic skin feels smooth, cool and dry. A neuroma may be palpable and may be tender. Where sensory nerve damage exists, the patient will point to the anaesthetic part; however, it is useful for the surgeon to map out the area of loss and to chart it as absent, abnormal or normal. The quality of sensation is difficult to assess objectively, but light touch, pinprick, two-point discrimination, pressure and temperature can be charted.

The patient cannot perform certain movements, though passive range may be full. Muscle tone and power are lost, and bulk is diminished. In testing individual muscles errors may occur, especially in the hand, because of anomalous innervation, trick movements or supplementary movements. To assess recovery, power may usefully be charted in five grades (p. 194).

X-rays are usually normal but in late cases there may be regional osteoporosis.

Diagnosis

With a suspected nerve injury, the following questions arise.

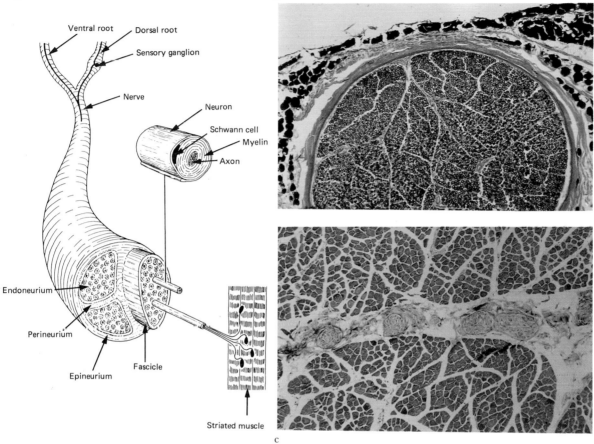

a

Ventral root   Dorsal root

Sensory ganglion

Nerve

Neuron

Schwann cell

Myelin

Axon

Endoneurium

Perineurium

Epineurium   Fascicle

Striated muscle

b

c

11.1 Nerve structure   (a) Diagram of the structural elements of a peripheral nerve. (b) Histological section through a large nerve. (c) High-power view of the same, showing blood vessels in the perineurium.

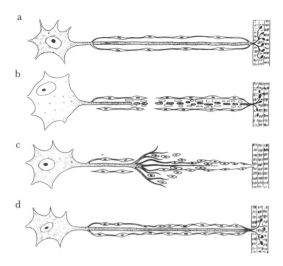

11.2 Nerve injury and repair (a) Normal axon and target organ (striated muscle). (b) Following nerve injury the distal part of the axon disintegrates and the myelin sheath breaks up. The nerve cell nucleus becomes eccentric and Nissl bodies are sparse. (c) New axonal tendrils grow into the mass of proliferating Schwann cells. One of the tendrils will find its way into the old endoneurial tube and (d) the axon will slowly regenerate.

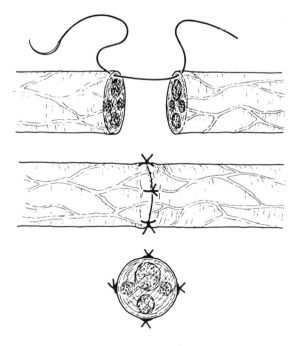

11.3 Nerve repair The stumps are correctly orientated and attached by fine sutures through the epineurium.

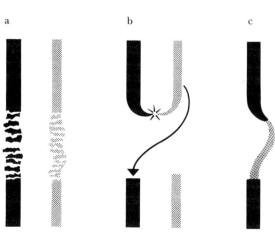

11.4 Pedicle graft (a) Severe damage to both the ulnar and the median nerves. (b) The damaged area has been excised and the two proximal ends joined together as a loop. (c) Four weeks later the ulnar part of the loop has been divided proximally and attached to the distal stump of the median nerve.

Is a nerve lesion present? A quick examination is carried out for each nerve, by inviting a characteristic movement or testing for sensibility in a specific area.

At what level is the lesion? Usually this is obvious from the injury; if it is not, individual muscles whose branches arise at successive levels must be tested. Special investigations are occasionally useful (see below).

What type of lesion is present? Clinical examination may suggest a neurotmesis; a palpable nerve bulb confirms it. Partial division is liable to produce hyperaesthesia or excess sweating. With neurapraxia, paralysis is not total and recovery begins after a few days or weeks.

Is the lesion recovering? The earliest evidence is Tinel's sign: the nerve is tapped lightly, starting peripherally; the point at which the patient feels pain or tingling in the distribution of the nerve indicates how far (if at all) recovery has progressed.

Repeated examination at intervals will show if (and when) the most proximally innervated muscles are recovering. Axonal regeneration is expected to occur at the rate of 1 mm per day.

Special investigations

Nerve blocking A small quantity of local anaesthetic may be injected around the injured nerve. If this is followed by greater sensory or motor loss the lesion is partial. Similarly, by injecting around undamaged nerves, overlap can be recognized.

Electrical tests Precise information about the nature, level and extent of recovery in nerve lesions can be obtained by: (1) the assessment of strength/duration curves; (2) electromyographic study of voluntary action potentials; and (3) the measurement of motor and sensory conduction velocities at various levels.

Treatment

NERVE EXPLORATION Closed injuries usually recover spontaneously and it is worth waiting until the most proximally supplied muscle should have regained function. Exploration is indicated: (1) if the nerve was seen to be divided and needs to be repaired; (2) if the type of injury (e.g. a knife wound) suggests that the nerve is likely to have been cut; (3) if recovery is inappropriately delayed and the diagnosis is in doubt.

The incision will be long, as the nerve must be widely exposed above and below the lesion before the lesion itself is cleared. The nerve must be handled gently with suitable instruments. Bipolar diathermy is used. Magnification helps; an operating microscope is ideal but a loupe or watchmaker's headpiece is better than nothing. A nerve stimulator is essential if scarring makes recognition uncertain.

PRIMARY REPAIR A divided nerve is best repaired as soon as this can be done safely. Primary suture at the time of wound toilet, though not easy (because the sheath is very thin), has considerable advantages: the nerve ends have not retracted much; their relative rotation is usually undisturbed; and there is no fibrosis. But if repair would involve groping about in the depths of a dirty wound it should be postponed, at least until the wound has healed. Other contraindications are severe traction injuries where direct suture is impossible, unfavourable operating conditions, and the presence of other injuries that require more urgent attention.

Associated fractures are stabilized and soft-tissue injuries repaired before attending to the nerve. A clean cut nerve is sutured without further preparation; a ragged cut may need paring of the stumps with a sharp blade, but this must be kept to a minimum. The stumps are anatomically orientated and fine (10/0) sutures are inserted in the epineurium. There should be no tension on the suture line. Opinions are divided on the value of fascicular repair with perineurial sutures.

A traction lesion – especially of the brachial plexus – may leave a gap too wide to close. These injuries are best dealt with in specialized centres, where primary grafting can be carried out.

If a tourniquet is used it should be a pneumatic one; it must be released and bleeding stopped before the wound is closed.

The limb is splinted in a position to ensure minimal tension on the nerve; if flexion needs to be excessive, a graft is required. The splint is retained for 3–6 weeks and thereafter physiotherapy is encouraged.

DELAYED REPAIR Late repair – i.e. weeks or months after the injury – may be indicated because (1) a closed injury was left alone but shows no sign of recovery at the expected time, (2) the diagnosis was missed and the patient presents late or (3) primary repair has failed. The options must be carefully weighed: if the patient has adapted to the functional loss, if it is a high lesion and reinnervation is unlikely within the critical 2-year period, or if there is a pure motor loss which can be treated by tendon transfers, it may be best to leave well alone. Excessive scarring and intractable joint stiffness may, likewise, make nerve repair questionable; yet in the hand it is still worthwhile simply to regain protective sensation.

The lesion is exposed, working from normal tissue above and below towards the scarred area. When the nerve is in continuity it is difficult to know whether resection is necessary or not. If the nerve is only slightly thickened and feels soft, and there is conduction across the lesion, resection is not advised; if the 'neuroma' is hard and there is no conduction on nerve stimulation, it should be resected, paring back the stumps until healthy fascicles are exposed. With a lateral 'neuroma', only the abnormal part is excised.

How to deal with the gap? The nerve must be sutured without tension. The stumps may be brought together by gently mobilizing the proximal and distal segments, by flexing nearby joints to relax the soft tissues, or (in the case of the ulnar nerve) by transposing the nerve trunk to the flexor aspect of the elbow. In this way, gaps of 2 cm in the median nerve, 4–5 cm in the ulnar nerve and 6–8 cm in the sciatic nerve can usually be closed, the limb being splinted in the 'relaxing' position for 4–6 weeks after the operation. Elsewhere, gaps of more than 1–2 cm usually require grafting or nerve transfer.

NERVE GRAFTING Free autogenous nerve grafts can be used to bridge gaps too large for direct suture. Cutaneous nerves that can be spared for use as grafts include the lateral cutaneous nerve of the thigh, the saphenous, the sural, and the medial cutaneous nerve of the forearm. Because their diameter is small, several strips may be used (cable graft). The graft should be long enough to lie without any tension, and it should be routed through a well-vascularized bed. The graft is attached at each end either by fine sutures or with fibrin glue (Narakas, 1988).

Vascularized grafts are used in special situations. If the ulnar and median nerves are both damaged (e.g. in Volkmann's ischaemia) a pedicle graft from the ulnar nerve may be used to bridge the gap in the median. The two proximal stumps are joined in a U-loop; 4 weeks later the ulnar part of the loop is divided more proximally and swung down, with its blood supply intact, to be sutured to the distal median stump. Even bolder is the concept of free vascularized grafts for certain brachial plexus lesions (Birch et al., 1988).

Research into using muscle grafts to bridge gaps is well advanced (Norris et al., 1988). A block of muscle is excised, dipped in liquid nitrogen, thawed and positioned in the gap. The myotubules act as channels along which axons can grow.

NEUROTIZATION A healthy but easily dispensable nerve can be transferred and sutured to a damaged nerve whose motor or sensory function is more important. This principle has been applied to brachial plexus injuries where the long thoracic, the accessory or the intercostal nerves are transferred to distal segments of the plexus that are irreparably detached from their proximal roots (Narakas and Hentz, 1988). The results are only moderately good, but the alternative is often amputation.

CARE OF PARALYSED PARTS While recovery is awaited the skin should be guarded against burns and the circulation assisted by massage. The joints should be moved through their full range twice daily to prevent stiffness. Splints may be necessary and 'lively splints' are the best; they hold the paralysed muscle in its shortened position by means of a spring which is weak enough to allow the unparalysed muscles to work against it.

Prognosis

TYPE OF LESION Neurapraxia always recovers fully; axonotmesis usually recovers well; neurotmesis does less well and traction injuries have the worst prognosis of all.

LEVEL OF LESION The higher the lesion, the worse the prognosis.

TYPE OF NERVE Purely motor or purely sensory nerves recover better than mixed nerves, because there is less likelihood of axonal confusion.

SIZE OF GAP Above the critical resection length, suture is not successful.

AGE In children the prognosis is better than in adults.

DELAY IN SUTURE This is a most important adverse factor. After a few months, recovery following suture becomes progressively less likely.

ASSOCIATED LESIONS Damage to vessels, tendons and other structures makes it more difficult to obtain recovery of a useful limb even if the nerve itself recovers.

SURGICAL TECHNIQUES Skill, experience and suitable facilities are needed to treat nerve injuries. If these are lacking, it is wiser to perform the essential wound toilet and then transfer the patient to a specialized centre.

Brachial plexus – birth injuries

Birth injury of the brachial plexus ('obstetrical palsy') is due to excessive traction and is usually associated with (1) difficult cephalic delivery of a large baby, especially where forceps have been used, or (2) breech delivery with problems during extraction of the head. The right side is affected more often than the left (Gilbert, Razabone and Amar-Khodja, 1988).

Clinical features

The diagnosis is usually obvious at birth: after a difficult delivery the baby has a floppy or flail arm. Further examination a day or two later will distinguish two types of injury: upper and lower root lesions.

Upper root lesions (Erb's palsy), due to injury of C5, C6 and (sometimes) C7. The abductors and external rotators of the shoulder and the supinators are paralysed. The arm is held to the

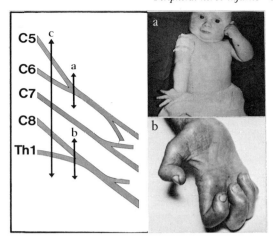

11.5 Brachial plexus Damage at **a** causes an Erb's palsy (upper photograph); this is more common than damage at **b** which causes Klumpke's palsy (lower photograph); **c** represents a lesion of the entire plexus.

side, internally rotated and pronated. There may also be loss of finger extension. Sensation is intact.

Lower root lesions (Klumpke's palsy), due to injury of C8 and T1. This is much less common, but more severe; examination may show that it is actually part of a complete plexus lesion. All finger muscles are paralysed and there may also be loss of sensation, vasomotor impairment and a unilateral Horner's syndrome. In complete lesions the entire limb is paralysed.

X-rays should be taken to exclude fractures of the shoulder or clavicle.

Management

Over the next few weeks one of several things may happen.

Paralysis may recover completely Many (perhaps most) of the upper root lesions recover spontaneously. The most reliable indicator is return of the biceps activity by the third month (Gilbert, Razabone and Amar-Khodja, 1988).

Paralysis may improve A total lesion may partially resolve, leaving the infant with either an upper or a lower root syndrome which is unlikely to change.

Paralysis may remain unaltered This is more likely with complete lesions and lower root palsies, especially in the presence of a Horner's syndrome.

CONSERVATIVE TREATMENT   While waiting for recovery, gentle physiotherapy keeps the joints mobile. Traditional methods of splintage in abduction are useless and may even produce further traction.

OPERATIVE TREATMENT   If there is no recovery whatever by 3 months, operative intervention should be considered. Unless the roots are avulsed, it may be possible to excise the scar and bridge the gap with free sural nerve grafts; if the roots are avulsed, neurotization may give a worthwhile result. This is highly demanding surgery which should be undertaken only in specialized centres (Gilbert, Razabone and Amar-Khodja 1988).

If fixed deformities develop, they may require operative correction at a later stage; for example, by osteotomy of the neck of the humerus for fixed internal rotation or division of soft tissues for fixed adduction and pronation.

Brachial plexus – later lesions

Most brachial plexus injuries are due to severe traction, usually following a fall on the side of the neck or the shoulder. Supraclavicular distraction may involve the nerve roots; severe shoulder injuries are associated with infraclavicular lesions; simple shoulder dislocation may give a partial paralysis, which usually recovers; fractures of the clavicle rarely damage the plexus, and then only if caused by a direct blow.

Clinical features

The presence of a nerve lesion is usually obvious, but associated injuries may make it difficult to establish exactly what has happened.

In upper plexus injuries (C5 and 6) the shoulder abductors and external rotators and the forearm supinators are paralysed. Sensory loss involves the outer aspect of the arm and

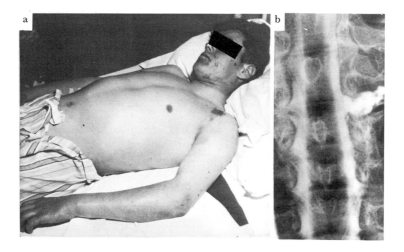

11.6 Brachial plexus   (a) Telltale abrasions on the face and shoulder show how this motorcyclist pulled his entire plexus apart. (b) The myelogram shows leakage of the dye, indicating root avulsion.

forearm. A Tinel sign in the neck may indicate the level of lesion.

Pure lower plexus injuries are rare. Wrist and finger flexors are weak, and the intrinsic hand muscles are paralysed; consequently a claw hand develops. Sensation is lost in the ulnar forearm and hand. There may be an associated Horner's syndrome, indicating avulsion of C8 and T1.

and numb. Sometimes the scapular muscles and one side of the diaphragm too are involved. A Horner's syndrome means that the C8 and T1 roots are damaged.

It is crucial to establish how far from the cord the lesion is. Preganglionic lesions are irreparable; postganglionic lesions may either recover (axonotmesis) or may be amenable to repair. Features suggesting root avulsion are (1) severe pain, (2) paralysis of scapular muscles or diaphragm, (3) Horner's syndrome, (4) severe vascular injury, (5) associated fractures of the cervical spine and (6) spinal cord dysfunction.

THE HISTAMINE TEST Intradermal injection of histamine usually causes a triple response in the surrounding skin. This local axon reflex is absent in the affected dermatome in postganglionic injuries. If the flare reaction persists in an anaesthetic area of skin, the lesion must be proximal to the posterior root ganglion – i.e. it is probably a root avulsion.

ELECTROMYOGRAPHY AND SENSORY CONDUCTION STUDIES may, similarly, help to localize the level of the injury.

MYELOGRAPHY alone may reveal evidence of root avulsion, but the most reliable investigation is *CT combined with myelography.*

Management

INITIAL TREATMENT usually takes place in a general unit where fractures and other associated injuries will be given priority. However, open injuries, including stab wounds, should be explored without delay and clean cut nerves repaired or grafted. Closed traction lesions should not be explored except in a specialized centre after full investigation: this includes cervical CT radiculography which enables preganglionic lesions to be diagnosed (such lesions

are not amenable to repair although neurotization may be possible).

LATER TREATMENT may be necessary in those patients too ill to undergo surgery or transfer in the early stages. Contraindications to further surgery are (1) severe associated injuries of the limb, (2) very long delay between injury and repair, (3) clear evidence of root avulsion, and possibly (4) advanced age and general infirmity. The final decision on the type of reconstruction is usually made only after surgical exploration of the plexus. A ruptured nerve root or trunk may be repaired or grafted. Upper plexus lesions have the best prognosis and the patient may regain shoulder or elbow function. Lower plexus lesions are much less favourable and hand function is seldom restored, though protective sensation may be a worthwhile goal. Complete lesions usually involve a combination of root avulsions and ruptures, and here there is little choice but to use whatever proximal nerves are available to link with the distal plexus by free grafts, giving priority to re-innervation of the musculocutaneous nerve (for elbow flexion) and the lateral cord (for shoulder abduction) (Hentz and Narakas, 1988).

'SALVAGE' OPERATIONS If there is no recovery – and, indeed, sometimes as an alternative to nerve suture in lesions with a poor prognosis – tendon transfers may be useful; for example, latissimus dorsi or pectoralis major transfer to elbow flexors. If the hand is minimally affected, it is worthwhile arthrodesing the shoulder so that the arm can be abducted by the scapular muscles; an alternative is transfer of the trapezius to the proximal humerus (Aziz, Singer and Wolff, 1990). Very occasionally a patient with a completely flail and insensitive limb may prefer amputation through the mid-humerus combined with arthrodesis of the shoulder.

Long thoracic nerve

The long thoracic nerve of Bell (C5, 6, 7) may be damaged in shoulder or neck injuries (usually an axonotmesis) or during operations such as first rib resection, transaxillary sympathectomy or radical mastectomy. However, serratus anterior palsy is also seen after comparatively benign events, such as carrying loads on the shoulder, and even viral illnesses or toxoid injections.

Clinical features

Paralysis of serratus anterior is the commonest cause of winging of the scapula. The patient may complain of aching and weakness on lifting the arm. Examination shows little abnormality until the arm is elevated in flexion or abduction. The classic test for winging is to have the patient pushing forwards against the wall or thrusting the shoulder forwards against resistance.

Treatment

Except after direct injury or division, the nerve usually recovers spontaneously, though this may take a year or longer. Persistent winging of the scapula occasionally requires operative stabilization by transferring pectoralis minor or major to the lower part of the scapula.

Spinal accessory nerve

The spinal accessory nerve (C3, 4) supplies the sternomastoid muscle and then runs obliquely across the posterior triangle of the neck to innervate the upper half of the trapezius. Because of its superficial course, it is easily injured in stab wounds and operations in the posterior triangle of the neck (e.g. lymph node biopsy). It is also sometimes involved, with the brachial plexus, in traction injuries.

Clinical features

Following an open wound or operation, the patient complains of pain in the shoulder and

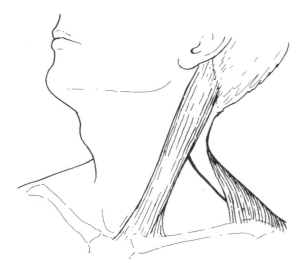

11.7 Accessory nerve   The accessory nerve is embedded in the fascia which covers the posterior triangle and is easily damaged during lymph node biopsy or excision (and in stab wounds).

weakness on abduction of the arm. Usually the true nature of the problem is not appreciated and diagnosis is delayed for weeks or months. Typically there is mild winging of the scapula on active abduction of the arm against resistance; unlike the deformity in serratus anterior palsy, this disappears on flexion or forward thrusting of the shoulder. In late cases there may be wasting of the trapezius and drooping of the shoulder.

Treatment

Stab injuries should be explored immediately and the nerve repaired. If the exact cause of injury is uncertain, it is prudent to wait for 4–6 weeks for signs of recovery. If this does not occur, the nerve should be explored (1) to confirm the diagnosis and (2) to repair the lesion by direct suture or grafting. While waiting for recovery the arm is held in a sling to prevent dragging on the neck muscles. Occasionally, persistent scapular instability is severe enough to require stabilization.

Suprascapular nerve

The suprascapular nerve, which arises from the upper trunk of the brachial plexus (C5, 6), runs through the suprascapular notch to supply the supra- and infraspinatus muscles. It may be injured in fractures of the scapula, by a direct blow, by sudden traction, or simply by carrying a heavy load over the shoulder.

Clinical features

There may be a history of injury, but patients sometimes present with unexplained pain in the suprascapular region and weakness of shoulder abduction – symptoms readily mistaken for a rotator cuff syndrome. There is usually wasting of the supraspinatus and diminished power of abduction and external rotation. Electromyography may help to establish the diagnosis.

Treatment

This is usually an axonotmesis which clears up spontaneously after 2–3 months. In the absence of trauma one might suspect a nerve entrapment syndrome, and decompression by division of the suprascapular ligament often brings improvement.

Axillary nerve

The axillary nerve (C5, 6) arises from the posterior cord of the brachial plexus, runs along subscapularis and across the axilla just inferior to the shoulder joint. It emerges behind the humerus, deep to the deltoid; after supplying the teres minor, it divides into a medial branch which supplies the posterior part of the deltoid and a patch of skin over the muscle and an anterior branch that curls round the surgical neck of the humerus to innervate the anterior two-thirds of the deltoid. The landmark for this important branch is 5 cm below the tip of the acromion.

The nerve is sometimes ruptured in a brachial plexus injury. More often it is merely bruised during shoulder dislocation or fractures of the humeral neck (axonotmesis). Iatrogenic injuries occur in transaxillary operations on the shoulder and with lateral deltoid-splitting incisions.

The patient cannot abduct the shoulder, due to deltoid weakness. There may be a tiny area of numbness over the deltoid.

Treatment

Following fractures or dislocations, spontaneous recovery is the rule. However, persistent isolated paralysis of the deltoid following a brachial plexus injury suggests complete division of the nerve; if there is no recovery after 3 months, the nerve should be explored and – if possible – repaired. If this fails, provided that trapezius and serratus anterior are functioning, shoulder arthrodesis can provide both stability and some degree of 'abduction'.

Radial nerve

The radial nerve may be injured at the elbow, in the upper arm or in the axilla.

Clinical features

Low lesions are usually due to fractures or dislocations at the elbow, or to a local wound. Iatrogenic lesions of the posterior interosseous nerve where it winds though the supinator muscle are sometimes seen after operations on the proximal end of the radius. The patient complains of clumsiness and, on testing, cannot extend the metacarpophalangeal joints of the hand. In the thumb there is also weakness of abduction and interphalangeal extension.

High lesions occur with fractures of the humerus or after prolonged tourniquet pressure. There is an obvious wrist drop, due to weakness of the radial extensors of the wrist, as well

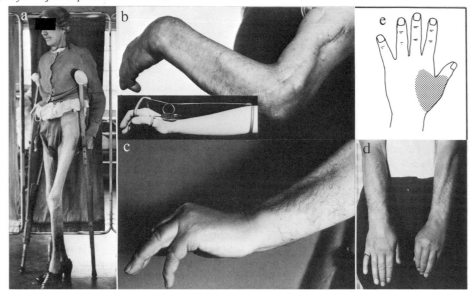

11.8 Radial nerve lesions   (a) Crutches should not be thrust high into the axilla, or palsy may follow; (b) complete division with drop wrist (*inset* – Brian Thomas' splint); (c) this patient demonstrates the inability to extend the fingers at the knuckle joints, but he can straighten the interphalangeal joints with his intrinsic muscles; (d) wasting; (e) sensory loss.

inability to extend the metacarpophalangeal joints. Sensory loss is limited to a small patch on the dorsum around the anatomical snuffbox.

Very high lesions   may be caused by trauma or operations around the shoulder. More often, though, they are due to chronic compression in the axilla; this is seen in drink and drug addicts who fall into a stupor with the arm dangling over the back of a chair ('Saturday-night palsy') or in thin elderly patients using crutches ('crutch palsy'). In addition to weakness of the wrist and hand, the triceps is paralysed and the triceps reflex is absent.

Treatment

Open injuries should be explored and the nerve repaired or grafted as soon as possible.

A closed lesion is usually an axonotmesis – and function eventually returns. One can therefore afford to wait. However, lesions associated with fractures, and any possible iatrogenic injury, should be explored if there is no recovery by 6 weeks.

While recovery is awaited, a Brian Thomas splint is worn; this is a 'lively' splint holding the metacarpophalangeal joints straight and the thumb straight and abducted, while still permitting active use of the hand.

If recovery does not occur, the disability can be largely overcome by tendon transfers: pronator teres to the short radial extensor of the wrist, flexor carpi radialis to the long finger extensors and palmaris longus to the long thumb abductor.

Ulnar nerve

Injuries of the ulnar nerve are usually either near the wrist or near the elbow, although open wounds may damage it at any level.

Clinical features

Low lesions   are often caused by cuts on shattered glass. There is numbness of the ulnar one and a half fingers. The hand assumes a typical posture in repose – the claw hand deformity – with hyperextension of the metacarpophalangeal joints of the ring and little fingers, due to weakness of the intrinsic muscles. Hypothenar and interosseous wasting may be obvious by comparison with the normal hand. Finger abduction is weak and the loss of thumb adduction makes pinch difficult. The patient is asked to grip a sheet of paper forcefully between thumbs and index fingers while the examiner tries to pull it away; powerful flexion of the thumb interphalangeal joint signals weakness of adductor pollicis and overcompensation by the flexor pollicis longus (Froment's sign).

Entrapment of the ulnar nerve in the pisohamate tunnel (Guyon's canal) is often seen in long-distance cyclists who lean with the pisiform pressing on the handlebars. Unexplained lesions of the distal (motor) branch of the nerve may be due to compression by a deep carpal ganglion.

High lesions occur with elbow fractures or dislocations. The hand is not markedly deformed because the ulnar half of flexor digitorum profundus is paralysed and the fingers are therefore less 'clawed'. Otherwise, motor and sensory loss are the same as in low lesions.

'Ulnar neuritis' may be caused by chronic entrapment of the nerve in the medial epicondylar (cubital) tunnel, especially where there is severe valgus deformity of the elbow, compression along the edge of an osteoarthritic

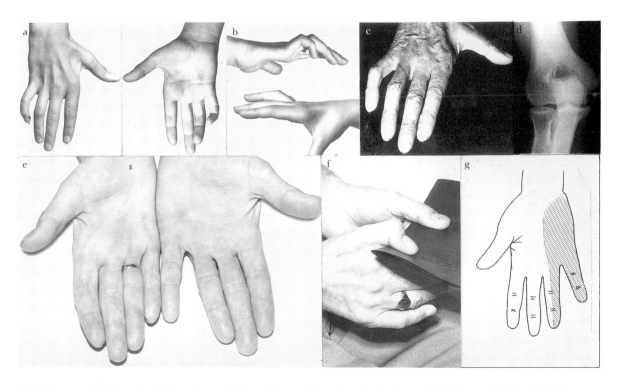

11.9 Ulnar nerve lesions   (a, b) Low ulnar palsy: intrinsic muscle wasting; in the ring and little fingers the knuckle joints are hyperextended (paralysed lumbricals) and the interphalangeal joints are flexed (paralysed interossei). (c) High ulnar palsy: profundus action is lost, so the terminal interphalangeal joints are not flexed (ulnar paradox). He had cut his elbow on some glass; (d) the x-ray shows the glass fragment. (e) When the patient tries to push his little fingers apart, weakness of one abductor digiti minimi is displayed. (f) Froment's sign – because adductor pollicis is weak, the flexor pollicis longus is being used. (g) Sensory loss.

joint, or prolonged pressure on the elbows in anaesthetized or bed-ridden patients. The patient complains of pain and paraesthesia in the ulnar nerve territory, aggravated by pressure behind the medial epicondyle. Ulnar sensation is often diminished but motor weakness and wasting are late features. The diagnosis is confirmed by demonstrating reduced conduction velocity.

Treatment

Exploration and suture of a divided nerve are well worthwhile, and anterior transposition at the elbow permits closure of gaps up to 5 cm. While recovery is awaited, the skin should be guarded against burns. 'Lively' splints keep the hand supple and useful.

Nerve entrapment may need decompression – either a simple splitting of the aponeurosis between the humeral and ulnar heads of the flexor carpi ulnaris or, if there is an obvious deformity or local obstruction, by transposing the nerve to the front of the elbow and resecting the intermuscular septum above the medial epicondyle.

If there is no recovery after nerve division, the hand may still retain reasonable function. The main disabilities are loss of metacarpophalangeal flexion and index finger abduction (which renders the index finger unstable during pinch). Metacarpophalangeal flexion can be improved by superficialis-to-extensor tendon transfers (Bunnell) or by tightening the volar capsule of each MCP joint (Zancolli). Index abduction is improved by transferring extensor pollicis brevis to the radial side of the finger.

Median nerve

The median nerve is commonly injured near the wrist or high up in the forearm.

Low lesions may be caused by cuts in front of the wrist or by carpal dislocations. The patient is unable to abduct the thumb, and sensation is lost over the radial three and a half digits. In long-standing cases the thenar eminence is wasted and trophic changes may be seen.

Nerve entrapment in the carpal tunnel is common. Symptoms are usually mild and intermittent: pain in the hand with tingling and numbness in the median nerve distribution – especially at night when the hand is tucked in with the wrist flexed and immobile. Conduction velocity is reduced across the wrist.

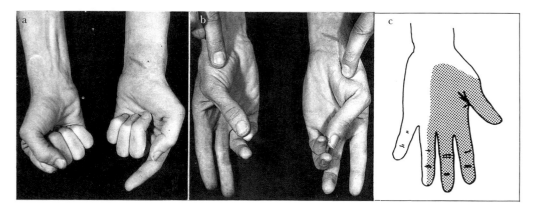

11.10 Cut median nerve   (a) The pointing index when trying to clench the fist. (b) Opponens wasting. (c) Sensory loss.

High lesions are generally due to forearm fractures or elbow dislocation, but stabs and gunshot wounds may damage the nerve at any level. The signs are the same as those of low lesions but, in addition, the long flexors to the thumb, index and middle fingers, the radial wrist flexors and the forearm pronator muscles are all paralysed. Typically the hand is held with the ulnar fingers flexed and the index straight (the 'pointing sign').*

In the rare *anterior interosseous nerve syndrome* this short motor branch of the median nerve may be trapped just below the elbow under the humeral part of the pronator teres muscle. The patient complains of pain in the forearm and feeble pinch due to weakness of thumb and index finger flexion. There is no sensory abnormality. Nerve conduction tests will confirm the diagnosis.

Treatment

If the nerve is divided, suture or nerve grafting should always be attempted. Extensive nerve mobilization may be necessary, the incision sometimes extending above the elbow. Postoperatively the wrist is splinted in flexion to avoid tension; when movements are commenced, wrist extension should be prevented.

Nerve entrapment at the wrist is treated by slitting the transverse carpal ligament to decompress the carpal tunnel. Entrapment of the anterior interosseous branch below the elbow may, likewise, require operative release.

Late lesions are sometimes seen. If there has been no recovery, the disability is severe because of sensory loss and deficient pincer action. If sensation recovers but not opposition, one of the superficialis tendons can be transferred to the distal end of the opponens pollicis.

---

* If your median nerve is cut through,
Your buttons are hard to undo.
The front of your thumb
And three fingers are numb,
And your fist points the way to the loo.

Lumbrosacral plexus

Any part of the plexus may be injured by sacroiliac dislocation or fractures of the sacrum. These lesions are usually incomplete and often missed; the patient may complain of no more than patchy muscle weakness and some difficulty with micturition. Sensation is diminished in the perineum or in one or more of the lower limb dermatomes. *Plexus injuries should always be looked for in patients with fractures of the pelvis.*

Recovery is usually quite good and no purpose is served by operative exploration.

INDIVIDUAL ROOTS may be compressed by a tumour, by a prolapsed intervertebral disc or by narrowing of the spinal canal. Pressure on L3 and L4 roots causes weakness of knee extension, depression of the knee reflex and loss of sensation over the anterior thigh and medial side of the leg. Pressure on L4 and L5 causes weakness of the hamstrings and, often, a hyperactive knee jerk due to the unopposed extensor contraction. Pressure on L5 causes weakness of big toe extension and altered sensation over the front of the leg and foot. Pressure on S1 causes weakness of plantarflexion and eversion, a depressed ankle jerk and altered sensation along the sole.

X-ray of the spine, contrast myelography and computed tomography may be needed to pinpoint the lesion.

The indications for operation and nerve root decompression are pain, progressive muscle weakness or sphincter dysfunction.

Lateral cutaneous nerve

The lateral cutaneous nerve of the thigh (L2, 3) may be compressed where it runs through the inguinal ligament just medial to the anterior superior iliac spine. The patient complains of numbness and paraesthesia over the anterolateral aspect of the thigh (*meralgia paraesthetica*). If troublesome the condition may be relieved by freeing the nerve or, in extreme cases, dividing it.

Femoral nerve

The femoral nerve may be injured by a gunshot wound, by pressure or traction during an operation or by bleeding into the thigh.

Clinical features

Quadriceps action is lacking and the patient is unable to extend the knee actively. There is numbness of the anterior thigh and medial aspect of the leg. The knee jerk is depressed.

Treatment

This is a fairly disabling lesion and, where possible, counter-measures should be undertaken. A thigh haematoma may need to be evacuated. A clean cut of the nerve may be treated successfully by suturing or grafting. The alternative would be a caliper to stabilize the knee, or tendon transfers of hamstrings to quadriceps.

Sciatic nerve

Division of the main sciatic nerve is rare except in gunshot wounds. Traction lesions may occur with traumatic hip dislocations and with pelvic fractures. Intraneural haemorrhage in patients receiving anticoagulants is a rare cause of intense pain and partial loss of function.

Iatrogenic lesions are sometimes discovered after total hip replacement – due either to direct trauma or possibly to thermal injury from extruded acrylic cement; in most cases, though, no specific cause can be found and injury is assumed to be due to traction.

Clinical features

In a complete lesion the hamstrings and all muscles below the knee are paralysed; the ankle jerk is absent. Sensation is lost below the knee, except on the medial side of the leg which is supplied by the femoral nerve. The patient walks with a drop foot and a high-stepping gait to avoid dragging the insensitive foot on the ground.

Sometimes only the deep part of the nerve is affected, producing what is essentially a lateral popliteal lesion (see below). Electrodiagnostic studies will help to establish the level of the injury.

If sensory loss extends into the thigh and the gluteal muscles are weak, suspect an associated lumbosacral plexus injury.

In late cases the limb is wasted and ischaemic, with fixed deformities of the foot and trophic ulcers on the sole.

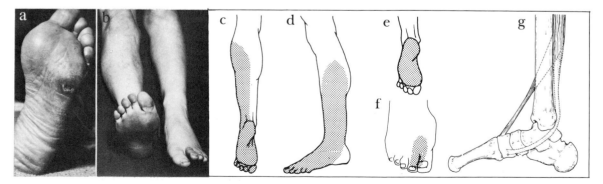

11.11 Sciatic nerve Two problems in sciatic nerve lesions are (a) trophic ulcers because of sensory loss and (b) foot drop. Sensory loss following division of (c) complete sciatic nerve, (d) lateral popliteal nerve, (e) posterior tibial nerve and (f) anterior tibial nerve. (g) Drop foot can be treated by rerouting tibialis posterior so that it acts as a dorsiflexor.

Treatment

If the nerve is known to be divided, suture or nerve grafting should be attempted even though it may take more than a year for leg muscles to be reinnervated. While recovery is awaited, a below-knee drop foot splint is fitted. Great care is taken to avoid damaging the insensitive skin and to prevent trophic ulcers.

The chances of recovery are generally poor and, at best, will be long delayed and incomplete. Partial lesions, in which there is protective sensation of the sole, can sometimes be managed by transferring tibialis posterior to the front in order to counteract the drop foot. If there is no recovery whatever, amputation may be preferable to a flail, deformed, insensitive limb.

Peroneal nerves

Injuries may affect either the common peroneal (lateral popliteal) nerve or one of its branches, the deep or superficial peroneal nerves.

Clinical features

The common peroneal nerve is often damaged at the level of the fibular neck by severe traction when the knee is forced into varus (e.g. in lateral ligament injuries and fractures around the knee, or during operative correction of gross valgus deformities), or by pressure from a splint or a plaster cast, from lying with the leg externally rotated, by skin traction, by an intraneural ganglion or by wounds. The patient has a drop foot, and can neither dorsiflex nor evert the foot. He walks with a high-stepping gait to avoid catching the toes. Sensation is lost over the front and outer half of the leg and the dorsum of the foot.

The deep peroneal nerve runs between the muscles of the anterior compartment of the leg and emerges at the lower border of the extensor retinaculum of the ankle. It may be threatened in an anterior compartment syndrome; causing pain and weakness of dorsiflexion and sensory loss in a small area of skin between the first and second toes. Sometimes the distal portion is cut during operations on the ankle, resulting in paraesthesia and numbness on the dorsum around the first web space.

The superficial peroneal nerve descends along the fibula, innervating the peroneal muscles and emerging through the deep fascia 5–10 cm above the ankle to supply to the skin over the dorsum of the foot and the medial four toes. The muscular portion may be involved in a lateral compartment syndrome. The patient complains of pain in the lateral part of the leg and numbness or paraesthesia of the foot; there may be weakness of eversion and sensory loss on the dorsum of the foot. The cutaneous branches alone may be trapped where the nerve emerges from the deep fascia, or stretched by a severe inversion injury of the ankle, causing pain and sensory symptoms without muscle weakness (Styf, 1989).

Chronic or intermittent compartment syndromes of the deep and superficial peroneal nerves are quite common in long-distance runners. Symptoms are brought on by exercise, which causes the muscles to swell within the anterior fascial compartment.

Treatment

Direct injuries of the common peroneal nerve and its branches should be explored and repaired or grafted wherever possible. While recovery is awaited a splint may be worn to control ankle weakness. Unfortunately, the results of nerve repair are not very good. However, if there is no recovery, the disability can be minimized by tibialis posterior tendon transfer or by foot stabilization.

An acute compartment syndrome calls for immediate decompression by splitting the fascia.

Chronic compartment syndromes, in which symptoms are triggered by exercise, may likewise need decompression. However, even after fasciectomy, patients may still have symptoms following very strenuous activity.

Entrapment syndromes often require no treatment, but if symptoms are disabling they can be relieved by local fasciectomy.

Tibial nerves

The tibial (medial popliteal) nerve is rarely injured except in open wounds. The distal part (posterior tibial nerve) is sometimes involved in injuries around the ankle.

Clinical features

The tibial nerve supplies the flexors of the ankle and toes. With division of the nerve, the patient is unable to plantarflex the ankle or flex the toes; sensation is absent over the sole and part of the calf. Because both the long flexors and the intrinsic muscles are involved, there is not much clawing. With time the calf and foot become atrophic and pressure ulcers may appear on the sole.

The posterior tibial nerve runs behind the medial malleolus under the flexor retinaculum, gives off a small calcaneal branch and then divides into *medial and lateral plantar nerves* which supply the intrinsic muscles and the skin of the sole. Fractures and dislocations around the ankle may injure any of these branches and the resultant picture depends on the level of the lesion. Thus, posterior tibial nerve lesions cause wide sensory loss and clawing of the toes due to paralysis of the intrinsics with active long flexors; but injury to one of the smaller branches causes only limited sensory loss and less noticeable motor weakness. A compartment syndrome of the foot (e.g. following metatarsal fractures) is easily missed if one fails to test specifically for plantar nerve function.

Entrapment of the posterior tibial nerve (the tarsal tunnel syndrome) may follow injury of the ankle or may occur spontaneously. The patient complains of burning pain in the foot and there may be diminished sensation in the sole. Pressure behind the medial malleolus and valgus manipulation of the ankle sometimes cause pain and paraesthesia. The diagnosis should be confirmed by nerve conduction tests.

Treatment

A complete nerve division should be sutured as soon as possible. A peculiarity of the tibial nerve is that injury or repair (especially delayed repair) may be followed by causalgia.

While recovery is awaited, a suitable orthosis is worn to prevent excessive dorsiflexion, and the sole is protected against pressure ulceration.

Tarsal tunnel entrapment may be relieved by fitting a medial arch support that holds the foot in slight varus. If this fails, surgical decompression is indicated.

Compartment syndromes and Volkmann's contracture

Capillary perfusion of a nerve may be markedly reduced by swelling within an osteofascial compartment. Direct trauma, prolonged compression or arterial injury may result in muscle swelling and a critical rise in compartment pressure; if unrelieved, this causes further impedance of blood flow, more prolonged ischaemia and so on into a vicious circle of events ending in necrosis of nerve and muscle. This may occur after proximal arterial injury, soft-tissue bleeding from fractures or operations, circular compression by tight dressings or plasters, and even direct pressure in a comatose person lying on a hard surface. Lesser, self-relieving effects are sometimes produced by muscle swelling due to strenuous exercise. Common sites are the forearm and leg; less common are the foot, upper arm and thigh. The acute compartment syndrome and its late effects (Volkmann's contracture) are described in Chapter 23.

Entrapment syndromes

Chronic nerve compression causes slowing of conduction and a variable degree of demyelination; in severe cases, this goes on to true wallerian degeneration and thinning of the nerve (Ochoa and Marotte, 1973).

Wherever peripheral nerves traverse fibro-osseous tunnels they are at risk of entrapment and compression, especially if the soft tissues increase in bulk (as they may in pregnancy, myxoedema or with rheumatoid arthritis) or if there is a local obstruction (e.g. a ganglion or osteophytic spur).

Peripheral neuropathy may render a nerve more sensitive to compression; a generalized disorder such as diabetes should therefore always be excluded. There is evidence, too, that proximal compression (e.g. discogenic root compression) may predispose the nerve to the effects of distal entrapment – the so-called *double-crush syndrome* (Upton and McComas, 1973).

Common sites for nerve entrapment are the *carpal tunnel* (median nerve) and the *cubital tunnel* (ulnar nerve); less common sites are the *tarsal tunnel* (posterior tibial nerve), the *inguinal ligament* (lateral cutaneous nerve of the thigh), the *suprascapular notch* (suprascapular nerve), the *neck of the fibula* (common peroneal nerve) and the *fascial tunnel of the superficial peroneal nerve*. A special case is the *thoracic outlet*, where the subclavian vessels and roots of the brachial plexus cross the first rib between the scalenus anterior and medius muscles. In these cases there may be vascular as well as neurological signs.

Many *unusual pain syndromes* have been attributed to nerve entrapment.

Clinical features

The patient complains of unpleasant tingling or pain or numbness. Symptoms are usually intermittent and sometimes related to specific postures which compromise the nerve. Thus, in the *carpal tunnel syndrome* they occur at night when the wrist is held still in flexion, and relief is obtained by moving the hand 'to get the circulation going'. In *ulnar neuropathy*, symptoms recur whenever the elbow is held in acute flexion for long periods. In the *thoracic outlet syndrome*, paraesthesia in the distribution of C8 and T1 may be elicited by pulling the arm downwards and backwards.

In long-standing cases there may be motor weakness and muscle wasting.

Electrodiagnostic examination helps to confirm the diagnosis, establish the level of compression and estimate the degree of nerve damage. Conduction is slowed across the compressed segment and EMG may show abnormal action potentials in muscles that are not obviously weak or wasted, or fibrillation in cases with severe nerve damage.

Treatment

Entrapment syndromes can usually be cured by operative decompression of the tunnel. However, in long-standing cases with muscle atrophy there may be endoneurial fibrosis and axonal degeneration; tunnel decompression may fail to give complete relief (Gelberman et al., 1988).

Iatrogenic injuries

During operation an important nerve may be injured by accidental scalpel or diathermy wounds, excessive traction, compression by instruments, snaring by sutures or heating and compression by extruded acrylic cement. Nerves most frequently involved are the spinal accessory or the trunks of the brachial plexus (during operations in the posterior triangle of the neck), the axillary and musculocutaneous nerves (during operations for recurrent dislocation of the shoulder), the posterior interosseous branch of the radial nerve (during approaches to the proximal end of the radius), the median nerve at the wrist (in tendon surgery), the cutaneous branch of the radial nerve (when operating for de Quervain's disease), the digital nerves (in operations for Dupuytren's contracture), the sciatic nerve (in hip arthroplasty), the common peroneal nerve (in operations around the knee) and the sural nerve (in operations on the calcaneum).

Tourniquet pressure is an important cause of nerve injury in orthopaedic operations. Damage is due to direct pressure rather than prolonged ischaemia (Ochoa, Fowler and Gilliat, 1972); injury is therefore more likely with very high cuff pressure (it need never be more than 75 mmHg above systolic pressure), a non-pneumatic tourniquet or a very narrow cuff.

However, ischaemic damage may occur at 'acceptable' pressures if the tourniquet is left on for more than 3 hours (Klenerman, 1980).

Manipulative pressure or traction – e.g. during reduction of a fracture or dislocation – may injure a nerve coursing close to the bone or across the joint. Shoulder abduction and varus angulation of the knee under anaesthesia are particularly dangerous. Even moderate pressure or traction can be harmful in patients with peripheral neuropathy – always a risk in alcoholics and diabetics (Bonney, 1986).

Injections are occasionally misdirected and delivered into a nerve – usually the radial or sciatic, or any nerve close to the site of venepuncture.

Irradiation may cause irreparable nerve damage, a mishap not always avoidable when cancer treatment demands such exposure.

Diagnosis

Following operations in 'high-risk' areas of the body, local nerve function should always be tested as soon as the patient is awake. Even then it may be difficult to distinguish true weakness or sensory change from the 'normal' post-operative discomfort and unwillingness to move.

Initially it may be impossible to tell whether the lesion is a neurapraxia or a neurotmesis. With closed procedures it is more likely to be the former, with open ones the latter. If there is no recovery after a few weeks, EMG may be helpful.

Prevention and treatment

Awareness is all. Knowing the situations in which there is a real risk of nerve injury is the best way to prevent the calamity. The operative exposure should be safe and well rehearsed; important nerves should be given a wide berth or otherwise kept under vision and out of harm's way; retraction should be gentle and intermittent; hidden branches (such as the posterior interosseous nerve in the supinator muscle) should be retracted with their muscular covering.

If a nerve is seen to be divided, it should be repaired immediately. If the injury is discovered only after the operation, it is wiser to wait for signs that might clarify the diagnosis; however, if nerve division seems likely, if there is a marked loss of function and no flicker of recovery by 6 weeks, the nerve should be explored. Even then, fibrosis may make diagnosis difficult; nerve stimulation will show whether there is conduction across the injured segment. Partial lesions, injuries that cause only minor disability and those that can be salvaged by effective tendon transfers are probably best left alone. More serious lesions may need excision and repair or grafting.

The patient should at all times be kept informed of the true state of affairs and the surgeon should record all findings meticulously.*

Pain

Many – perhaps most – musculoskeletal disorders are accompanied by pain. Whatever the nature of the underlying condition, pain usually requires treatment in its own right; sometimes it becomes the main focus of attention even after the initiating factors have disappeared or subsided.

Pain perception

Pain is confounding. The same receptors that appreciate discomfort also respond to tickling with feelings of pleasure. The electrical discharge in 'mild' pain is no different from that in 'severe' pain. That the degree of discomfort is related to the magnitude of the physical stimulus cannot be doubted, but ultimately both the severity of the pain and its character are experienced subjectively and cannot be measured.

---

* Keep away from nerves or see them clearly,
For if you cut them it may cost you dearly;
But if you have, you must confess –
In the long run it will cost you less.

Pain receptors (nociceptors) in the form of free nerve endings are found in almost all tissues. They are stimulated by mechanical distortion, by chemical, thermal or electrical irritation, or by ischaemia. Musculoskeletal pain associated with trauma or inflammation is due to both tissue distortion and chemical irritation (local release of kinins, prostaglandins and serotonin). Visceral nociceptors respond to stretching and anoxia. In nerve injuries the regenerating axons may be hypersensitive to all stimuli.

Pain transmission occurs via both myelinated axons (the large-diameter A-δ fibres), which carry well-defined and well-localized sensation, and the far more numerous unmyelinated axons (small-diameter C fibres) which are responsible for crude, poorly defined pain. From the dorsal horn synapses in the cord, fibres run via the spinothalamic tracts to the thalamus and cortex (where pain is appreciated and localized) as well as the reticular system, which may be responsible for reflex autonomic and motor responses to pain.

Pain modulation Pain impulses may be suppressed or inhibited by (1) simultaneous sensory impulses travelling via adjacent axons or (2) impulses descending from the brain. Thus, it is posited that pain impulses are 'sorted out' – some of them blocked, some allowed through – in the dorsal horn of the cord (the 'gate-control' theory of Melzak and Wall, 1965). This could explain why counter-stimulation sometimes reduces pain perception. In addition, certain morphine-like compounds (endorphins and enkephalins), normally elaborated in the brain and spinal cord, can inhibit pain sensibility. These neurotransmitters are activated by a variety of agents, including severe pain itself, other neurological stimuli, psychological messages and placebos.

Pain threshold is the level of stimulus needed to induce pain. There is no fixed 'threshold' for any individual; pain perception is the result of all the factors mentioned above, operating against a complex and changing psychological background. The threshold is lowered by fear, anxiety, depression, lack of self-esteem and mental or physical fatigue; and it is elevated by relaxation, diversion, reduction of anxiety and general psychological support. The manage-ment of pain involves not only the elimination of noxious stimuli, or the administration of painkillers, but also the care of the whole person.

Acute pain

Severe acute pain, as seen typically after injury, is accompanied by an autonomic 'fight or flight' reaction: increased pulse rate, peripheral vasoconstriction, sweating, rapid breathing, muscle tension and anxiety. Similar features are seen in pain associated with acute neurological syndromes or in malignant disease. Lesser degrees of pain may have negligible side effects.

Treatment is directed at (1) removing or counteracting the painful disorder; (2) splinting the painful area; (3) making the patient feel comfortable and secure; (4) administering analgesics, anti-inflammatory drugs or – if necessary – narcotic preparations; and (5) alleviating anxiety.

Chronic pain

Chronic pain usually occurs in degenerative and arthritic disorders or in malignant disease and is accompanied by vegetative features such as fatigue and depression.

Treatment again involves alleviation of the underlying disorder if possible and general analgesic therapy, but there is an increased need for rehabilitative and psychologically supportive measures.

Chronic pain syndrome

In a minority of patients with chronic pain there is an apparent mismatch between the bitterness of complaint and the degree of physical abnormality. The most common example is the patient with discogenic disease and prolonged, unresponsive, disabling low back pain. Labels such as 'functional overlay', 'compensitis', 'supratentorial reaction' and 'illness behaviour' are introduced and both patient and doctor are overtaken by a sense of hopelessness. Sometimes there are well-marked features of depression, or complaints of widespread somatic illness (pain in various parts of the body, muscular weakness, paraesthesiae, palpitations and impotence).

Treatment is always difficult and should, ideally, be managed by a team that includes a specialist in pain control, a psychotherapist, a rehabilitation specialist and a social worker. Pain may be alleviated by a variety of measures: (1) analgesics and anti-inflammatory drugs; (2) local injections to painful areas; (3) local counterirritants; (4) acupuncture; (5) transcutaneous nerve stimulation; (6) sympathetic block; and, occasionally, (7) surgical interruption of pain pathways. These methods, as well as psychosocial assessment and therapy, are best applied in a dedicated pain clinic.

Reflex sympathetic dystrophy

A number of clinical syndromes appear under this heading, including *algodystrophy*, *Sudeck's atrophy*, the *shoulder–hand syndrome* and – particularly after a nerve injury – *causalgia*. What they have in common is pain, vasomotor instability, trophic skin changes and osteoporosis. Precipitating causes are trauma (often trivial), operation or arthroscopy, a peripheral nerve lesion, myocardial infarction or stroke. The cause is unknown but peripheral sympathetic overactivity is an important component.

Clinical features

Following some precipitating event, the patient complains of persistent pain in the affected area – usually the hand or foot, sometimes the knee, hip or shoulder. In the mild or early case there may be no more than slight swelling, with tenderness and stiffness of the nearby joints. More suspicious are local redness and warmth, sometimes changing to cyanosis with a blotchy, cold and sweaty skin. X-rays are usually normal but radionuclide scanning at this stage shows increased activity.

Later, or in more severe cases, trophic changes become apparent: a smooth shiny skin with scanty hair and atrophic brittle nails. Swelling and tenderness persist and there may be marked loss of movement. X-rays now show patchy osteoporosis, which may be quite diffuse.

In the most advanced stage, there may be severe joint stiffness and fixed deformities. The acute symptoms may subside after a year or 18 months, but some degree of pain often persists indefinitely.

Causalgia is a severe form of sympathetic dystrophy, usually seen after nerve injury. Pain is intense, often 'burning' or 'penetrating' and exacerbated by touching, jarring or sometimes even by a loud noise. Symptoms may start distally and progress steadily up the limb to involve an entire quadrant of the body.

Treatment

Treatment should be started as early as possible; if the condition is allowed to persist for more than a few months it may become irreversible.

The mainstay of treatment is sympathetic blockade, which often gives complete relief. This can be done by one or more local anaesthetic injections to the stellate or the appropriate lumbar sympathetic ganglia, or by regional block with guanethidine given intravenously to the affected limb (Hannington-Kiff, 1979).

Mild cases often respond to a simple regimen of reassurance, anti-inflammatory drugs and physiotherapy. If there is no improvement after 2 weeks, and as a first measure in all severe cases, a sympathetic block is administered; guanethidine is often adequate for the upper limb but ganglion block is better for the lower limb. Subcutaneous calcitonin has also been used with good effect, and some patients respond to acupuncture or transcutaneous electrical nerve stimulation.

References and further reading

Aids to the Examination of the Peripheral Nervous System (1976) MRC Memorandum no. 45. London: HM Stationery Office

Aziz, W., Singer, R.M. and Wolff, T.W. (1990) Transfer of the trapezius for flail shoulder after brachial plexus injury. *Journal of Bone and Joint Surgery* **72B**, 701–704

Birch, R., Dunkerton, M., Bonney, G. and Jamieson, A.M. (1988) Experience with the free vascularized ulnar nerve graft in repair of supraclavicular lesions of the brachial plexus. *Clinical Orthopaedics and Related Research* **237**, 96–104

Bonney, G. (1986) Iatrogenic injuries of nerves. *Journal of Bone and Joint Surgery* **68B**, 9–13

Gelberman, R.H., Rydevik, B.L., Pess, G.M., Szabo, R.M. and Lundborg, G. (1988) Carpal tunnel syndrome. A scientific basis for clinical care. *Orthopedic Clinics of North America* **19**, 115–124

Gilbert, A., Razabone, R. and Amar-Khodja, S. (1988) Indications and results of brachial plexus surgery in obstetrical palsy. *Orthopedic Clinics of North America* **19**, 91–105

Hannington-Kiff, J.G. (1979) Relief of causalgia in limbs by regional intravenous guancthidine. *British Medical Journal* **2**, 367–368

Hentz, V.R. and Narakas, A. (1988) The results of micro-neurosurgical reconstruction in complete brachial plexus palsy. *Orthopedic Clinics of North America* **19**, 107–114

Klenerman, L. (1980) Tourniquet time – how long? *Hand* **12**, 231–234

Lundborg, G. (1988) Intraneural microcirculation. *Orthopedic Clinics of North America* **19**, 1–12

Melzak, R. and Wall, P.D. (1965) Pain mechanisms: a new theory. *Science* **150**, 971–979

Mubarak, S.J. and Hargens, A.R. (1981) *Compartment Syndromes and Volkmann's Contracture*, W.B. Saunders, Philadelphia

Narakas, A. (1988) The use of fibrin glue in repair of peripheral nerves. *Orthopedic Clinics of North America* **19**, 187–199

Narakas, A.O. and Hentz, V.R. (1988) Neurotization in brachial plexus injuries. Indication and results. *Clinical Orthopaedics and Related Research* **237**, 43–56

Norris, R.W., Glasby, M.A., Gattuso, J.M. and Bowden, R.E.M. (1988) Peripheral nerve repair in humans using muscle autografts. *Journal of Bone and Joint Surgery* **70B**, 530–533

Ochoa, J., Fowler, T.J. and Gilliat, R.W. (1972) Anatomical changes in peripheral nerves compressed by pneumatic tourniquet. *Journal of Anatomy* **113**, 433–455

Ochoa, J. and Marotte, L. (1973) The nature of the nerve lesion caused by chronic entrapment in the guinea-pig. *Journal of Neurological Science* **19**, 491–495

Omer, G.E. (1968) Evaluation and reconstruction of the forearm and hand after traumatic peripheral nerve injuries. *Journal of Bone and Joint Surgery* **50A**, 1454–1478

Seddon, H.J. (1942) A classification of nerve injuries. *British Medical Journal* **2**, 237–239

Seddon, H.J. (1975) *Surgical Disorders of the Peripheral Nerves* 2nd edn, Churchill Livingstone, Edinburgh and London

Styf, J. (1989) Entrapment of the superficial peroneal nerve. *Journal of Bone and Joint Surgery* **71B**, 131–135

Upton, A.R.M. and McComas, A.J. (1973) The double crush in nerve entrapment syndromes. *Lancet* **2**, 359–361

Orthopaedic operations

12

To operate on bone requires the tools of a carpenter, but orthopaedic surgery is not carpentry; biological imperatives ensure that it never can be. *The art and skill of orthopaedic surgery is directed not to constructing a particular arrangement of parts but to restoring function to the whole.*

Preparation

PLANNING Operations upon bone must be carefully planned in advance, when accurate measurements can be made and bones can be compared for symmetry with those of the opposite limb.

STERILITY The need for sterility is even greater in bone surgery than in soft-tissue surgery; any wound infection represents a setback, but bone infection can be a disaster.

EQUIPMENT The minimum requirements for orthopaedic operations are drills (for boring holes), osteotomes (for cutting cancellous bone), saws (for cutting cortical bone), chisels (for shaping bone), gouges (for removing bone) and plates, screws and screwdrivers (for fixing bone).

Many operations such as joint replacement, spinal fusion and the various types of internal fixation require special implants and instruments to ensure that these implants are correctly aligned and fixed. It is well-nigh criminal to attempt these operations without gaining familiarity with the equipment and practising the operation on dry specimens. 'Preparatory

242

surgery' is still sadly neglected; it should be normal practice conducted in every hospital offering an orthopaedic service.

THE 'BLOODLESS FIELD' Many operations on limbs can be done more rapidly and accurately if bleeding is prevented by a tourniquet. This should always be a pneumatic cuff, applied over bulky soft tissues to minimize nerve pressure, inflated to not more than 100 mmHg above the systolic pressure and removed within 2 hours; whenever practicable it should be removed before the wound is closed, so that bleeding can be controlled and a 'silent' postoperative haematoma prevented. Excessive or prolonged pressure can cause permanent nerve or muscle damage (Klenerman, 1980).

Basic procedures

DRILLING Drilling may be necessary simply to evacuate a bone abscess, or a series of holes may facilitate cutting through cortex with an osteotome. Most commonly, however, the drill is used to prepare seat-holes for screws; the holes should also be tapped before inserting the screws.

CUTTING Cancellous bone can be cut with an osteotome; the tapered edge cleaves soft bone, but may shatter cortical bone. The tubular shaft, therefore, has to be weakened by drilling a series of holes before applying the osteotome. Less hazardous, and more accurate, is a motorized saw.

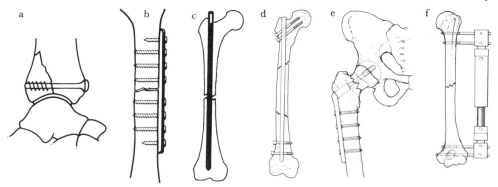

12.1 Some ways of fixing bone (a) With a single screw – this is a lag screw (threaded only distally) and therefore achieving interfragmentary compression. (b) Plate and screws. (c) Intramedullary nail. (d) Locked intramedullary nail. (e) Dynamic hip screw. (f) External fixator.

MODELLING The bone surface can be shaped with a chisel; concave surfaces are worked more easily with a gouge.

REAMING To ream means (literally) to widen. A joint socket, or the medullary cavity of a tubular bone, may need reaming before it will accept a prosthesis or a nail of suitable size.

Osteoporotic bone seldom needs reaming; if any is required it should be done with great care to avoid shattering the bone.

FIXING Bone fragments can be firmly joined by simple *screwing* (especially if a small piece has to be fixed back in position), by *attaching a bridging plate* to the bone with a row of screws, by passing a *long nail* down the medullary canal, by using an *external fixator*, by transfixing the fragments with *pins or wires*, by *stapling* the pieces together (only in soft bone), by securing the pieces with *malleable wire*, or by a *combination* of these methods. All these will eventually loosen or break unless natural union occurs.

Operations on bones

Osteotomy

Osteotomy may be used to correct deformity, to change the shape of the bone, or to relieve pain in arthritis. Preoperative planning is essential,

with precise measurements of the patient and the x-rays. The following must be determined.

The exact site of bone division For corrective osteomy this should be as near as possible to the site of deformity. For joint realignment, local geometry dictates the level.

The amount of correction required The intended angular or rotational shift must be measured in degrees.

The method of correction To change an angular deformity a wedge of bone may have to be removed ('closing wedge') or inserted ('opening wedge'). The size of the wedge should be calculated accurately and reproduced on a template for use during the operation.

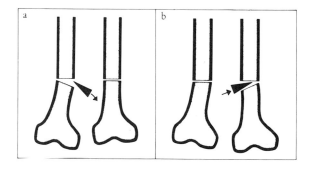

12.2 Osteotomy A bent bone can be straightened (a) by removing a wedge of bone, or (b) by inserting one: (a) is sometimes called a 'closing wedge osteotomy' – it is easier, but leaves the bone shorter; (b) is an 'opening wedge' – it maintains length but may be more difficult to do.

The method of fixation Sometimes plaster splintage alone will suffice. Usually internal or external fixation is preferred. The bone must be splinted or protected from weightbearing until union is complete.

Complications

(1) The commonest complication is over- or undercorrection of the deformity: hence the importance of preoperative planning. (2) Non-union may occur if fixation is inadequate; raw bone surfaces must be firmly apposed and securely splinted. (3) Joint stiffness may occur if the limb is not exercised. (4) As with all bone operations, infection is a calculated risk.

Bone grafts

Bone grafts can provide linkage or splintage as well as osteogenesis. To provide linkage (e.g. in filling cavities or replacing crushed bone) cancellous grafts are best. To provide splintage (e.g. in treating non-union or arthrodesing a joint) cortical bone is often needed. Osteogenesis is brought about partly by the activity of cells surviving on the surface of the graft but mainly by the stimulation of osteoprogenitor cells in the host bed – an effect that is due to the presence of a bone morphogenetic protein in the graft matrix (Urist, 1970).

AUTOGRAFTS (AUTOGENOUS GRAFTS) In these, bone is moved from one place to another in the same individual. They are the most commonly used grafts and are satisfactory provided that sufficient bone of the sort required is available and that, at the recipient site, there is a clean vascular bed.

Vascularized grafts are theoretically ideal. Bone is transferred complete with its blood supply, which is anastomosed to vessels at the recipient site. The technique is difficult and time consuming, requiring microsurgical skill. Available donor sites include the iliac crest (complete with one of the circumflex arteries), the fibula (with the peroneal artery) and the lower radius.

Cancellous autografts can be obtained from the thicker portions of the ilium, the greater trochanter, the proximal metaphysis of the tibia, the lower radius, the olecranon, or from an excised femoral head. Cortical grafts can be harvested from any convenient long bone or from the iliac crest; they usually need to be fixed with screws, sometimes reinforced by a plate, and can be placed on the host bone, or inlaid, or slid along the long axis of the bone.

Vascularized grafts remain completely viable and become incorporated by a process analogous to fracture healing. All other autografts undergo necrosis, though a few surface cells remain viable. The graft stimulates an inflammatory response with the formation of a fibrovascular stroma; through this, blood vessels and osteoprogenitor cells can pass from the recipient bone to the graft. Apart from providing a stimulus for bone growth (osteoinduction), the graft also provides a passive scaffold for the new growth (osteoconduction). Cancellous grafts become incorporated more quickly and more completely than cortical grafts.

ALLOGRAFTS (HOMOGRAFTS) With these, bone is transferred from one individual (alive or dead) to another of the same species. They can be stored in a bone bank and, as supplies can be plentiful, are particularly useful when large defects have to be filled.

Fresh allografts, though dead, are not immunologically acceptable. They induce an inflammatory response in the host and this may lead to rejection. However, the antigenicity can be reduced by freezing or freeze-drying, or by ionizing radiation.

The process of incorporation (when it occurs) is similar to that with autografts but slower and less complete (Heiple, Chase and Herndon, 1963). Demineralization is another way of reducing antigenicity and it may also enhance the osteoinductive properties of the graft (Urist, 1970). The best way of ensuring the incorporation of foreign grafts of all kinds is to impregnate the graft with marrow obtained from the host (Nade and Burwell, 1977; Salama, 1983).

Allografts are plentiful and can be stored for long periods. However, sterility must be ensured. This can be done by exposure to ethylene oxide or by ionizing radiation, but their physical properties and potential for osteoinduction are considerably altered by doses that are high enough to ensure sterility (Friedlaender, 1987; Aspenberg, Johnsson and Thorngren, 1990). Freezing the grafts and storing them at −70°C is much less harmful but the graft must then be harvested under sterile conditions and the donor must be cleared for malignancy, veneral disease, hepatitis and HIV; this requires prolonged (several months) testing of the donor before the graft is used.

Recent advances in the use of large osteocartilaginous grafts obtained from fresh cadavers have opened the possibility of replacing entire joints. The bone must be removed under aseptic conditions; cartilage preservation is enhanced by immersion in glycerol, and the entire graft is then deep frozen until it is needed. Here, again, the donor must be screened for hepatitis and HIV.

OTHER VARIETIES (XENOGRAFTS) are from another mammalian species, such as pigs or cows. After treatment for antigenicity they should, theoretically, behave like allografts, but in practice they are much less effective unless host marrow is added to the graft. 'Artificial bone' made of hydroxyapatite composites can be used in the same way to fill a cavity or bridge a small gap.

Applications

Vascularized grafts tend to be used only in exceptional circumstances such as congenital pseudarthrosis of the tibia or non-union of a fractured femoral neck.

Cortical or corticocancellous grafts are needed where bone has been lost as a result of trauma or has been removed because it contained a tumour. When reinforced by metallic implants, large gaps can be filled.

Cancellous grafts have a wide variety of uses, including: (1) filling cavities; (2) augmenting the compression side of a long-bone fracture which is being fixed internally; (3) filling the space after the crushing of a metaphysis; (4) occupying the spaces left when revising a loose prosthesis; (5) as part of the treatment for

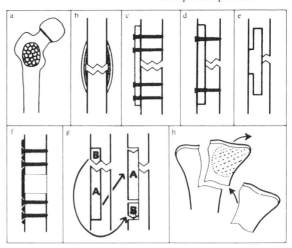

12.3 Bone grafts (a) Chip grafts to fill a cavity; (b) onlay strips of cancellous bone (Phemister technique); (c) onlay cortical graft; (d) inlay cortical graft; (e) latch graft; (f) cancellous block graft plus plating (Nicoll technique); (g) sliding graft – the portion marked A is slid up to bridge the fracture; (h) large cadaveric osteocartilaginous graft obtained fresh and sterile from an organ donor.

atrophic non-union of a fracture; (6) to augment a deficient acetabulum during hip surgery; and (7) as part of a fusion operation, particularly of the spine.

Leg length equalization

Inequality of leg length may result from many causes, including congenital anomalies, malunited fractures, epiphyseal injuries, infections and paralysis. Inequality greater than 2.5 cm needs treatment; this may involve shortening the longer leg, lengthening the shorter leg, or both.

Shortening the longer leg

In children, epiphyseal arrest is an effective method of shortening; it can be temporary, using staples fixed across the growth plate, or permanent, using bone grafts. One method of grafting is to excise a rectangular block of bone including the physis, rotate it through 90 degrees and then reinsert it. In deciding when to operate, Menelaus' (1966) formula, though approximate, is useful; he assumes that each year the lower femoral and upper tibial epiphyses contribute 1.0 cm and 0.6 cm, respectively, in length; and that these epiphyses fuse at 16 years of age in boys and 14 years in girls.

In adults it is obviously necessary to excise a segment of bone, preferably from the femur, since tibial shortening is more complicated and is cosmetically unattractive; up to 7.5 cm of femoral shortening can be achieved without permanent loss of function. The safest technique is to excise a segment from between the lesser trochanter and the femoral isthmus (a step cut may be preferred), to approximate the cut ends, and to fix them together with an intramedullary nail locked at the proximal end (Kenwright and Albinana, 1991).

Shortening should, of course, be applied only if the patient's residual height will still be acceptable. It should also be remembered that, since the longer leg is usually the normal one, if a serious complication such as non-union ensues, the patient may 'not have a leg to stand on'.

Lengthening the shorter leg

Lengthening, the commonest method of equalizing leg length, is most easily accomplished by wearing a raised shoe, but this is often inadequate or unacceptable. Surgical lengthening can be achieved by distracting the growth plate (chondrodiatasis), or distracting the callus forming after an osteotomy (callotasis), or both. These techniques have become much safer since it has been appreciated how slow distraction must be if neural or vascular damage is to be avoided. Distraction is achieved via a unilateral external fixator or using a circular fixator with tensioned wires transfixing the bone (Ilizarov, 1992).

Chondrodiatasis involves controlled, symmetrical distraction of the growth plate and can be used for the femur, the tibia or both (with the tibia 2 cm of the fibular shaft needs to be excised); gains of between a third and a half of the original bone length have been achieved (de Bastiani et al., 1986); with either bone the distal epiphysis is used. Screws or transfixion wires are attached to the epiphysis and to the

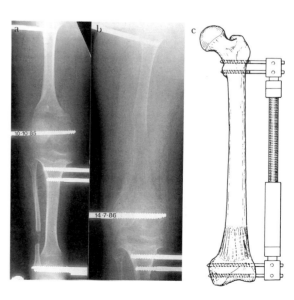

12.4 Leg length equalization The longer leg can be shortened by (a) excising a segment of bone or by (b) arresting epiphyseal growth. The simplest way to lengthen the shorter leg is, of course, to wear a raised shoe or boot (c).

12.5 Leg length equilization – chondrodiatasis The shorter leg can, in a child, be lengthened by (a, b) chondrodiatasis; the interval between the two films is 9 months. (Courtesy of Mr M. Saleh.) The drawing (c) shows where the growth plate has been 'stretched'.

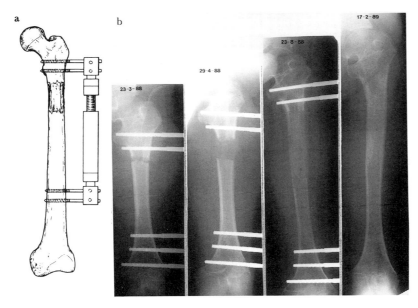

12.6 Leg length equalization – callotasis At any age, lengthening can be achieved by callotasis (callus 'stretching') after osteotomy. (a) Shows one technique. (b) 10 cm was gained in this achondroplastic patient. (Courtesy of Mr M. Saleh.)

diaphysis, and distraction proceeds at 0.25 mm twice daily. More rapid distraction may split the growth plate, leading to bony bridging across it. Partial weightbearing is allowed from the start. Distraction ceases when the desired gain has been achieved but the fixator is not yet removed. After a period of stabilization, often 3–4 weeks, dynamic loading with full weightbearing is permitted and the apparatus is then removed. Subsequent epiphyseal growth may not be normal and so it is wise not to begin treatment until 2 years before the end of the child's growth. Complications include fracture of the physis, asymmetrical growth, subluxation of the knee and infection.

Callotasis can be performed at any age. It involves dividing the bone, waiting until callus starts to appear (usually about 10 days) and then distracting the callus. The technical details are important. First the screws or wires of the fixator are inserted, then the periosteum is incised, but carefully preserved; shallow drill holes are made through the cortex, which is then gently broken or divided, leaving the medulla intact if possible (corticotomy). Then the fixator is applied and, as soon as callus appears, distraction is started and proceeds at 0.25 mm four times daily (twice as fast as with chondrodiatasis). X-rays are taken at 4-weekly

intervals to ensure that there is a continuous cloud of callus between the bone ends. As with chondrodiatasis, distraction is followed by a static period of stabilization after which dynamic loading with weightbearing is permitted. When the bone looks radiologically sound the fixator can be removed, though with unilateral fixators the screws are usually left in place until it is certain that the patient has no untoward symptoms. Throughout treatment, physiotherapy to preserve joint movement is advisable.

Bone transport Callotasis can be used for transporting a segment from one part of a bone to another. This may be used to close a gap and, if necessary, to lengthen the bone at the same time.

Operations to increase stature

Bilateral leg lengthening is a feasible procedure for achondroplastics and other individuals of short stature, but detailed consultation is an essential preliminary. The prospective patient must understand that treatment is painful, prolonged, and may be associated with a substantial number of complications such as pin-track sepsis, angulatory deformity or fracture.

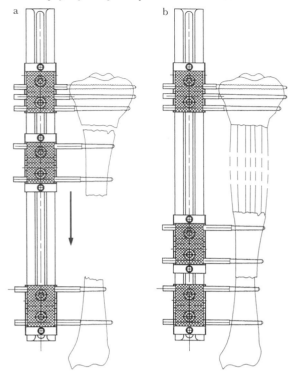

12.7 Bone transport   (a) Bone loss or excision may leave a gap in the shaft. Proximal osteotomy and callotasis allows a segment of the diaphysis to be moved distally (b), thus restoring continuity.

Morever, gain in height is not the same as 'normality'. Nevertheless, successful treatment is so rewarding ('People no longer look at me in the street'; 'I can now get things off a shelf without having to climb up') that it should not be withheld if the patient is otherwise normal and is psychologically prepared. Referral to a specialized centre is wise.

The techniques of lengthening described above are used and two bones at a time can be dealt with. Simultaneous lengthening of the ipsilateral femur and tibia has been advocated as a means of ensuring that the patient will complete the treatment programme, but it is kinder to lengthen both tibiae at one procedure and both femora at another. Gains in height averaging 30 cm have been achieved by combining the bone lengthening with soft-tissue releases (Vilarrubias, Ginebreda and Jimeno, 1990).

Operations on joints

Arthrotomy

Arthrotomy (opening a joint) may be indicated: (1) to inspect the interior or perform a synovial biopsy; (2) to drain a haematoma or an abscess; (3) to remove a loose body or damaged structure (e.g. a torn meniscus); and (4) to excise inflamed synovium. The intra-articular tissues should be handled with great care, and if postoperative bleeding is expected (e.g. after synovectomy) a drain should be inserted – postoperative haemarthrosis predisposes to infection. Following the operation the joint should be rested for a few days, but thereafter movement must be encouraged.

Realignment

This is essentially an osteotomy designed to redistribute stress to a less damaged part of the joint. In early osteoarthritis of the hip or knee it is often effective in relieving pain.

Arthrodesis

The most reliable operation for a painful or unstable joint is arthrodesis; where stiffness does not seriously affect function, this is often the treatment of choice. Examples are the spine, the tarsus, the ankle, the wrist and the interphalangeal joints. Arthrodesis is useful also for a knee that is already fairly stiff (provided

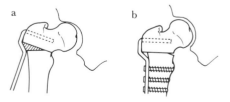

12.8 Joint realignment   (a) The joint space is not congruent; (b) an osteotomy has realigned it – now it is nearly equal throughout.

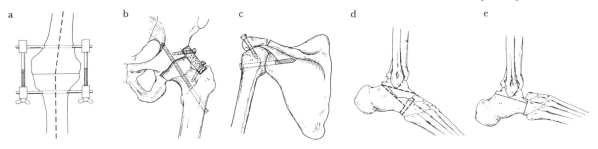

12.9 Arthrodesis (a) Compression arthrodesis; (b) screw plus bone graft; (c) similar technique using the acromion. (d, e) Subtalar–mid-tarsal fusion.

the other knee has good movement) and for a flail shoulder. More controversial is arthrodesis of the hip. Though it is a reasonable alternative to arthroplasty or osteotomy for joint disease in young patients, there is an understandable resistance to sacrificing all movement in such an important joint. It is difficult to convey to the patient that a fused hip can still 'move' by virtue of pelvic tilting and rotation; the best approach is to introduce the patient to someone who has had a successful arthrodesis.

The principles of arthrodesis are straightforward: (1) both joint surfaces are denuded of cartilage; (2) they are apposed in the optimum position and held by some form of internal or external fixation; (3) bone grafts are added in the larger joints to promote osseous bridging; and (4) the limb is usually splinted until union is complete.

The main *complication* is non-union with the formation of a pseudarthrosis. Rigid fixation lessens this risk, and, where feasible (e.g. the knee and ankle), the bony parts are squeezed together by compression clamps.

Arthroplasty

Arthroplasty, the surgical refashioning of a joint, aims to relieve pain and to retain or restore movement. The following are the main varieties.

EXCISION ARTHROPLASTY Sufficient bone is excised to create a gap at which movement can occur (e.g. Girdlestone's hip arthroplasty). In

some situations (e.g. after excising the trapezium) a shaped Silastic 'spacer' can be inserted.

PARTIAL REPLACEMENT One articular component only is replaced (e.g. Moore's prosthesis for a fractured femoral neck); or one compartment of a joint is replaced (e.g. the medial or the lateral half of the tibiofemoral joint). The prosthesis is kept in position either by acrylic cement or by a cementless fit between implant and bone.

TOTAL REPLACEMENT Both articular bone ends are replaced by prosthetic implants; for biomechanical reasons, the convex component is usually metal and the concave high-density polyethylene. They are fixed to the host bone, either with acrylic cement or by a cementless press-fit technique. The rationale, indications and complications of total joint replacement are discussed in detail on p. 424.

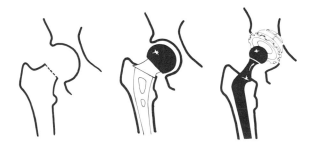

12.10 Arthroplasty The main varieties as applied to the hip joint: (a) excision arthroplasty (Girdlestone); (b) partial replacement – an Austin Moore prosthesis has been inserted after removing the femoral head; (c) total replacement.

Microsurgery and limb replantation

Microsurgical techniques are used in repairing nerves and vessels, transplanting bone with a vascular pedicle, substituting a less essential digit (e.g. a toe) for a more essential one (e.g. a thumb) and – occasionally – for reattaching a severed limb or digit. Essential prerequisites are an operating microscope, special instruments, microsutures, a chair with arm supports and – not least – a surgeon well practised in microsurgical techniques.

For replantation, the severed part should be kept cool during transport. Shortly before operation it is soaked in aqueous chlorhexidine solution. Two teams now dissect, identify and mark each artery, nerve and vein of the stump and the limb. Following careful debridement the bones are shortened to reduce tension and fixed together by wires, nails or plates. Next the vessels are sutured – veins first and (if possible) two veins for each artery. A vessel of 1 mm diameter needs seven or eight circumferential sutures! Nerves and tendons next need suturing; the excision of less important muscles is another way of reducing tension. Only healthy

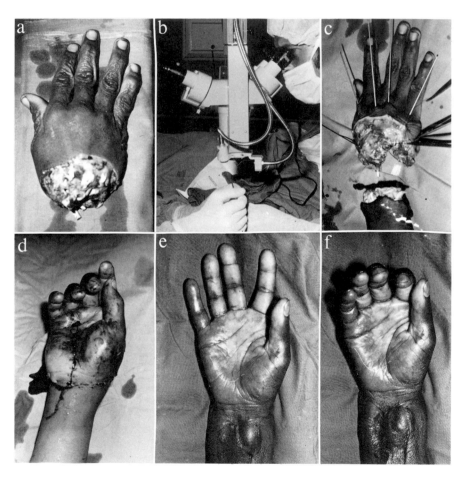

12.11 Microsurgery and limb replantation   (a) The problem – a severed hand. (b) The solution – replantation with microsurgical techniques. (c) The bones of the severed hand have been fixed with Kirschner wires as a preliminary to suturing vessels and nerves. (d) The appearance at the end of the operation (e, f) The limb 1 year later; the fingers extend fully and bend about half-way. But the hand survived, has moderate sensation and the patient was able to return to work (as a guillotine operator in a paper works!).

ends of approximately equal diameter should be joined; tension, kinking and torsion must be prevented. Dextran 70 (Macrodex) at the end of the operation and heparin for a few days afterwards are useful. Decompression of skin and fascia, as well as thrombectomy, may be needed in the postoperative period.

Replantation surgery is time consuming, expensive and often unsuccessful. It should be carried out only in centres specially equipped, and by teams specially trained, for this work.

Amputations

Indications

Colloquially the indications are three Ds – Dead, Dangerous and Damn nuisance.

DEAD (OR DYING) usually from *peripheral vascular disease*, but sometimes following *severe trauma, burns* or *frostbite*. Peripheral vascular disease alone accounts for almost 90% of all amputations.

DANGEROUS because it harbours a *malignant tumour*, or *potentially lethal sepsis* (especially gas gangrene), or because of a *crush injury*, where releasing the compression may result in renal failure (the crush syndrome).

DAMN NUISANCE or worse than no limb at all – because of *pain, gross malformation, recurrent sepsis* or *severe loss of function*. The combination of deformity and loss of sensation is particularly trying, and in the lower limb is likely to result in pressure ulceration.

Varieties

A *provisional amputation* may be necessary because primary healing is unlikely. The limb is amputated as distal as the causal conditions will allow. Skin flaps sufficient to cover the deep tissues are cut and sutured loosely over a pack. Re-amputation is performed when the stump condition is favourable.

Definitive end-bearing amputation is performed when weight is to be taken through the end of a stump. Therefore the scar must not be terminal, and the bone end must be solid, not hollow, which means it must be cut through or near a joint. Examples are through-knee and Syme's amputations.

Definitive non-end-bearing amputations are the commonest variety. All upper limb and most lower limb amputations come into this category. Because weight is not to be taken at the end of the stump, the scar can be terminal.

Amputations at the sites of election

Most lower limb amputations are for ischaemic disease and are performed through the site of election below the most distal palpable pulse. Sometimes, especially in below-knee amputations, the level can be modified by measurement of the transcutaneous oxygen pressure (Christensen and Clarke, 1986). The 'sites of election' are determined by the demands of prosthetic design and local function. Too short a stump may tend to slip out of the prosthesis. Too long a stump may have inadequate circulation and can become painful, or ulcerate; moreover, it complicates the incorporation of a joint in the prosthesis. For all that, the skill of the modern prosthetist has made it possible to amputate at almost any site.

Principles of technique

A tourniquet is used unless there is arterial insufficiency. Skin flaps are cut so that their combined length equals one and a half times the width of the limb at the site of amputation. As a rule anterior and posterior flaps of equal length are used for the upper limb and for above-knee amputations; below the knee a long posterior flap is usual.

Muscles are divided distal to the proposed site of bone section; subsequently, opposing groups are sutured over the bone end to each other and to the periosteum, thus providing better muscle control as well as better circulation. Nerves are divided proximal to the bone cut.

The bone is sawn across at the proposed level. In below-knee amputations the front of the tibia

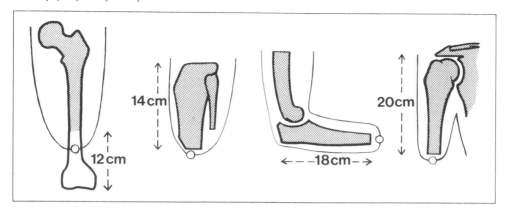

12.12 Amputations The traditional sites of election; the scar is made terminal because these are not end-bearing stumps.

is usually bevelled and the fibula cut 3 cm shorter, but some surgeons prefer to cut both bones at the same level, aiming at a 'square' stump.

The main vessels are tied, the tourniquet is removed and every bleeding point meticulously ligated. The skin is sutured carefully without tension. Suction drainage is advised and the stump firmly bandaged.

Aftercare

If a haematoma forms, it is evacuated at 5–6 days from operation. Repeated firm bandaging or a temporary pylon helps to make the stump conical. The muscles must be exercised, the joints kept mobile and the patient taught to use his prosthesis.

Amputations other than at the sites of election

FOREQUARTER AMPUTATION This mutilating operation should be done only when there is hope of eradicating malignant disease or palliating otherwise intractable pain.

DISARTICULATION AT THE SHOULDER This is rarely indicated, and if the head of the humerus can be left, the appearance is much better. If 2.5 cm of humerus can be left below the anterior axillary fold, it is possible to hold the stump in a prosthesis.

BELOW THE ELBOW The shortest stump that will stay in a prosthesis is 2.5 cm, measured from the front of the flexed elbow. However, an even shorter stump may be useful as a hook to hang things from. Longer stumps are an advantage only if modern prostheses, which allow pronation and supination, are available.

AMPUTATIONS IN THE HAND These are discussed on p. 332.

HINDQUARTER AMPUTATION This operation is performed only for malignant disease. Sir Gordon Gordon-Taylor's (Gordon-Taylor et al., 1952) technique should be followed in detail.

DISARTICULATION THROUGH THE HIP This is rarely indicated and is difficult to fit with a prosthesis. If the femoral head, neck and trochanters can be left, it is possible to fit a tilting-table prosthesis in which the upper femur sits flexed; if, however, a good prosthetic service is available, a disarticulation and moulding of the torso to a wedge shape is preferable.

THIGH AMPUTATIONS A longer stump offers the patient better control of the prosthesis, but at least 12 cm must be left below the stump for the knee mechanism. With less than 18 cm from the top of the greater trochanter it is difficult to keep the stump in the socket.

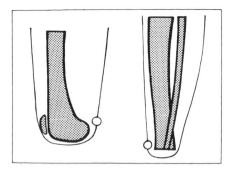

12.13 Amputations Through-knee and Syme's amputations are end-bearing; consequently the scars are not terminal.

AROUND THE KNEE The Stokes–Gritti operation (in which the trimmed patella is apposed to the trimmed femoral condyle) is rarely performed because the bone may not unite securely, the end-bearing stump is rarely satisfactory and there is no room for a sophisticated knee mechanism.

Amputation through the knee is becoming increasingly popular, especially for vascular insufficiency. A long anterior or equal medial and lateral flaps are used. The patella is left *in situ* and the patellar ligament sutured to the cruciate ligaments. A temporary pylon can be fitted within a few days. Through-knee amputations are also of value in children, because the lower femoral growth disc is preserved.

A very short below-knee amputation (less than 3 cm) is worse than a through-knee amputation and should be avoided.

BELOW-KNEE AMPUTATIONS Healthy below-knee stumps can be fitted with excellent prostheses allowing good function and nearly normal gait. Even a 5–6 cm stump may be fittable in a thin patient; more makes fitting easier, but there is no advantage in prolonging the stump beyond the conventional 14 cm. With a long posterior flap and suction drainage, healing can often be achieved even when the blood supply is impaired.

ABOVE THE ANKLE Syme's amputation is sometimes very satisfactory, provided the circulation of the limb is good. It gives excellent function in children and is well accepted by men, but women find it cosmetically undesirable. The indications are few, and the operation is diffi-cult to do well. Because the stump is designed to be end-bearing, the scar is brought away from the end by cutting a long posterior flap. The flap must contain not only the skin of the heel but also all the fibrofatty tissue, to provide a good pad for weightbearing, and therefore in cutting the flap the bone must be picked clean. The bones are divided just above the malleoli to provide a broad area of cancellous bone, to which the flap should stick firmly, otherwise the soft tissues tend to wobble about. Pirogoff's amputation is similar in principle to Syme's but is rarely performed. The back of the os calcis is stuck onto the cut end of the tibia and fibula.

PARTIAL FOOT AMPUTATION The problem is that the tendo Achillis tends to pull the foot into equinus; this can be prevented by splintage, tenotomy or tendon transfers. The foot may be amputated at any convenient level; for example, through the mid-tarsal joints (Chopart), through the tarsometatarsal joints (Lisfranc), through the metatarsal bones or through the metatarsophalangeal joints. It is best to disregard the classic descriptions and to leave as long a foot as possible provided it is plantigrade and that an adequate flap of plantar skin can be obtained. The only prosthesis needed is a specially moulded slipper worn inside a normal shoe.

IN THE FOOT Where feasible, it is better to amputate through the base of the proximal phalanx rather than through the metatarsophalangeal joint. With diabetic gangrene, septic arthritis of the joint is not uncommon; the entire ray (toe plus metatarsal bone) should be amputated.

Prostheses

All prostheses must fit comfortably; they should also function well and look presentable. The patient accepts and uses a prosthesis much better if it is fitted soon after operation; delay is unjustifiable now that modular components are available and only the socket need be made individually. Powered prostheses are being developed.

In the upper limb, the distal portion of the prosthesis is detachable and can be replaced by

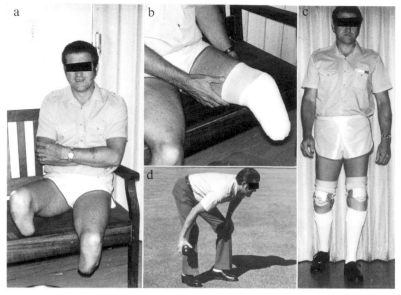

12.14 Amputations – fitting the prosthesis (a) This man had severe congenital deformities which necessitated bilateral below-knee amputations. (b) A cast was made of each stump, and from this the stump socket was fashioned and fitted into a prosthesis. (c) The prosthesis (held on in this case by straps above the knee) is called 'patellar-tendon-bearing', but most of the weight is taken on the femoral condyles. (d) After rehabilitation he has excellent balance and has resumed a near-normal life.

a 'dress hand' or by a variety of useful gadgets.

In the lower limb, weight can be transmitted through the ischial tuberosity, the patellar tendon, the upper tibia or the soft tissues; combinations are permissible and near-total-contact sockets are available for below-knee stumps. The prosthesis is held on by braces, or a belt or a tight thigh corset; for above-knee stumps a suction socket is available.

Complications of amputation stumps
Early complications

In addition to the complications of any operation (especially secondary haemorrhage from infection), there are two special hazards: breakdown of skin flaps and gas gangrene.

BREAKDOWN OF SKIN FLAPS   This may be due to ischaemia, to suturing under excessive tension or (in below-knee amputations) to an unduly long tibia pressing against the flap.

GAS GANGRENE   Clostridia and spores from the perineum may infect a high above-knee amputation (or re-amputation), especially if performed through ischaemic tissue.

Late complications

SKIN   Eczema is common, and tender purulent lumps may develop in the groin. A rest from the prosthesis is indicated.

Ulceration is usually due to poor circulation, and re-amputation at a higher level is then necessary. If, however, the circulation is satisfactory and the skin around an ulcer is healthy, it may be sufficient to excise 2.5 cm of bone and resuture.

MUSCLE   If too much muscle is left at the end of the stump, the resulting unstable 'cushion' induces a feeling of insecurity which may prevent proper use of a prosthesis; if so, the excess soft tissue must be excised.

ARTERY   Poor circulation gives a cold, blue stump which is liable to ulcerate. This problem chiefly arises with below-knee amputations and often re-amputation is necessary.

NERVE   A cut nerve always forms a bulb and occasionally this is painful and tender. Excising 3 cm of the nerve above the bulb sometimes succeeds. Alternatively, the epineural sleeve of the nerve stump is freed from nerve fascicles for 5 mm and then sealed with a synthetic tissue adhesive (Martini and Fromm, 1989).

'Phantom limb' is the term used to describe the feeling that the amputated limb is still present. The patient should be warned of the possibility; eventually the feeling recedes or disappears.

A painful phantom limb is very difficult to treat. Intermittent percussion to the end of the stump has been recommended for phantom limb and for painful nerve bulb; it sounds brutal but success is claimed.

JOINT   The joint above an amputation may be stiff or deformed. A common deformity is fixed flexion and fixed abduction at the hip in above-knee stumps (because the adductors and ham-string muscles have been divided). It should be prevented by exercises. If it becomes established, subtrochanteric osteotomy may be necessary. Fixed flexion at the knee makes it difficult to walk properly and should also be prevented.

BONE   A spur often forms at the end of the bone, but is usually painless. If there has been infection, however, the spur may be large and painful and it may be necessary to excise the end of the bone with the spur.

If the bone is transmitting little weight, it becomes osteoporotic and liable to fracture. Such fractures are best treated by internal fixation.

Implant materials

Metal

Metal used in implants (screws, plates, prostheses) should be tough, strong, non-corrodible, biologically inert and easily sterilizable. Those commonly used are stainless steel, cobalt–chromium alloys and titanium alloys.

No one material is ideal for all purposes. Stainless steel, because of its relative plasticity, can be cold worked; not only is it easier to manufacture such implants, but also cold working is a way of hardening and strengthening the material. Moreover, its tensile plasticity (ductility) makes it possible to bend stainless steel plates to required shapes during an operation without seriously disturbing their strength.

Cobalt-based alloys (Vitallium, Vinertia) must be cast or wrought. The implants are therefore difficult to manufacture, but they are stronger, more rigid and less liable to corrosion than steel.

Titanium alloys can be worked and shaped like steel, and are corrosion-resistant; however, in metal-on-metal prostheses they are liable to adhesive wear and sludge formation.

IMPLANT FAILURE
Metal implants may not be strong enough to resist local bending forces, and fatigue fractures

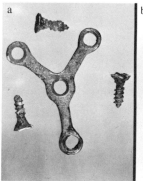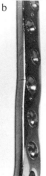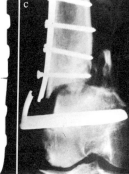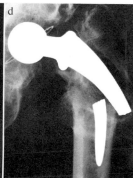

12.15 Implant failure   (a) An ancient metal implant, showing corrosion of the plate and screws; (b) the tiny defect in this plate, due to stress corrosion cracking, is just visible in the x-ray; (c) complete implant failure; (d) the implant is not necessarily to blame – this man was being taken home after a small celebration; he alighted from the car, unhappily without waiting for it to stop.

of plates and screws are common. In some cases, tough, even strong implants fail because they are wrongly placed or inadequately fixed and cannot withstand repetitive bending movement; if used to treat a fracture, protection may be needed until the bone has joined.

CORROSION

Corrosion is rarely a problem except with plates and screws, where it may be initiated by abrasive damage to polished oxide surfaces, or minute surface cracks due to fatigue failure. Crevice corrosion weakens the metal ('stress corrosion cracking') and may cause a local inflammatory reaction and osteoclastic bone resorption; the result is breakage or loosening of the implant.

All metallic implants corrode to some extent; the corrosion products are biologically active and they permeate every tissue of the body (Black, 1988). Whether this might prove harmful only time will tell, but clearly there is justification for removing fracture implants when they are no longer needed.

DISSIMILAR METALS

Dissimilar metals immersed in solution in contact with one another may set up galvanic corrosion with accelerated destruction of the more reactive (or 'base') metal. In the early days of implant surgery when highly corrodible metals were used, the same thing happened in the body. However, the passive alloys now used for implants do not exhibit this phenomenon (titanium being particularly resistant to chemical attack), and the traditional fear of using dissimilar metals in bone implants is probably exaggerated.

FRICTION AND WEAR

The coefficient of friction is constant for any two surfaces regardless of their size. However, shape has a marked influence on this property. In a ball-and-socket joint the frictional moment is related to the degree of congruity and the size of the ball (the larger the ball, the greater the frictional resistance). The type of material also is important; metal-on-metal may cause adhesive wear ('seizing'), whereas metal-on-plastic has a low coefficient of friction and is therefore better for joint replacements.

Metal wear particles may cause local inflammation and scarring, and occasionally a toxic or allergic reaction; most importantly, however, they may cause implant loosening following their uptake by macrophages and subsequent activation of osteoclastic bone resorption (Scales, 1991; Witt and Swann, 1991). Metal wear particles have also been demonstrated in lymph nodes and other organs far distant from the implant; the significance of this finding is uncertain.

INFECTION

Metal does not cause infection, but implants may encourage the persistence of infection (1) by offering an acceptable substrate for bacterial growth and (2) by impeding drainage.

MALIGNANCY

A few cases of malignancy at the site of metal implants have been reported, but the number is so small in comparison with the number of implants that the risk can probably be discounted (Apley, 1989).

High-density polyethylene

High-density polyethylene (HDPE) is an inert thermoplastic polymer modified to provide increased strength and wear resistance. In contact with polished metal it has a low coefficient of friction and it therefore seemed ideal for joint replacement. This has proved to be true in hip reconstruction with a simple ball-and-socket articulation. However, it has one major disadvantage – a tendency to viscoelastic deformity (stretching) and creep; this occurs particularly at the knee, probably because of its complex and demanding load characteristics. HDPE is also easily abraded, and hard chips of bone or acrylic cement trapped on its surface cause it to disintegrate. Even in the absence of severe surface abrasion, wear products may find their way into the bone/cement interface and stimulate bone resorption and prosthesis loosening.

Silicon compounds

There is a wide variety of silicon polymers, of which silicone rubber (Silastic) is particularly useful. It is firm, tough, flexible and inert, and is used to make hinges for replacing finger and toe joints, and for spacers to replace resected

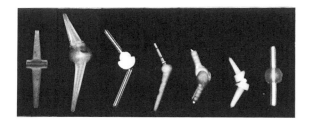

12.16 Implants Many of the implants used to replace finger joints are made partly or wholly of Silastic. A small sample of the models available is illustrated – reading from left to right: Swanson, Nicolle, Devas, St Georg, Mathys, ICLH, Helal universal.

bone (e.g. the head of the radius or the trapezium). Silastic wears well but may fracture if the implant surface is nicked or torn by a sharp instrument or piece of bone. The presence of silicon in the body may induce a giant cell synovitis; sometimes bone erosion and 'cyst' formation are seen at some distance from the actual implant.

Ceramics

Ceramic materials are being used, either alone or bonded to metal, for joint replacement prostheses. They are hard and strong, and porous ceramic implants could allow bone ingrowth as a means of fixation, but they are also brittle and have not found wide acceptance.

Carbon

This eminently biocompatible material is looking for a purpose. As graphite it has wear and lubricant properties that might fit it for joint replacement. As carbon fibre it is sometimes used to replace ligaments; it induces the formation of longitudinally aligned fibrous tissue which substitutes for the natural ligament. However, the carbon fibres tend to break up and if particles find their way into the synovial cavity they induce a synovitis. Carbon composites are also used to manufacture plates and joint prostheses; these have a lower modulus of elasticity than metal and may therefore be more compatible with the bone to which they are attached.

Acrylic cement

In joint replacements the prostheses are often fixed to the bone with acrylic cement (polymethylmethacrylate), which acts as a grouting material (Charnley, 1970). It is applied to the bone as a partially polymerized dough, in which the prosthesis is embedded. With sufficient pressure the pasty material is forced into the bony interstices and, when fully polymerized, the hard compound prevents all movement between prosthesis and bone. It can withstand large compressive loads but is easily broken by tensile stress.

When the partially polymerized cement is forced into the bone there is often a drop in blood pressure; this is attributed to the uptake of residual monomer, which can cause peripheral vasodilatation, but there may also be fat embolization from the bone marrow. This is seldom a problem in fit patients with osteoarthritis, but in elderly people who are also osteoporotic, monomer and marrow fat may enter the circulation very rapidly when the cement is compressed and the fall in blood pressure can be alarming (and occasionally fatal).

With good cementing technique osseointegration can and does take place on the acrylic surface. However, if the initial cement application is not perfect, a fibrous layer forms at the cement/bone interface, its thickness depending on the degree of cement penetration into the bone crevices. In this flimsy membrane fine granulation tissue and foreign body giant cells can be seen. This relatively quiescent tissue remains unchanged under a wide range of biological and mechanical conditions, but if there is excessive movement at the cement/bone interface, or if polyethylene or metallic wear products track down into the cement/bone interface, an aggressive reaction produces bone resorption and disintegration of the interlocking surface; occasionally this is severe enough to justify the term 'aggressive granulomatosis' or 'aggressive osteolysis' (Eskola et al., 1990). Bone resorption and cement loosening may also be associated with low-grade infection which can manifest for the first time many years after the operation; whether the infection in these cases precedes the loosening or vice versa is still not known for certain.

Hydroxyapatite

The mineral phase of bone exists largely in the form of crystalline hydroxyapatite (HA). It is not surprising, therefore, that this material has been used to reproduce the osteoinductive and osteoconductive properties of bone grafts. Porous hydroxyapatite obtained from coral exoskeleton is rapidly incorporated in living bone (Holmes, Bucholz and Mooney, 1986) ˙ and synthetic implants consisting of hydroxyapatite, tricalcium phosphate and fibrillar collagen, when mixed with host marrow, have been used successfully as graft substitutes in humans (Kocialkowski, Wallace and Price, 1990). HA can also be plasma sprayed onto titanium alloy implants; the HA coating is a highly acceptable substrate for bone cells and promotes rapid osseointegration (Stephenson et al., 1991). This principle has been applied in the use of uncemented hip replacement prostheses; however, a final verdict on its value must await long-term follow-up studies.

References and further reading

Apley, A.G. (1989) Editorial. Malignancy and joint replacement. *Journal of Bone and Joint Surgery* **71B**, 1

Aspenberg, P., Johnsson, E. and Thorngren, K.-G. (1990) Dose-dependent reduction of bone inductive properties by ethylene oxide. *Journal of Bone and Joint Surgery* **72B**, 1036–1037

Black, J. (1988) Editorial. Does corrosion matter? *Journal of Bone and Joint Surgery* **70B**, 517–519

Charnley, J. (1970) *Acrylic Cement in Orthopaedic Surgery*, Churchill Livingstone, Edinburgh and London

Christensen, K.S. and Clarke, M. (1986) Transcutaneous oxygen measurement in peripheral occlusive disease. *Journal of Bone and Joint Surgery* **68B**, 423–426

de Bastiani, G., Aldegheri, R., Brivio, L.R. and Trivella, G. (1986) Chondrodiatasis – controlled symmetrical distraction of the epiphyseal plate. *Journal of Bone and Joint Surgery* **68B**, 550–556

Eskola, A., Santavirta, S., Konttinen, Y.T., Hoikka, V., Tallroth, K. and Lindholm, T.S. (1990) Cementless revision of aggressive granulomatous lesions in hip replacement. *Journal of Bone and Joint Surgery* **72B**, 212–216

Friedlaender, G.E. (1987) Bone grafts. *Journal of Bone and Joint Surgery* **69A**, 786–790

Gordon-Taylor, G., Wiles, P., Patey, D.H., Turner-Warwick, W. and Monro, R.S. (1952) The inter-innomino-abdominal operation. *Journal of Bone and Joint Surgery* **34B**, 14–21

Heiple, K.G., Chase, S.W. and Herndon, C.H. (1963) A comparative study of the healing process following different types of bone transplantation. *Journal of Bone and Joint Surgery* **45A**, 1593–1616

Holmes, R.E., Bucholz, R.W. and Mooney, V. (1986) Porous hydroxyapatite as a bone-graft substitute in metaphyseal defects. *Journal of Bone and Joint Surgery* **68A**, 904–911

Ilizarov, G.A. (1992) *Transosseous Osteosynthesis*, Springer, Berlin, Heidelberg, New York

Imamaliev, A.S. (1969) The preparation, preservation and transplantation of articular bone ends. In *Recent Advances in Orthopaedics* (ed. A.G. Apley), Churchill, London, pp. 209–263

Kenwright, J. and Albinana, J. (1991) Problems encountered in leg shortening. *Journal of Bone and Joint Surgery* **73B**, 671–675

Klenerman, L. (1980) Tourniquet time – how long? *Hand* **12**, 231–234

Kocialkowski, A., Wallace, W.A. and Price, H.G. (1990) Clinical experience with a new artifical bone graft. *Injury* **21**, 142–144

Martini, A. and Fromm, B. (1989) A new operation for the prevention and treatment of amputation neuromas. *Journal of Bone and Joint Surgery* **71B**, 379–382

Mears, D.C. (1979) *Materials in Orthopedic Surgery*, Williams & Wilkins, Baltimore

Menelaus, M.B. (1966) Correction of leg length discrepancy by epiphyseal arrest. *Journal of Bone and Joint Surgery* **48B**, 336–339

Nade, S. and Burwell, R.G. (1977) Decalcified bone as a substrate for osteogenesis. *Journal of Bone and Joint Surgery* **59B**, 189–196

O'Brien, B.McC. (1977) *Microvascular Reconstructive Surgery*, Churchill Livingstone, Edinburgh

Perkins, G. (1961) *Orthopaedics*, Athlone Press, London

Robinson, K.P. (1976) Amputations of the lower limb. *British Journal of Hospital Medicine* **16**, 629–637

Salama, R. (1983) Xenogenic bone grafting in humans. *Clinical Orthopaedics and Related Research* **174**, 113–121

Saleh, M. and Sharrard, W.J.W. (1989) Leg lengthening in achondroplasia. In *External Fixation and Functional Bracing* (eds. R. Coombs, S.Green and A. Sarmiento), Orthotext, London

Scales, J.T. (1991) Black staining around titanium alloy prostheses – an orthopaedic enigma. *Journal of Bone and Joint Surgery* **73B**, 534–535

Stephenson, P.K., Freeman, M.A.R., Revell, P.A. et al. (1991) The effect of hydroxyapatite coating on ingrowth of bone into cavities in an implant. *Journal of Arthroplasty* **6**, 51–58

Symposium on limb ablation and limb replacement (1967) *Annals of the Royal College of Surgeons of England* **40**, 203–288

Urist, M.R. (1970) Bone formation in implants of partially and wholly demineralized bone matrix. *Clinical Orthopaedics and Related Research* **71**, 271–278

Vilarrubias, J.M., Ginebreda, I. and Jimeno, E. (1990) Lengthening of the lower limbs and correction of lumbar hyperlordosis in achondroplasia. *Clinical Orthopaedics and Related Research* **250**, 143–149

Witt, J.D. and Swann, M. (1991) Metal wear and tissue response in failed titanium alloy total hip replacements. *Journal of Bone and Joint Surgery* **73B**, 559–563

Part 2 — Regional Orthopaedics

The shoulder

13

Examination

Symptoms

Pain is the commonest symptom. It may derive from any of the joints of the shoulder complex, from the surrounding tendons, or – as referred pain – from some distant site such as the neck, the mediastinum or the diaphragm. Cardiac ischaemia may cause localized pain in either shoulder. It is important to ask *where* the pain is felt, and *when*. True shoulder pain or pain from the musculotendinous cuff is felt anterolaterally over the deltoid muscle, sometimes radiating down the arm; pain on top of the shoulder suggests acromioclavicular dysfunction; pain in the supraclavicular region is usually referred from the cervical spine. The relationship to posture may be significant: pain in flexion, abduction and internal rotation – typically when cleaning or painting a wall – is characteristic of rotator cuff impingement; pain in full abduction and external rotation – the 'tennis serve position' – suggests instability of the shoulder.

Stiffness may be progressive and severe – so much so as to merit the term 'frozen shoulder'.

Deformity may consist of prominence of the acromioclavicular joint or winging of the scapula.

Loss of function is expressed as inability to reach behind the back and difficulty with combing the hair or dressing.

Signs

The patient should always be examined from in front and from behind. Both upper limbs, the neck and the chest must be visible.

● LOOK

Skin Scars or sinuses are noted; don't forget the axilla!

Shape Asymmetry of the shoulders, winging of the scapula, wasting of the deltoid or short rotators and acromioclavicular dislocation are best seen from behind; joint swelling or wasting of the pectoral muscles is more obvious from in front. A joint effusion may 'point' in the axilla. Compare the two sides for swelling of the acromioclavicular or sternoclavicular joint. Wasting of the deltoid suggests a nerve lesion; wasting of the supraspinatus may be due to either a full-thickness tear or a suprascapular nerve lesion.

Position If the arm is held internally rotated, think of posterior dislocation of the shoulder.

● FEEL

Skin Because the joint is well covered, inflammation rarely influences skin temperature.

The *soft tissues* and *bony points* are carefully palpated, following a mental picture of the anatomy. A helpful routine is to start with the sternoclavicular joint, then follow the clavicle laterally to the acromioclavicular joint, and so onto the anterior edge of the acromion and

261

around the acromion to the back of the joint. With the shoulder held in extension, the supraspinatus tendon can be pinpointed just under the anterior edge of the acromion; below this, the bony prominence bounding the bicipital groove is easily felt, especially if the arm is gently rotated so that the hard ridge slips medially and laterally under the palpating fingers. Tenderness and crepitus can often be accurately localized to a particular structure.

● MOVE

Active movements are observed first from in front and then from behind, with the patient either standing or sitting. Sideways elevation of the arms normally occurs in the plane of the scapula – i.e. about half-way between the coronal and sagittal planes – with the arm rising through an arc of 180 degrees. However, by convention, abduction is performed in the coronal plane and flexion/extension in the sagittal plane.

Abduction starts at 0 degrees; the early phase of movement takes place almost entirely at the glenohumeral joint, but as the arm rises the scapula begins to rotate on the thorax and in the last 60 degrees of abduction movement is almost entirely scapulothoracic. This rhythmic transition from glenohumeral to scapulothoracic movement is disturbed by disorders in the joint or by dysfunction of the stabilizing ten-

dons around the joint. Thus, abduction may be (1) difficult to initiate, (2) diminished in range or (3) altered in rhythm, the scapula moving too early and creating a shrugging effect. If movement is painful, the arc of pain must be noted; pain in the mid-range of abduction suggests a minor rotator cuff tear or supraspinatus tendinitis; pain at the end of abduction is often due to acromioclavicular arthritis.

Flexion and extension are examined, asking the patient to raise the arms forwards and then backwards. To test adduction he is asked to move the arm across the front of his body. Rotation is tested: first, with the arms close to the body and the elbows flexed to 90 degrees, the hands are separated as widely as possible (external rotation) and brought together again across the body (internal rotation); then the patient is asked to clasp his fingers behind his neck (external rotation in abduction); then to reach up his back with his fingers (internal rotation in adduction).

Passive movements These can be deceptive because, even with a stiff shoulder, the arm can be raised to 90 degrees by scapulothoracic movement. To test true glenohumeral abduction the scapula must first be anchored; this is done by the examiner pressing firmly down on the top of the shoulder with one hand while the other hand moves the patient's arm. Grasping the angle of the scapula as a method of anchorage is less satisfactory.

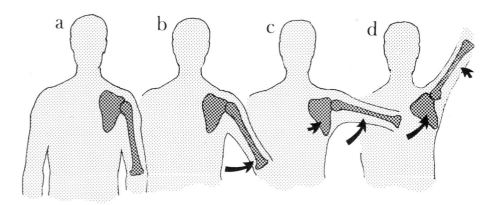

13.1 Scapulohumeral movement (a–c) During the early phase of abduction, most of the movement takes place at the glenohumeral joint. As the arm rises, the scapula begins to rotate on the thorax (c). In the last phase of abduction, movement is almost entirely scapulothoracic (d).

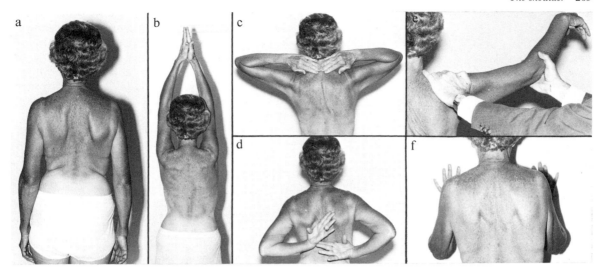

13.2 Examination Small alterations in scapulothoracic and glenohumeral rhythm are best seen from behind. (a) Symmetry of the neck, shoulders and scapulae is assessed. (b) Full abduction (or 'circumduction'), a combination of scapular and glenohumeral movements. (c) Abduction and external rotation. (d) Adduction and internal rotation (slightly limited on the right). (e) True glenohumeral movement is gauged by pressing down firmly on the scapula to stop scapulothoracic movement. (f) When the patient presses against a wall the scapula should remain flat; if serratus anterior is weak it stands out prominently ('winging').

Power The deltoid is examined for bulk and tautness while the patient abducts against resistance. To test serratus anterior (long thoracic nerve, C5, 6, 7) the patient is asked to push forcefully against a wall with both hands; if the

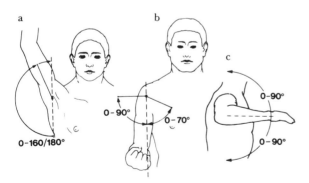

13.3 Normal range of movement (a) Abduction is from 0 to 160 (or even 180) degrees, but only 90 degrees of this takes place at the glenohumeral joint (in the plane of the scapula, 20 degrees anterior to the coronal plane); the remainder is scapular movement. (b) External rotation is usually almost 90 degrees, but internal is rather less because the trunk gets in the way. (c) With the arm abducted to a right angle, internal rotation can be assessed without the trunk getting in the way.

muscle is weak, the scapula is not stabilized on the thorax and stands out prominently (winged scapula). Pectoralis major is tested by having the patient thrust both hands firmly into the waist.

OTHER JOINTS

Clinical assessment is completed by examining the cervical spine (as a common source of referred pain) and testing for generalized joint laxity (a frequent accompaniment of shoulder instability).

IMAGING

At least two views should be obtained: an anteroposterior in the plane of the shoulder, and an axillary projection with the arm in abduction to show the relationship of the humeral head to the glenoid. Look for evidence of subluxation, or dislocation, joint space narrowing, bone erosion and calcification in the soft tissues. The acromioclavicular joint is best shown by an anteroposterior projection with the tube tilted upwards 20–30 degrees.

Double contrast arthrography, CT and MRI are useful methods for diagnosing rotator cuff tears or atypical forms of shoulder instability.

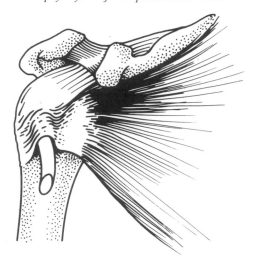

13.4 Anatomy   A tough ligament stretches from the coracoid to the acromion process; the humeral head moves beneath this arch during abduction and the rotator cuff may be irritated or damaged as it glides in this confined space.

ARTHROSCOPY

Shoulder arthroscopy is now well established as a means of diagnosing intra-articular lesions, detachment of the labrum or capsule, and impingement or tears of the rotator cuff. In some cases the disorder can be dealt with surgically at the same time (Ogilvie-Harris and Wiley, 1986).

Rotator cuff syndrome (impingement syndrome)

The rotator cuff is a sheet of conjoint tendons closely applied over the top of the shoulder capsule and inserting into the greater tuberosity of the humerus. It is made up of subscapularis in front, supraspinatus above and infraspinatus and teres minor behind – the 'rotator' muscles, which have an important function in stabilizing the head of the humerus by pulling it firmly into the glenoid whenever the deltoid lifts the arm forwards or sideways. Arching over the cuff is a fibro-osseous canopy – the coracoacromial

arch – formed by the acromion process postero-superiorly, the coracoid process anteriorly and the coracoacromial ligament joining them. Separating the tendons from the arch, and allowing them to glide, is the subacromial bursa. Of the four cuff tendons, the supraspinatus is the most exposed; it runs over the top of the shoulder under the anterior edge of the acromion and the adjacent acromioclavicular joint, with the intra-articular portion of the biceps tendon closely applied to its deep surface.

Pathology

The rotator cuff syndrome is a painful disorder which is thought to arise from impingement of the tendons (mainly supraspinatus) under the coracoacromial arch (Neer, 1972). Normally the cuff rubs against the anterior edge of the acromion and the coracoacromial ligament when the arm is abducted, flexed and internally rotated (the 'impingement position'), and this is prevented by elevating the arm in external rotation (the position of freedom). Perhaps significantly, the site of impingement is also the 'critical area' of hypovascularity in the supraspinatus tendon about 1 cm proximal to its insertion into the greater tuberosity (Rathbun and Macnab, 1970); this diminished vascularity is common and is a key feature of the pathological process.

Severe or chronic impingement may be caused by: (1) bony ridges or 'osteophytes' on the anteroinferior edge of the acromion; (2) osteoarthritic thickening of the acromioclavicular joint; (3) swelling of the cuff or the subacromial bursa in inflammatory disorders such as gout or rheumatoid arthritis; or (4) prolonged or excessive use of the arm in the 'impingement position' (e.g. cleaning windows, painting walls or polishing large flat surfaces).

The mildest injury is a type of friction, which may give rise to a localized inflammatory reaction or tendinitis. This is usually self-limiting, but with prolonged impingement – and especially in older people – minute tears can develop and these may be followed by scarring, fibrocartilaginous metaplasia or calcification in the tendon. Healing is accompanied by a vascular reaction and local congestion (in

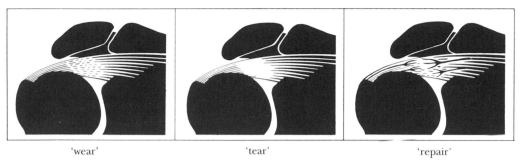

'wear'   'tear'   'repair'

13.5 The pathology of rotator cuff lesions

itself painful) which may contribute to further impingement in the constricted space under the coracoacromial arch whenever the arm is elevated.

Sometimes – perhaps where healing is more tardy or following a sudden strain – the microscopic disruption extends, becoming a partial or full-thickness tear of the cuff; shoulder function is then more seriously compromised and active abduction may be impossible. The tendon of the long head of biceps, lying adjacent to the supraspinatus, also may be involved and is often ruptured.

WEAR, TEAR AND REPAIR   The pathological processes described above may be summed up as 'wear', 'tear' and 'repair'. In the young patient 'repair' is vigorous; consequently, healing is relatively rapid but (because the repair process itself causes pain) it is accompanied by considerable distress. The older patient has more 'wear' but less vigorous 'repair'; healing will be slower but pain less severe. Thus acute tendinitis (which affects younger patients) is intensely painful but rapidly better; chronic tendinitis (a middle group) is only moderately painful but takes many months to recover and may be complicated by partial tears; and a complete tear (which usually occurs in the elderly) becomes painless soon after injury, but never mends. Degenerative changes are extremely common and small tears of the cuff are found at autopsy in almost everyone aged over 60.

SECONDARY ARTHROPATHY   Large tears of the cuff eventually lead to serious disturbance of shoulder mechanics. The humeral head migrates upwards, abutting against the acromion process, and passive abduction is severely re-stricted. Abnormal movement predisposes to osteoarthritis of the acromioclavicular joint and eventually, of the glenohumeral joint (Neer's 'cuff tear arthropathy': Neer, Craig and Fukuda, 1983). Occasionally this may progress to a rapidly destructive arthropathy (McCarty et al., 1981) (see below).

Clinical features

As suggested above, the clinical features depend on the stage of the disorder, the age of the patient and the vigour (or otherwise) of the healing response.

SUBACUTE TENDINITIS   The patient, usually under 40 years of age, develops shoulder pain after vigorous or strenuous activity – e.g. competitive swimming or a weekend of house decorating. The shoulder looks normal but is acutely tender along the anterior edge of the acromion; point tenderness is most easily elicited by palpating this spot with the shoulder held in extension, thus placing the supraspinatus tendon in an exposed position anterior to the acromion process. On active abduction scapulohumeral rhythm is disturbed and pain is aggravated as the arm traverses an arc between 60 and 120 degrees (the 'painful arc'). Repeating the movement with the arm in full external rotation throughout may be much easier and relatively painless; this is virtually pathognomonic of supraspinatus tendinitis. Painful impingement may also be demonstrated by holding the arm at 90 degrees of flexion and then forcibly rotating the shoulder internally. The condition is usually reversible and it settles down once the initiating activity is avoided.

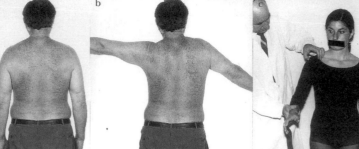

13.6 Supraspinatus tendinitis (a, b) In abduction, scapulohumeral rhythm is disturbed on the right and the patient has a painful arc starting at about 60 degrees. (c) Supraspinatus tenderness is felt along the anterior edge of the acromion.

CHRONIC TENDINITIS The patient, usually aged between 40 and 50, may give a history of recurrent attacks of subacute tendinitis, the pain settling down with rest or anti-inflammatory treatment, only to recur when more demanding activities are resumed. Characteristically pain is worse at night; the patient cannot lie on the affected side and often finds it more comfortable to sit up out of bed. Pain and slight stiffness of the shoulder may restrict even simple activities such as hair grooming or dressing. Examination shows features similar to those of subacute tendinitis: a painful arc of movement, disturbed scapulohumeral motion, tenderness over the cuff insertion and a positive 'impingement sign'. In addition there may be signs of bicipital tendinitis: tenderness along

the bicipital groove and crepitus on moving the biceps tendon.

A disturbing feature is coarse crepitations or palpable snapping over the rotator cuff when the shoulder is passively rotated; this may signify a partial tear or marked fibrosis of the cuff.

Although supraspinatus usually takes the brunt of the insult, the subscapularis or posterior tendons are sometimes more severely involved. If there is doubt about the site of the lesion, this can be resolved by injecting the various tendons with lignocaine and noting when the pain is abolished (Kessel and Watson, 1977).

CUFF DISRUPTION The most advanced stage of the disorder is progressive fibrosis and disrup-

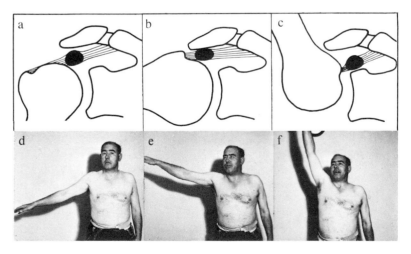

13.7 Painful arc (a–f) The patient registers pain only over a limited arc of abduction, and the diagrams show why. The middle diagram (b) explains the term 'impingement' syndrome.

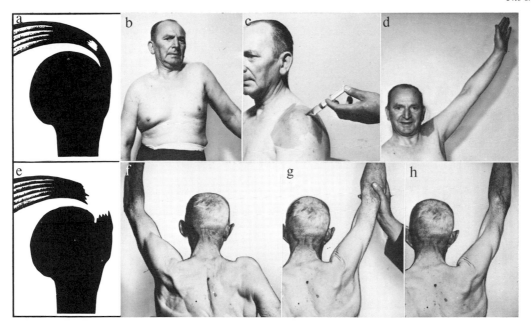

13.8 Torn supraspinatus (a–d) Partial tear of left supraspinatus: the patient can abduct actively once pain has been abolished with local anaesthetic.
(e–h) Complete tear of right supraspinatus: active abduction is impossible even when pain subsides (f), or has been abolished by injection; but once the arm is passively abducted (g), the patient can hold it up with his deltoid muscle (h).

tion of the cuff. *Partial tears* may occur within the substance or on the deep surface of the cuff and are not easily detected, even on direct inspection of the cuff. They are deceptive also in that continuity of the remaining cuff fibres permits active abduction with a painful arc, making it difficult to tell whether chronic tendinitis is complicated by a partial tear. The patient is usually aged over 45 and gives a history of refractory shoulder pain with increasing stiffness and weakness. Sometimes there is a palpable click on performing 'pot-stirring' rotation of the shoulder. The diagnosis may be confirmed by ultrasonography, MRI or shoulder arthroscopy.

A *complete tear* may follow a long period of chronic tendinitis, but occasionally it occurs 'out of the blue' after a sprain or jerking injury of the shoulder. There is sudden pain and the patient is unable to abduct the arm. Passive abduction also may, in the early stages, be limited or prevented by pain. These signs are common to both partial and complete tears; to distinguish between them, pain is abolished by injecting a local anaesthetic. If active abduction is now possible the tear must be only partial.

If some weeks have elapsed since the injury the two types are easily differentiated. With a complete tear, pain has by then subsided and the clinical picture is unmistakable: active abduction is impossible and attempting it produces a characteristic shrug; but passive abduction is full and once the arm has been lifted above a right angle the patient can keep it up by using his deltoid (the 'abduction paradox'); when he lowers it sideways it suddenly drops (the 'drop arm sign').

With time there may be some recovery of active abduction, though power is weaker than normal. There is usually wasting of the supraspinatus and infraspinatus, and on testing the biceps there may be an old tear of the long head tendon (see below). There is often tenderness of the acromioclavicular joint.

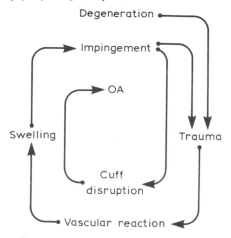

Degeneration

Impingement

OA

Swelling

Trauma

Cuff
disruption

Vascular reaction

The vicious spiral of rotator cuff lesions

In long-standing cases of partial or complete rupture, secondary osteoarthritis of the shoulder may supervene and movements are then severely restricted.

Imaging

X-rays are usually normal in the early stages of the cuff syndrome, but with chronic tendinitis there may be erosion, sclerosis or cyst formation at the site of cuff insertion on the greater tuberosity. Thinning of the acromion process, with upward displacement of the humeral head suggests a long-standing cuff tear. Osteoarthritis of the acromioclavicular joint is common in older patients. Sometimes there is calcification of the supraspinatus, but this is usually a red herring and not the cause of pain (see below).

Arthrography may reveal a cuff tear, the opaque medium extending from the joint into the subacromial space.

Ultrasonography is a possible technique for demonstrating large cuff tears.

MRI is an effective means of visualizing the structures around the shoulder joint (Seegar, 1989). Tears of the supraspinatus can be demonstrated; it is useful also in excluding other disorders such as glenohumeral instability.

Diagnosis of shoulder pain

In assessing the patient with shoulder pain, six groups of conditions must be considered.

REFERRED PAIN FROM DISTANT LESIONS Cervical disc syndromes often cause pain in the shoulder, over the scapula and down the arm; the cervical spine should always be examined and a neurological assessment is essential. Less common disorders which should be excluded are neuralgic amyotrophy (see p. 218) and mediastinal pathology, including ischaemic heart disease.

DISORDERS OF THE GLENOHUMERAL JOINT Movements are more uniformly restricted and x-rays usually reveal the underlying pathology – for

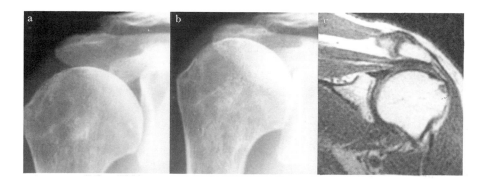

13.9 Chronic tendinitis – imaging   (a, b) When the patient attempts to abduct, the head of the humerus rides upwards to abut against the acromion process. Note the marked erosion of the acromioclavicular joint. (c) MRI shows thickening of the supraspinatus and an erosion at its insertion. The acromioclavicular joint is swollen and clearly abnormal.

THE PAINFUL SHOULDER

Referred pain syndromes
Cervical spondylosis
Mediastinal pathology
Cardiac ischaemia

Joint disorders
Glenohumeral arthritis
Acromioclavicular arthritis

Bone lesions
Infection
Tumours

Rotator cuff disorders
Tendinitis
Rupture
Frozen shoulder

Instability
Dislocation
Subluxation

Nerve injury

BONE LESIONS in the proximal humerus or scapula. X-ray changes are usually diagnostic.

LESIONS OF THE ROTATOR CUFF Acute calcific tendinitis and adhesive capsulitis ('frozen shoulder') are often confused with the classic rotator cuff (or 'impingement') syndrome. They are distinct disorders (see below) though their clinical features often overlap with those of the impingement syndrome.

INSTABILITY OF THE SHOULDER Recurrent glenohumeral subluxation may cause baffling symptoms, and sometimes the condition is complicated by the development of impingement.

NERVE INJURY Injury of the spinal accessory or suprascapular nerves may result in pain and weakness around the shoulder, sometimes resembling a rotator cuff disorder. These conditions are excluded by careful neurological examination.

Treatment of impingement syndrome

CONSERVATIVE TREATMENT The uncomplicated impingement syndrome (or tendinitis) is often self-limiting and symptoms settle down once the harmful activity is eliminated. Patients should be instructed in shoulder activities and ways of avoiding the 'impingement position'. Physiotherapy, including ultrasound and active exercises in the 'position of freedom', may tide the

example, rheumatoid arthritis, tuberculosis or osteoarthritis.

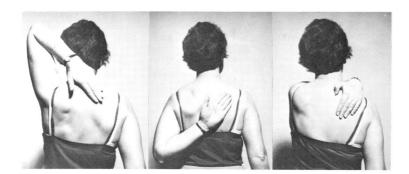

13.10 'Brachial neuralgia' – the scratch test 'Shoulder' pain may be due to disorders proximal to the joint (e.g. cervical spondylosis or cardiac ischaemia), disorders distal to the joint (e.g. arthritis of the elbow or carpal tunnel syndrome), or disorders of the shoulder itself (e.g. the rotator cuff syndromes, glenohumeral arthritis, acromioclavicular arthritis or bone disease). If the patient can scratch the opposite scapula in these three ways. the shoulder joint and its tendons are unlikely to be at fault.

patient over the painful healing phase. A short course of non-steroidal anti-inflammatory tablets sometimes brings relief. If all these methods fail, and before disability becomes marked, the patient should be given one or two injections of methylprednisolone into the subacromial space. In most cases this regimen of treatment will relieve the pain, and it is then important to continue with suitable modifications of shoulder activity for at least 6 months. Healing is slow, and a hasty return to full activity will often precipitate further attacks of tendinitis.

SURGICAL TREATMENT   If pain and other signs of impingement do not subside after 6 months of conservative treatment, or if symptoms recur persistently after each period of treatment, an operation is advisable. Certainly this is preferable to prolonged and repeated treatment with anti-inflammatory drugs and local corticosteroids. The indication is more pressing if there are signs of a partial rotator cuff tear. The object is to 'decompress' the rotator cuff by excising the coracoacromial ligament, undercutting the anterior part of the acromion process and, if necessary, reducing any obstructing mass at the acromioclavicular joint (Neer, 1972). Through an anterior incision the deltoid muscle is split and the part arising from the anterior edge of the acromion is dissected free, exposing the coracoacromial ligament, the acromion and the acromioclavicular joint. The

coracoacromial ligament is excised and the anteroinferior portion of the acromion is removed by an undercutting osteotomy. The cuff is then inspected: if there is a defect, it is repaired. Excrescences on the undersurface of the acromioclavicular joint are pared down. If the joint is hypertrophic, the outer 1 cm of clavicle is removed; this last step exposes even more of the cuff and permits reconstruction of larger defects. An important step is careful reattachment of the deltoid to the acromion, if necessary by suturing though drill holes in the acromion; failure to obtain secure attachment may lead to postoperative pain and weakness. After the operation, shoulder movements are commenced as soon as pain subsides. Arthroscopic decompression is being developed as an alternative to open operation (Gartsman, 1990).

Large cuff tears are difficult to reconstruct and this may require proximal mobilization of the rotator muscles. Postoperatively the repair is protected by splinting the arm in abduction for 4–6 weeks. The results of surgery are only moderately satisfactory.

Acute rupture of the cuff may be the primary indication for surgery, especially in younger patients. However, in those over 65 years of age, and in long-standing cases that are painless, operation is contraindicated.

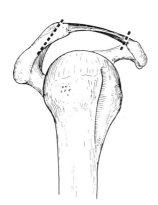

13.11 Impingement syndrome – surgical treatment The entire coracoacromial arch is removed and an oblique undercutting osteotomy enlarges the space beneath the acromion.

Lesions of the biceps tendon

Tendinitis

Bicipital tendinitis usually occurs together with rotator cuff impingement; rarely, it presents as an isolated problem in young people after unaccustomed shoulder strain. Tenderness is sharply localized to the bicipital groove. Two manoeuvres that often cause pain are: (1) resisted flexion with the elbow straight and the forearm supinated (Speed's test); and (2) resisted supination of the forearm with the elbow bent (Yergason's test).

Rest, local heat and deep transverse frictions usually bring relief, but, if recovery is delayed, a corticosteroid injection will help. For refractory cases, anterior acromioplasty is occasionally indicated.

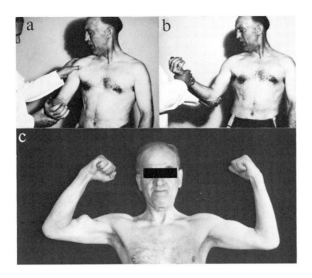

13.12 Biceps tendon Tendinitis: localized tenderness (a), and pain on flexion against resistance (b).
(c) Ruptured long head of right biceps: compared with the normal side, the belly of biceps is lower and rounder.

Calcification of the rotator cuff

Acute calcific tendinitis

Acute shoulder pain may follow deposition of calcium hydroxyapatite crystals, usually in the 'critical zone' of the supraspinatus tendon slightly medial to its insertion, occasionally elsewhere in the rotator cuff. The condition is not unique to the shoulder, and similar lesions are seen in tendons and ligaments around the ankle, knee, hip and elbow.

The cause is unknown but it is thought that local ischaemia leads to fibrocartilaginous metaplasia and active shedding of crystals by the chondrocytes (Uthoff and Sarkar, 1978). Calcification alone is probably not painful; symptoms, when they occur, are due to the florid vascular reaction which produces swelling and tension in the tendon. Resorption of the calcific material is rapid and it may soften or disappear entirely within a few weeks.

Rupture

Rupture of the *tendon of the long head of biceps* usually accompanies rotator cuff disruption, but sometimes the biceps lesion is paramount. The patient is always aged over 50. While lifting he feels something snap and the shoulder, which previously may have been painless, aches for a time. The upper arm looks bruised and, when the patient flexes the elbow, the belly of the biceps forms a prominent lump in the lower part of the arm. Isolated tears in elderly patients need no treatment. However, if the rupture is part of a rotator cuff lesion – and especially if the patient is young and active – this is an indication for anterior acromioplasty; at the same time the distal tendon stump can be sutured to the bicipital groove. Postoperatively the arm is lightly splinted with the elbow flexed for 4 weeks.

Avulsion of the distal attachment of the biceps is uncommon. The muscle retracts from the elbow and active elbow flexion is painful. If the patient is seen soon afterwards, reattachment of the tendon to the radial tuberosity may be quite feasible. In late cases, where the muscle has retracted some distance, operation is contraindicated.

Clinical features

An adult, often young, complains of aching, sometimes following overuse. Hourly the pain increases in severity, rising to an agonizing climax. After a few days, pain subsides and the shoulder gradually returns to normal. In some patients the process is less dramatic and recovery slower. During the acute stage the arm is held immobile; the joint is usually too tender to permit palpation or movement.

On *x-ray*, calcification just above the greater tuberosity is always present. As pain subsides the dense blotch gradually disappears.

Treatment

If symptoms are not very severe the arm is rested in a sling and the patient is given a short course of indomethacin. If pain is more intense a single injection of corticosteroid (methylprednisolone 40 mg) and local anaesthetic (lignocaine 1%) is given into the hypervascular area. If this is not rapidly effective, or if symptoms soon recur, relief can be obtained by an operation at which the calcific material is scooped out.

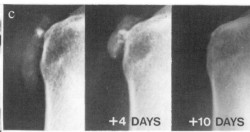
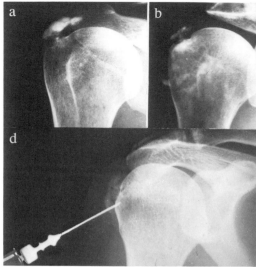

13.13 Acute calcification of supraspinatus (a) Dense mass in the tendon. (b) Following the 'reaction' some calcium has escaped into the subdeltoid bursa; (c) spontaneous dispersal. (d) An attempt at treatment by aspiration; this procedure is much more likely to succeed if image-intensification and television control are used.

Chronic calcification

Asymptomatic calcification of the rotator cuff is common and often appears as an incidental finding in shoulder x-rays. When it is seen in association with the impingement syndrome, it is tempting to attribute the symptoms to the only obvious abnormality – supraspinatus calcification. However, the connection is doubtful and treatment should be directed at the impingement lesion rather than the calcification.

Adhesive capsulitis (frozen shoulder)

The term 'frozen shoulder' should be reserved for a well-defined disorder characterized by progressive pain and stiffness of the shoulder which usually resolves spontaneously after about 18 months. The process often starts as a chronic tendinitis but inflammatory changes spread to involve the entire cuff and the underlying capsule. As the inflammation subsides, the tissues contract, the capsule may stick to the humeral head and the infra-articular synovial gusset may be obliterated by adhesions.

The cause is unknown. It has been suggested that this is an autoimmune response to the products of local tissue breakdown. Though usually 'idiopathic', a similar condition is sometimes seen following hemiplegia or myocardial infarction.

Clinical features

The patient, aged 40–60, may give a history of trauma, often trivial, followed by aching in the shoulder and arm. Pain gradually increases in severity and often prevents sleeping on the affected side. After several months it begins to subside, but as it does so stiffness becomes more and more of a problem, continuing for another 6–12 months after pain has disappeared. Gradually movement is regained, but it may not return to normal.

Usually there is nothing to see except slight wasting; there may also be some tenderness, but movements are always limited and in a severe case the shoulder is extremely stiff.

X-rays reveal decreased bone density in the humerus; arthrography shows a contracted joint.

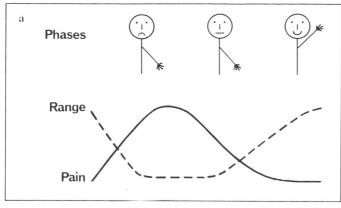

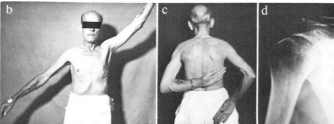

13.14 Frozen shoulder (a) Natural history of frozen shoulder. The face tells the story.

(b, c, d) Patient in phase 2: limited abduction (b); limited internal rotation (c); localized rarefaction (d).

Differential diagnosis

POST-TRAUMATIC STIFFNESS After any severe shoulder injury, stiffness may persist for some months. It is maximal at the start and gradually lessens, unlike the pattern of a frozen shoulder.

DISUSE STIFFNESS If the arm is nursed over-cautiously (e.g. following a forearm fracture) the shoulder may stiffen. Again, the characteristic pattern of a frozen shoulder is absent.

REFLEX SYMPATHETIC DYSTROPHY Shoulder pain and stiffness may follow myocardial infarction or a stroke. The features are similar to those of a frozen shoulder and it has been suggested that the latter is a form of reflex sympathetic dystrophy. In severe cases the whole upper limb is involved, with trophic and vasomotor changes in the hand (the 'shoulder–hand syndrome').

Treatment

Conservative treatment aims at relieving pain and preventing further stiffening while recovery is awaited. It is important not only to administer analgesics and anti-inflammatory drugs but also to reassure the patient that recovery is certain.

Heat sometimes helps, though often ice-packs are more soothing. Exercises are encouraged, the most valuable being 'pendulum' exercises in which the patient leans forward at the hips and moves his arm as if stirring a giant pudding (this is really a form of assisted active movement, the assistance being supplied by gravity). However, the patient is warned that moderation and regularity will achieve more than sporadic masochism. Injections of corti-costeroid and local anaesthetic sometimes help.

Once acute pain has subsided, manipulation under anaesthesia often hastens recovery; methylprednisolone and lignocaine are injected, then external rotation is restored, and finally abduction is gently but firmly regained.

Active exercises should recommence immediately afterwards. Alternatively, movement can be increased by distending the joint with a large volume (50–200 ml) of sterile saline. Arthrography demonstrates that distension or manipulation achieve their effect by rupturing the capsule.

Chronic instability of the shoulder

The shoulder achieves its uniquely wide range of movement at the cost of stability. The humeral head is held in the shallow glenoid socket by the glenoid labrum, the glenohumeral ligaments, the coracohumeral ligament, the overhanging canopy of the coracoacromial arch and the surrounding muscles. Failure of any of these mechanisms may result in chronic instability of the joint. This can take the form of either recurrent *dislocation* or recurrent *subluxation*. In 95% of cases the displacement is *anterior*; in the remainder it is either *posterior* or *multidirectional.*

Pathology

Anterior dislocation usually follows an acute injury in which the arm is forced into abduction, external rotation and extension. In *recurrent dislocation* the labrum and capsule are often detached from the anterior rim of the glenoid (the classic Bankart lesion); however, in some cases the labrum remains intact and the capsule and glenohumeral ligaments are either stripped away or stretched anteriorly and inferiorly. In addition there may be an indentation on the posterolateral aspect of the humeral head – the Hill–Sachs lesion, a compression fracture due to the humeral head being forced against the anterior glenoid rim each time it dislocates.

Anterior subluxation may follow and alternate with episodes of dislocation. However, in some cases the shoulder never dislocates completely and in these the labral tear and bone defect may be absent.

Posterior dislocation is rare; when it occurs it is usually due to a violent jerk in an unusual position, following an epileptic fit or a severe electric shock. The posterior capsule is stripped from the bone or stretched, and there may be an indentation on the anterior aspect of the humeral head. Recurrent instability is almost always a *posterior subluxation*, with the humeral head riding back on the posterior lip of the glenoid.

Multidirectional instability is associated with capsular and ligamentous laxity, and sometimes with weakness of the shoulder muscles. Little force is required to displace the joint and it may subluxate even with mildly stressful daily activities.

Anterior instability

This is far and away the commonest type of instability, accounting for over 95% of cases.

Clinical features

The patient is usually a young man who gives a history of his shoulder 'coming out', perhaps during a sporting event. The first episode of *acute dislocation* is a landmark and he may be able to describe the mechanism precisely: an applied force with the shoulder in abduction, external rotation and extension. The diagnosis may have been verified by x-ray and the injury treated by closed reduction and 'immobilization' in a bandage or sling for several weeks. This may be the first of many similar episodes: *recurrent dislocation* develops in over 50% of patients under the age of 25 and in about 20% of older patients (Hovelius et al., 1983).

Recurrent subluxation is less obvious. The patient may describe a 'catching' sensation, followed by 'numbness' or 'weakness' – the so-called dead arm syndrome – whenever the shoulder is used in the overhead position (e.g. by throwing a ball, serving at tennis or swimming). Pain with the arm in abduction may suggest a rotator cuff syndrome; it is as well to remember that recurrent subluxation may actually cause supraspinatus tendinitis.

On examination, between episodes of dislocation, the shoulder looks normal and movements are full. Clinical diagnosis rests on the *apprehension sign*. With the patient seated or lying, the examiner cautiously lifts the arm into abduction, external rotation and then extension; at the crucial moment the patient senses that the humeral head is about to slip out anteriorly and his body tautens in apprehension. The test should be repeated with the examiner applying pressure to the front of the shoulder; with this manoeuvre, the patient feels more secure and the apprehension sign is negative.

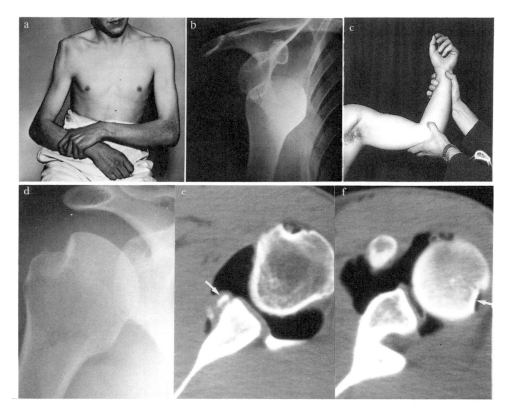

13.15 Anterior instability (a, b) Anterior dislocation of the shoulder. This may be followed by recurrent dislocation and (c) a positive 'apprehension test'. (d) The plain x-ray shows a large depression in the posterosuperior part of the humeral head (the Hill–Sachs sign). (e, f) MRI shows both a Bankart lesion, with a flake of bone detached from the anterior edge of the glenoid, and the Hill–Sachs lesion (arrows).

Examination of the other joints may reveal generalized ligamentous laxity.

Dislocation is easily diagnosed in anteroposterior and lateral views of the shoulder. The Hill–Sachs lesion (when it is present) is best shown by an anteroposterior x-ray with the shoulder internally rotated, or in the axillary view. Subluxation is seen in the axillary views.

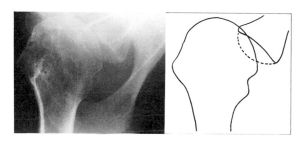

13.16 Recurrent subluxation X-ray showing anterior subluxation; the humeral head is riding on the lip of the glenoid.

Treatment

If dislocation recurs at long intervals, the patient may choose to put up with the inconvenience and simply try to avoid vulnerable positions of the shoulder. There is no convincing evidence that recurrent dislocation predisposes to osteoarthritis.

The indications for operative treatment are: (1) frequent dislocations, especially if these are painful; and (2) recurrent subluxation or a fear of dislocation sufficient to prevent participation in everyday activities, including sport.

Operations are of three types: (1) those that repair the torn glenoid labrum and capsule (the Bankart procedure); (2) those that shorten the anterior capsule and subscapularis by an overlapping repair (the Putti–Platt operation); and (3) those that reinforce the antero-inferior capsule by redirecting other muscles across the front of the joint (e.g. the Bristow operation – Helfet, 1958).

If the labrum and anterior capsule are detached, and there is no marked joint laxity, the Bankart operation combined with anterior capsulorrhaphy is recommended. The joint is exposed by the deltopectoral approach, the labrum is sutured to drill holes in the glenoid rim and, if necessary, the capsule is tightened by an overlapping tuck without shortening the subscapularis (Thomas and Matsen, 1989). The Putti–Platt operation, in which the subscapularis is overlapped and shortened, also gives good results but at the cost of significant loss of external rotation (Hovelius et al., 1983; Regan et al., 1989). The Bristow operation, in which the coracoid process with its attached muscles is transposed to the front of the neck of the scapula, gives less loss of external rotation.

Posterior instability

Clinical features

Posterior dislocation is rare, and when it does occur it is often missed. There may be a history of fairly violent injury, and dislocation may be associated with fractures of the proximal humerus. On examination the arm is held in internal rotation and attempts at external rotation are resisted. The anteroposterior x-ray may show a typical 'globular' appearance of the proximal humerus (the humeral head seen end-on because it is internally rotated); if the arm can be abducted, an axillary view will show the dislocation quite clearly.

Recurrent instability usually takes the form of subluxation when the arm is used in flexion and internal rotation. The diagnosis may be confirmed by x-rays (axillary views) or CT scanning.

Treatment

Recurrent subluxation can usually be treated conservatively, by encouraging muscle strengthening exercises and teaching the patient how to control the position of the shoulder (Fronek, Warren and Bowen, 1989). The results of operative treatment are less predictable than in anterior instability; surgery should be considered only if (1) the condition is genuinely disabling, (2) there is no gross joint laxity, and (3) the patient is emotionally well adjusted. Posterior capsular reconstruction can be augmented by a posterior bone block; postoperatively the shoulder is held abducted and externally rotated in a spica for 6 weeks.

Multidirectional instability

Sometimes anterior or posterior instability changes gradually to inferior and then multi-directional instability (Neer and Foster, 1980).

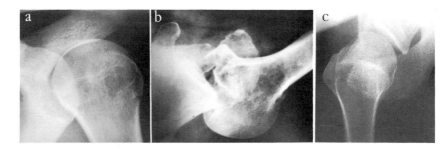

13.17 Posterior instability (a) In the anteroposterior view the humeral head looks globular but may mistakenly be called normal. (b) The lateral view shows the obvious subluxation with impaction of the humeral head; (c) the defect in the anterior part of the head.

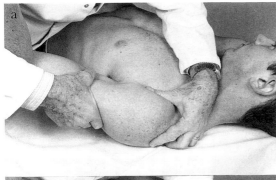

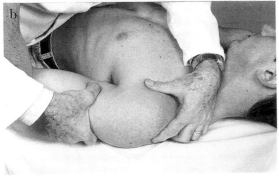

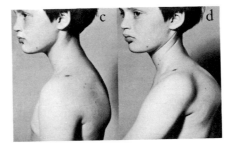

13.19 Habitual subluxation   The clue is the unconcerned expression.

13.18 Multidirectional instability   (a) The anterior and (b) the posterior drawer tests are best performed with the patient lying supine. The amount of movement is compared with that on the unaffected side.

The condition is difficult to diagnose with certainty, but anterior and posterior drawer tests performed with the patient lying supine are helpful (Gerber and Ganz, 1984). Often there is generalized joint laxity and the patient may show a tendency to voluntary subluxation. Surgical treatment is seldom indicated; muscle strengthening exercises and training in joint control are helpful.

Atraumatic dislocation or subluxation

Displacement of the humeral head can occur even without trauma if there are congenital anatomical abnormalities or ligamentous laxity. The patient can *voluntarily* subluxate or dislocate the shoulder painlessly and can reduce it again; emotionally disturbed patients may find the temptation to do so irresistible. Sometimes

displacement occurs so frequently as to justify the term *habitual*. Operative treatment is seldom successful and is best avoided.

Tuberculosis (see also Chapter 2)

Tuberculosis of the shoulder is uncommon. It usually starts as an osteitis but is rarely diagnosed until arthritis has supervened. This may proceed to abscess and sinus formation, but in some cases the tendency is to fibrosis and ankylosis. If there is no exudate the term 'caries sicca' is used; however, one suspects that many such cases, formerly diagnosed on the basis of coexisting pulmonary tuberculosis rather than joint biopsy or bacteriological examination, are actually examples of frozen shoulder.

Clinical features

Adults are mainly affected. They complain of a constant ache and stiffness lasting many months or years. The striking feature is wasting of the muscles around the shoulder, especially the deltoid. In neglected cases a sinus may be present over the shoulder or in the axilla. There is diffuse warmth and tenderness, and all movements are limited and painful. Axillary lymph nodes may be enlarged.

X-ray   Generalized rarefaction is present, usually with some erosion of the joint surfaces. There may be abscess cavities in the humerus or glenoid, with little or no periosteal reaction.

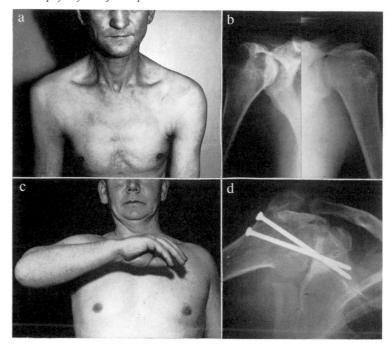

13.20 Tuberculosis (a) Marked wasting of right deltoid. (b) Bone rarefaction and joint damage in arthritis, compared with the normal.

(c, d) After arthrodesis of the glenohumeral joint scapulothoracic movement remains, permitting useful abduction.

Treatment

In addition to systemic treatment with anti-tuberculous drugs, the shoulder should be rested until acute symptoms have settled. Thereafter movement is encouraged and, provided the articular cartilage is not destroyed, the prognosis for painless function is good. If there are repeated flares, or if the articular surfaces are extensively destroyed, the joint should be arthrodesed.

The glenohumeral joint, with its lax capsule and folds of synovium, shows marked soft-tissue inflammation. Often there is an accumulation of fluid and fibrinoid particles which may rupture the capsule and extrude into the muscle planes. Cartilage destruction and bone erosion are often severe.

The subacromial bursa and the synovial sheath of the long head of biceps become inflamed and thickened; often this leads to rupture of the rotator cuff and the biceps tendon.

Rheumatoid arthritis (see Chapter 3)

The acromioclavicular joint, the shoulder joint and the various synovial pouches around the shoulder are frequently involved in rheumatoid disease.

The acromioclavicular joint develops an erosive arthritis which may go on to capsular disruption and instability.

Clinical features

The patient may be known to have generalized rheumatoid arthritis; occasionally, however, acromioclavicular erosion discovered on an x-ray of the chest is the first clue to the diagnosis.

Pain and swelling are the usual presenting symptoms; the patient has increasing difficulty with simple tasks such as combing the hair or washing the back. Though it may start on one side, the condition usually becomes bilateral.

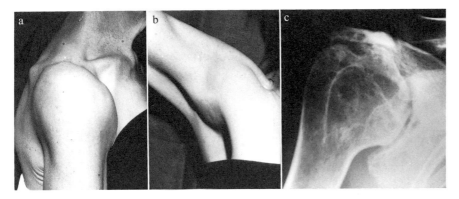

13.21 Rheumatoid arthritis   (a) Large synovial effusions cause easily visible swelling; small ones are likely to be missed – especially if they present, like this one (b), in the axilla. (c) X-rays show erosion of the joint and of the periarticular bone.

Synovitis of the joint results in swelling and tenderness anteriorly, superiorly or in the axilla.

Tenosynovitis produces features similar to those of cuff lesions, including tears of supraspinatus or biceps. Joint and tendon lesions usually occur together and conspire to cause the marked weakness and limitation of movement that are features of the disease.

X-ray changes are typical of rheumatoid arthritis; in addition, there may be superior subluxation of the humeral head due to complete disruption of the cuff.

Treatment

If general measures do not control the synovitis, a mixture of methylprednisolone and nitrogen mustard may be injected into the joint, the subacromial bursa and the bicipital tendon sheath; this should not be repeated more than two or three times.

If synovitis persists, operative synovectomy is carried out; at the same time, cuff tears may be repaired. Excision of the lateral end of the clavicle may relieve acromioclavicular pain.

In advanced cases pain and stiffness can be very disabling. Provided the rotator cuff is not completely destroyed and there is still adequate bone stock, joint replacement may be carried out. This operation provides good pain relief and moderate shoulder function.

If the rotator cuff is destroyed, or bone erosion very advanced, arthrodesis may be preferable; despite its apparent limitations, it gives improved function because scapulothoracic movement is usually undisturbed.

Osteoarthritis

Osteoarthritis is usually secondary to local trauma or long-standing rotator cuff lesions. Often chondrocalcinosis is present as well but it is not known whether this predisposes to osteoarthritis or appears as a sequel to joint degeneration.

Clinical features

The patient is usually aged 50–60 and may give a history of injury or a previous painful arc syndrome. There is usually little to see, but shoulder movements are restricted in all directions.

X-rays show distortion of the joint, bone sclerosis and osteophyte formation; the articular 'space' may be narrowed or may show calcification.

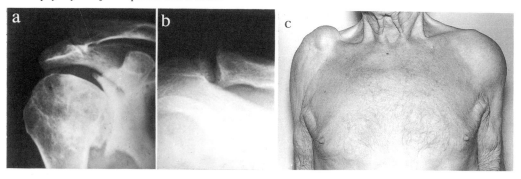

13.22 Osteoarthritis (a) Osteoarthritis of the glenohumeral joint, which is less common than (b) osteoarthritis of the acromioclavicular joint. (c) This amount of swelling from the acromioclavicular joint is distinctly unusual.

Treatment

Analgesics and anti-inflammatory drugs relieve pain, and exercises, may improve mobility. Most patients manage to live with the restrictions imposed by stiffness, provided pain is not severe.

In advanced cases, if pain becomes intolerable shoulder arthroplasty is justified. It may not improve mobility much, but it does relieve pain. The alternative is arthrodesis.

OSTEOARTHRITIS OF THE ACROMIOCLAVICULAR JOINT is common in old people and causes a painful swelling over the top of the shoulder. If analgesics are ineffectual, pain may be relieved by excision of the lateral end of the clavicle.

Rapidly destructive arthropathy (Milwaukee shoulder)

Occasionally, in the presence of long-standing or massive cuff tears, patients develop a rapidly progressive and destructive form of osteoarthritis in which there is severe erosion of the glenohumeral joint, the acromion process and the acromioclavicular joint. McCarty et al. (1981) attributed the changes to hydroxyapatite crystal shedding from the torn rotator cuff and a synovial reaction involving the release of lysosomal enzymes (including collagenases) which lead to cartilage breakdown. The same condition is seen in other joints such as the hip and knee.

Clinical features

The patient is usually aged over 60 and may have suffered with shoulder pain for many years. Over a period of a few months the

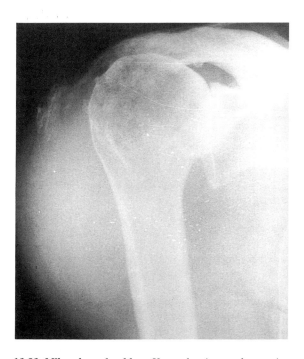

13.23 Milwaukee shoulder X-ray showing a destructive arthropathy with marked swelling and calcification in the soft tissues around the shoulder.

shoulder becomes swollen and increasingly unstable. On examination there is marked crepitus in the joint and loss of active movements.

X-rays show severe erosion of the articular surfaces and subluxation of the joint.

Treatment

There is no satisfactory treatment for this condition. Resurfacing arthroplasty may relieve pain but will not improve function, because the rotator cuff is disrupted and the joint is unstable.

Disorders of the scapula and clavicle

Congenital elevation of the scapula (Sprengel's deformity)

The scapulae normally complete their descent from the neck by the third month of fetal life; occasionally one remains unduly high. Associated deformities of the cervical spine are common and sometimes there is a family history of scapular deformity.

Deformity is the only symptom and may be noticed at birth. The shoulder on the affected side is elevated; the scapula looks and feels abnormally high, smaller than usual and somewhat prominent. Occasionally both scapulae are affected. Movements are painless but abduc-tion may be somewhat limited by fixation of the scapula. Associated deformities such as fusion of cervical vertebrae, kyphosis or scoliosis may be present. X-rays may reveal such anomalies, and sometimes a bony bridge between the scapula and the cervical spine (the omovertebral bar).

In the *Klippel–Feil syndrome* there is bilateral failure of scapular descent associated with marked anomalies of the cervical spine and failure of fusion of the occipital bones. Patients look as if they have no neck; there is a low hairline, bilateral neck webbing and gross limitation of neck movement. (This condition should not be confused with *bilateral shortness of the sternomastoid muscle*, in which the head is poked forward and the chin thrust up; the absence of associated congenital lesions is a further distinguishing feature.)

Treatment

Mild cases are best left untreated. Marked limitation of abduction or severe deformity may necessitate operation. In children under 6 years of age, the scapula can be repositioned by releasing the muscles along the vertebral and superior borders of the scapula, excising the supraspinous portion of the scapula and the omovertebral bar, pulling the scapula down, then reattaching the muscles to hold it firmly in its new position (Lebovic, Ehrlich and Zaleske, 1990). In older children this carries a risk of brachial nerve compression or traction between the clavicle and first rib; here it is safer merely to excise the supraspinous scapula in order to improve the appearance.

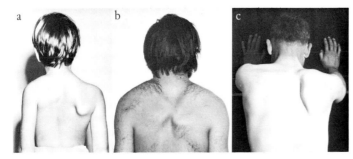

13.24 Scapular disorders (a) Sprengel shoulder; (b) Klippel–Feil syndrome; (c) winged scapula.

Scapular instability

Winging of the scapula causes asymmetry of the shoulders, but may not be obvious until the patient tries to contract the serratus anterior against resistance. *Weakness or paralysis of the serratus anterior* may arise from (1) lesions of the fifth, sixth and seventh cervical nerve roots (injury or viral neuropathy), (2) injury to the brachial plexus (a blow to the top of the shoulder, severe traction on the arm or carrying heavy loads on the shoulder), (3) direct damage to the long thoracic nerve (e.g. during radical mastectomy), and (4) in the girdle type of muscular dystrophy.

Disability is usually slight and is best accepted. However, if function is noticeably impaired, it is possible to stabilize the scapula by transferring the sternal portion of pectoralis major and attaching it via a fascia lata graft to the lower pole of the scapula; or the scapula can be fixed to the rib cage.

A less obvious, but sometimes more disabling, form of scapular instability may follow *injury to the spinal accessory nerve* (e.g. following operations in the posterior triangle of the neck). The trapezius muscle is an important stabilizer of the shoulder and loss of this function results in weakness and pain on active abduction against resistance. Early recognition may permit nerve repair or grafting.

Grating scapula

The patient complains of grating or clicking on moving the arm. It is painless but annoying. Usually no cause is found, though bony, muscular and bursal abnormalities have been blamed. Tangential x-ray views of the scapula should be obtained to exclude an osteochondroma on the undersurface of the scapula; if present, the lesion can be excised. Otherwise no treatment is necessary.

Hyperostosis of the clavicle

Several individually rare disorders are associated with pain and swelling over the clavicle or the sternoclavicular joint. They are often confused, though certain characteristic features permit appropriate differentiation in the majority of cases.

CONDENSING OSTEITIS OF THE CLAVICLE is usually seen in women of 30–50 years who present with pain in or near the sternoclavicular joint. The medial end of the clavicle may be thickened, x-rays reveal sclerosis and radionuclide scanning shows increased activity in the affected bone. The condition is thought to result from mechanical stress due to lifting activities (Cone et al., 1983). No treatment is necessary.

STERNOCOSTOCLAVICULAR HYPEROSTOSIS is similar to condensing osteitis, but is usually bilateral and may be associated with pustules on the palms and soles (Resnick, 1980). Sclerosis affects the medial end of the clavicle, the adjacent sternum and the upper ribs. It may be an infective lesion, though organisms are seldom cultured.

SEPTIC ARTHRITIS OF THE STERNOCLAVICULAR JOINT is rare except in drug abusers following intravenous injections. Local signs may be misleadingly mild but x-rays may show erosion of the sternoclavicular joint and the adjacent bone. Treatment is by antibiotics and local drainage of infected material.

CHRONIC RECURRENT MULTIFOCAL OSTEOMYELITIS usually occurs in children, and the clavicle is one of the sites of predilection. It usually involves the middle third of the bone and results in fusiform swelling and radiological

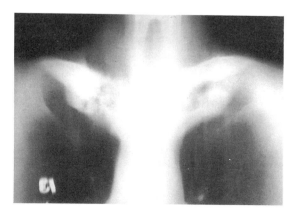

13.25 Sternoclavicular hyperostosis Tomogram showing irregularity and hyperostosis of the sternoclavicular joint.

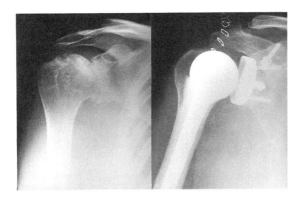

13.26 Arthroplasty X-ray appearances before and after total joint replacement.

signs of thickening and sclerosis. There is no obvious infective organism, but the histology is typical of an inflammatory lesion (Bjorksten and Boquist, 1980). There is no effective treatment and the condition may persist for many years.

Operations

Arthroplasty of the shoulder

In recent years shoulder arthroplasty has gradually gained acceptance, though the results are less satisfying than those of hip or knee replacement.

The indications for arthroplasty are: (1) severe joint injury with multiple fractures of the proximal humerus; (2) destructive lesions of the humeral head, including osteonecrosis; (3)

rheumatoid arthritis; and (4) osteoarthritis. The greater the integrity of the surrounding soft tissues (and especially the rotator cuff), the more stable will the new joint be, and thus the better the outcome of the operation. Joint replacement is contraindicated in patients with severe cuff disruption, though even here it is sometimes done to relieve pain.

If the glenoid is unaffected (e.g. in four-part fractures of the proximal humerus), a humeral endoprosthesis alone may suffice. If the glenoid is affected, it is replaced by a metal-backed polyethylene surface which is fixed with methylmethacrylate cement.

The complications of shoulder replacement are those of joint replacement in general (see p. 426). Despite the fact that the scapula affords only moderately secure socket fixation, loosening of the glenoid cup is not a serious problem.

Outcome depends largely on the indications for surgery. Arthroplasty for fractures, avascular necrosis or proximal humeral tumours gives good pain relief and shoulder movement, though power is always diminished. Where there is more extensive joint destruction and disruption of the soft tissues (e.g. in rheumatoid arthritis), pain relief is still excellent but the range of movement is only moderately improved (Kelly, Foster and Fisher, 1987).

Arthrodesis

Arthrodesis of the shoulder is now seldom performed, but it is still a useful operation for severe shoulder dysfunction due to (1) paralysis

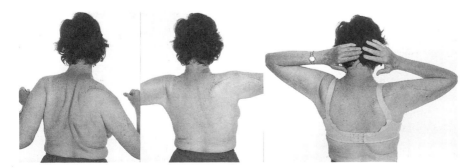

13.27 Arthrodesis The useful function after a successful arthrodesis.

of the scapulohumeral muscles, (2) infective disorders of the glenohumeral joint (including tuberculous arthritis) or (3) advanced erosive arthritis with massive disruption of the rotator cuff. A prerequisite is stable and powerful scapulothoracic movement, because with an arthrodesis shoulder 'movement' is achieved entirely by rotation of the scapula on the thorax.

Through a posterior incision the joint is disarticulated, the surfaces are rawed, then fixed together by a heavy nail, screws or a plate. The acromion is osteotomized and hinged into a bed chiselled out of the humerus. The shoulder is held in a plaster spica for 3–6 months. The optimal position is abduction 50 degrees, flexion 25 degrees and internal rotation sufficient to allow the hand to reach the mouth.

Despite the restriction of glenohumeral movement, postoperative function is surprisingly good – and guaranteed to be painless.

Notes on applied anatomy

The anatomy of the shoulder is uniquely adapted to allow freedom of movement and maximum reach for the hand. Five 'articulations' are involved: (1) the true (synovial) glenohumeral joint, (2) the pseudojoint between the humerus and the coracoacromial arch, (3) the sternoclavicular joint, (4) the acromioclavicular joint and (5) the scapulothoracic articulation.

The shallow glenohumeral articulation has little inherent stability because the glenoid surface area is only one-quarter that of the humeral articular surface. The extent to which the socket is deepened by the labrum may seem trivial, but it must be significant because labral tears are associated with dislocation. Stability depends upon muscle control. The tendons of the short rotators – subscapularis in front, supraspinatus above, infraspinatus and teres minor behind – blend with the capsule of the shoulder to form the rotator cuff. During abduction these muscles draw the head of the humerus firmly into its socket while the deltoid

elevates the arm. As abduction proceeds, the external rotators twist the arm so that the greater tuberosity clears the projecting acromion, and scapulothoracic movement permits further reach to 180 degrees. In fact, abduction at the glenohumeral joint cannot exceed 90 degrees because no further articular surface of the humeral head is available; but external rotation of the humerus liberates more surface and permits full abduction, in which the scapulothoracic articulation plays its part. The scapulothoracic and glenohumeral joints move synchronously, though in the first 30 degrees of abduction little scapulothoracic movement is visible; of the remaining 150 degrees of abduction, about 90 degrees is at the glenohumeral joint. The sternoclavicular joint participates in movements close to the trunk (e.g. shrugging or bracing the shoulders); the acromioclavicular joint moves in the last 60 degrees of abduction.

References and further reading

Bjorksten B. and Boquist, L. (1980) Histopathological aspects of chronic recurrent multifocal osteomyelitis. *Journal of Bone and Joint Surgery* **62B**, 376–380

Cone, R.D., Resnick, D., Goergen, T.G. et al. (1983) Condensing osteitis of the clavicle. *American Journal of Roentgenology* **141**, 387–388

Froneck, J., Warren, R.F. and Bowen, M. (1989) Posterior subluxation of the glenohumeral joint. *Journal of Bone and Joint Surgery* **71A**, 205–210

Gartsman, G.M. (1990) Arthroscopic acromioplasty for lesions of the rotator cuff. *Journal of Bone and Joint Surgery* **72A**, 169–180

Gerber, C. and Ganz, R. (1984) Clinical assessment of instability of the shoulder. *Journal of Bone and Joint Surgery* **66B**, 551–556

Helfet, A.J. (1958) Coracoid transplantation for recurring dislocation of the shoulder. *Journal of Bone and Joint Surgery* **40B**, 198–202

Hensinger, R.N., Lang, J.E. and MacEwen, G.D. (1974) Klippel–Feil syndrome. *Journal of Bone and Joint Surgery* **56A**, 1246–1253

Hovelius, L., Erikkson, K., Fredin, H. et al. (1983) Recurrence after initial dislocation of the shoulder. *Journal of Bone and Joint Surgery* **65A**, 343–349

Kelly, I.G., Foster, R.S. and Fisher, W.D. (1987) Near total shoulder replacement in rheumatoid arthritis. *Journal of Bone and Joint Surgery* **69B**, 723–726

Kessel, L. and Watson, M. (1977) The painful arc syndrome. *Journal of Bone and Joint Surgery* **59B**, 166–172

Lebovic, S.J., Ehrlich, M.G. and Zaleske, D.J. (1990) Sprengel deformity. *Journal of Bone and Joint Surgery* **72A**, 192–197

McCarty, D.J., Halverson, P.B., Carrera, G.F., Brewer, B.J. and Kozin, F. (1981) Milwaukee shoulder: association of microspheroids containing hydroxyapatite crystals, active collagenase and neutral protease with rotator cuff defects. *Arthritis and Rheumatism* **24**, 464–473

McLaughlin, H.L. (1962) Rupture of the rotator cuff (an Instructional Course Lecture). *Journal of Bone and Joint Surgery* **44A**, 979–983

MacNab, I. (1973) Rotator cuff tendinitis. *Annals of the Royal College of Surgeons of England* **53**, 271–287

Neer, C.S. (1972) Anterior acromioplasty for the chronic impingement syndrome in the shoulder. *Journal of Bone and Joint Surgery* **54A**, 41–50

Neer, C.S. and Foster, C.R. (1980) Inferior capsular shift for involuntary inferior and multidirectional instability of the shoulder. A preliminary report. *Journal of Bone and Joint Surgery* **62A**, 897–908

Neer, C.S., Craig, E.V. and Fukuda, H.F. (1983) Cuff tear arthropathy. *Journal of Bone and Joint Surgery* **65A**, 1232–1244

Ogilvie-Harris, D.J. and Wiley, A.M. (1986) Arthroscopic surgery of the shoulder. *Journal of Bone and Joint Surgery* **68B**, 201–207

Rathbun, J.B. and MacNab, I. (1970) The microvascular pattern of the rotator cuff. *Journal of Bone and Joint Surgery* **52B**, 540–553

Regan, W.D. Jr, Webster-Bogaert, S., Hawkins, R.J. and Fowler, P.J. (1989) Comparative functional analysis of the Bristow, Magnuson–Stack and Putti–Platt procedures for recurrent dislocation of the shoulder. *American Journal of Sports Medicine* **17**, 42–48

Resnick, D. (1980) Sternocostoclavicular hyperostosis. *American Journal of Roentgenology* **135**, 1278–1280

Richardson, A.T. (1975) The painful shoulder. *Proceedings of the Royal Society of Medicine* **68**, 731–736

Seeger, L.L. (1989) Magnetic resonance imaging of the shoulder. *Clinical Orthopaedics and Related Research* **244**, 48–59

Thomas, S.C. and Matsen, F.A. III (1989) An approach to the repair of avulsion of the glenohumeral ligaments in the management of traumatic anterior glenohumeral instability. *Journal of Bone and Joint Surgery* **71A**, 506–513

Uthoff, H.K. and Sarkar, S.D. (1978) Calcifying tendinitis – its pathogenetic mechanism and rationale for its treatment. *International Orthopaedics* **2**, 187–194

Wolfgang, G.L. (1974) Surgical repair of tears of the rotator cuff of the shoulder. *Journal of Bone and Joint Surgery* **56A**, 14–26

Examination

Symptoms

Pain   localized to the medial or lateral condyle is usually due to tendinitis. Pain arising in the joint is more diffuse. Remember that the elbow is a common site of referred pain from the cervical spine.

Stiffness,   if it is mild, may hardly be noticed. If it is severe, it can be very disabling; the patient may be unable to reach up to the mouth (loss of flexion) or the perineum (loss of extension); limited supination makes it difficult to carry large objects.

Swelling   may be due to injury or inflammation; a soft lump on the back of the elbow suggests an olecranon bursitis.

Instability   is not uncommon in the late stage of rheumatoid arthritis.

Ulnar nerve symptoms   (tingling, numbness and weakness of the hand) may occur in elbow disorders because of the nerve's proximity to the joint.

Signs

● LOOK
Both upper limbs must be completely exposed. The patient holds his arms alongside his body with palms forwards. Varus or valgus deformity is then obvious, but it cannot be accurately assessed unless the elbow extends fully. He then holds his arms out sideways at right angles to the body with palms upwards and elbows straight. In this position, wasting or lumps are easily seen.

● FEEL
The back of the joint is palpated for warmth, subcutaneous nodules, synovial thickening and fluid (fluctuation on each side of the olecranon); the back and sides are felt for tenderness and to determine whether the bony points are correctly placed.

The joint line can be located laterally by feeling for the head of the radius (pronating and supinating the forearm makes this easier), but medially it is difficult to find.

The ulnar nerve is fairly superficial behind the medial condyle and here it can be rolled under the fingers to feel if it is thickened or hypersensitive.

● MOVE
Flexion and extension are compared on the two sides. Then, with the elbows tucked into the sides and flexed to a right angle, the radioulnar joints are tested for pronation and supination.

● X-RAY
The position of each bone is noted, then the joint line and space. Next, the individual bones are inspected for evidence of old injury or bone destruction. Finally, loose bodies are sought.

NOTE   Where appropriate, other parts are examined: the neck (for cervical disc lesions), the shoulder (for cuff lesions) and the hand (for nerve lesions).

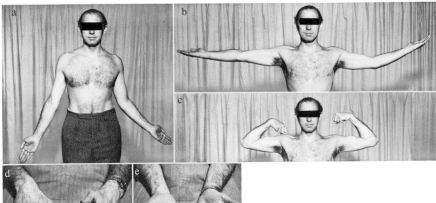

14.1 Examination The signs demonstrated are of osteoarthritis in the left elbow: (a) valgus deformity, (b) limited extension, (c) limited flexion, (d, e) limited pronation and supination.

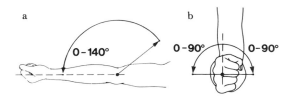

14.2 Normal range of movement (a) The extended position is recorded as 0 degrees and any hyperextension as a minus quantity; flexion is full when the arm and forearm make contact. (b) From the neutral position the radioulnar joint rotates 90 degrees into pronation and 90 into supination.

Elbow deformities

Cubitus valgus

The normal carrying angle of the elbow is 10–15 degrees of valgus; anything more than this is regarded as a valgus deformity, which is usually quite obvious when the patient stands with arms to the sides and palms facing forwards.

The commonest cause is non-union of a fractured lateral condyle; the deformity may be associated with marked prominence of the medial condylar outline.

The importance of cubitus valgus is the liability to delayed ulnar palsy; years after the causal injury the patient notices weakness of the hand, with numbness and tingling of the ulnar

fingers. The deformity itself needs no treatment, but for delayed ulnar palsy the nerve should be transposed to the front of the elbow.

Cubitus varus ('gun-stock' deformity)

The deformity is most obvious when the elbow is extended and the arms are elevated. The most common cause is malunion of a supracondylar fracture. The deformity can be corrected by a wedge osteotomy of the lower humerus.

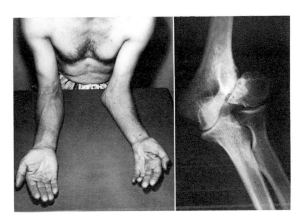

14.3 Cubitus valgus This man's valgus deformity, the sequel to an un-united fracture of the lateral condyle, has resulted in ulnar nerve palsy.

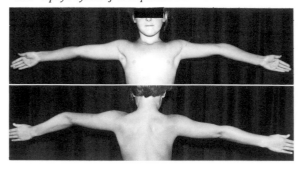

14.4 Cubitus varus This ugly deformity, the sequel to a supracondylar fracture, was later corrected by osteotomy.

Dislocated head of radius

Congenital dislocation of the radial head may be anterior or posterior and is usually bilateral. The patient may notice the lump, which is easily palpable and can be felt to move when the forearm is rotated. X-rays show that the dislocated head is dome-shaped. If the lump limits elbow flexion it can be excised (beware of the posterior interosseous nerve).

Unilateral anterior dislocation may be acquired (if a Monteggia fracture-dislocation was left unreduced) and in time the head becomes dome-shaped. Open reduction and stabilization with a Kirschner wire is worth considering.

Subluxation of the radial head is commonly associated with bone dysplasias in which the ulna is disproportionately shortened. It causes little disability, but if it becomes troublesome the radial head can be excised after all growth has ceased.

Osteochondritis dissecans

The capitulum is one of the common sites of osteochondritis dissecans. This is probably due to repeated stress following prolonged or unaccustomed activity. The pathological changes are identical to those in the knee (see p. 450).

The patient – usually a young boy – complains of aching which is aggravated by activity and relieved by rest. On examination there may be swelling, signs of an effusion, tenderness over the capitulum and slight limitation of movement. If the fragment has separated, there may be intermittent locking.

X-rays show the characteristic features of osteochondritis. The end result may be permanent flattening of the capitulum.

Treatment is usually symptomatic. However, if the fragment has separated and is lying free in the joint, it should be removed.

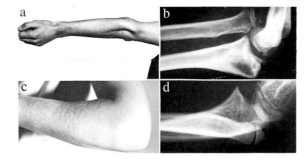

14.5 Dislocated head of radius (a, b) Anterior dislocation, from an old Monteggia fracture; (c, d) posterior dislocation – the radial head is dome-shaped, suggesting that the dislocation was congenital.

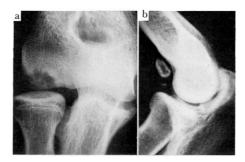

14.6 Osteochondritis dissecans (a) The capitulum is fragmented and slightly flattened. (b) Sometimes the fragment separates and lies in the joint.

Loose bodies

Loose bodies in the elbow may be due to: (1) osteochondritis dissecans; (2) acute trauma (an osteocartilaginous fracture); (3) osteoarthritis (separation of osteophytes); or (4) synovial chondromatosis (a cluster of mainly cartilaginous 'pebbles').

The patient may complain of sudden locking and unlocking of the joint. Symptoms of osteoarthritis may coexist.

A loose body is rarely palpable. When degenerative changes have occurred, extremes of movement are limited. *X-rays* nearly always reveal the loose body or bodies; in the special case of osteochondritis dissecans there is a rarefied cystic area in the capitulum and enlargement of the radial head.

If loose bodies are troublesome, they should be removed.

Tuberculosis
(see also Chapter 2)

Although the disease begins as synovitis or osteomyelitis, tuberculosis of the elbow is rarely seen until arthritis supervenes. The onset is insidious with a long history of aching and stiffness. The most striking physical sign is the marked wasting. While the disease is active the joint is held flexed, looks swollen, feels warm and diffusely tender; movement is considerably limited and accompanied by pain and spasm.

X-rays show generalized rarefaction and often an apparent increase of joint space because of bone erosion.

Treatment In addition to general antituberculous treatment, the elbow is rested – at first in a splint and positioned at 90 degrees of flexion and mid-rotation, later simply by applying a collar and cuff. Surgical debridement is rarely needed.

Rheumatoid arthritis
(see also Chapter 3)

The elbow is involved in more than 50% of patients with polyarticular rheumatoid arthritis, and in the majority of cases the condition is bilateral. In the early stages the synovitis causes pain and tenderness, especially over the radio-humeral joint line. Later, the whole elbow may become swollen and stiff. If, however, bone destruction is severe, instability and capsular rupture are more frequent sequels.

X-rays reveal bone erosion, with gradual destruction of the radial head and widening of the trochlear notch of the ulna. Sometimes large synovial extensions penetrate the articular surface and appear as cysts in the proximal radius or ulna.

Treatment

In addition to general treatment, the elbow should be splinted during periods of active synovitis. Local injections of corticosteroids or radiocolloids may reduce pain and swelling dramatically.

OPERATIVE TREATMENT If, despite adequate conservative treatment, synovitis persists – and more particularly if this is associated with erosion of the radial head – synovectomy is worthwhile. This is usually performed through

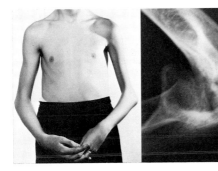

14.7 Tuberculosis of the elbow Muscle wasting is marked and bone destruction extensive.

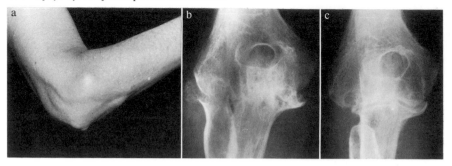

14.8 Rheumatoid arthritis   (a) This rheumatoid patient has nodules over the olecranon and a bulge over the radiohumeral joint; (b) his x-rays show deformity of the radial head and marked erosion of the rest of the elbow. (c) Excision of the radial head combined with synovectomy relieved the pain and the joint looks much healthier.

a lateral approach, with excision of the radial head. There are two reasons for this: the radiocapitellar surfaces are almost invariably eroded, and radial head excision permits wider access to the hypertrophic synovium. The operation relieves pain and may slow the progress of the disease, but after 5–6 years erosion of the humeroulnar joint often causes increasing instability and recurrence of pain.

Progressive bone destruction and instability may call for reconstructive surgery. There is a dilemma: arthrodesis is very disabling and is unlikely to be accepted by the patient; yet joint

replacement is difficult to perform, uncertain in its outcome and fraught with complications such as infection, instability and dislocation, ulnar neuropathy and aseptic loosening of the implants. Nevertheless, total elbow replacement (either an unconstrained resurfacing or a semiconstrained arthroplasty) is gaining acceptance (Souter, 1989).

Osteoarthritis

(see also Chapter 5)

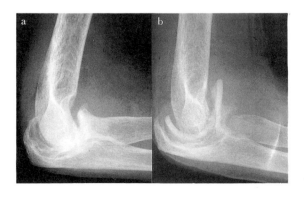

14.9 Arthroplasty   (a) Before and (b) after an interposition arthroplasty with a sheet of Silastic. The patient was well pleased with the relief of pain.

Osteoarthritis of the elbow is uncommon and usually denotes some recognizable underlying pathology – a previous fracture or ligamentous injury, loose bodies in the joint, long-standing occupational stress, inflammatory arthritis or gout. 'Primary' osteoarthritis – especially when it is part of a polyarticular disorder – strongly suggests calcium pyrophosphate deposition disease (see Chapter 4).

The *clinical features* are those of osteoarthritis elsewhere: pain; stiffness, especially following periods of inactivity; local tenderness; thickening of the joint; crepitus; and restriction of movement. Osteophytic hypertrophy may cause ulnar nerve palsy.

X-rays show narrowing of the joint space with

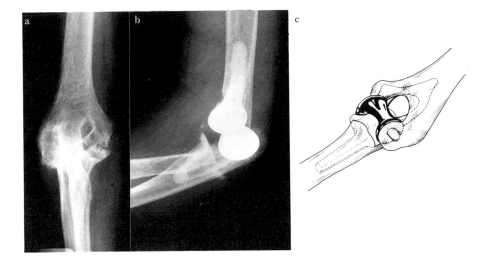

14.10 Total elbow replacement (a) Severe rheumatoid arthritis of the elbow. (b) X-ray after joint replacement. (c) The Souter arthroplasty: a metal humeral prosthesis and polyethylene ulnar implant.

sclerosis and osteophytes. One or more loose bodies may be seen; chondrocalcinosis and periarticular calcification are typical of pyrophosphate arthropathy.

Treatment is usually limited to pain control and the use of non-steroidal anti-inflammatory preparations. Loose bodies, if they cause locking, should be removed. If there are signs of ulnar neuritis, the nerve should be transposed.

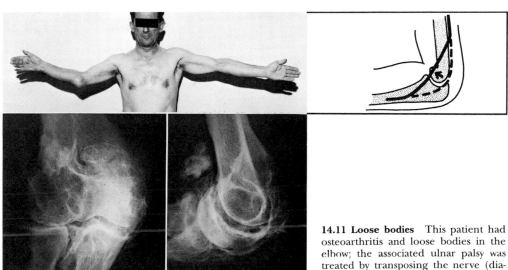

14.11 Loose bodies This patient had osteoarthritis and loose bodies in the elbow; the associated ulnar palsy was treated by transposing the nerve (diagram).

Neuropathic arthritis

(see also Chapter 5)

Neuropathic arthritis of the elbow is seen in syringomyelia. Sometimes neurological features predominate and the diagnosis may be known; occasionally the patient presents with progressive instability of the elbow. The joint may be markedly swollen and hypermobile, with coarse crepitation on passive movement, or it may be completely flail. Treatment consists of splintage to maintain stability.

Other causes of flail elbow include an old gunshot wound and neglected rheumatoid arthritis.

Stiffness of the elbow

BOTH ELBOWS
The commonest cause of bilateral stiffness is rheumatoid arthritis; other causes include arthrogryposis and ankylosing spondylitis. If both elbows are completely stiff at impractical angles, disability is severe; arthroplasty or joint replacement, to enable at least one hand to reach the mouth, may be needed.

ONE ELBOW
Congenital synostosis of the superior radio-ulnar joint (with loss of rotation) is only moderately inconvenient, but if the humerus shares in the synostosis the disability is considerable; a more useful angle can be achieved by

osteotomy, although the stiffness is of course unaffected.

Post-traumatic stiffness

Temporary stiffness may follow any elbow injury; although manipulation under anaesthesia may improve movement at other joints, at the elbow it often makes matters worse and should not be attempted. Permanent limitation of movement is likely after severe fractures into the joint in adults, or when injury has been complicated by myositis ossificans.

To minimize post-traumatic stiffness, an injured elbow should be rested and forced movements absolutely prohibited. At the first suggestion of myositis ossificans, complete rest in a plaster gutter is imperative; non-steroidal anti-inflammatory drugs may help to prevent further ossification. When the calcified area has become well defined (and this may take several years) it can be removed, sometimes with benefit.

Tennis elbow (lateral epicondylitis)

Pain and tenderness over the lateral epicondyle of the elbow is a common complaint among tennis players – but even more common in non-players (Coonrad and Hooper, 1973). The

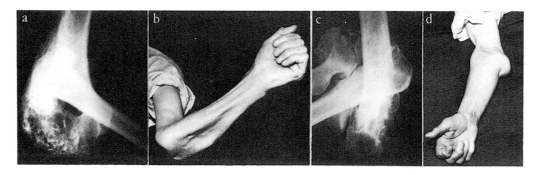

14.12 Flail elbow   (a, b) Following gunshot wound; (c, d) neuropathic arthritis.

exact cause is unknown, but the condition is probably a chronic tendinitis of the common extensor origin, rather similar to the 'overuse' or 'attrition' lesions of the rotator cuff at the shoulder. Like supraspinatus tendinitis, it may result in small tears, fibrocartilaginous metaplasia, microscopic calcification and a painful vascular reaction in the tendon fibres close to the lateral epicondyle.

Clinical features

Pain comes on gradually, often after a period of unaccustomed elbow activity. It is usually localized to the lateral epicondyle, but in severe cases it may radiate widely. It is aggravated by movements such as pouring out tea, turning a stiff doorhandle, shaking hands or lifting with the forearm pronated.

The elbow looks normal, and flexion and extension are full and painless. Characteristically there is localized tenderness just below the lateral epicondyle; pain can be reproduced by passively stretching the wrist extensors or actively extending the wrist with the elbow straight.

The *x-ray* is usually normal, but occasionally shows calcification at the tendon origin.

Treatment

Many methods of treatment are available; a useful sequence is as follows.

1. INJECTION   The tender area is injected with a mixture of 1% lignocaine and methylprednisolone. If the condition is improved, but not cured, the injection is repeated 3 weeks later.

2. PHYSIOTHERAPY Deep transverse frictions, though sometimes effective, are painful; a more comfortable alternative is ultrasound.

3. MANIPULATIONS   The elbow is forcibly extended with the forearm prone and the wrist fully palmarflexed.

4. REST   If the patient will submit to resting the arm in a sling or, better still, in plaster, for several weeks, recovery is usual.

5. OPERATION   A few cases are sufficiently persistent or recurrent for operation to be indicated. The origin of the common extensor muscle is detached from the lateral epicondyle. Additional procedures such as division of the orbicular ligament or removal of a 'synovial fringe' are sometimes advocated; they probably make very little difference to the outcome.

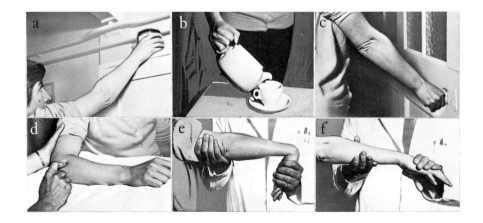

14.13 Tennis elbow Symptoms: (a, b, c) movements that cause pain – in all three the extensor carpi radialis brevis is in action.
Signs: (d) localized tenderness; (e) pain on passive stretching; (f) pain on resisted dorsiflexion.

Other overuse syndromes

Golfer's elbow is comparable to tennis elbow except that the flexor origin (not the extensor) is affected. Treatment is similar.

Javelin throwers using the over-arm action may avulse the tip of the olecranon; with the round-arm action the medial ligament may be avulsed.

Baseball pitchers may suffer extensive elbow damage with hypertrophy of the lower humerus which no longer fits into the olecranon, and loose-body formation. The junior equivalent (little leaguer's elbow) is partial avulsion of the medial epicondyle.

Bursitis

The olecranon bursa sometimes becomes enlarged as a result of pressure or friction; if the enlargement is a nuisance the fluid may be aspirated.

The commonest non-traumatic cause is gout; there may be a sizeable lump with calcification on x-ray. A chronically enlarged bursa may need excision. In rheumatoid arthritis, also, the bursa may become enlarged, but more often subcutaneous nodules develop just distal to the olecranon process; painful nodules sometimes need to be excised.

Nerve lesions

Ulnar nerve

Ulnar palsy is often the sequel to elbow disorders such as osteoarthritis, valgus deformity or constriction of the nerve by a fibrous band at the proximal end of the flexor carpi ulnaris muscle (ulnar tunnel). Occasionally, the nerve repeatedly dislocates forwards.

The usual presenting symptom is numbness or weakness in the hand. Clawing may develop and the interossei (especially the first) are wasted. The nerve may be tender in the region of the elbow.

The nerve can be freed by dividing the roof of the ulnar tunnel if this is the cause; but transposition to the front of the elbow is more reliable. Through a long incision curving behind the medial epicondyle, the ulnar nerve is mobilized for several centimetres. The common flexor origin is then detached and the nerve is transposed to the front of the elbow, deep to the muscle belly and in the same plane as the median nerve. The distal part of the medial intermuscular septum must be excised to prevent kinking of the nerve. The common flexor tendon is reattached, and at the end of the operation the elbow is immobilized flexed for 3 weeks.

Posterior interosseous nerve

Posterior interosseous nerve lesions just below the elbow can give rise to palsy. Tumour (e.g. lipoma), ganglion, fibrosis and traumatic neuritis have all been described. The treatment is operative decompression.

Notes on applied anatomy

The elbow needs to be able to convey the hand upwards to the head and mouth, downwards to the perineum and legs, and also to a wide variety of working positions at bench, desk, wall or table. A varied combination of flexion and extension with pronation and supination is clearly needed.

The hinge at which flexion and extension take place is a complex one. The humeroulnar component needs not only flexibility but also stability, for pushing (or using crutches); this combination is provided by the conformity of the pulley (the trochlea) with the olecranon.

In the coronal plane the axis of the hinge is tilted so that, in full extension, the elbow is in a few degrees of valgus. This 'carrying' angle may be altered by malunion of a fracture or by epiphyseal damage; increased valgus is likely to stretch the ulnar nerve as it passes behind the medial condyle. Distal to the condyle the nerve is closely applied to the elbow capsule, and there also it may be affected if the joint is osteoarthritic. If transposition of the ulnar nerve to the front is needed, it is important to divide the lower end of the medial intermuscular septum, otherwise the nerve may be kinked.

On the lateral side of the elbow the posterior interosseous nerve passes between the two parts of the supinator muscle, and there it is vulnerable when the head of the radius is being approached surgically. In front of the elbow lies the brachialis muscle and also the median nerve in company with the great vessels; these relationships make an anterior approach to the elbow somewhat uninviting.

Pronation and supination seldom take place at the radioulnar joints alone, nearly always there is movement also at the shoulder and a small amount of abduction and adduction occurs between the olecranon and the trochlea. The humeroradial joint is held in position by the strong annular (orbicular) ligament which embraces the head and neck of the radius but is not attached to it. The capsule of the elbow is attached to the annular ligament but also is not attached to the radius. The circular and slightly concave upper surface of the radius ensures that in all positions of rotation it retains adequate contact with the capitulum.

Elbow injuries are common in children, and a knowledge of the ossific centres is important. That for the capitulum appears at the age of 2 years, the medial epicondylar epiphysis appears at 5 and the trochlear epiphysis at 10. The centre for the lateral condyle does not appear until the age of 12, so avulsion before that age will not show on x-ray. Any doubts as to whether these centres are normal on an x-ray are best resolved by comparison with a film of the uninjured elbow.

References and further reading

Capener, N. (1966) The vulnerability of the posterior interosseous nerve of the forearm. *Journal of Bone and Joint Surgery* **48B**, 770–773 [see also 3 following articles in that issue]

Coonrad, R.W. and Hooper, W.R. (1973) Tennis elbow: course, natural history; conservative and surgical management. *Journal of Bone and Joint Surgery* **55A**, 1177–1187

Godshall, R.W. and Hansen, C.A. (1971) Traumatic ulnar neuropathy in adolescent baseball pitchers. *Journal of Bone and Joint Surgery* **53A**, 359–361

MacNicol, M.F. (1979) The results of operation for ulnar neuritis. *Journal of Bone and Joint Surgery* **61B**, 159–164

Roles, N.C. and Maudsley, R.H. (1972) Radial tunnel syndrome. *Journal of Bone and Joint Surgery* **54B**, 499–508

Souter, W.A. (1989) Surgery for rheumatoid arthritis. 1. Upper limb. Surgery of the elbow. *Current Orthopaedics* **3**, 9–13

The wrist

15

Examination

Symptoms

Pain may be localized to the radial side (especially in tenovaginitis of the thumb tendons), to the ulnar side (possibly from the radioulnar joint) or to the dorsum (the usual site in disorders of the carpus).

Stiffness is often not noticed until it is severe.

Swelling may signify involvement of either the joint or the tendon sheaths.

Deformity is a late symptom except after trauma.

Loss of function After pain, the commonest symptom is diminished function in the hand – a firm grip is possible only with a strong, stable, painless wrist that also has a reasonable range of movement.

Signs

Examination of the wrist is not complete without also examining the elbow, forearm and hand. Both upper limbs should be completely exposed.

● LOOK

The skin is inspected for scars. Both wrists and forearms are compared to see if there is any deformity. If there is swelling, note whether it is diffuse or localized to one of the tendon sheaths.

296

● FEEL

Undue warmth is noted. Tender areas must be accurately localized and the bony landmarks compared with those of the normal wrist. The site of tenderness may be diagnostic in (1) de Quervain's disease (tip of radial styloid), (2) scaphoid fracture (anatomical snuffbox), (3)

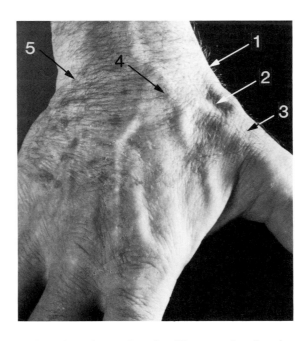

15.1 Tender points at the wrist The exact site of tenderness may be diagnostic for: (1) de Quervain's disease: (2) scaphoid fracture; (3) carpometacarpal osteoarthritis; (4) tenosynovitis of extensor carpi radialis brevis; (5) tenosynovitis of extensor carpi ulnaris.

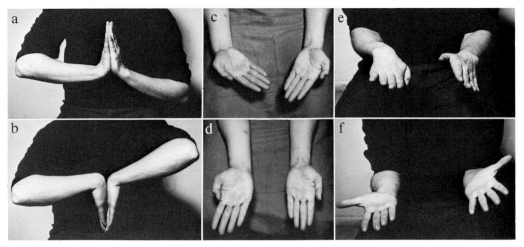

15.2 Examination   All movements of the left wrist are limited: (a) dorsiflexion, (b) palmarflexion, (c) ulnar deviation, (d) radial deviation, (e) pronation, (f) supination.

Kienböck's disease (over the lunate), (4) carpometacarpal osteoarthritis (base of first metacarpal) and (5) localized tenosynovitis of any of the wrist tendons.

● MOVE

To compare passive dorsiflexion of the wrists the patient places his palms together in the position of prayer, then elevates his elbows. Palmarflexion is examined in a similar way. Radial and ulnar deviation are measured in either the palms-up or the palms-down position. With the elbows at right angles and tucked in to the sides, pronation and supination are assessed. Active movements should be tested against resistance; loss of power may be due to

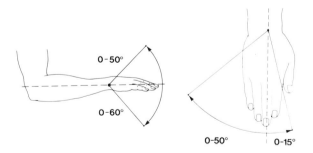

15.3 Normal range of movement   From the neutral position dorsiflexion is slightly less than palmarflexion. Most hand functions are performed with the wrist in ulnar deviation; normal radial deviation is only about 15 degrees.

pain, tendon rupture or muscle weakness. Grip strength can be gauged by having the patient squeeze the examiner's hand; mechanical instruments allow more accurate assessment of both power grip and pinch.

While testing passive movements, the presence of abnormal 'clicks' should be noted; they may signify one or other form of carpal instability.

● X-RAY

Anteroposterior and lateral views are routinely obtained, and often both wrists must be x-rayed for comparison. Special views may be necessary to show scaphoid fractures or carpal instability. Note the position of the carpal bones and look for evidence of joint space narrowing, especially at the carpometacarpal joint of the thumb.

Wrist deformities

Congenital and childhood deformities

Congenital deformities are uncommon and, either because they are merely part of a generalized disorder or because hand function is still incompletely developed, often neglected. Some of the least rare disorders are described below.

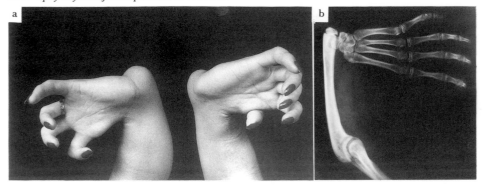

15.4 Radial club hand   (a) Bilateral. (b) X-ray of a unilateral case – the entire radius is absent.

Carpal fusions

Coalescence of two or more of the carpal bones is the commonest congenital abnormality; it is usually inherited as an autosomal dominant trait and may be bilateral. Often it is associated with other abnormalities. It seldom causes problems and no treatment is necessary.

Radial club hand

The infant is born with the wrist in marked radial deviation. There is absence of the whole or part of the radius and usually also the thumb or the entire first two rays of the hand. It may occur as an isolated abnormality or as part of a generalized dysplasia.

Treatment in the neonate consists of gentle manipulation and splintage. Operations to stabilize and centralize the carpus may be cosmetically attractive, but they seldom improve function; the untreated deformity may already be in the hand-to-mouth position. If function deteriorates, centralization of the carpus over the ulna is recommended, preferably before the age of 3 years.

Madelung's deformity

In this deformity the lower radius curves forwards, carrying with it the carpus and hand but leaving the lower ulna sticking out as a lump on the back of the wrist. It may be congenital or post-traumatic. The congenital disorder may appear as an isolated entity or as part of a generalized dysplasia; although the abnormality is present at birth, the deformity is rarely seen before the age of 10 years, after which it increases until growth is complete. Function is usually excellent.

Treatment   If deformity is severe the lower end of the ulna may be excised (Darrach's procedure); this is sometimes combined with osteotomy of the radius.

Ulnar club hand

In this rare deformity ulnar deviation is present at birth and is due to partial or complete

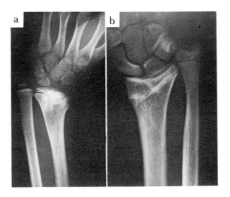

15.5 Madelung's deformity   (a) Damage to radial growth disc, which might cause (b) Madelung's deformity.

absence of the ulna; in addition the ulnar rays of the hand may be missing. As the child grows the radial head may dislocate.

Treatment consists of stretching and splintage during the first few months. If deformity is marked, excision of the ulnar anlage and osteotomy of the radius may improve the appearance.

Distal ulnar dysplasia

In older children with hereditary multiple exostoses there is often disproportionate shortening of the ulna; its distal end becomes carrot-shaped and the radius is bowed. The same deformity is sometimes seen in dyschondroplasia, and occasionally without any obvious bone disease.

Treatment is seldom necessary. If deformity is marked, ulnar lengthening (with or without osteotomy of the radius) may be advisable.

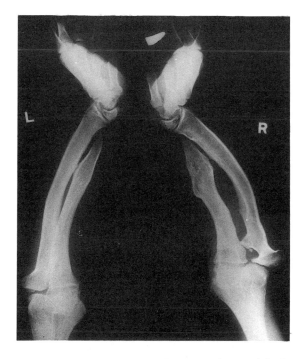

15.6 Distal ulnar dysplasia The x-ray characteristically shows a tapering, carrot-shaped distal end of ulna. This bilateral case was due to hereditary multiple exostoses; there is bilateral bowing of the radius and on the right side the radial head has dislocated.

Acquired deformities

Various deformities may follow injury or disease of the wrist.

Physeal injury

Fracture-separation of the distal radial epiphysis may result in partial fusion of the physis, with asymmetrical growth deformity of the wrist. The bony bridge crossing the physis, if it is small, may be excised and replaced by a fat graft. Once growth slows down the deformity can be corrected by a suitable osteotomy, if necessary combined with soft-tissue release.

Forearm fractures

After a Colles' fracture radial deviation and posterior angulation are common. These deformities cause little disability but may look ugly.

Subluxation of the distal radioulnar joint may result in prominence of the ulnar head and loss of pronation or supination. This can sometimes be treated by reconstructing the distal articulation; otherwise the head of the ulna may need to be excised. In young patients abnormal angulation of the radius may lead to progressive carpal collapse and loss of grip strength. A radial osteotomy is then necessary.

Rheumatoid deformities

The typical rheumatoid deformity is radial deviation of the wrist, with or without radio-ulnar subluxation. With erosion of the radiocarpal joint, forward subluxation of the carpus develops (see below).

Drop wrist

With radial nerve palsy the wrist drops into flexion and active extension is lost. If the nerve does not recover, tendon transfers may successfully restore function.

Kienböck's disease

Robert Kienböck, in 1910, described what he called 'traumatic softening' of the lunate bone. This is a form of ischaemic necrosis that usually follows chronic stress or injury. It has been suggested that relative shortening of the ulna ('negative ulnar variance') predisposes to compression of the lunate against the distal edge of the radius, but this has not been proven convincingly (Gelberman et al., 1975). The condition is not uncommon in cerebral palsy.

Pathology

As in other forms of ischaemic necrosis, the pathological changes proceed in four stages: *stage 1*, ischaemia without naked-eye or radiographic abnormality; *stage 2*, trabecular necrosis with reactive new bone formation and increased radiographic density, but little or no distortion of shape; *stage 3*, collapse of the bone; and *stage 4*, disruption of radiocarpal congruence and secondary osteoarthritis.

Clinical features

The patient, usually a young adult, complains of ache and stiffness; only occasionally is there a history of acute trauma. Tenderness is localized over the lunate and grip strength is diminished. In the later stages wrist movements are limited and painful.

X-rays at first show no abnormality, but radioscintigraphy may reveal increased activity. Later there is either mottled or diffuse density of the bone. In stage 3 the bone looks squashed and irregular, and in stage 4 there are osteoarthritic changes in the wrist.

Treatment

In early cases, splintage of the wrist for 6–12 weeks relieves pain and possibly reduces lunate compression. If bone healing catches up with ischaemia, the lunate – though dense – may remain virtually undistorted. However, if pain persists, and even more so if the bone begins to flatten, operative treatment is indicated.

OPERATIVE TREATMENT While the wrist architecture is only minimally disturbed (i.e. up to early stage 3), it seems rational to aim for a redistribution of carpal stress by either shortening the radius or performing a distal wedge osteotomy that allows the medial edge of the radius to tilt away from the lunate. Excellent results have been reported with radial shortening, even for stage 3 disease (Nakamura, Imaeda and Miura, 1990; Weiss et al., 1991). Ulnar lengthening, with the same objective, seems to be mechanically less satisfactory.

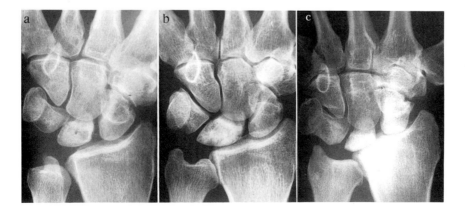

15.7 Kienböck's disease: three patients (a) In stage 2 – the bone shows mottled increase of density, but is still normal in shape. (b) In stage 3 – density is more marked and the lunate looks slightly squashed. (c) In stage 4 – the bone has collapsed and there is radiocarpal osteoarthritis. In all three the ulna looks a little short.

Once the bone has collapsed, the options are limited. Lunate replacement by a silicone prosthesis, once popular, gives poor long-term results and is no longer advocated (Alexander et al., 1990). Other procedures, such as intercarpal fusion or excision of the proximal row of the carpus, may improve function but in the long term will not prevent the occurrence of osteoarthritis. If osteoarthritis does supervene, the alternatives are (1) splintage and stoic acceptance or (2) arthrodesis of the wrist.

Carpal instability

Rheumatoid arthritis characteristically causes joint erosion and instability of the wrist.

Post-traumatic instability is less obvious; the precipitating injury may be slight and is sometimes forgotten.

Pathology

Abnormal movement between individual carpal bones or between the carpus and the forearm bones may result in a variety of anatomical abnormalities, some of them static and some becoming apparent only when the wrist is moved and stressed.

A number of classifications, based on different perceptions of carpal mechanics, have been proposed (Linscheid et al., 1972; Alexander and Lichtman, 1984; Taleisnik, 1988; Weber, 1988). Basic to an understanding of the pathomechanics is the recognition that the wrist functions as a system of intercalated segments or links, stabilized by the intercarpal ligaments and the scaphoid which acts as a bridge between the proximal and distal rows of the carpus. If the ligaments are torn, or the scaphoid is fractured, the segments may collapse – either as a static deformity or perhaps only on contraction of the surrounding muscles. Normally the longitudinal axes of the radius, lunate, capitate and third metacarpal form a straight line; if the middle segments collapse, this line becomes zig-zag. In *dorsal intercalated segmental instability* (DISI) the distal

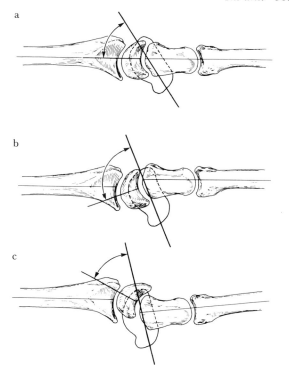

15.8 Carpal instability The relationships of the carpal bones in (a) the normal wrist, (b) DISI and (c) VISI.

articular surface of the lunate tilts (rotates) dorsally and the scaphoid tilts volarwards; this may be associated with unstable scaphoid fractures or scapholunate dissociation. In *volar intercalated segmental instability* (VISI) the distal surface of the lunate is rotated in a palmar direction; here the ligamentous disruption is mainly between the lunate and triquetrum.

For practical purposes, three types of instability are distinguished: lateral, medial and proximal.

LATERAL CARPAL INSTABILITY This usually takes the form of *scapholunate dissociation* – the commonest type of carpal instability. It may follow perilunar dislocation but it also occurs as an isolated injury. It is often associated with dorsal segmental instability (DISI) and volar rotation of the scaphoid.

Scaphocapitate and *scaphotrapezial disruption* are rare forms of lateral instability.

MEDIAL CARPAL INSTABILITY There is usually a *triquetrolunate dissociation* and volar rotation of the lunate (VISI); the scapholunate relationship remains intact.

PROXIMAL CARPAL INSTABILITY Here the instability is at the radiocarpal joint. The commonest form is *ulnar translocation* of the carpus. It may follow an injury to the wrist, but it is also one of the characteristic deformities of rheumatoid arthritis. The carpus migrates ulnarwards and rotates towards the radial side. Dorsal and volar *radiocarpal subluxation* are uncommon, except in advanced erosive arthritis. Malunion of distal radial fractures sometimes results in secondary dynamic instability without either scapholunate or triquetrolunate dissociation.

Clinical features

There may be a history of injury – usually a fall on the outstretched hand. In rheumatoid arthritis, wrist deformity appears insidiously.

The patient complains of pain or weakness in the wrist, and certain movements may cause clicking or snapping. Tenderness may be localized to a specific site in the wrist. Clicking may be elicited by rotating the wrist during axial compression; if this is consistently associated with pain, instability should be suspected.

X-ray

Diagnosis usually hinges on the x-ray. At least four views are needed: posteroanterior, with the wrist pronated, in both ulnar and medial deviation; anteroposterior, with the wrist supinated; and a true lateral view to show the relationships of the radial, lunate and capitate axes.

In *scapholunate dissociation* the anteroposterior x-ray shows an abnormal gap between the scaphoid and lunate (the Terry-Thomas sign); the rotated scaphoid looks foreshortened, with a cortical ring of density. The lateral view may show dorsal rotation of the lunate and volar rotation of the scaphoid (DISI).

In *triquetrolunate dissociation* there may be a

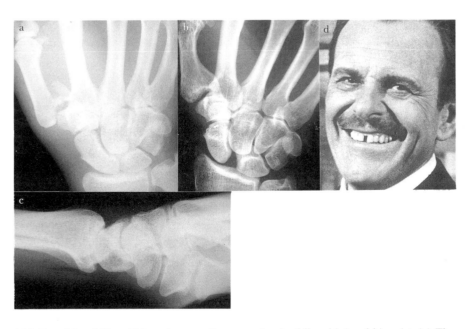

15.9 Carpal instability This patient was first seen after he fell and injured his wrist. (a) The x-ray showed a Bennett's fracture of the base of the first metacarpal and no other injury was apparent. A year later he was still complaining of pain in the wrist; x-rays at this stage (b, c) showed a gap between the scaphoid and lunate (the Terry-Thomas sign), rotation of the scaphoid and – in the lateral view – dorsal tilting of the lunate. (d) The actor, Terry-Thomas (reproduced by permission; © United Artists Inc.).

gap, and the dorsally rotated triquetrum appears triangular in shape; the lateral view may show the lunate tilted towards the palm (VISI).

Ulnar translocation and *wrist subluxation* are usually obvious; there may, in addition, be signs of previous fracture or rheumatoid arthritis.

Treatment

The best 'treatment' is to make the correct diagnosis at the time of injury, to reduce the carpal displacement (if necessary by operation), and to hold the position (either with plaster or with Kirschner wires) until the ligaments heal.

In chronic instability, ligament repair is impractical. Conservative treatment is mainly palliative and consists of local splintage, corticosteroid injections (occasionally) and analgesic or anti-inflammatory preparations if pain is marked.

Operative treatment is indicated if discomfort and weakness seriously interfere with daily activities. Sometimes a limited intercarpal arthrodesis is feasible. However, if the radiocarpal joint is involved, wrist arthrodesis is probably more suitable.

Tuberculosis (see also Chapter 2)

At the wrist, tuberculosis is rarely seen until it has progressed to a true arthritis. Pain and stiffness come on gradually and the hand feels weak. The forearm looks wasted; the wrist is swollen and feels warm. Involvement of the flexor tendon compartment may give rise to a large fluctuant swelling that crosses the wrist into the palm (compound palmar ganglion). In a neglected case there may be a sinus. Movements are restricted and painful.

X-rays show localized osteoporosis and irregularity of the radiocarpal and intercarpal joints, and sometimes bone erosion.

Diagnosis

The condition must be differentiated from rheumatoid arthritis. Bilateral arthritis of the wrist is nearly always rheumatoid in origin, but when only one wrist is affected the signs resemble those of tuberculosis. X-rays and serological tests may establish the diagnosis, but often a biopsy is necessary.

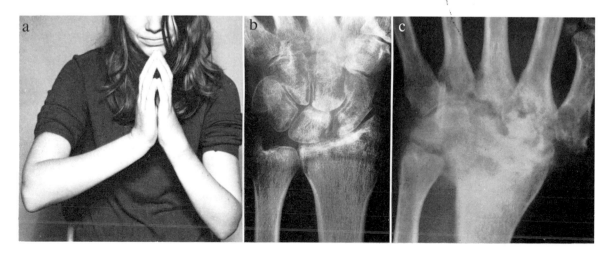

15.10 Tuberculosis (a) This girl presented with chronic ache and swelling of her left wrist; the forearm was wasted and extension absent; (b) her x-ray shows the washed-out appearance of osteoporosis around the wrist. (c) A different patient who had severe tuberculous arthritis; the disease is no longer active (hence the dense appearance), but destruction has been extensive.

Treatment

Antituberculous drugs are given and the wrist is splinted. If an abscess forms, it must be drained. If the wrist is destroyed, systemic treatment should be continued until the disease is quiescent and the wrist is then arthrodesed.

Rheumatoid arthritis

(see also Chapter 3)

After the metacarpophalangeal joints, the wrist is the most common site of rheumatoid arthritis. Tenosynovitis may lead to tendon ruptures; this, together with erosion of the radiocarpal and intercarpal joints, often leads to instability. An unstable wrist means a weak hand; deformities of the metacarpophalangeal joints are almost invariably associated with complementary deformities of the wrist.

Clinical features

Pain, swelling and tenderness usually start on the ulnar side and are due either to tenosynovi-tis of the extensor carpi ulnaris or to erosion of the radioulnar joint. With extension to the radiocarpal joint, the wrist gradually drifts into radial deviation and volar subluxation. *X-rays* reveal osteoporosis and erosion of the ulnar styloid and of the radiocarpal and intercarpal joints.

Pain and instability at the wrist contribute significantly to the loss of power grip in the hand, and radial deviation of the carpus may predispose to 'compensatory' ulnar drift of the fingers.

Treatment

In the early stage (synovitis or tenosynovitis) splintage and intrasynovial injection of hydrocortisone and nitrogen mustard are usually effective. In the second stage (early joint erosion with minimal instability) synovectomy and soft-tissue stabilization may prevent further destruction and deformity; this may be combined with excision of the ulnar head and transposition of the extensor carpi radialis longus to the ulnar side of the wrist (to counteract its tendency to radial drift). In stage 3, articular destruction and radiocarpal dislocation may require either arthrodesis or an arthroplasty with a Silastic prosthesis.

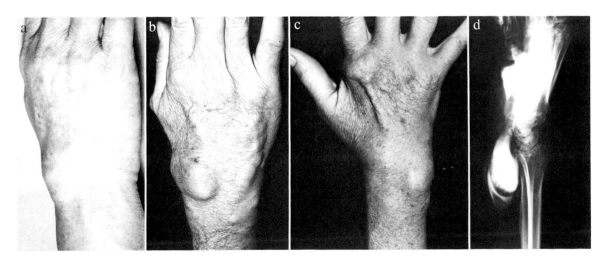

15.11 Rheumatoid arthritis (1)   (a) Synovitis of the wrist; (b) here there is also tenosynovitis of the extensor carpi ulnaris; (c) synovitis of the inferior radioulnar joint; (d) contrast radiography showing a large protrusion from the flexor sheath.

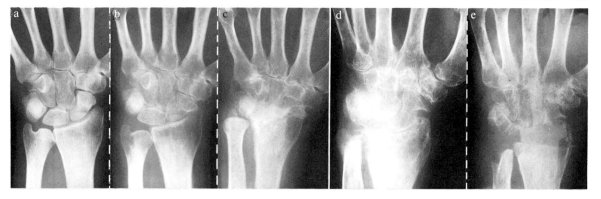

15.12 Rheumatoid arthritis (2)   (a) At first the x-rays show only soft-tissue swelling; (b) 7 years later, this patient shows early bone changes – periarticular osteoporosis and diminution of the joint space; (c) 5 years later still, bony erosions and joint destruction are marked. (d) Another patient with severe disease, who has been treated by (e) excising the diseased surfaces and inserting a Silastic spacer – reasonable stability was restored; this can be done only if the joint has not been too severely distorted.

Osteoarthritis

Osteoarthritis of the wrist is uncommon except as the sequel to injury. Any fracture into the joint may predispose to osteoarthritis, but the commonest is a fractured scaphoid, especially with non-union or avascular necrosis. Post-traumatic carpal instability and Kienböck's disease are less frequent causes.

Clinical features

The patient may have forgotten the original injury. Years later he complains of pain and stiffness. At first these occur intermittently after use; later they become more constant, and recurrent 'wrist sprains' are common.

The appearance is usually normal and there is no wasting. Movements at the wrist and radioulnar joints are limited and painful.

X-rays show irregular narrowing at the radio-carpal joint, with bone sclerosis; the proximal portion of the scaphoid or the lunate may be irregular and dense.

Treatment

Rest, in a polythene splint, is often sufficient treatment. Excision of the radial styloid process is helpful when osteoarthritis has followed scaphoid injury. Arthrodesis of the wrist is rarely necessary.

Carpometacarpal osteoarthritis

Osteoarthritis of the trapeziometacarpal joint is quite common in postmenopausal women. It is often accompanied by Heberden's nodes of the finger joints; in these circumstances it is often bilateral and part of a generalized osteoarthritis.

Clinical features

Except in cases obviously due to local trauma (e.g. a Bennett's fracture), the patient is usually middle-aged and may have osteoarthritis elsewhere. Pain is felt fairly diffusely on the radial side of the wrist, but tenderness and bony thickening are sharply localized to the trapeziometacarpal joint. In advanced cases the thumb metacarpal is adducted, the trapeziometacarpal joint is subluxated and the base of the metacarpal is unusually prominent.

X-rays show narrowing of the trapeziometa-carpal joint. Radioscintigraphy is useful in early

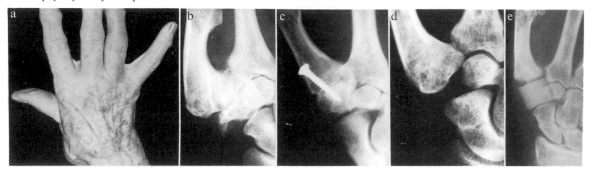

15.13 Osteoarthritis of the carpometacarpal thumb joint   (a) Typical deformity in an advanced case, with (b) narrow joint space and osteophytes. If operation is needed, the possibilities are (c) arthrodesis, (d) excision of the trapezium, or (e) replacement arthroplasty using a Silastic spacer.

cases when the diagnosis is in doubt; increased activity precedes the more obvious x-ray changes.

Treatment

Most patients can be treated by anti-inflammatory preparations, local corticosteroid injections and temporary splintage. If these measures fail to control pain, or if instability becomes marked, operative treatment may be necessary.

Excision of the trapezium (excisional arthroplasty) gives pain relief and return of function, though thumb pinch is always weak. Prosthetic replacement of the trapezium by a silicone implant inserted into the metacarpal bone gives good results, provided local deformity is not marked. An alternative is arthrodesis of the carpometacarpal joint.

Carpal tunnel syndrome

In the normal carpal tunnel there is barely room for all the tendons and the median nerve; consequently, any swelling is likely to result in compression and ischaemia of the nerve. Usually the cause eludes detection; the syndrome is, however, common at the menopause, in rheumatoid arthritis, in pregnancy and in myxoedema. Computed tomography has shown that women have smaller tunnels than men,

and those with carpal tunnel syndrome have the smallest tunnels of all.

There is some evidence that proximal compression of the nerve roots (e.g. by cervical discogenic disease) may act as a predisposing factor to peripheral entrapment.

Clinical features

Pain and paraesthesia occur in the distribution of the median nerve in the hand. Night after night the patient is woken in the early hours with burning pain, tingling and numbness. Hanging the arm over the side of the bed, or shaking the arm, may relieve the symptoms. During the day little pain is felt except with such activities as knitting or holding a newspaper, where the arms are kept immobile. In advanced cases there may be clumsiness and weakness.

The condition is eight times more common in women than in men. The usual age group is 40–50 years; in younger patients it is not uncommon to find related factors such as pregnancy or rheumatoid disease.

Both hands, or only the dominant hand, may be involved. Abnormal physical signs are usually absent; ideally the condition should be diagnosed before signs are obvious. The pattern of sensory changes can sometimes be reproduced by holding the wrist fully palmarflexed for 1 minute or by compressing the arm with a sphygmomanometer cuff. In late cases there is wasting of the thenar muscles and weakness of

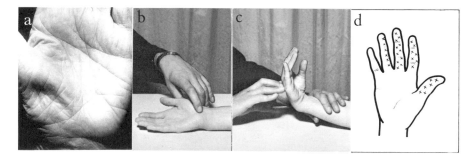

15.14 Carpal tunnel syndrome (a) Wasting of the thenar eminence is seldom obvious and rarely as marked as in this patient. (b) Pressure on the tunnel or (c) forced palmarflexion may induce pain or tingling. (d) The 'map test' – asking the patient to mark out the affected area – may show that it corresponds to the sensory distribution of the median nerve.

thumb abduction. Electrical studies show slowing of nerve conduction across the wrist.

Diagnosis

The symptoms of carpal tunnel syndrome are easily mistaken for those of cervical spondylosis involving C6 and C7. X-ray signs of cervical disc degeneration are common in older people and this adds to the confusion. The classic complaint of pain and paraesthesia at night together with nerve conduction changes help to establish the diagnosis.

Treatment

In the vast majority of cases, operative division of the anterior carpal ligament offers a quick and simple cure. Conservative treatment may be preferable during pregnancy; the wrist is splinted at night to prevent it folding into flexion.

de Quervain's disease (stenosing tenovaginitis)

Painful thickening of the tendon sheath containing extensor pollicis brevis and abductor pollis longus was described by Fritz de Quervain almost 100 years ago. The condition is due to excessive or prolonged friction where the tendons emerge from the sheath at the distal end of the radius. The sheath becomes inflamed and thickened, but the tendons are normal.

Clinical features

The condition is most common in women aged 40–50, who complain of pain on the radial side of the wrist. There may be a history of unaccustomed activity such as pruning roses or wringing out clothes. Sometimes there is a visible swelling over the distal end of the radius,

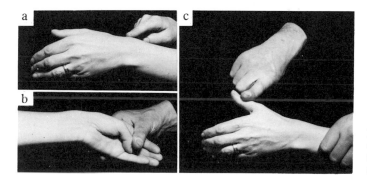

15.15 de Quervain's disease (a) The patient can point to the painful area; (b) forced adduction is painful; (c) pain on active extension against resistance.

and the tendon sheath feels thick and hard. Tenderness is most acute at the very tip of the radial styloid. Abduction of the thumb against resistance and passive adduction of the thumb across the palm (Finkelstein's test) are both painful.

Diagnosis

The condition must be distinguished from an *ununited scaphoid fracture* and *osteoarthritis of the trapeziometacarpal joint*, both of which cause pain and tenderness somewhat distal to the radial styloid.

Treatment

The early case can be relieved by a corticosteroid injection into the tendon sheath, sometimes combined with plaster splintage of the wrist. Resistant cases need an operation, which consists of slitting the thickened tendon sheath. Sometimes there is duplication of tendons and even of the sheath, in which case both sheaths need to be divided. Care should be taken to prevent injury to the dorsal sensory branches of the radial nerve, which may cause intractable dysaesthesia.

Swellings around the wrist

Ganglion

The ubiquitous ganglion most commonly appears on the back of the wrist. It arises not by synovial herniation from a joint or tendon sheath but from cystic degeneration within the substance of the capsule or fibrous sheath. The distended cyst contains a glairy, viscous fluid.

The patient, often a young adult, presents with a painless lump, though occasionally there is slight ache and weakness. The lump is well defined, cystic and not tender; it can sometimes be transilluminated and may feel more tense when the tendons are put into action. The back of the wrist is the commonest site, but ganglia in front may compress a nerve or penetrate between the fibres, causing numbness or weakness.

Treatment is usually unnecessary. The lump can safely be left alone; it often disappears spontaneously. If it becomes troublesome, and certainly if there is any pressure on a nerve, operative removal is justified. Even then it may recur with embarrassing persistence; it is not easy to ensure that every shred of abnormal tissue is removed.

Tenosynovitis

Swelling of the tendon sheaths on the dorsum of the wrist is often seen in rheumatic disease. Sometimes this is associated with tendon ruptures and loss of active extension of the metacarpophalangeal joints. The diagnosis is seldom in doubt. If operative synovectomy is performed, the stretched sheath should be carefully preserved and passed deep to the tendons to reline the dorsum of the wrist.

Compound palmar ganglion

Chronic inflammation distends the common sheath of the flexor tendons both above and below the flexor retinaculum. Rheumatoid arthritis and tuberculosis are the commonest causes. The synovial membrane becomes thick and villous. The amount of fluid is increased and it may contain fibrin particles moulded by repeated movement to the shape of melon seeds. The tendons may eventually fray and rupture.

Pain is unusual but paraesthesia due to median nerve compression may occur. The swelling is hourglass in shape, bulging above and below the flexor retinaculum; it is not warm or tender; fluid can be pushed from one part to the other (cross-fluctuation).

If the condition is tuberculous, general treatment is begun (p. 49). The contents of the ganglion are evacuated, streptomycin is instilled and the wrist rested in a splint. If these measures fail the entire flexor sheath is dissected out. Complete excision is also the best treatment when the cause is rheumatoid disease.

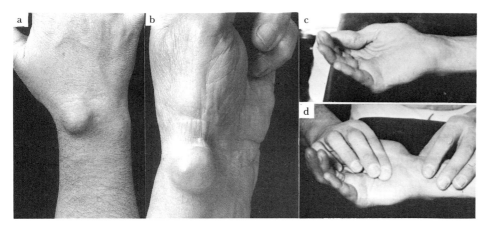

15.16 Wrist swellings   (a, b) Common sites of simple ganglion. (c, d) Compound palmar ganglion with cross-fluctuation.

Notes on applied anatomy

In most positions of the forearm the styloid process of the radius is more distal than that of the ulna, but with the forearm supinated the two processes are at approximately the same level. The relationship may be altered as a result of injury or with Kienböck's disease. Just distal to the radial styloid is the scaphoid, immediately beneath the anatomical snuffbox, which is one of the key areas for localizing tenderness.

Tenderness at the distal end of the snuffbox may incriminate the carpometacarpal joint of the thumb. More proximal tenderness may be from tenovaginitis of the extensor pollicis brevis and abductor pollicis longus; within their fibrous sheath these tendons may be duplicated or triplicated, and, unless this is appreciated, surgical decompression may be inadequate. Dorsal to the snuffbox the oblique course of extensor pollicis longus exposes it to damage by a careless incision.

The mosaic of the carpal bones is arranged in two rows, with the pisiform as the odd man out. The scaphoid, trapezium and thumb combine to function almost as a separate entity, a 'jointed strut', with independent movement; degenerative arthritis of the wrist occurs almost exclusively in the joints of this strut (Fisk, 1970).

Wrist dorsiflexion takes place at both the radiocarpal joint (the first two-thirds) and at the midcarpal joint (the final third). Palmarflexion is predominantly at the radiocarpal joint. Abduction (radial deviation) of the wrist is much less than adduction. When the wrist is fully dorsiflexed the scaphoid, which straddles the midcarpal joint, swivels backwards. Even so, it is vulnerable and liable to fracture. When it does, the more ulnar deviated the wrist, the more proximal is the fracture.

Stability of the carpus depends not only upon bony conformity, joint capsules and overlying tendons but also upon a series of tough ligaments. The volar radiocarpal ligament is the most important of these and, if torn, leads to carpal instability. It is precisely when a scaphoid fracture is associated with carpal instability that complications, such as non-union, are likely to occur.

On their volar aspect the carpal bones form a concavity roofed over by the carpal ligament; in the tunnel lie the flexor tendons and sheath together with the median nerve. The palmar branch of the nerve (supplying the all-important thenar muscles) is in danger if, during a decompression operation, the carpal ligament is divided too far radially. On the radial side of the wrist, branches of the radial nerve are vulnerable; and on the ulnar side, the close relationship of the ulnar nerve to the pisiform must be borne in mind.

References and further reading

Alexander, C.E. and Lichtman, D.M. (1984) Ulnar carpal instabilities. *Orthopedic Clinics of North America* **15**, 307–320

Alexander, A.H., Turner, M.A., Alexander, C.E. and Lichtman, D.M. (1990) Lunate silicone replacement arthroplasty in Kienböck's disease: a long-term follow-up. *Journal of Hand Surgery* **15A**, 401–407

Andren, L. and Eiken, O. (1971) Athrographic studies of wrist ganglions. *Journal of Bone and Joint Surgery* **53A**, 299–302

Fisk, G.R. (1970) Carpal instability and the fractured scaphoid. *Annals of the Royal College of Surgeons of England* **46**, 63–76

Gelberman, R.H., Salamon, P.B., Jurst, J.M. et al. (1975) Ulnar variance with Kienböck's disease. *Journal of Bone and Joint Surgery* **57A**, 674–676

Kienböck, R. (1910, translated in 1980) Concerning traumatic malacia of the lunate and its consequences. *Clinical Orthopaedics* **149**, 4–8

Lamb, D.W. (1972) The treatment of radial club hand. *Hand* **4**, 22–30

Linscheid, R.L., Dobyns, J.H., Beabout, J.W. and Bryan, R.S. (1972) Traumatic instability of the wrist. *Journal of Bone and Joint Surgery* **54A**, 1612–1632

Nakamura, R., Imaeda, T. and Miura, T. (1990) Radial shortening for Kienböck's disease: factors affecting the operative result. *Journal of Hand Surgery* **15B**, 40–45

Ranawat, C.S., Defiore, J. and Straub, L.R. (1975) Madelung's deformity. *Journal of Bone and Joint Surgery* **57A**, 772–775

Roca, J., Beltran, J.E., Fairen, M.F. and Alvarez, A. (1976) Treatment of Kienböck's disease using a silicone rubber implant. *Journal of Bone and Joint Surgery* **58A**, 373–376

Taleisnik, J. (1988) Carpal instability. *Journal of Bone and Joint Surgery* **70A**, 1262–1268

Weber, E.R. (1988) Wrist mechanics and its association with ligamentous instability. In *The Wrist and its Disorders* (ed. D.M. Lichtman), W.B. Saunders, Philadelphia, pp. 41–52

Weiss, A.-P.C., Welland, A.J., Moore, J.R. and Wilgis, E.F.S. (1991) Radial shortening for Kienböck's disease. *Journal of Bone and Joint Surgery* **73A**, 384–391

The hand

16

Examination

The hand is (in more senses than one) the medium of introduction to the outside world. Deformity and loss of function are quickly noticed – and often bitterly resented.

Symptoms

Pain is usually felt in the palm or in the finger joints. A poorly defined ache may be referred from the neck, shoulder or mediastinum.

Deformity may appear suddenly (due to tendon rupture) or slowly (suggesting bone, joint or other pathology).

Swelling may be localized, or may occur in many joints simultaneously. Characteristically, rheumatoid arthritis causes swelling of the proximal joints, and osteoarthritis the distal joints.

Loss of function is particularly troublesome in the hand. The patient may have difficulty handling eating utensils, holding a cup or glass, grasping a doorknob (or a crutch), dressing or (most trying of all) attending to personal hygiene.

Sensory change and motor weakness provide well-defined clues to neurological disorders.

Signs

Both upper limbs should be bared for comparison. Examination of the hand needs patience and meticulous attention to detail. Always ask which is the dominant hand.

● LOOK
The skin may be scarred, altered in colour, dry or moist, and hairy or smooth. Wasting and deformity, and the presence of any lumps, should be noted. The resting posture is an important clue to nerve or tendon damage. Swelling may be in the subcutaneous tissue, in a tendon sheath or in a joint. The nails may show signs of atrophy or disease (e.g. psoriasis).

● FEEL
The temperature and texture of the skin are noted and the pulse is felt. If a nodule is felt, the underlying tendon should be moved to discover if it is attached. Swelling or thickening may be in the subcutaneous tissue, a tendon sheath, a joint or one of the bones. Tenderness should be accurately localized to one of these structures.

● MOVE

Active movements With palms facing upwards the patient is asked to curl the fingers into full flexion; a 'lagging finger' is immediately obvious. Individual movements are then examined, first at the metacarpophalangeal joints and then at each interphalangeal joint in turn. The patient is asked to touch the tip of each finger with the tip of the thumb.

Passive movements are examined in a similar manner, noting and, if necessary, recording the range of movement at each joint.

GRIP STRENGTH
Grip strength is assessed by asking the patient to squeeze the examiner's fingers; it may be diminished because of muscle weakness, finger stiffness or wrist instability. Strength can be

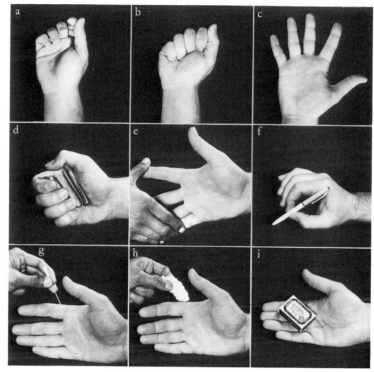

16.1 Examination Positions: (a) resting position, (b) full flexion, (c) full extension.

Strength: (d) power grip, (e) finger abduction, (f) pinch grip.

Sensation: (g) pinprick, (h) light touch, (i) stereognosis.

measured more accurately by having the patient squeeze a partially inflated sphygmomanometer cuff (normally a pressure of 150 mmHg can be achieved easily) or a mechanical dynamometer. Pinch grip also should be measured.

NEUROLOGICAL ASSESSMENT

If symptoms such as numbness, tingling or weakness exist – and in all cases of trauma – a full neurological examination of the upper limbs should be carried out, testing power, reflexes and sensation. Further refinement is achieved by testing two-point discrimination, sensibility to heat and cold, and stereognosis.

FUNCTIONAL TESTS

Ultimately it is function that counts; patients learn to overcome their defects by ingenious modifications and trick movements. Specific activities can be tested by giving the patient a variety of tasks to perform: holding a pencil, turning a key, picking up a pin, gripping a small-handled tool and holding a glass. Each finger has its special task: the thumb and index finger are used for pinch. The index finger is

also an important sensory organ; slight loss of movement matters little, but if sensation is abnormal the patient probably won't use the finger at all. The middle finger controls the position of objects in the palm. The ring and little fingers are used for power grip; any loss of movement here will affect function markedly.

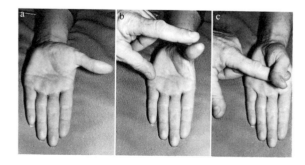

16.2 Movements of the thumb With the hand held flat on the table and palm upwards, the patient is asked (a) to stretch the thumb away from the hand (extension), (b) to lift it towards the ceiling (abduction) and (c) to squeeze down onto the examiner's finger (adduction).

Space & stability

Open & close

Pinch & touch

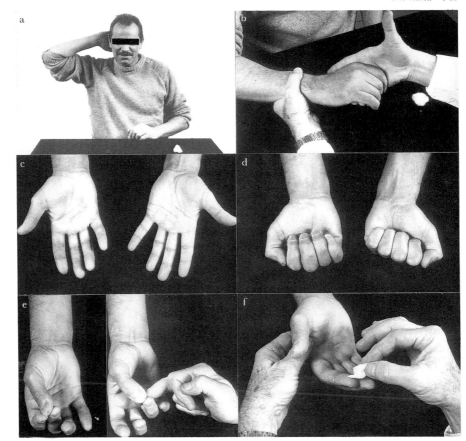

16.3 Rapid assessment When approximate assessment of hand function suffices, three pairs of manoeuvres provide the necessary information. (a, b) Can the patient move his shoulder and position his hand accurately in space (e.g. touch the back of his head), and can he stabilize the wrist during power grip? (c, d) Can the patient spread the extended fingers and thumb apart (enabling large objects to be held), and make a tight fist (needed for holding handles)? (e, f) Can the patient reach his fingertips and then pinch? And can he feel you touching each digit?

RAPID ASSESSMENT

In most cases a rapid assessment can be carried out, and this will indicate whether a more detailed examination is required (see Fig. 16.3).

Deformities of the hand

Congenital deformities

The hand and foot are much the commonest sites of congenital deformities of the musculo-skeletal system; the incidence is no less than 1 in 2500 live births.

Early recognition is important, and definitive treatment should be timed to fit in with the developing skills and functional demands of the child. If surgery is contemplated, it should be carried out as soon as technically feasible and certainly before the age of 3 years. Psychological support for parents and children is important if problems of social adaptation and self-esteem are to be avoided.

Some deformities are due to well-recognized genetic or chromosome disorders; some are due to environmental factors – a viral infection,

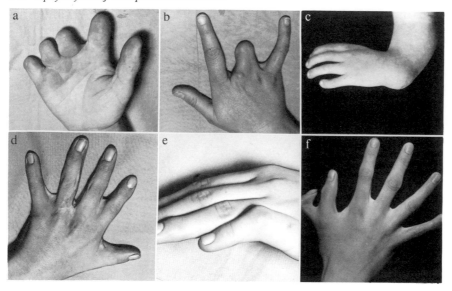

16.4 Congenital deformities   (a) Congenital amputations; (b) missing digits; (c) radial club hand; (d) syndactyly; (e) camptodactyly; (f) extra digits.

nuclear radiation or harmful drug administration during the first 3 months of pregnancy.

The disorders are conveniently divided into five groups: *failure to develop, failure of differentiation, focal defects, overgrowth or undergrowth* and *generalized malformations.*

Failure of development

TRANSVERSE FAILURE   Absence of parts ('congenital amputations') may occur at any level; the commonest is missing fingers.

AXIAL FAILURE   Radial ray, ulnar ray or central defects produce a variety of syndromes.

Radial club hand   is due to partial or complete absence of the radius and thumb; there is marked radial deviation of the wrist. An absent thumb can be treated by pollicization, using the index finger. The full-blown radial club hand should at first be splinted, with the intention of operating before the age of 3 years. During infancy a soft-tissue correction permits improved splintage; between 1 and 3 years the carpus may be centralized over the ulna. Later correction (e.g. with an Ilizarov fixator) should be considered only if it does not prevent the hand from reaching the mouth.

Central defects   affect the second, third and fourth rays. There may be a cleft, with only the middle ray missing. If all three central rays are absent, the hand resembles a lobster claw. Function is often excellent, and reconstructive surgery should be undertaken only if this offers some definite improvement.

Failure of differentiation

Syndactyly (congenital webbing)   may be corrected by separating the fingers and repairing the defects with skin grafts.

Camptodactyly   is a fixed flexion deformity of the proximal interphalangeal joint (usually of the little finger). It is hereditary and often bilateral, but deformity is rarely obvious before the age of 10 years. No treatment is needed.

Clinodactyly (bent finger)   also affects the little finger and is inherited as an autosomal dominant trait. Treatment is unnecessary.

Focal defects

Polydactyly (extra digits)   is the commonest hand malformation. The extra finger should be amputated, if only for cosmetic reasons.

Constriction bands may occur in the fingers (as elsewhere in the limbs). Distal oedema may be severe. The constricted skin is excised and repaired by Z-plasty or grafting.

Overgrowth and undergrowth

A giant finger is unsightly, but attempts at operative reduction are fraught with complications. Hypoplastic fingers are occasionally treated by bone lengthening.

Generalized malformations

The hand may be involved in generalized disorders such as Marfan's syndrome ('spider hand') or achondroplasia ('trident hand').

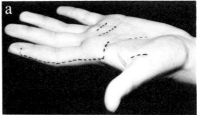

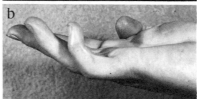

16.5 Deformities – skin (a) Skin incisions should never cross the creases on the flexor surface; those shown are safe; (b) postoperative contracture of a badly placed scar.

Acquired deformities

Deformity of the hand may be due to disorders of the skin, subcutaneous tissues, muscles, tendons, joints, bones or neuromuscular function. Often there is a history of trauma, or infection or concomitant disease; at other times the patient is unaware of any cause.

Problems arise for three reasons: (1) the cosmetic effect may be disturbing; (2) function may be impaired; and (3) the deformed part often gets in the way during normal activities.

Assessment and management of hand deformities demands a detailed knowledge of functional anatomy and, in particular, of the normal mechanisms of balanced movement in the wrist and fingers.

Skin contracture

Cuts and burns of the palmar skin are liable to heal with contracture. Surgical incisions should never cross skin creases; they should be parallel with them or in the mid-axial line of the fingers (an exception is Bruner's zig-zag incision). Established contractures may require excision of the scar and Z plasty of the remaining skin.

Contracture of the superficial palmar fascia (palmar aponeurosis)

The superficial palmar fascia fans out from the wrist towards the fingers, sending extensions across the metacarpophalangeal joints to the fingers. Hypertrophy and contracture of the palmar fascia may lead to puckering of the palmar skin and fixed flexion of the fingers (Dupuytren's contracture: see p. 320).

Muscle contracture

Ischaemic contracture of the forearm muscles may follow circulatory insufficiency due to injuries at or below the elbow (Volkmann's ischaemic contracture: p. 552). There is shortening of the long flexors; the fingers are held in flexion and can be straightened only when the wrist is flexed. Sometimes the picture is complicated by associated damage to the ulnar or median nerve (or both). If disability is marked, some improvement may be obtained by releasing the shortened muscles at their origin above the elbow, or else by excising the dead muscles and restoring finger movement with tendon transfers.

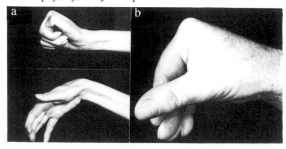

16.6 Deformities – muscle   (a) Ischaemic contracture of the long flexors in the forearm; with the wrist in extension, the fingers involuntarily curl into flexion; when the wrist flexes, the pull on the finger flexors is released. (b) Flexion deformity due to ischaemic contracture of the intrinsic hand muscles (the 'intrinsic-plus' hand).

Shortening of the intrinsic muscles of the hand produces a characteristic deformity: flexion at the metacarpophalangeal joints with extension of the interphalangeal joints and adduction of the thumb (the 'intrinsic-plus' hand). Slight degrees of deformity may not be obvious, but can be diagnosed by the 'intrinsic-plus' test: with the metacarpophalangeal joints pushed passively into hyperextension (thus putting the intrinsics on stretch), it is difficult or impossible to flex the interphalangeal joints passively. The causes of intrinsic shortening or contracture are: (1) spasm (e.g. in cerebral palsy); (2) volar subluxation of the metacarpophalangeal joints (e.g. in rheumatoid arthritis); (3) scarring after trauma or infection; and (4) shrinkage due to

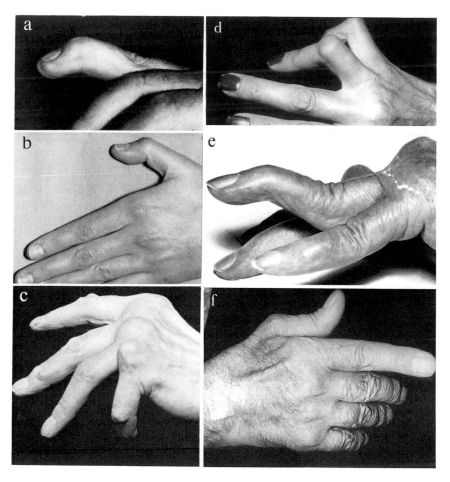

16.7 Deformities – tendons   (a) Mallet finger. (b) Mallet thumb. (c) Dropped fingers due to rupture of extensor tendons. (d) Boutonnière. (e) Swan-neck deformity. (f) The so-called 'W-thumb', which results from rupture of the extensor pollicis brevis.

distal ischaemia. Moderate contracture can be treated by resecting a triangular segment of the intrinsic 'aponeurosis' at the base of the proximal phalanx (Littler's operation).

Tendon lesions

'Mallet finger' ('baseball finger')   This results from injury to the extensor tendon of the terminal phalanx. It may be due to direct trauma but more often follows tendon rupture when the finger tip is forcibly bent during active extension, perhaps while tucking the blankets under a mattress or trying to catch a ball. The terminal joint is held flexed and the patient cannot straighten it, but passive movement is normal. With the extensor mechanism unbalanced, the proximal interphalangeal joint may become hyperextended. An acute mallet finger should be splinted with the joint in extension for 6 weeks. Old lesions need treatment only if the deformity is marked, hand function seriously impaired and the joint still mobile. An ellipse of skin and extensor tendon is excised over the terminal knuckle, the defect is tightly sutured and the joint is held extended with a Kirschner wire for 4 weeks.

Ruptured extensor pollicis longus ('mallet thumb')   The long thumb extensor may rupture after fraying where it crosses the wrist (e.g. after a Colles' fracture, or in rheumatoid arthritis). The distal phalanx drops into flexion; it can be passively but not actively extended. Direct repair is unsatisfactory and a tendon transfer, using the extensor indicis, is needed.

Dropped finger   Sudden loss of finger extension at the metacarpophalangeal joint is usually due to tendon rupture at the wrist (e.g. in rheumatoid arthritis). If direct repair is not possible, the distal portion can be attached to an adjacent finger extensor.

Boutonnière deformity   This lesion (which the French call 'le buttonhole') presents as a flexion deformity of the proximal interphalangeal joint. It is due to interruption or stretching of the central slip of the extensor tendon where it inserts into the base of the middle phalanx; the usual causes are direct trauma or rheumatoid disease. The lateral slips

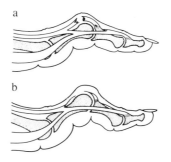

16.8 Deformities – boutonnière   (a) When the middle slip of the extensor tendon first ruptures there is no more than an inability to extend the proximal interphalangeal joint. If it is not repaired, (b) the lateral slips slide towards the volar surface, the knuckle 'buttonholes' the extensor hood, and the distal joint is drawn into hyperextension.

separate and the head of a proximal phalanx thrusts through the gap like a finger through a buttonhole. Initially deformity is slight and passively correctible; later the soft tissues contract, resulting in fixed flexion of the proximal and hyperextension of the distal interphalangeal joint.

In the early post-traumatic case, splinting the proximal interphalangeal joint in full extension for 6 weeks usually leads to union; the alternative is direct suture of the central slip.

In later cases where the joint is still passively correctible, one lateral slip can be transposed to the base of the middle phalanx, or the healthy portion of the middle slip can be lengthened and reattached, the joint being held straight with a Kirschner wire for 4 weeks. Long-standing fixed deformities are extremely difficult to correct and may be better left alone.

Boutonnière deformity of the thumb metacarpophalangeal joint is common in rheumatoid arthritis (see Chapter 3).

Congenital laxity of the volar plate of the metacarpophalangeal joint may cause a pseudo-boutonnière deformity, which is relieved by tightening the plate.

Swan-neck deformity   This is the reverse of boutonnière deformity; the proximal interpha-

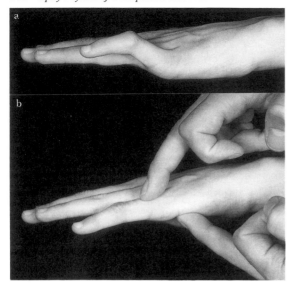

16.9 Pseudo-boutonnière deformity   (a) The little finger is typically cocked up at the metacarpal joint and flexed at the proximal interphalangeal joint. (b) If the metacarpophalangeal joint is stabilized, the patient can easily straighten the finger.

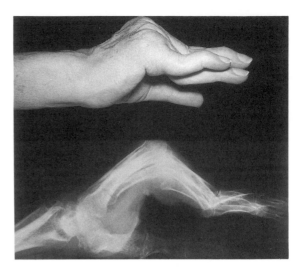

16.10 Swan-neck deformity   The typical appearance and x-ray.

langeal joint is hyperextended and the distal interphalangeal joint flexed. The deformity can be reproduced voluntarily by lax-jointed individuals. The clinical disorder has many causes, with one thing in common: imbalance of extensor versus flexor action at the proximal interphalangeal joint. Thus it may occur (1) *if the proximal interphalangeal extensors overact* (e.g. due to intrinsic muscle spasm or contracture, or after disruption of the distal extensor attachment or volar subluxation of the metacarpophalangeal joint, both of which cause extensor force to be concentrated on the proximal interphalangeal joint); or (2) *if the proximal interphalangeal flexors are inadequate* (paralysis or division of the flexor superficialis). If the deformity is allowed to persist, secondary contracture of the intrinsic muscles, and eventually of the proximal interphalangeal joint itself, make correction increasingly difficult and ultimately impossible.

While the deformity is still correctible, the cause can usually be established by three simple manoeuvres: (1) test for isolated superficialis action; (2) test for intrinsic contracture (p. 316); (3) stabilize the metacarpophalangeal

joint and see if this corrects the deformity. Treatment depends on the cause, and may involve operative release of shrunken intrinsics, reduction and stabilization of the metacarpophalangeal joint, and tightening of the volar proximal interphalangeal structures. If a mallet deformity is present, this must be corrected as well. An isolated injury or rupture of the superficialis tendon seldom warrants repair.

A tight, fixed deformity will not yield to any form of dynamic correction. If function is severely impaired the joint can be arthrodesed in a more acceptable position.

Joint disorders

Rheumatoid arthritis causes multiple deformities of both hands. The most typical is ulnar deviation of the fingers, but this may be combined with boutonnière and swan-neck deformities.

Osteoarthritis of the distal and middle finger joints is common in postmenopausal women and may cause deformity. If disability is severe the joint may be arthrodesed. Osteoarthritis of the thumb carpometacarpal joint may result in subluxation, with adduction of the first metacarpophalangeal joint. Treatment is essentially that of the underlying disorder, but if metacarpal adduction is severe the thenar muscles may have to be released.

Gout produces large tophi and severe joint deformity. In addition to systemic treatment, evacuation of tophaceous material is sometimes advisable.

Trauma may result in recurrent or persistent dislocation or subluxation. The best known, '*game-keeper's thumb*', is due to disruption of the ulnar collateral ligament of the thumb metacarpophalangeal joint with instability.

Stiff joints may follow trauma, infection or injudicious splintage. A stiff finger, whether bent or straight, is a nuisance. Physiotherapy may help, but in long-standing cases, if operative release is unsuccessful, the finger may have to be amputated.

Bone lesions

A variety of bone lesions (acute infection, tuberculosis, malunited fractures, infantile rickets, tumours) may cause metacarpal or phalangeal deformity. X-rays usually show the abnormality. In addition to treating the pathological lesion, deformity may need correction by osteotomy with internal fixation.

Neuromuscular disorders

Cerebral palsy and stroke may cause spastic paresis with severe hand deformities. The 'intrinsic-plus' posture is easily recognized. Another common disability is 'thumb-in-palm'; the tendency to adduct and flex the thumb into the palm is increased by activity, especially finger flexion. Releasing the adductor pollicis from the third metacarpal may improve the appearance, but normal thumb pinch is rarely restored.

Other neurological disorders, such as poliomyelitis, leprosy, syringomyelia and peroneal muscle atrophy, may cause hand deformities. If there is only partial involvement, tendon transfer may be feasible.

Peripheral nerve lesions cause characteristic deformities: the drop wrist and drop fingers of

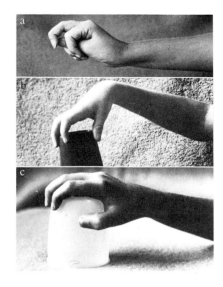

16.11 The hand in cerebral palsy (a) Typically, when the wrist is extended the fingers flex and the thumb tucks into the palm; the hand unclasps only (b) when the wrist is flexed. After muscle release (c) the hand may be able to open with the wrist in a functional position.

radial nerve palsy, the flat simian thumb and pointing index finger of median nerve palsy, and the claw hand of ulnar nerve palsy.

INTRINSIC PARALYSIS (the 'intrinsic-minus' or 'claw' hand) Weakness or paralysis of the intrinsic muscles results in metacarpophalangeal extension and partial flexion of the interphalangeal joints of the fingers and thumb (a type of 'claw hand'); finger abduction and adduction are impossible. If all the intrinsics are affected (e.g. after poliomyelitis) the thumb lies flat at the side of the hand and cannot be opposed. In ulnar nerve palsy only the ring and little fingers are clawed, because the index and middle lumbricals are supplied by the median nerve; thumb opposition is retained but thumb pinch is unstable because index-finger abduction is weak, and loss of thumb adduction is compensated for by exaggerated interphalangeal flexion during strong pinch (Froment's sign; p. 231).

The objectives of treatment are: (1) stabilization of the metacarpophalangeal joints in flexion; this can be achieved by a many-tailed

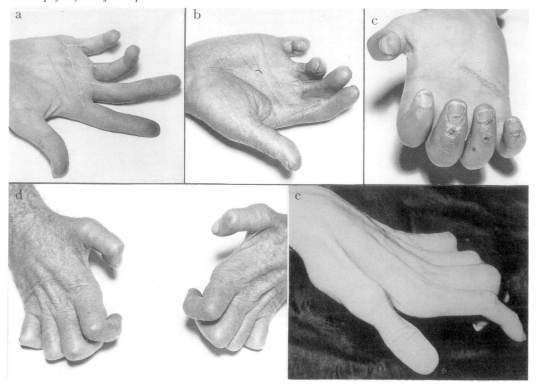

16.12 Examples of claw hand   (a) Following badly placed incisions; (b) ulnar nerve palsy. (c) Volkmann's contracture. (d) Bilateral clawing in peroneal muscular atrophy; (e) associated with the nerve lesions of leprosy.

tendon transfer (splitting a flexor superficialis tendon) or, if a suitable motor is not available, by tightening the volar metacarpophalangeal capsules; (2) restoration of index abduction to provide stable pinch (e.g. by extensor tendon transfer to the first dorsal interosseous); and (3) restoration of thumb opposition (if it is lost) by a tendon transfer looped around a pisiform pulley and attached to the proximal phalanx of the thumb. *Before any of these operations, stiff finger joints must be made mobile.*

Dupuytren's contracture

This is a nodular hypertrophy and contracture of the superficial palmar fascia (palmar aponeurosis). The condition is inherited as an autosomal dominant trait and is most common in people of European (especially Anglo-Saxon) descent. There is a high incidence in epileptics receiving phenytoin therapy and in patients with AIDS; associations with alcoholic cirrhosis, diabetes and pulmonary tuberculosis have also been described.

Recent work (Murrell, Francis and Howlett, 1989) has revealed a marked increase in fibroblast density, a disorganized pattern of collagen distribution and microvascular constriction in the fibrous cords of Dupuytren's contracture. The authors hypothesize that the fibrotic changes are due to the action of oxygen-free radicals produced in relatively ischaemic tissues where increased xanthine oxidase activity would promote the formation of superoxide from the oxidation of hypoxanthine and xanthine.If this is so, a xanthine oxidase inhibitor (allopurinol) should alleviate the condition.

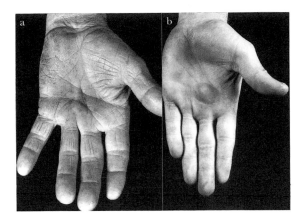

16.13 Dupuytren's contracture (a) In the early case there is usually only a palmar nodule but no deformity. This must be distinguished from (b) an implantation dermoid which produces a more superficial nodule in the skin.

Pathology

The palmar aponeurosis thickens, usually opposite the ring finger. Early on, there is proliferation of immature fibroblasts; later the fascia thickens and shrinks, its distal prolongations pulling the fingers into flexion and its cutaneous attachments puckering the palmar skin.

The digital nerve is displaced or enveloped, but not invaded, by fibrous tissue.

Occasionally the plantar aponeurosis also is affected.

Clinical features

The patient – usually a middle-aged man – complains of a nodular thickening in the palm. Gradually this extends distally to involve the ring or little finger. Pain may occur but is seldom a marked feature. Often both hands are involved, one more than the other. The palm is puckered, nodular and thick. If the subcutaneous cords extend into the fingers they may produce flexion deformities at the metacarpophalangeal and proximal interphalangeal joints. Sometimes the dorsal knuckle pads are thickened (Garrod's pads).

Similar nodules may be seen on the soles of the feet. There is a rare, curious association with fibrosis of the corpus cavernosum (Peyronie's disease).

Diagnosis

Dupuytren's contracture must be distinguished from skin contracture (where the previous

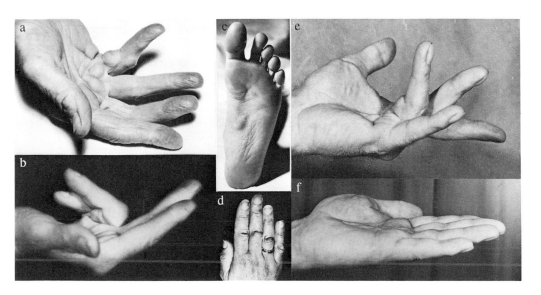

16.14 Dupuytren's contracture (a) Moderately severe, with diagnostic nodules and pits; (b) severe contracture. (c) Dupuytren's nodule in the sole; (d) Garrod's pads. (e, f) Before and after subcutaneous fasciotomy.

laceration is usually obvious) and tendon contracture (where the 'cord' moves on passive flexion of the finger).

Treatment

Operation is indicated if the deformity is a nuisance or rapidly progressing. The aim is reasonable, not complete, correction.

Only the thickened part of the fascia is excised (complete fasciectomy is unnecessary and fraught with complications). The affected area is approached through a longitudinal or a Z-shaped incision and, after carefully freeing the nerves, the hypertrophic cords are excised. Skin closure may be facilitated by multiple Z-plasties. After operative correction a splint is applied, and removed daily for wax baths and exercises. After 6 weeks it is used only as a night splint for a further 3–6 months.

In severe finger contractures, fasciectomy may have to be preceded by closed fasciotomy to obtain some correction and permit adequate skin toilet; great care is needed to prevent injury to the nerves and vessels.

Amputation is occasionally advisable if there is severe contraction of the joint capsule.

Trigger finger (digital tenovaginitis)

A flexor tendon may become trapped at the entrance to its sheath; on forced extension it passes the constriction with a snap ('triggering'). The usual cause is thickening of the fibrous tendon sheath (often following local trauma or unaccustomed activity), but a similar hold-up may occur in rheumatoid tenosynovitis.

Clinical features

Any digit (including the thumb) may be affected, but the ring and middle fingers most commonly. The patient notices that the finger clicks as he bends it; when the hand is unclenched, the affected finger remains bent but with further effort it suddenly straightens with a snap. A tender nodule can be felt in front of the affected sheath.

INFANTILE TRIGGER THUMB Babies sometimes develop tenovaginitis of the thumb flexor sheath. The diagnosis is often missed, or the condition is wrongly taken for a 'dislocation'. Very occasionally the child grows up with the thumb permanently bent.

Treatment

Early cases may be cured by an injection of methylprednisolone carefully placed at the entrance of the tendon sheath. Refractory cases need operation: through a transverse incision in the distal palmar crease, or in the metacarpophalangeal crease of the thumb, the fibrous sheath is incised until the tendon moves freely. In babies it is worth waiting a few months, as spontaneous recovery often occurs.

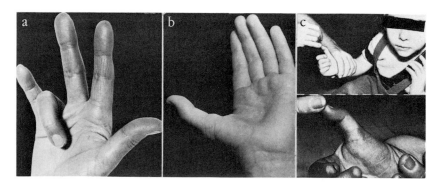

16.15 Stenosing tenovaginitis (a) Trigger finger; (b) trigger thumb – the only variety which occurs in children, in whom (c) the thumb may be stuck bent.

Rheumatoid arthritis

(see also Chapter 3)

The hand, more than any other region, is where rheumatoid arthritis carves its story. In *stage 1* there is synovitis of joints (metacarpophalangeal and proximal interphalangeal) and of tendon sheaths (flexor and extensor). In *stage 2*, joint and tendon erosions prepare the ground for mechanical derangement. And in *stage 3*, joint instability and tendon rupture cause progressive deformity and loss of function.

Clinical features

STAGE 1   Pain, stiffness and swelling of the fingers are early symptoms; often the wrist also is painful and swollen. Carpal tunnel compression from flexor tenosynovitis sometimes causes the first symptom. Examination may reveal swelling of the metacarpophalangeal joints, the proximal interphalangeal joints (giving the fingers a spindle shape) or the wrists; both hands are affected, more or less symmetrically. Swelling of tendon sheaths is usually seen on the dorsum of the wrist, on its ulnar side (extensor carpi ulnaris) and on the volar aspect of the proximal phalanges. The joints are tender and crepitus may be felt on moving the tendons. Joint mobility and grip strength are diminished.

STAGE 2   As the disease progresses, early deformities make their appearance: slight radial deviation of the wrist and ulnar deviation of the fingers; correctible swan-necking; an isolated boutonnière; the sudden appearance of a drop finger or mallet thumb (from extensor tendon rupture).

STAGE 3   In the later stage, long after inflammation may have subsided, established deformities are the rule: the carpus settles into radial tilt and volar subluxation; there is marked ulnar drift of the fingers and volar dislocation of the metacarpophalangeal joints, often associated with multiple swan-neck and boutonnière deformities. When these abnormalities become fixed, functional loss may be so severe that the patient can no longer dress or feed herself.

X-rays

During *stage 1* the x-rays show only soft-tissue swelling and osteoporosis around the joints. In *stage 2*, joint 'space' narrowing and small periarticular erosions appear; these are com-

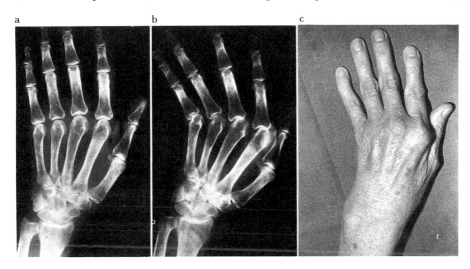

a   b   c

16.16 Rheumatoid arthritis – ulnar drift   (a) Early ulnar drift. (b) The same patient 2 years later – the progressive finger deformity is accompanied by (perhaps preceded by) an equal and opposite wrist deformity, in which the entire carpus moves ulnarwards and rotates radialwards. (c) The clinical appearance shows the zig-zag deformity.

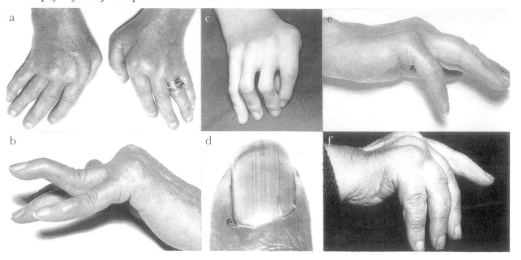

16.17 Rheumatoid arthritis – hands   (a) Ulnar drift; (b) swan-neck deformity; (c) boutonnière deformities; (d) 'nail-fold lesion' due to arteritis; (e) dropped finger; (f) three dropped fingers.

monest at the metacarpophalangeal joints and in the styloid process of the ulna. In *stage 3*, articular destruction may be marked, affecting the metacarpophalangeal proximal interphalangeal and wrist joints almost equally. Joint deformity and dislocation are common.

Treatment

IN STAGE 1   treatment is directed essentially at controlling the systemic disease and the local synovitis. In addition to general measures (p. 57), splints may reduce pain and swelling

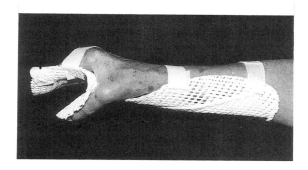

16.18 Rheumatoid arthritis – treatment Lightweight splints are worn to rest the joints, not to correct deformity.

and improve mobility. *These splints are not corrective but are designed to rest inflamed joints and tendons*; in mild cases they are worn only at night, in more active cases during the day as well. Persistent synovitis of a few joints or tendon sheaths may benefit from local injections of the 'anti-inflammatory cocktail' containing methylprednisolone (40 mg), nitrogen mustard (1 ml of a 0.02% solution) and 1% lignocaine (1 ml); only small quantities are injected (e.g. 0.5 ml for a metacarpophalangeal joint or flexor tendon sheath and 1 ml for the wrist). This should not be repeated more than two or three times. A boggy flexor tenosynovitis may not respond to this limited therapeutic assault; operative synovectomy may be needed. If carpal tunnel symptoms are present, the transverse carpal ligament is divided.

IN STAGE 2   it becomes increasingly important to prevent deformity. Uncontrolled synovitis of joints or tendons requires operative synovectomy followed by physiotherapy. Excision of the distal end of the ulna, synovectomy of the common extensor sheath and the wrist, and reconstruction of the soft tissues on the ulnar side of the wrist may arrest joint destruction and progressive deformity. Early instability and ulnar drift at the metacarpophalangeal joints can be corrected by excising the inflamed

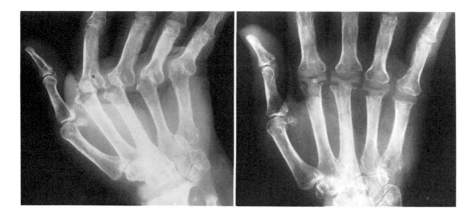

16.19 Rheumatoid arthritis – treatment In advanced rheumatoid arthritis the meta-carpophalangeal joints may be completely dislocated, as they were in this patient; joint replacement with flexible Silastic spacers corrected her deformity and restored stability.

synovium, tightening the capsular structures, releasing the ulnar pull of the intrinsic tendons and hitching the proximal phalanx back into position by reinforcing the extensor attachment to the base of the finger. A mobile boutonnière also can be treated operatively (p. 317). Isolated tendon ruptures are repaired or bypassed by appropriate tendon transfers. All these procedures are followed by dynamic splintage and physiotherapy.

IN STAGE 3 deformity is combined with articular destruction; soft-tissue correction alone will not suffice. For the metacarpophalangeal and interphalangeal joints of the thumb, arthrodesis gives predictable pain relief, stability and functional improvement. The metacarpophalangeal joints of the fingers can be excised and replaced with Silastic 'spacers', which improve stability and correct deformity. Replacement of interphalangeal joints gives less predictable results; if deformity is very disabling (e.g. a fixed swan-neck) it may be better to settle for arthrodesis in a more functional position. At the wrist, painless stability can be regained by replacing the joint with a Silastic prosthesis or, if need be, by arthrodesis in slight flexion and ulnar deviation.

Osteoarthritis

Osteoarthritis of the distal interphalangeal joints is very common in postmenopausal women. It often starts with pain in one or two

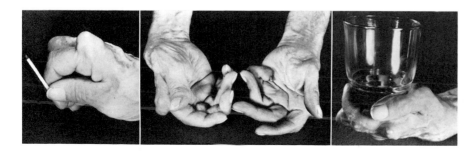

16.20 Rheumatoid arthritis – does it need treatment? Not always. Why interfere if deformities have been present for years and the hand still works? Despite gross deformity this patient can manipulate tiny objects and large ones.

fingers; the distal joints become swollen and tender, the condition usually spreading to all the fingers of both hands. On examination there is bony thickening around the distal interphalangeal joints (Heberden's nodes) and some restriction of movement. Not infrequently some of the proximal interphalangeal joints are involved (Bouchard's nodes) and the carpo-metacarpal joint of the thumb may show similar changes.

X-rays reveal narrowing of the joint spaces and osteophyte formation.

Treatment is symptomatic; pain and tenderness gradually subside and the patient is left with painless, knobbly fingers.

Acute infections of the hand

Infection of the hand is frequently limited to one of several well-defined compartments: under the nail fold (paronychia); the pulp space (whitlow), subcutaneous tissues elsewhere; the tendon sheaths; and the deep fascial spaces. Usually the cause is a staphylococcus which has been implanted by fairly trivial injury. However, contaminated cuts, with unusual organisms, account for about 10% of cases.

Pathology

Here, as elsewhere, the response to infection is an acute inflammatory reaction with oedema, suppuration, raised tissue tension and, ultimately, tissue necrosis. Even apparently trivial infections may give rise to lymphangitis and septicaemia.

Clinical features

Usually there is a history of trauma, but it may have been so trivial as to pass unnoticed. A few hours or days later the finger (or hand) becomes painful and swollen. There may be throbbing and sometimes the patient feels ill and feverish.

On examination the finger or hand is red and swollen, and usually exquisitely tender over the site of tension. However, in immune-compromised patients, in the very elderly and in babies, local signs may be mild. With superficial infection the patient can usually be persuaded to flex an affected finger; with deep infections active flexion is not possible. The arm should be examined for lymphangitis and swollen glands, and the patient more generally for signs of septicaemia. X-rays of the hand may show features of osteomyelitis or septic arthritis; with severe infections there may be bone necrosis. If pus becomes available, this should be sent for bacteriological examination.

In making the diagnosis, three conditions must be excluded: acute tendon rupture (which may resemble a tenosynovitis), insect bites (which closely mimic subcutaneous infections) and acute gout (which is easily mistaken for septic arthritis).

Treatment

Superficial hand infections are common; if their treatment is delayed or inadequate, infection may rapidly extend, with serious consequences. The essentials of treatment are as follows.

ANTIBIOTICS   As soon as the diagnosis is made, antibiotic treatment is started – usually with cloxacillin and, in severe cases, with fusidic acid as well, or, for bite wounds, metronidazole. This may later be changed when bacterial sensitivity is known.

REST AND ELEVATION   In a mild case the hand is rested in a sling. In a severe case the patient is admitted to hospital and the arm is elevated in a roller towel while the patient is kept under observation. Analgesics are given for pain.

DRAINAGE   If there are signs of an abscess – throbbing pain, marked tenderness and toxaemia – the pus should be drained. A tourniquet and either general or regional block anaesthesia are essential. The incision should be made at the site of maximal tenderness, but never across a skin crease. When pus is encountered it must be carefully mopped away and a search made for deeper pockets of infection. It may be necessary to snip away necrotic skin. A

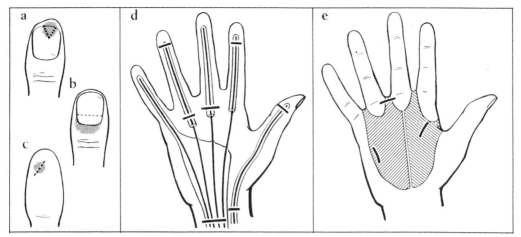

16.21 Infections   (a) To drain an apical abscess it is often best to excise a triangle of nail. (b) Acute paronychia is most efficiently drained by excising the proximal part of the nail. (c) A pulp abscess should be drained over the point of maximal tenderness. (d) Synovial sheath infections can be drained by incisions near their proximal or distal ends, or both. (e) Incisions for web abscess and for the rare infections of the mid-palmar and thenar spaces (partly redrawn from *The Infected Hand* by D. A. Bailey, published by H. K. Lewis, London).

drain is unnecessary. The wound should be covered with a single layer of paraffin gauze and the area generously packed with fluffed gauze swabs. The pus obtained is sent for culture.

SPLINTAGE   At the end of the operation the hand is splinted with the wrist slightly extended, the metacarpophalangeal joints 90 degrees flexed, the interphalangeal joints fully extended and the thumb adducted (the 'position of safety'). A removable splint will permit wound dressing and handbaths (where necessary) and exercises. The forearm is elevated in a roller towel.

POSTOPERATIVE MANAGEMENT   If the tissues were contaminated or necrotic, operative drainage is followed by daily handbaths using plain soap and water. While the hand is free, active movements are carried out under the guidance of a 'hand therapist'. After each treatment session, the dressings and splintage are re-applied.

PREVENTING STIFFNESS   The worst outcome is a stiff hand. Prevention is far better than cure. The three cardinal rules are: (1) splint in the position of safety; (2) elevate; and (3) start movements as soon as possible.

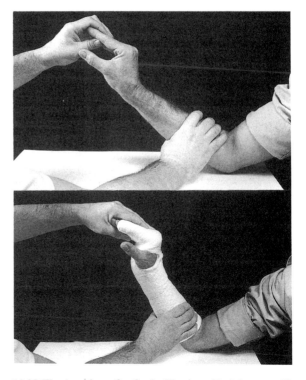

16.22 The 'position of safety'   The knuckle joints are 90 degrees flexed, the finger joints extended and the thumb abducted. This is the position in which the ligaments are at their longest and splintage is least likely to result in stiffness.

Infections at special sites

Nail fold (paronychia)

Infection under the nail fold is the commonest hand infection and is seen most often in children. The area is swollen, red and tender. If pus is present it can often be released simply by lifting the nail fold from the nail; otherwise it must be incised. If there is pus under the nail, the proximal third of the nail has to be removed.

Chronic paronychia may be due to (1) inadequate drainage, or (2) fungal infection, which requires specific treatment.

Pulp (whitlow)

Pulp space infection causes throbbing pain. The fingertip is swollen, red and acutely tender. Early drainage is essential. Under antibiotic cover a small incision over the site of maximal tenderness is usually sufficient. If treatment is delayed, x-rays may show a sequestrum which should be removed.

Other subcutaneous infections

Anywhere in the hand a blister or superficial cut may become infected, causing redness, swelling and tenderness. A local collection of pus should be drained through a small incision over the site of maximal tenderness (but never crossing a skin crease or the web edge). It is important to exclude a deeper pocket of pus in a nearby tendon sheath or in one of the deep fascial spaces.

Tendon sheaths (suppurative tenosynovitis)

Suppurative tenosynovitis is uncommon but dangerous. Unless treatment is swift and effective, the patient may end up with a useless finger due to tendon necrosis or adhesions. The affected digit is painful and swollen; it is held bent, is very tender and the patient will not move it or permit it to be moved. Pus must be drained through two incisions – one at the proximal end of the sheath and one at the distal end; using a fine catheter the sheath is then irrigated with Ringer's lactate solution.

Tendon-sheath infection in the thumb or little finger may spread proximally to the synovial bursa. This has to be drained through a further incision just above the wrist.

Finger movements are started only when the infection has cleared.

Fascial spaces

Infection from a web space or from an infected tendon sheath may spread to either of the deep fascial spaces of the palm. The palm is ballooned, so its normal concavity is lost; swelling may extend to the dorsum of the hand. There is extensive tenderness and the whole hand is held still. For drainage an incision is made directly over the abscess and sinus forceps inserted; if the web space is infected it, too, should be incised; a thenar space abscess is best approached through the first web space.

Occasionally, deep infection extends proximally; pus may track up the forearm where it can be drained by anteromedial or anterolateral incisions.

Open injuries of the hand

Over 75% of work injuries affect the hands; inadequate treatment costs the patient (and society) dear in terms of functional disability.

Clinical assessment

The spectrum of open injuries embraces tidy or 'clean' cuts, lacerations, crushing and injection injuries, burns and pulp defects. Examination should be gentle and painstaking. Skin damage is important, but it should be remembered that even a tiny, clean cut may conceal nerve or tendon damage. Sensation is tested and re-tested. Active movements are elicited to assess tendon damage, but if this is too painful the resting attitude of the fingers is a useful guide.

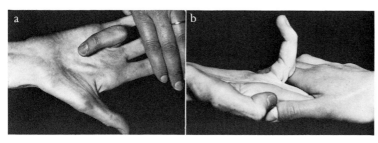

16.23 Testing superficialis To detect superficialis competence, first anchor the profundus, which is a 'mass action' muscle. (a) The superficialis is normal; it alone is flexing the annularis – the tip is flail. (b) The superficialis is not working; only by using profundus (with difficulty) can the annularis be flexed; consequently the tip is not flail (Apley, 1956).

X-ray examination may show fractures or foreign bodies.

It is important to know the patient's occupation and whether he is right- or left-handed.

Primary treatment

PREOPERATIVE CARE   The patient may need treatment for pain and shock. if the wound is contaminated, antibiotics should be given as soon as possible. Prophylactics against tetanus and gas gangrene may also be needed. The hand is lightly splinted and the wound covered with a sterile dressing.

WOUND EXPLORATION AND DEBRIDEMENT   Under general or regional block anaesthesia, the wound area is cleaned and explored. A pneumatic tourniquet is helpful but not essential; it should certainly not be used with crush injuries, where muscle viability is in doubt. Skin is too precious to waste and only obviously dead skin should be excised. For adequate exposure the wound may need enlarging, but incisions must not cross a skin crease or an interdigital web. Through the enlarged wound, loose debris is picked out, dead muscle is excised and the tissues are thoroughly irrigated with Ringer's lactate solution.

Amputation   Amputation of a finger as a primary procedure should be avoided unless the damage involves many tissues and is clearly irreparable. Even when a finger has been amputated by the injury, the possibility of reattachment should be considered.

Burns   with only partial skin loss are cleaned, and covered with non-stick dressings backed by wool; the limb is elevated. The dressing is left undisturbed for 10–14 days but finger movements are encouraged. (Treatment by exposure, practised in some burns units, demands a specially clean environment.) With whole-thickness skin loss, devitalized tissue is excised, the wound cleaned and dressed, and 5 days later skin-grafted. Electric burns may cause extensive damage and thrombosis which become apparent only after several days.

Injection injuries of oil, grease, solvents, hydraulic fluid or paint under pressure are damaging because of tension, toxicity or both. The thumb or index finger is usually involved. Substances can gain entry even through intact skin. Air or lead paint may show on x-ray. Immediate decompression and removal of the foreign substance offers the best hope, but most reported series feature a high incidence of finger or partial hand amputation.

TISSUE REPAIR   *Fractures* are reduced and held with Kirschner wires, unless there is some specific contraindication. *Joint capsule and ligaments* are repaired with fine sutures. *Severed nerves* are likewise sutured with the finest, non-reactive material.

For *cut extensor tendons* primary repair is easy and safe; the only contraindication is a dirty wound.

Flexor tendon repair is a more contentious issue. Primary repair should not be attempted if the wound is contaminated or if the cut ends can be found only by extensive dissection. Division of the superficialis tendon alone causes little disability and does not require repair. All other lacerations of one or both tendons at any level should ideally be treated by primary suture – but only if the cut is clean, operation is early and the surgeon sufficiently expert. Certainly cuts proximal to the flexor sheath or distal to the superficialis insertion can be sutured.

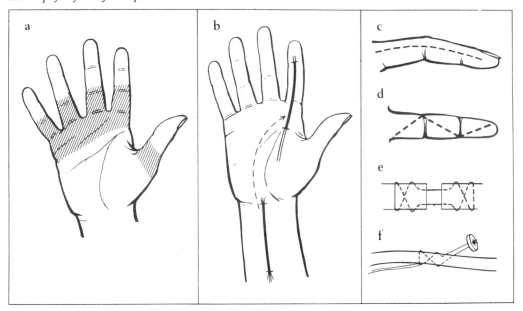

16.24 Tendon injuries   (a) Zones of the hand (redrawn from *Injuries of the Hand* by R. J. Furlong, published by Churchill, London). The intermediate zone (shaded) contains two tendons and two sheaths. (b) The principle of tendon grafting to replace a cut profundus. (c) Mid-axial incision. (d) Bruner's zig-zag incision. (e) One method of tendon suture. (f) Bunnell's pull-out technique.

Those within the flexor sheath (between the distal palmar crease and the proximal interphalangeal joint) are liable to form adhesions if sutured, so unless the skills and facilities are of a high order these injuries are best left alone, to be dealt with 3–6 weeks later by secondary suture or tendon grafting.

The cut tendon is exposed through a mid-axial incision in the finger or a zig-zag extension of the skin wound. As much of the tendon sheath as possible is preserved. Various methods of tendon suture have been developed, the object being to appose the cut ends with as little damage as possible to the extrinsic and intrinsic blood supply (Kleinert et al., 1973).

CLOSURE   The tourniquet is removed and meticulous haemostasis obtained. Haematoma formation leads to poor healing and tendon adhesions. Unless the wound is contaminated, the skin is closed – either by direct suture without tension or, if there is skin loss, by skin grafting. Free grafts are conveniently taken from the front of the forearm; but it may be necessary later to replace them with full-thick-ness grafts. If tendon or bare bone is exposed, this must be covered by a flap graft taken from either a local or a distant site. Sometimes a severely mutilated finger is sacrificed and its skin used as a rotation flap.

Pulp and fingertip injuries   Split-skin or full-thickness grafts are conventional, but in most children and selected adults spontaneous healing (carefully supervised) offers an equally good appearance, with better sensation.

DRESSING AND SPLINTAGE   The wound is covered with several thicknesses of dry gauze and ample wool. A firm bandage ensures even pressure, and a light plaster slab holds the wrist and hand in the desired position: after primary flexor tendon suture, the wrist and fingers are bandaged in flexion, so as to take tension off the suture lines; in all other cases the hand is splinted in the 'position of safety' (the wrist slightly extended, the metacarpophalangeal joints almost 90 degrees flexed, the interphalangeal joints extended and the thumb abducted). This is the position in which the metacarpophalangeal and interphalangeal ligaments are fully stretched and fibrosis therefore least likely to cause contractures. *Failure to appreciate this point is the commonest cause of irrecoverable stiffness after injury.*

Postoperative management

IMMEDIATE AFTERCARE The hand is kept elevated and at rest. Antibiotics are continued as necessary. If a primary flexor tendon repair has been performed, the bulky dressing is removed on the third day and replaced by an elastic splint which maintains wrist and metacarpophalangeal flexion but permits active interphalangeal extension. In all other cases the dressing is left undisturbed for 3 weeks, unless the fingers become unduly swollen or blue or numb.

ASSESSMENT At 3 weeks the dressings are taken off. It is now possible to estimate, from the state of healing and a knowledge of the operative findings, what the future function of the hand is likely to be.

The sensory and the various motor functions are separately assessed. With this information, and a knowledge of the patient's work and hobbies, the nature of further treatment can be decided; it may be conservative (rehabilitation) or operative.

REHABILITATION When the wound has healed, active exercises and wax baths are started. The hand is increasingly used for more and more arduous and complex tasks, especially those that resemble the patient's normal job, until he is fit to start work; if necessary, his work is modified temporarily. Even if further surgery is required, tendon or nerve repair is postponed until the skin is healthy, there is no oedema and the joints have regained a normal range of passive movement.

Secondary operations

The primary treatment of hand injuries should always be carried out with an eye to any future reconstructive procedures that might be necessary. These are of three kinds: secondary repair or replacement of damaged structures, amputation of fingers, or reconstruction of a mutilated hand.

SECONDARY REPAIR

SKIN If the skin cover has broken down or is unsuitable for surgery it is replaced by a graft. As always, the skin creases must be respected. Contractures are dealt with by Z-plasty or skin replacement. When important volar surfaces are insensitive, a flap of skin complete with its nerve supply may be transposed (sensory flap).

TENDONS Primary sutures may have been contraindicated by wound contamination, undue delay between injury and repair, massive skin loss or inadequate operating facilities. In these circumstances secondary repair or tendon grafting is necessary.

Distal to superficialis insertion Only the profundus tendon can have been cut. The disability of an unbalanced terminal phalanx may require surgery. If the cut is more than 1 cm from the tendon insertion, end-to-end suture may be possible; otherwise the joint can be stabilized in 30 degrees of flexion by a tenodesis, using the distal stump of the tendon. If the cut is more distal, the best solution is to advance the profundus tendon and reattach it to the terminal phalanx (taking care not to damage the volar plate of the terminal joint). The alternative is arthrodesis in 30 degrees of flexion.

Within the flexor sheath In a clean wound with adequate skin cover, delayed primary repair can be done up to 6 weeks after injury – but far better within the first 3 weeks. The area is exposed through a zig-zag extension of the previous wound. The fibrous flexor sheath is excised, leaving the important pulleys opposite the base of the proximal phalanx and the waist of the middle phalanx. Tendon strips may have been retracted and are brought into view by flexing the fingers or 'milking' the proximal parts distally; sometimes a proximal stump needs to be retrieved through a separate palmar incision. *If both tendons are divided*, both should be repaired if possible; if not, the superficialis tendon should be excised proximal to the vinculum through a separate incision in the palm. *If superficialis alone is severed* and function is good, it should likewise be excised. *If profundus alone is cut*, it should be repaired; if this is not feasible, it can be excised leaving superficialis intact, and arthrodesis of the terminal joint carried out later.

Free tendon grafts, using palmaris longus, are much less satisfactory and a full range of flexion is never obtained.

Proximal to the flexor sheath   tendon injuries can be treated by direct suture; the suture line is protected by wrapping the lumbrical muscle around it.

Within the carpal tunnel The area must be adequately exposed to permit careful matching of cut tendons and nerves; many a patient has ended up with the palmaris longus joined to the median nerve! Some of the transverse carpal ligament should be left intact to prevent bowstringing.

NERVES   Cut median or ulnar nerves are repaired in the usual way. Digital nerves also are sutured if the finger has satisfactory motor function, but suture distal to the knuckle often fails. Useful sensation can sometimes be restored by using a sensory cross-finger pedicle graft.

JOINTS   Joint stiffness is best treated by active exercises. Stiff knuckle joints are sometimes helped by capsulotomy. Flail joints are stabilized by tenodesis or arthrodesis.

BONES   Malunion, especially if rotational, may require treatment. Non-union is exceedingly rare, but grafting may be required.

AMPUTATION

INDICATIONS   A finger is amputated only if it remains painful or unhealed, or a nuisance (i.e. if the patient cannot flex it, or cannot straighten it or cannot feel with it), and then only if repair is impossible or uneconomic.

TECHNIQUE   The aim is a mobile digit covered by healthy skin with normal sensation. A palmar flap is best and must always be ample in size; a tight flap usually gives pain.

In the thumb every millimetre is worth preserving; even a stiff or deformed thumb is worth keeping. The index and little fingers are amputated as distally as possible, provided there is voluntary control of the proximal phalanx; if not, oblique amputation through the metacarpal shaft gives a good cosmetic result.

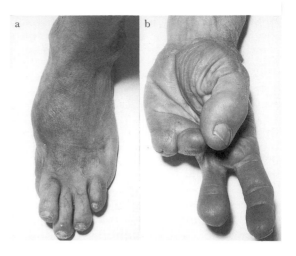

16.25 Late reconstruction   (a) The hallux of this foot has been transplanted to replace the traumatically amputated thumb of (b), where it can be seen to function well.

The middle and ring fingers should not be amputated through the knuckle joint, or the hand will be ugly and small objects fall through it. If the proximal phalanx can be left, the hand is still ugly but stronger. Alternatively, the entire finger with most of its metacarpal may be amputated; the hand is weakened but the amputation is less noticeable.

LATE RECONSTRUCTION

A severely mutilated hand should be dealt with by a hand expert. Three possibilities may be considered in exceptional cases.

1. If all the fingers have been lost but the thumb is present, a new finger can sometimes be constructed with cancellous bone, covered by a tube flap of skin.
2. If the thumb has been lost the three possibilities are: pollicization (rotating a finger to oppose the other fingers); osteoplastic reconstruction (which requires several operations but may provide a good grip); and toe transplant (usually from the hallux).
3. If the thumb and all the fingers have been lost, making a cleft between two metacarpal bones may permit pincer action.

Notes on applied anatomy

The hand serves three basic functions: *sensory perception, precise manipulation* and *power grip.* The first two involve the thumb, index and middle fingers; without normal sensation and the ability to oppose these three digits, manipulative precision will be lost. The ring and little fingers provide power grip, for which they need full flexion though sensation is less important.

With the wrist flexed the fingers and thumb fall naturally into extension. With the wrist extended the fingers curl into flexion and the tips of the thumb, index and middle fingers form a functional tripod; this is the *position of function,* because it is best suited to the actions of prehension.

Finger flexion is strongest when the wrist is powerfully extended; normal grasp is possible only with a painless, stable wrist. Spreading the fingers produces abduction to either side of the middle finger; bringing them together, adduction. Abduction and adduction of the thumb occur in a plane at right angles to the palm (i.e. with the hand lying palm upwards, abduction points the thumb to the ceiling). By a combination of movements the thumb can also be opposed to each of the other fingers. Functionally, the thumb is 40% of the hand.

JOINTS *The carpometacarpal joints* The second and third metacarpals have very little independent movement; the fourth and fifth have more, allowing greater closure of the ulnar part of the hand during power grip. The metacarpal of the thumb is the most mobile and the first carpometacarpal joint is a frequent target for degenerative arthritis.

The metacarpophalangeal joints flex to about 90 degrees, the range increasing progressively from the index to the little finger. The collateral ligaments are lax in extension (permitting abduction) and tight in flexion (preventing abduction). *If these joints are immobilized they should always be in flexion, so that the ligaments are at full stretch and therefore less likely to shorten if they should fibrose.*

The interphalangeal joints are simple hinges, each flexing to about 90 degrees. Their collateral ligaments send attachments to the volar plate and these fibres are tight in extension and lax in flexion; *immobilization of the interphalangeal joints, therefore, should always be in extension.*

MUSCLES AND TENDONS Two sets of muscles control finger movements: the long extrinsic muscles (extensors, deep flexors and superficial flexors), and the short intrinsic muscles (interossei, lumbricals and the short thenar muscles). The extrinsics act synergistically, extending the metacarpophalangeal and flexing the interphalangeal joints; the intrinsics do the reverse – they flex the metacarpophalangeal and extend the interphalangeal joints. They do this only when the dorsal and palmar interossei act together; otherwise the dorsal interossei abduct and the palmar adduct the fingers from the axis of the middle finger. Spasm or contracture of the intrinsics produces the *intrinsic-plus* posture – flexion at the metacarpophalangeal joints, extension at the interphalangeal joints and adduction of the thumb. Paralysis of the intrinsics produces the *instrinsic-minus* posture – hyperextension of the metacarpophalangeal and flexion of the interphalangeal joints ('claw hand').

Tough fibrous sheaths enclose the flexor tendons as they traverse the fingers; starting just proximal to the metacarpophalangeal joints (level with the distal palmar crease) they extend

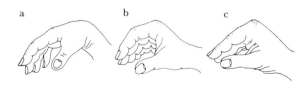

16.26 Three positions of the hand (a) The position of relaxation, (b) the position of function (ready for action) and (c) the position of safety, with the ligaments taut.

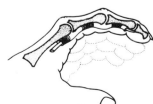

16.27 The flexor sheaths The flexor tendons run in fibrous tunnels from the metacarpal heads to the distal finger joints.

to the distal interphalangeal joints. They serve as runners and pulleys, so preventing the tendons from bowstringing during flexion. Scarring within the fibro-osseous tunnel prevents normal flexion.

The long extensor tendons are prevented from bowstringing at the wrist by the extensor retinaculum; here they are liable to frictional trauma. Over the metacarpophalangeal joints each extensor tendon widens into an expansion which inserts into the proximal phalanx and then splits in three; a central slip inserts into the middle phalanx, the two lateral slips continue distally, join and end in the distal phalanx. Division of the middle slip causes a flexion deformity of the proximal interphalangeal joint (boutonnière); rupture of the distal conjoined slip causes flexion deformity of the distal interphalangeal joint (mallet finger).

NERVES Most of the muscles and the palmar skin of the first three digits (which work together as a functional tripod) are supplied by the median nerve, the muscles and palmar skin of the ring and little fingers by the ulnar nerve, and the long extensors and dorsal skin by the radial nerve. The ulnar nerve also supplies the intrinsics.

SKIN The palmar skin is relatively tight and inelastic; skin loss can be ill-afforded and wounds sutured under tension are liable to break down. The acute sensibility of the digital palmar skin cannot be achieved by any skin graft. By contrast, dorsal skin is lax and mobile, skin wounds are easier to close and skin loss can be readily made good by grafts.

Just deep to the palmar skin is the palmar aponeurosis, the embryological remnant of a superficial layer of finger flexors; attachment to the bases of the proximal phalanges explains part of the deformity of Dupuytren's contracture. Incisions on the palmar surface are also liable to contracture unless they are placed in the line of the skin creases or along the mid-lateral borders of the fingers.

References and further reading

Apley, A.G. (1956) Test for the power of flexor digitorum sublimis. *British Medical Journal* 1, 25–26

Boyes, J.H. (ed.) (1971) *Bunnell's Surgery of the Hand*, 5th edn, Lippincott, Philadelphia

James, J.I.P. (1970) The assessment and management of the injured hand. *Hand* 2, 97–105

Kleinert, H.E., Kutz, J.E., Atasoy, E. and Stormo, A. (1973) Primary repair of flexor tendons. *Orthopedic Clinics of North America* 4, 865–876

Kleinert, H.E., Schepels, S. and Gill, T. (1985) Flexor tendon injuries. *Surgical Clinics of North America* 61, 267–286

Lamb, D.W. (1977) Radial club hand. *Journal of Bone and Joint Surgery* 59A, 1–13

Muira, T., Kino, Y. and Nakamura, R. (1976) Reconstruction of the mutilated hand. *Hand* 8, 78–85

Murrell, G.A.C., Francis, M.J.O. and Howlett, C.R. (1989) Dupuytren's contracture. *Journal of Bone and Joint Surgery* 71B, 367–373

Pulvertaft, R.G. (1973) Twenty-five years of hand surgery. *Journal of Bone and Joint Surgery* 55B, 32–55

Stack, H.G. (1973) *The Palmar Fascia*, Churchill Livingstone, Edinburgh

Wynn Parry, C.B. (1981) *Rehabilitation of the Hand*, 4th edn, Butterworths, London

The neck

17

Examination

Symptoms

The common symptoms of neck disorder are pain and stiffness.

Pain is felt in the neck itself, but it may also be referred to the shoulders or arms. Always enquire if any posture or movement makes it worse; or better.

Stiffness may be either intermittent or continuous. Sometimes it is so severe that the patient can scarcely move the head.

Deformity usually appears as a wry neck; occasionally the neck is fixed in flexion.

Numbness, tingling and weakness in the upper limbs may be due to pressure on a nerve root; weakness in the lower limbs may result from cord compression in the neck.

Headache sometimes emanates from the neck, but if this is the only symptom other causes should be suspected.

'Tension' It is important to listen to the patient's nuances of metaphor and mode of complaint. The neck and back are common 'target zones' for psychosomatic illness.

Signs

No examination of the neck is complete without examination of both upper limbs.*

* Two arms = one neck; if both arms are affected, suspect the neck.

● LOOK
Any deformity is noted. Wry neck, due to muscle spasm, may suggest a disc lesion, an inflammatory disorder or cervical spine injury; but it also occurs with intracranial lesions and disorders of the eyes or semicircular canals. Neck stiffness is usually fairly obvious.

● FEEL
The neck is examined for tender areas or lumps. Muscle spasm may be felt. The anterior structures (trachea, thyroid, oesophagus) should be carefully palpated.

● MOVE
Forward flexion, extension, lateral flexion and rotation are tested, and then shoulder movements. Range of motion normally diminishes with age, but even then movement should be smooth and painfree.

NEUROLOGICAL EXAMINATION
Neurological examination of the upper limbs is mandatory in all cases; in some the lower limbs also should be examined. Muscle power, reflexes and sensation should be carefully tested; even small degrees of abnormality may be significant.

PULSES
The radial pulse is felt with the arm at rest and on traction; it may weaken or disappear if the thoracic outlet is abnormally tight. The subclavian artery also is palpated; it is much easier to feel if a cervical rib is present.

● X-RAY
The anteroposterior view should show the regular, undulating outline of the lateral masses; their symmetry may be disturbed by

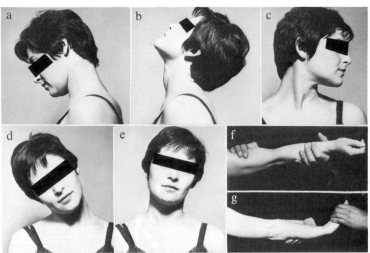

17.1 Examination (a) Flexion, (b) extension, (c) rotation, (d, e) sideways tilt; (f, g) testing power in the elbow and wrist extensors. In this patient with signs of a prolapsed disc, flexion and tilting to the left are limited.

destructive lesions or fractures. A projection through the mouth is required to show the upper two vertebrae. In the lateral view the cervical curve shows four parallel lines: one along the anterior surfaces of the vertebral bodies, one along their posterior surfaces, one along the posterior borders of the lateral masses and one along the bases of the spinous processes; any malalignment suggests subluxation.

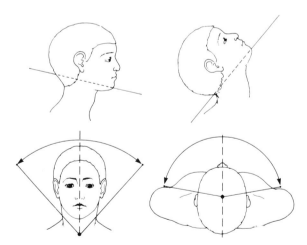

17.2 Normal range of movement In full flexion the chin normally touches the chest; in full extension the imaginary line joining the chin to the posterior occipital protuberance (the occipitomental line) forms an angle of at least 45 degrees with the horizontal, and usually over 60 degrees in young people. Lateral flexion and rotation are equal in both directions.

The disc spaces are inspected and the posterior interspinous spaces compared; if one is wider than the rest, it suggests subluxation or vertebral tilting. Osteophytes are sought; in oblique views their relationship to the intervertebral foramina can be seen. Flexion and extension views are required to demonstrate instability.

COMPUTED TOMOGRAPHY (CT)
In the cervical spine, computed tomography may be invaluable; it shows the shape of the spinal canal and the integrity of the bony structures. Encroaching lesions are sometimes better displayed by combined CT and myelography.

Deformities of the neck

Torticollis

In torticollis the chin is twisted upwards and towards one side. The condition may be either *congenital* or *secondary* to other local disorders.

Infantile (congenital) torticollis

The sternomastoid muscle on one side is fibrous and fails to elongate as the child grows; consequently, progressive deformity develops.

The cause is unknown; the muscle may have suffered ischaemia from a distorted position *in utero* (the association with breech presentation and hip dysplasia is supporting evidence), or it may have been injured at birth.

CLINICAL FEATURES A history of difficult labour or breech delivery is common. In 20% of patients a lump is noticed in the first few weeks of life; it is well defined and involves one or both heads of the sternomastoid. At this stage there is neither deformity nor obvious limitation of movement and within a few months the lump has disappeared.

Deformity does not become apparent until the child is 1–2 years old. The head is tilted to one side, so that the ear approaches the shoulder; the sternomastoid on that side may feel tight and hard. There may also be asymmetrical development of the face. These features become increasingly obvious as the child grows.

DIAGNOSIS Other causes of wry neck (bony anomalies, discitis, lymphadenitis) should be excluded. The history and the typical facial appearance are helpful clues.

TREATMENT If the diagnosis is made during infancy, daily muscle stretching may prevent the incipient deformity. Established wry neck needs operative correction. The contracted muscle is divided (usually at its lower end but sometimes at the upper end or at both ends) and the head is manipulated into the neutral position. After operation, correction must be maintained, at first by a skull-cap tied under the axilla. Subsequently a polythene collar is worn until the child automatically holds the head correctly. Stretching exercises also are continued.

Secondary torticollis

A tilt or twist of the neck may develop as a result of skin scarring (especially after burns), inflamed neck glands or ocular disorders. The commonest cause in adults is a prolapsed intervertebral disc with secondary muscle spasm. Other causes are vertebral injuries, tuberculosis, pyogenic infection, ankylosing spondylitis, osteoid osteoma, intraspinal tumours and intracranial tumours of the poste-

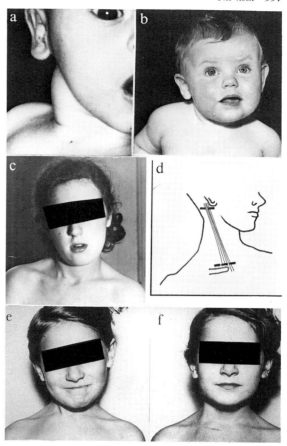

17.3 Torticollis Natural history: (a) sternomastoid tumour in a young baby; (b) early wry neck; (c) deformity with facial hemiatrophy in the adolescent.

Surgical treatment: (d) two sites at which the sternomastoid may be divided; (e, f) before and a few months after operation.

rior fossa. The diagnosis may emerge only after extensive investigations.

SPASMODIC TORTICOLLIS is a bizarre type of dystonia associated with involuntary, twisting or clonic movements of the neck. Spasms are often triggered by emotional disturbance or attempts at correction. The exact cause is unknown, but some cases are associated with lesions of the basal ganglia. Correction is extremely difficult; various drugs, including anticholinergics, have been used, though with little success. More recently, the injection of botulinum toxin into the sternomastoid has produced marked im-

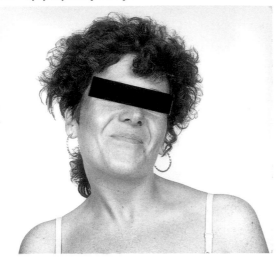

17.4 Spasmodic torticollis Attempted correction was forcibly resisted. This patient looks happy, but the deformity can be very distressing.

provement for periods of 3 months (Marsden and Quinn, 1990; D'Costa and Abbott, 1991). Psychotherapy may be more rewarding.

Vertebral anomalies

A variety of cervical vertebral anomalies have been described. Most are extremely rare. Only two examples are considered here: odontoid hypoplasia and vertebral synostosis.

Odontoid hypoplasia

Though rare, this anomaly is important because it may predispose to atlantoaxial instability (Cope and Olson, 1987). The abnormality is usually discovered incidentally in cervical spine x-rays but patients sometimes present in early adulthood with neck discomfort and transient neurological symptoms. The most frequent association exists in patients with developmental disorders such as Down's syndrome, Morquio's disease and all skeletal dysplasias involving the spine. Odontoid erosion should also be

sought in patients with severe rheumatoid disease, particularly if they are to undergo operations under general anaesthesia.

The diagnosis is usually obvious on x-ray (particularly tomography). Flexion–extension views should be obtained to assess the degree of instability.

If discomfort is marked, and even more so if neurological features are present, atlantoaxial arthrodesis is advisable.

Cervical vertebral synostosis (Klippel–Feil syndrome)

This is a rare developmental disorder representing a failure of segmentation; often cervical vertebral fusion is associated with other, visceral, anomalies (see p. 157).

Children with synostosis have a characteristic appearance: the neck is short or non-existent and there may be webbing; the hairline is low; and neck movements are limited. About 1 in 3 children with synostosis also has Sprengel's deformity of the scapula. X-rays reveal fusion of two or more cervical vertebrae; scoliosis is common. Many of these children have urinary tract abnormalities or congenital heart disease.

Treatment is unnecessary but parents should be warned of the risks of contact sports.

Prolapsed cervical disc

Cervical disc prolapse may be precipitated by local strain or injury, especially sudden unguarded flexion and rotation. In many cases (perhaps in all) there is a predisposing abnormality of the disc with increased nuclear tension. Prolapsed material may press on the posterior longitudinal ligament or dura mater, causing neck pain and stiffness as well as pain referred to the upper limb. Pressure on the nerve roots causes paraesthesia, and sometimes weakness, in one or both arms. Prolapse usually occurs immediately above or below the sixth cervical vertebra, so the nerve roots affected are C6 or C7.

Clinical features

The original attack, unlike that of a lumbar disc prolapse, can seldom be related to definite and severe strain. Subsequent attacks may be sudden or gradual in onset, and with trivial cause. The patient may complain of (1) pain and stiffness of the neck, the pain often radiating to the scapular region and sometimes to the occiput; and (2) pain and paraesthesia in one upper limb (rarely both), often radiating to the outer elbow, back of the wrist and to the index and middle fingers. Weakness is rare. Between attacks the patient feels well, although the neck may feel a bit stiff.

The neck may be held tilted forwards and sideways. The muscles are tender and movements are restricted.

The arms should be examined for neurological deficit. The C6 root innervates the biceps jerk, the biceps muscle and wrist dorsiflexion, and sensation of the lateral forearm, thumb and index finger; C7 innervates the triceps and radial jerks, the triceps muscle, wrist flexors and finger extensors, and sensation in the middle finger.

X-rays may reveal straightening out of the normal cervical lordosis (due to muscle spasm) and narrowing of the affected disc space. *CT* is helpful in showing a herniated disc, especially when combined with *myelography*. However, the best method of displaying the spinal canal and its contents is *MRI*.

Differential diagnosis

Acute cervical prolapse should be differentiated from the following.

NEURALGIC AMYOTROPHY Pain is sudden and severe, and situated over the shoulder rather than in the neck itself. Multiple neurological levels are affected.

CERVICAL SPINE INFECTIONS Pain is unrelenting and local spasm severe. X-rays show erosion of the vertebral end-plates.

CERVICAL TUMOURS Neurological signs are progressive and x-rays reveal bone destruction.

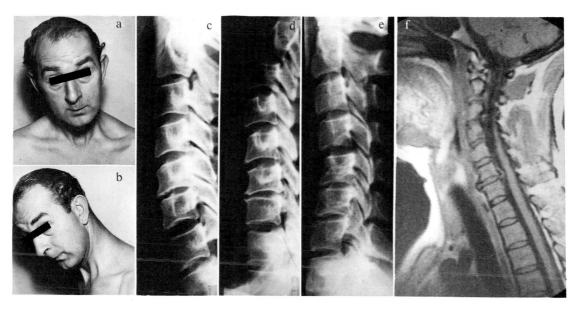

17.5 Cervical disc lesions (a, b) Acute wry neck due to a prolapsed disc. (c) A reduced disc space at C5/6 is not necessarily significant when the cervical lordosis is normal; in (d) the lordosis is obliterated and in (e) it is reversed – both suggest a prolapsed disc. (f) MRI showing a prolapsed disc at C5/6.

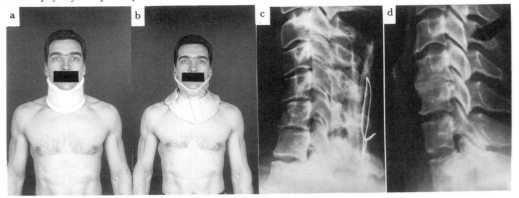

17.6 Cervical disc – treatment   (a) Standard cervical collar. (b) More rigid variety. Operative treatment may consist of (c) posterior fusion with bone grafts, or (d) anterior fusion, in which the disc is removed and the intervertebral height restored by a bone graft.

SUPRASPINATUS TENDON LESIONS   Although the distribution of pain may resemble that of a prolapsed cervical disc, tenderness is localized to the rotator cuff and shoulder movements are abnormal.

Treatment

Heat and analgesics are soothing but, as with lumbar disc prolapse, there are only three satisfactory ways of treating the prolapse itself.

REST   A collar will prevent unguarded movement; it may be made of felt, sponge-rubber or polythene.

REDUCE   Traction may enlarge the disc space, permitting the prolapse to subside. The head of the couch is raised and weights (up to 8 kg) are tied to a harness fitting under the chin and occiput. Traction is applied intermittently for no more than 30 minutes at a time.

REMOVE   If symptoms are refractory and severe enough, the disc may be removed through an anterior approach; bone grafts are inserted to fuse the affected area and to restore the normal intervertebral height (see below for the technique of anterior cervical fusion). Anterior decompression gives excellent long-term relief from radicular symptoms (Jonin et al., 1986).

Cervical spondylosis

Spondylosis is the most common disorder of the cervical spine. The intervertebral discs degenerate and flatten. Bony spurs appear at the anterior and posterior margins of the vertebral bodies; those that develop posteriorly may encroach upon the intervertebral foramina, causing pressure on the dural root sleeves and the nerve roots themselves.

Clinical features

The patient, usually aged over 40, complains of neck pain and stiffness. The symptoms come on gradually and are often worse on first getting up. The pain may radiate widely: to the occiput, the scapular muscles and down one or both arms. Paraesthesia, weakness and clumsiness are occasional symptoms. Typically there are exacerbations of more acute discomfort, and long periods of relative quiescence.

The appearance is normal. Tenderness is felt in the posterior neck muscles and scapular region; all movements are limited and painful.

In one or both upper limbs numbness or weakness may occasionally be found and one of the reflexes may be depressed.

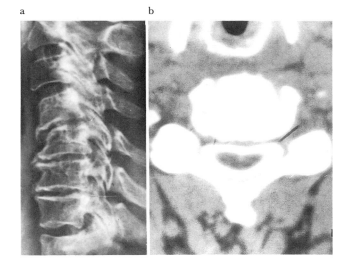

a   b

17.7 Cervical spondylosis (a) Typical x-ray showing multiple disc degeneration and osteophytes. (b) MRI showing encroachment upon the intervertebral foramina.

X-rays show narrowing of one or more intervertebral spaces, with spur formation (or lipping) at the anterior and posterior margins of the disc. These bony spurs (often referred to as 'osteophytes') may encroach upon the intervertebral foramina. If surgery is contemplated, *CT* or *MRI* should be employed to give the most accurate outline of the spinal canal and its contents.

Diagnosis

Other disorders associated with neck or arm pain and sensory symptoms must be excluded. Cervical spine lipping is very common in people over 40 years of age, most of whom are asymptomatic; this can be misleading in patients with other disorders.

CARPAL TUNNEL SYNDROME   Pain and paraesthesia are usually confined to the hand and are worse at night. Nerve conduction is slowed across the wrist. If symptoms fail to improve after carpal tunnel decompression, the patient should be investigated for cervical spondylosis and nerve root irritation.

SUPRASPINATUS TENDON LESIONS   Pain may resemble that of a prolapsed cervical disc, but shoulder movements are abnormal.

CERVICAL TUMOURS   With tumours of the spinal cord, nerve roots or lymph nodes, symptoms are usually continuous, and the x-ray may show the lesion.

THORACIC OUTLET SYNDROME   Symptoms resemble those of cervical spondylosis. The patient may have pain and sensory abnormality mainly down the ulnar border of the forearm. Symptoms are aggravated by arm traction and by elevation and external rotation of the shoulders. And, importantly, neck movements are neither painful nor restricted. X-rays may reveal a cervical rib.

Treatment

Heat and massage are often soothing, but restricting neck movements in a collar is the most effective treatment during painful attacks. Physiotherapy is the mainstay of treatment, patients usually being maintained in relative comfort by various measures including exercises, gentle passive manipulation and intermittent traction.

Operation is seldom indicated, but if only one intervertebral level is affected and symptoms are relieved only by a rigid and irksome support, anterior fusion is appropriate. For multiple level spondylosis, the long-term results of fusion are not significantly better than those following conservative treatment.

TECHNIQUE OF ANTERIOR CERVICAL FUSION The
patient lies supine with the neck supported on
a sandbag and the head turned to the side. At
the appropriate disc level a transverse incision is
made to one side of the midline. The plane
between the trachea and the carotid sheath
leads to the anterior surface of the spine. The
central portion of the affected disc together
with the adjacent bone is excised; the gap is
filled with a corticocancellous bone graft. After
the operation the patient wears a brace for 3–4
months.

Pyogenic infection

Pyogenic infection of the cervical spine is
uncommon, and therefore often misdiagnosed
in the early stages when antibiotic treatment is
most effective.

The organism – usually a staphylococcus –
reaches the spine via the blood stream. Initially,
destructive changes are limited to the intervertebral disc space and the adjacent parts of

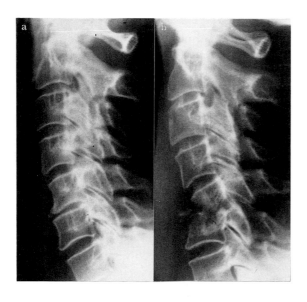

17.8 Pyogenic infection (a) The first x-ray, taken soon
after the onset of symptoms, shows narrowing of the C5/6
disc space but no other abnormality. (b) Three weeks later
there is dramatic destruction and collapse; the speed at
which these have occurred distinguishes pyogenic from
tuberculous infection.

the vertebral bodies. Later, abscess formation
occurs and pus may extend into the spinal canal
or into the soft-tissue planes of the neck.

Clinical features

Vertebral infection may occur at any age. The
patient complains of pain in the neck, often
severe and associated with muscle spasm and
marked stiffness. However, systemic symptoms
are often mild. On examination, neck movements are severely restricted. Blood tests may
show a leucocytosis and an increased ESR.

X-rays at first show either no abnormality or
only slight narrowing of the disc space; later
there may be more obvious signs of bone
destruction.

Treatment

Treatment is by antibiotics and rest. The cervical spine is 'immobilized' by traction; once the
acute phase subsides, a collar may suffice.
Operation is seldom necessary; as the infection
subsides the intervertebral space is obliterated
and the adjacent vertebrae fuse. If there is frank
abscess formation, this will require drainage.

Tuberculosis

Cervical spine tuberculosis is very rare. As with
other types of infection, the organism is blood-
borne and the infection localizes in the intervertebral disc and the anterior parts of the
adjacent vertebral bodies. As the bone crumbles, the cervical spine collapses into kyphosis.
A retropharyngeal abscess forms and points
behind the sternomastoid muscle at the side of
the neck. In late cases cord damage may cause
neurological signs varying from mild weakness
to tetraplegia.

Clinical features

The patient – usually a child – complains of
neck pain and stiffness. In neglected cases a
retropharyngeal abscess may cause difficulty in

swallowing or swelling at the side of the neck. On examination the neck is extremely tender and all movements are restricted. In late cases there may be obvious kyphosis, a fluctuant abscess in the neck or a retropharyngeal swelling. The limbs should be examined for neurological defects.

X-rays show narrowing of the disc space and erosion of the adjacent vertebral bodies.

Treatment

Treatment is by antituberculous drugs (p. 49) and 'immobilization' of the neck in a cervical brace or plaster cast for 6–18 months. Operative treatment may become necessary (1) to drain a retropharyngeal abscess, (2) to decompress a threatened cord, or (3) to fuse an unstable spine. Debridement of necrotic bone and anterior fusion with bone grafts may also be offered (4) as an alternative to prolonged immobilization in a brace or cast.

Rheumatoid arthritis

The cervical spine is severely affected in 30% of patients with rheumatoid arthritis. Three types of lesion are common: (1) erosion of the atlantoaxial joints and the transverse ligament, with resulting instability; (2) erosion of the atlanto-occipital articulations, allowing the odontoid peg to ride up into the foramen magnum (cranial sinkage); and (3) erosion of the facet joints in the mid-cervical region, sometimes ending in fusion but more often leading to subluxation. In addition, vertebral osteoporosis is common, due either to the disease or to the effect of corticosteroid therapy, or both. Considering the amount of atlantoaxial displacement that occurs (often greater than 1 cm), neurological complications are uncommon. However, they do occur – especially in long-standing cases – and are produced by mechanical compression of the cord, by local granulation tissue formation or (very rarely) by thrombosis of the vertebral arteries.

Clinical features

The patient is usually a woman with advanced rheumatoid arthritis. She has neck pain, and movements are markedly restricted. Symptoms and signs of root compression may be present in the upper limbs; less often there is lower limb weakness and upper motor neuron signs due to cord compression. Some patients, though completely unaware of any neurological deficit, are found on careful examination to have mild sensory disturbance or pyramidal tract signs (e.g. abnormally brisk reflexes).

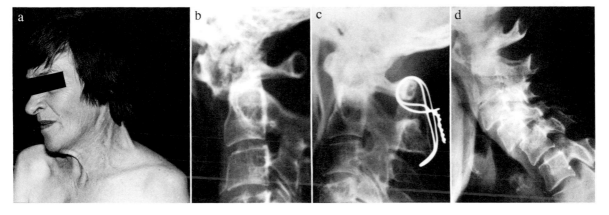

17.9 Rheumatoid arthritis (a) Movement is severely restricted; attempted rotation causes pain and muscle spasm. (b) Atlantoaxial subluxation is common; erosion of the joints and the transverse ligament has allowed the atlas to slip forward about 2 cm; (c) reduction and posterior fusion with wire fixation. (d) This patient has subluxation, not only at the atlantoaxial joint but also at two levels in the mid-cervical region.

X-rays show the features of an erosive arthritis, usually at several levels. *Atlantoaxial instability* is visible in lateral films taken in flexion and extension; in flexion the anterior arch of the atlas rides forwards, leaving a gap of 5 mm or more between the back of the anterior arch and the odontoid process; on extension the subluxation is reduced. *Atlanto-occipital erosion* is more difficult to see, but a lateral tomograph shows the relationship of the odontoid to the foramen magnum. Normally the odontoid tip is less than 5 mm above McGregor's line (a line from the posterior edge of the hard palate to the lowest point on the occiput); in erosive arthritis the odontoid tip may be 10–12 mm above this line. Flexion views may also show *anterior subluxation in the mid-cervical region.*

Treatment

Despite the startling x-ray appearances, serious neurological complications are uncommon. Pain can usually be relieved by wearing a collar.

The indications for operative stabilization of the cervical spine are (1) severe and unremitting pain, and (2) neurological signs of root or cord compression. Arthrodesis is by bone grafting followed by a halo–body cast, or by internal fixation (posterior wiring or a rectangular fixator) and bone grafting. Postoperatively a cervical brace is worn for 3 months; however, if instability is marked and operative fixation

insecure, a halo–jacket may be necessary. In patients with very advanced disease and severe erosive changes, postoperative morbidity and mortality are high (Ranawat et al., 1979). This is an argument for operating at an earlier stage for 'impending neurological deficit', as diagnosed from x-ray signs of severe atlantoaxial subluxation, upward migration of the odontoid or subaxial vertebral subluxation together with CT, myelographic or MR images of cord or brainstem compression (Clark, Goetz and Menezes, 1989).

Neuralgic amyotrophy (acute brachial neuritis)

This unusual cause of severe cervicobrachial pain and weakness is believed to be a viral infection of the cervical nerve roots; there is often a history of an antecedent viral infection and sometimes a small epidemic occurs among inmates of an institution.

The history alone often suggests the diagnosis. Pain in the shoulder and arm is intense and sudden in onset. It may extend into the neck and down as far as the hand; usually it lasts a few days but may continue for weeks. Other symptoms are paraesthesia in the arm or hand, and weakness of the muscles of the shoulder, forearm and hand.

Wasting of the deltoid or the small muscles of the hand may be obvious after a few days, and winging of the scapula is common. Isolated paralysis of the serratus anterior (which nearly always affects the right side) may be related, since the neurological involvement is often patchy (Foo and Swann, 1983). Shoulder movement is limited by pain but this limitation is invariably transient. Sensory loss in one or more of the cervical dermatomes is not uncommon. The feature that distinguishes neuralgic amyotrophy from an acute cervical disc herniation is the involvement of multiple nerve root levels.

There is no specific treatment; pain is controlled with analgesics. The prognosis is usually good but full neurological recovery may take months or years (Bacevich, 1976).

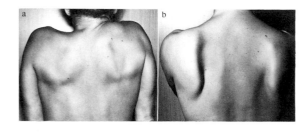

17.10 Neuralgic amyotrophy (a, b) This young nurse complained of acute neck and shoulder pain on the left. She has weakness of levator scapulae and slight winging of the left scapula. The neurological defect usually returns to normal but occasionally wasting and weakness are permanent.

Thoracic outlet syndrome ('cervical rib')

Neurological and vascular symptoms and signs in the upper limbs may be produced by compression of the lower trunk of the brachial plexus (C8 and T1) and subclavian vessels between the clavicle and the most proximal rib.

The subclavian artery and lower brachial trunk pass through a triangle based on the first rib and bordered by scalenus anterior and medius. Even under normal circumstances these neurovascular structures bend acutely when the arm rests by the side; an extra rib (or its fibrous equivalent extending from a large costal process), or an anomalous scalene muscle, sharpens the angle by forcing the vessel and nerve still higher. Even with normal ribs and muscles a post-fixed brachial plexus is excessively angulated.

These anomalies are all congenital; yet symptoms are rare before the age of 30. This is probably because, with declining youth, the shoulders sag, increasing the bend of the neurovascular bundle; indeed drooping shoulders alone may cause the syndrome.

As a result of increased angulation the first thoracic nerve may be stretched or compressed, causing sensory changes along the postaxial forearm and hand, with weakness of the intrinsic hand muscles. The subclavian artery is rarely compressed but may be narrowed by irritation of its sympathetic supply, or its wall damaged leading to the formation of small emboli.

Clinical features

There are no general symptoms or neck symptoms. The patient, usually a female in her 30s, may complain of: (1) pain and/or paraesthesia in the ulnar forearm and hand, worse after household chores or after carrying shopping; (2) weakness or clumsiness; and (3) excessive sweating, or blueness and coldness of the fingers.

If a female, the patient is often long-necked with sloping shoulders (like a Modigliani painting); if a male, he is more likely to be thick-necked and muscular.

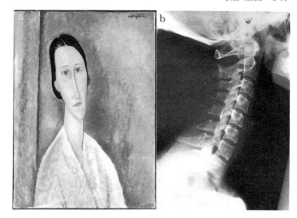

17.11 Thoracic outlet syndrome (a) Madame Zborowska. Oil on canvas. Amadeo Modigliani. 1918 (The Tate Gallery, London). (b) X-ray of a 'long-necked' woman: all the vertebrae down to T1 are above the clavicle.

A lump (the abnormally elevated subclavian artery) may be palpable above the clavicle. It pulsates, is tender and pressure on it may increase symptoms. Apart from this, neurological signs predominate. There may be mild clawing of one or both hands, slight wasting of the interosseous and hypothenar muscles and weakness of the intrinsics. Reflexes are usually normal. Sensation may be diminished in the C8 and T1 distribution.

Vascular signs are uncommon, but there may be cyanosis and increased sweating. Special manoeuvres are used to test for pulse obliteration. In one, the pulse fades when the arm is elevated to 90 degrees and externally rotated while the neck is turned to the opposite side. In another, the same effect is produced by pulling the arm downwards and backwards while pushing the neck away. It should be remembered that pulse amplitude changes with arm posture in most normal people.

Neck and shoulder movements are normal, a helpful observation in excluding a diagnosis of cervical disc disease or musculotendinous cuff disorder.

X-ray may show a 'long' neck – i.e. the first thoracic vertebra stands clear in views of the cervical spine. Occasionally a well-formed cervical rib is seen, but more often there is merely enlargement of the transverse process of the seventh cervical vertebra.

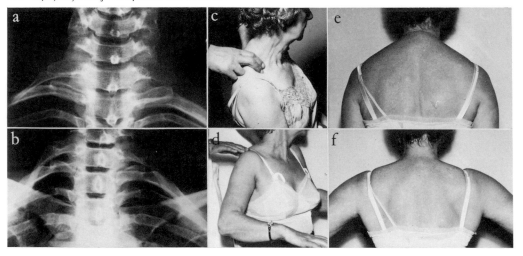

17.12 Cervical ribs (a) Unilateral; (b) bilateral. (c) A pulsating lump (the elevated subclavian artery) is usually palpable. (d) Teaching the patient shrugging exercises; before exercises the shoulders sag (e) – the aim is to restore the posture shown in (f).

Differential diagnosis

Many disorders resemble cervical rib syndrome.

CERVICAL SPINE LESIONS In disc prolapse or spondylosis, pain is more vaguely distributed, and neck movements are limited. In tuberculosis and secondary deposits the x-ray appearance is characteristic.

CARPAL TUNNEL SYNDROME Until this common disorder was widely recognized, many cases were wrongly called cervical rib syndrome. Even when x-rays show a rib, the symptoms may still be due to median nerve compression in the carpal tunnel. The nocturnal pain and its distribution are characteristic.

ULNAR TUNNEL SYNDROME The symptoms and signs are sharply confined to the distribution of the ulnar nerve, and the neck is unaffected.

ACROPARAESTHESIA There is sensory disturbance in both hands and sometimes the feet. When only the hands are affected the diagnosis is usually wrong, and the patient is probably suffering from a carpal tunnel syndrome.

PANCOAST SYNDROME Apical carcinoma of the bronchus may infiltrate the structures at the root of the neck, causing pain, numbness and

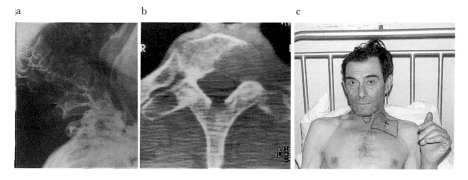

17.13 Malignant deposits Typical destructive changes in (a) the plain x-ray and (b) a CT scan. (c) This man, with a hard mass in the root of the neck and weakness of the left hand, had an apical carcinoma of the bronchus – Pancoast syndrome.

weakness of the hand. A hard mass may be palpable in the neck and x-ray of the chest shows a characteristic opacity.

SPINAL CORD LESIONS Syringomyelia or other spinal cord lesions may cause wasting of the hand, but other neurological features establish the diagnosis.

CUFF LESIONS With supraspinatus tendon lesions pain sometimes radiates to the arm and hand but shoulder movement is abnormal and painful.

Treatment

Most patients can be managed by conservative treatment: exercises to strengthen the shrugging muscles, postural training and instruction in ways of preventing shoulder droop or muscle fatigue, and analgesics when necessary.

Operative treatment is indicated if pain is severe, if muscle wasting is obvious or if there are vascular disturbances. The thoracic outlet is decompressed by removing the first rib (or the cervical rib). This is best accomplished by the transaxillary approach, but care must be taken to prevent injury to the brachial plexus and subclavian vessels, or perforation of the pleura (Roos, 1966).

Notes on applied anatomy

In the upright posture the neck has a gentle anterior convexity; this natural lordosis may straighten but is never quite reversed, even in flexion, unless it is abnormal.

Eight pairs of nerve roots from the cervical cord pass through the relatively narrow intervertebral foramina, the first between the occiput and C1, and the eighth between C7 and the first thoracic (T1) vertebra; thus each segmental root from the first to the seventh lies above the vertebra of the same number. Thus a lesion between C5 and C6 might compress the sixth root.

The intervertebral discs lie close to the nerve roots as they emerge through the foramina; even a small herniation often causes root symptoms rather than neck pain. Moreover, disc degeneration is associated with spur formation on both the posterior aspect of the vertebral body and the associated facet joint; the resulting encroachment on the intervertebral foramen traps the nerve root. It is important to remember, however, that 'root pain' alone (i.e. pain in the shoulder and arm) does not necessarily signify nerve-root irritation; it may be referred from the facet joint or the soft structures around it. Only paraesthesiae and sensory or motor loss are unequivocal evidence of nerve root compression.

At the atlanto-occipital joint, the movement that occur are nodding and tilting (lateral flexion); there is no rotation, and when this movement takes place (at the atlantoaxial joint) the atlas and the skull move as one. In the rest of the cervical spine, movements that occur are flexion, extension and tilting to either side; the facets permit subluxation or dislocation to occur without fracture, a displacement that the strong posterior ligaments normally prevent.

References and further reading

Bacevich, B.B. (1976) Paralytic brachial neuritis. *Journal of Bone and Joint Surgery* **58A**, 262–263

Clark, C.R., Goetz, D.D. and Menczes, A.H. (1989) Arthrodesis of the cervical spine in rheumatoid arthritis. *Journal of Bone and Joint Surgery* **71A**, 381–392

Cope, R. and Olson, S. (1987) Abnormalities of the cervical spine in Down's syndrome: diagnosis, risks and review of the literature, with particular reference to the Special Olympics, *Southern Medical Journal* **80**, 30–36

D'Costa, D.F. and Abbott, R.J. (1991) Low dose botulinum toxin in spasmodic torticollis. *Journal of the Royal Society of Medicine* **84**, 650–651

Editorial (1972) Signs and symptoms in cervical spondylosis. *Lancet* **2**, 70–72

Foo, C.L. and Swann, M. (1983) Isolated paralysis of the serratus anterior. *Journal of Bone and Joint Surgery* **65B**, 552–556

Jonin, M., Lesoin, F., Lozes, G., Thomas, C.E., Rousseaux, M. and Clarisse, J. (1986) Herniated cervical discs: analysis of a series of 230 cases. *Acta Neurochirurgica* **79**, 107–113

Marsden, C.D. and Quinn, N.P. (1990) The dystonias. *British Medical Journal* **300**, 139–144

Ranawat, C.S., O'Leary, P., Pellici, P. et al. (1979) Cervical spine fusion in rheumatoid arthritis. *Journal of Bone and Joint Surgery* **61A**, 1003–1010

Roos, D.B. (1966) Transaxillary approach for first rib resection to relieve thoracic outlet syndrome. *Annals of Surgery* **163**, 354–358

The back

18

Examination

Symptoms

The usual symptoms of back disorders are pain, stiffness and deformity in the back, and pain, paraesthesia or weakness in the lower limbs. The mode of onset is very important: did it start suddenly, perhaps after a lifting strain; or gradually without any antecedent event? Are the symptoms constant, or are there periods of remission? Are they related to any particular posture? Has there been any associated illness or malaise?

Pain, either sharp and localized or chronic and diffuse, is the commonest presenting symptom. Backache is usually felt low down and on either side of the midline, often extending into the upper part of the buttock.

Sciatica is a term used to describe pain radiating from the buttock into the thigh and calf – more or less in the distribution of the sciatic nerve. However, it is rarely due to sciatic nerve pathology. It is a type of *referred pain,* usually from the dural sleeve of a lumbar or sacral nerve root or from an abnormal vertebral joint. Kellgren (1977), in a classic experiment, showed that almost any structure in a spinal segment can, if irritated sufficiently, give rise to pain spreading into the lower limbs. In practice, however, pain referred from the root dura is characteristically more intense, aggravated by coughing or straining, and often accompanied by symptoms of root pressure such as numbness or paraesthesia.

348

Stiffness may be sudden in onset and almost complete (after a disc prolapse) or continuous and predictably worse in the mornings (suggesting arthritis or ankylosing spondylitis).

Deformity is usually noticed by others, but the patient may become aware of shoulder asymmetry or of clothes not fitting well.

Numbness or paraesthesia is felt anywhere in the lower limb, but can usually be mapped fairly accurately over one of the dermatomes. It is important to ask if it is aggravated by standing or walking and relieved by sitting down – the classic symptom of spinal stenosis.

Urinary retention or incontinence can be due to pressure on the cauda equina. *Faecal incontinence* or urgency, and *impotence,* may also occur.

Other symptoms important in back disorders are *urethral discharge, diarrhoea* and *sore eyes* – the features of Reiter's disease.

Signs

The patient is examined first standing, then lying face downwards, then lying face upwards. Adequate exposure is essential; patients should strip to their underclothes.

Signs with the patient standing

● LOOK

Skin Scars, pigmentation, abnormal hair or unusual skin creases may be seen.

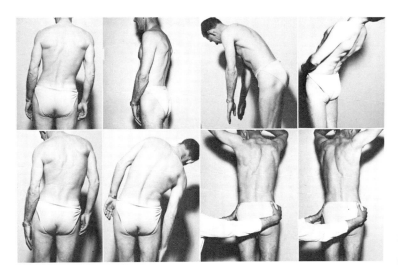

18.1 Examination (1) This patient has a prolapsed lumbar disc. He stands with a tilt. Forward flexion and tilting to the left are limited – other movements full.

Shape and posture Asymmetry of the chest, trunk or pelvis may be obvious, or may appear only when the patient bends forwards. Lateral deviation of the spine is described as a list to one or other side; lateral curvature is scoliosis.

Seen from the side the thoracic spine may seem unduly bent (kyphosis); if it is sharply angulated the prominence is called a kyphos or gibbus. The lumbar spine may be unusually flat or excessively lordosed.

If the patient consistently stands with one knee bent (even though his legs are equal in length) this suggests nerve root tension on that side; flexing the knee relaxes the sciatic nerve and reduces the pull on the nerve root.

● FEEL

The spinous processes and the interspinous ligaments are palpated, noting any prominence or a 'step'. *Tenderness* should be localized to (1) bony structures, (2) the intervertebral tissues or (3) the surrounding muscles.

● MOVE

Flexion is tested by asking the patient to try to touch his toes. Even with a stiff back he may be able to do this by flexing the hips; so watch the lumbar spine to see if it really moves, or, better still, measure the spinal excursion. The *mode of flexion* (whether it is smooth or hesitant) and the way in which the patient comes back to the upright position are also important. In lumbar instability the patient tends to regain the upright position by pushing on his knees. To test *extension* ask the patient to lean backwards; with a stiff spine he may cheat by bending the knees. The 'wall test' will unmask a minor flexion deformity; standing with the back flush against a wall, the heels, buttocks, shoulders and occiput should all make contact with the surface. Lateral flexion is tested by asking the patient to bend sideways, sliding his hand down the outer side of his leg; the two sides are compared. *Rotation* is examined by asking him to twist the trunk to each side in turn while the pelvis is anchored by the examiner's hands; this is essentially a thoracic movement and is not limited in lumbosacral disease. Rib excursion is assessed by measuring the *chest circumference* in full expiration and then in full inspiration; the normal difference is about 7 cm.

Muscle power in the feet and ankles is conveniently tested with the patient standing. Ask him to stand up on his toes (plantarflexion) and then to rock back on his heels (dorsiflexion); small differences between the two sides are easily spotted.

Signs with the patient lying face downwards

Bony outlines and small lumps can be felt more easily with the patient lying face down. Deep *tenderness* is easy to localize but difficult to ascribe to a particular structure.

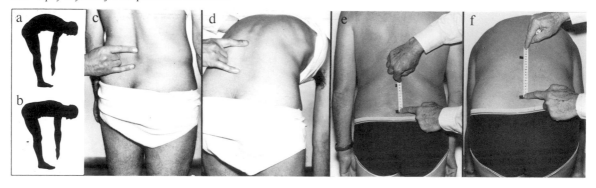

18.2 Examination (2)   In both diagrams the hands nearly reach the toes; to distinguish spine flexion (a) from hip flexion (b), watch the lumbar lordosis undoing as the patient bends. Alternatively (c, d), note the separation of fingers placed on the spinous processes. Better still (e, f), *measure* the lumbar excursion; with the patient upright, two bony points 10 cm apart are selected – in full flexion they should separate by at least a further 5 cm.

The popliteal and posterior tibial *pulses* are felt, hamstring *power* is tested and *sensation* on the back of the limbs assessed. The *femoral stretch test* (for lumbar root tension) is carried out by flexing the patient's knee and lifting the hip into extension; pain may be felt in the front of the thigh and in the back.

Signs with the patient lying on his back

The patient is observed as he turns – is there pain or stiffness? A rapid appraisal of the thyroid, chest (and breasts), abdomen (and scrotum) is worth while and, if there is even a hint of generalized disease, is essential. Hip and knee mobility are assessed before testing for cord or root involvement.

The *straight leg raising test* discloses lumbosacral root tension. With the knee held absolutely straight, the leg is lifted from the couch until the patient experiences pain – not merely in the thigh (which is common and not significant) but also in the buttock and calf (Lasègue's test); the angle at which this occurs is noted. Normally it should be possible to raise the limb to 80–90 degrees; people with lax ligaments can go even further. At the point where the patient

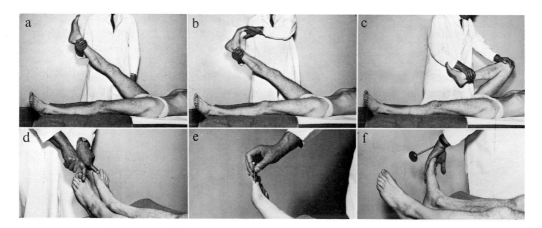

18.3 Examination (3)   The legs are examined for nerve root involvement. (a) Straight leg raising is limited, and (b) the sciatic stretch is positive; but (c) flexion of the hip with the knee bent is painless, demonstrating that the hip is not at fault. (d) Muscle power, (e) skin sensation and (f) the tendon reflexes are tested.

experiences discomfort, passive dorsiflexion of the foot may cause an additional stab of pain. If the knee is slightly flexed, buttock pain is suddenly relieved; pain may then be reinduced without extending the knee by simply pressing on the lateral popliteal nerve, to tighten it like a bowstring. Sometimes straight leg raising on the unaffected side produces pain on the affected side. This 'crossed sciatic tension' is indicative of severe root irritation, usually due to a central prolapsed disc, and suggests risk to the sacral nerve roots that control bladder function.

A *full neurological examination* of the lower limbs is then carried out.

The *pulses* are felt and the extremities are carefully examined for *trophic changes*.

Unless the signs point clearly to a spinal disorder, *rectal and vaginal examination* may also be necessary.

Imaging

Plain x-rays begin with anteroposterior and lateral views of the spine; for the lumbar region, oblique views of the spine, an anteroposterior x-ray of the pelvis and a posteroanterior view of the sacroiliac joints are often needed as well.

In the anteroposterior view the spine should look perfectly straight and the soft-tissue shadows should outline the normal muscle planes. Curvature (scoliosis) is obvious, and bulging of the psoas muscle plane may indicate a paravertebral abscess. Individual vertebrae may show alterations in structure (e.g. asymmetry or collapse) and the intervertebral spaces may be edged by bony spurs (suggesting disc degeneration) or bridged by fine bony syndesmophytes. The sacroiliac joints may show erosion or ankylosis.

In the lateral view the normal thoracic kyphosis and lumbar lordosis should be regular and uninterrupted. Anterior shift of an upper segment upon a lower (spondylolisthesis) may be associated with defects of the posterior arch which show best in oblique views. Individual vertebrae, which should be rectangular, may be wedged or biconcave. Bone density and trabecular markings also are best seen in lateral films.

Radioisotope scanning may pick up areas of increased activity, suggesting a fracture, a 'silent' metastasis or a local inflammatory lesion.

Computed tomography is invaluable in the diagnosis of structural bone changes (e.g. vertebral fracture) and intervertebral disc prolapse. When combined with *myelography* it gives valuable information about the contents of the spinal canal.

MR imaging may do away with the need for myelography. The spinal canal and disc spaces are clearly outlined in various planes.

Discography and *facet joint arthrography* are sometimes performed in the investigation of chronic back pain. Disc degeneration or facet joint arthritis may be seen but is not necessarily the cause of the symptoms.

Vertebral deformities

Variations and *abnormalities of segmentation* are common; they include harmless anomalies such as lumbarization of the first sacral segment, 'sacralization' of one or both transverse processes of the fifth lumbar vertebra and asymmetry of the apophyseal joints, as well as such conditions as hemivertebra, which may give rise to severe spinal deformity (see below).

The most serious type of *congenital defect* is spina bifida, which is dealt with in detail in Chapter 10.

'Spinal deformity' (as opposed to deformities of individual vertebrae) affects the entire shape of the back and manifests as abnormal curvature, in either the coronal plane (scoliosis) or the sagittal plane (kyphosis and lordosis).

Scoliosis

Scoliosis is an apparent lateral curvature of the spine. 'Apparent' because, although the torso does indeed have a sinuous appearance when seen from behind, and true lateral curvature of the spine is a real enough entity, the commonest form of scoliosis is actually a triplanar deformity with lateral, anteroposterior and rotational components (Dickson et al., 1984).

Postural scoliosis

In postural scoliosis the deformity is secondary or compensatory to some condition outside the spine, such as a short leg, or pelvic tilt due to contracture of the hip; when the patient sits (thereby cancelling leg asymmetry) the curve disappears. Local muscle spasm associated with a prolapsed lumbar disc may cause a skew back; although sometimes called 'sciatic scoliosis' this, too, is a spurious deformity.

Structural scoliosis

In structural scoliosis there is a non-correctible deformity of the affected spinal segment, an essential component of which is vertebral rotation; the spinous processes swing round towards the concavity of the curve. Dickson and his coworkers (1984) have pointed out that this is really a lordoscoliosis associated with rotational buckling of the spine. The initial deformity is probably correctible, but once it exceeds a certain point of mechanical stability the spine

buckles and rotates into a fixed deformity which does not disappear with changes in posture. Secondary curves nearly always develop to counterbalance the primary deformity; they, too, may later become fixed.

Once fully established, the deformity is liable to increase throughout the growth period. Thereafter, further deterioration is slight, though curves greater than 50 degrees may go on increasing by 1 degree per year.

Most cases have no obvious cause (*idiopathic scoliosis*); other varieties are *osteopathic* (due to bony anomalies), *neuropathic* (associated with some muscle dystrophies) and a *miscellaneous* group of connective-tissue disorders.

Clinical features

Deformity is usually the presenting symptom: an obvious skew back or a rib hump in thoracic curves, and asymmetrical prominence of one hip in thoracolumbar curves. Balanced curves sometimes pass unnoticed until an adult presents with *backache*. Where school screening programmes are conducted, children will be referred with very minor deformities.

There may be a *family history* of scoliosis or a record of some *abnormality during pregnancy or childbirth*; the early *developmental milestones* should be noted.

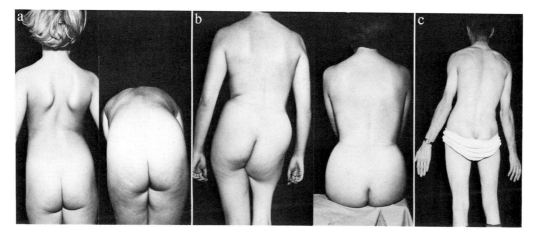

18.4 Mobile scoliosis   (a) Postural scoliosis disappears on flexion. (b) Short leg scoliosis disappears when the patient sits. (c) Sciatic scoliosis disappears when the underlying cause (a prolapsed disc) has been treated.

The trunk should be completely exposed and the patient examined from in front, from the back and from the side.

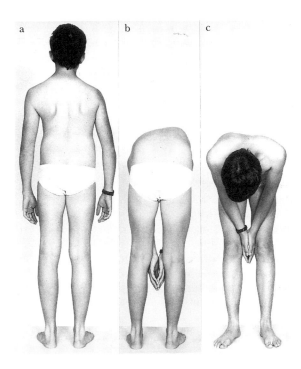

18.5 Fixed scoliosis (structural) Even if asymmetry is not noticed when the patient is standing (a), it shows clearly on flexion (b, c).

Skin pigmentation and congenital anomalies such as sacral dimples or hair tufts are sought. The *spine* may be obviously deviated from the midline, or this may become apparent only when the patient bends forward. The level and direction of the major curve convexity are noted (e.g. 'right thoracic' means a curve in the thoracic spine and convex to the right). In balanced deformities the occiput is over the midline; in unbalanced curves it is not. The hip sticks out on the concave side and the scapula on the convex. The breasts and shoulders also may be asymmetrical. With thoracic scoliosis, rotation causes the rib angles to protrude, thus producing an asymmetrical rib hump on the convex side of the curve.

The diagnostic feature of fixed (as distinct from postural or mobile) scoliosis is that forward bending makes the curve more obvious. Spinal mobility should be assessed and the effect of lateral bending on the curve noted.

Side-on posture should also be observed. There may appear to be excessive kyphosis or lordosis.

Leg length is measured. If one side is short, the pelvis is levelled by standing the patient on wooden blocks and the spine is re-examined.

General examination includes a search for the possible cause and an assessment of cardio-pulmonary function (which is reduced in severe curves).

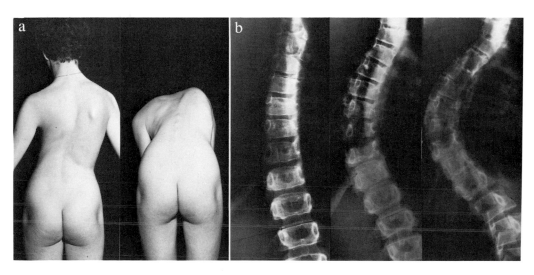

18.6 Fixed scoliosis (a) A fixed (structural) curve is more obvious on flexion. (b) Over a period of 4 years this curve has increased – most rapidly in the last 12 months, during the prepubertal spurt of growth.

X-rays

Plain films: full length posteroanterior and lateral x-rays of the spine and iliac crests must be taken with the patient erect. Structural curves show vertebral rotation: in the postero-anterior x-ray, vertebrae towards the apex of the curve appear to be asymmetrical and the spinous processes are deviated towards the midline; the upper and lower ends of the curve are identified as the levels where vertebral symmetry is regained. The degree of curvature is measured by drawing lines on the x-ray at the upper border of the uppermost vertebra and the lower border of the lowermost vertebra of the curve; the angle subtended by these lines is the *angle of curvature* (Cobb's angle). The primary structural curve is usually balanced by compensatory curves above and below, or by a second 'primary' curve, also with vertebral rotation (sometimes there are multiple 'primary' curves). What is not readily appreciated from these films is the degree of lordosis in the primary curve(s) and kyphosis in the compensatory curves (Archer and Dickson, 1989); indeed, it is postulated that flattening or reversal of the normal thoracic kyphosis superimposed on coronal plane asymmetry leads, with growth, to progressive idiopathic scoliosis. Lateral bending views are taken to assess the degree of curve correctibility.

Skeletal maturity is assessed in several ways (this is important because the curve often progresses most during the period of rapid skeletal growth and maturation). The iliac apophyses start ossifying shortly after puberty; ossification extends medially and, once the iliac crests are completely ossified, further progression of the scoliosis is minimal (Risser's sign). This stage of development usually coincides with fusion of the vertebral ring apophyses. 'Skeletal age' may also be estimated from x-rays of the wrist and hand.

Special imaging, including CT and myelography, may be necessary to define a vertebral abnormality or cord compression.

Special investigations

Pulmonary function tests are performed in all cases of severe chest deformity. A marked reduction in vital capacity is associated with diminished life expectancy and carries obvious risks for surgery.

Patients with muscular dystrophies or connective tissue disorders require full *biochemical* and *neuromuscular* investigation of the underlying condition.

Prognosis and treatment

Prognosis is the key to treatment: the aim is to prevent severe deformity. Generally speaking, the younger the child and the higher the curve the worse is the prognosis. Management differs for the different types of scoliosis, which are considered below.

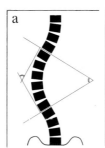
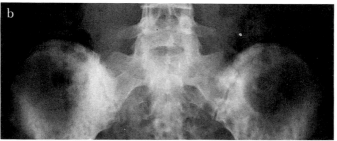

18.7 Scoliosis – measurement and maturity   (a) Measuring the primary curve; the disc spaces are wider on the convex side – lines drawn at each end of the primary curve show the angle of deformity (Cobb's angle). (b) When the iliac apophyses are completely ossified, spinal maturity has been reached; there may be further increase of curvature, but it will be slight.

Idiopathic scoliosis

About 80% of all scoliosis is idiopathic. The deformity is sometimes familial, and the population incidence of serious curves (over 30 degrees and therefore needing treatment) is 3 per 1000, though trivial curves are very much more common. The age at onset defines three groups: adolescent, juvenile and infantile.

Infantile thoracic

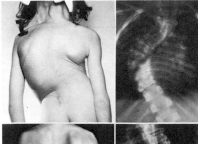

60% male.
90% convex to left.
Associated with ipsilateral plagiocephaly. May be resolving or progressive.
Progressive variety becomes severe.

Adolescent thoracic

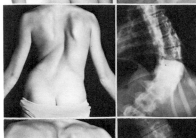

90% female.
90% convex to right.
Rib rotation exaggerates the deformity.
50% develop curves of greater than 70 degrees.

Thoracolumbar

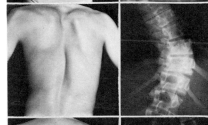

Slightly more common in females.
Slightly more common to right.
Features mid-way between adolescent thoracic and lumbar.

Lumbar

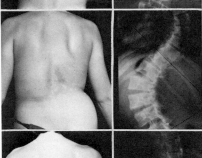

More common in females.
80% convex to left.
One hip prominent but no ribs to accentuate deformity.
Therefore not noticed early, but backache in adult life.

Combined

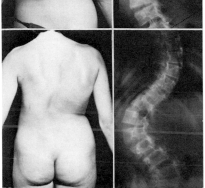

Two primary curves, one in each direction.
Even when radiologically severe, clinical deformity relatively slight because always well balanced.

18.8 Fixed scoliosis – idiopathic curve patterns

Adolescent idiopathic scoliosis

(presenting aged 10 or over)

This, the commonest group, occurs mostly (90%) in girls. Primary thoracic curves are usually convex to the right, lumbar curves to the left; intermediate (thoracolumbar) and combined (double primary) curves also occur. Progression is not inevitable; indeed, most curves under 20 degrees either resolve spontaneously or remain unchanged. However, once a curve starts to progress, it usually goes on doing so throughout the remaining growth period (and, to a much lesser degree, beyond that). Reliable predictors of progression are (1) a very young age, (2) marked curvature and (3) an incomplete Risser sign at presentation (Lonstein and Carlson, 1984). In prepubertal children, rapid progression is liable to occur during the growth spurt.

TREATMENT The aims of treatment are (1) to prevent a mild deformity from becoming severe, and (2) to correct an existing deformity that is unacceptable to the patient. A period of preliminary observation may be needed before deciding between conservative and operative treatment. At 4-monthly intervals the patient is examined, photographed and x-rayed so that curves can be measured and checked for progression.

If the patient is approaching skeletal maturity and the deformity is acceptable (which usually means it is less than 30 degrees and well balanced), treatment is probably unnecessary unless sequential x-rays show definite progression. *Exercises* are often prescribed; they have no effect on the curve but they do maintain muscle tone and may inspire confidence in a favourable outcome. If a curve between 20 and 30 degrees is progressing, some form of *support* may, in addition, be needed. The *Milwaukee brace* is principally a thoracic support consisting of a pelvic corset connected by adjustable steel supports to a cervical ring carrying occipital and chin pads; its purpose is to reduce the lumbar lordosis and encourage active stretching and straightening of the thoracic spine. The *Boston brace* is a snug-fitting underarm brace which provides lumbar or low thoracolumbar support. Corrective pads may be added to these devices to apply pressure at a particular site. A well-made brace can be worn 23 hours out of 24 and does not preclude full daily activities, including sport and exercises.

Operative treatment is indicated (1) for curves of more than 30 degrees that are cosmetically unacceptable, especially in prepubertal children who are liable to develop marked progression during the growth spurt, and (2) for milder deformity that deteriorates significantly despite conservative treatment. Balanced, dou-

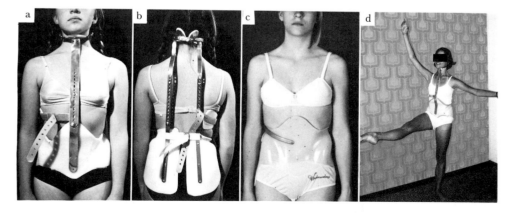

18.9 Fixed scoliosis – conservative treatment (a, b) The Milwaukee brace fits snugly over the pelvis below; chin and head pads promote active postural correction; a thoracic pad presses on the ribs at the apex of the curve. (c) The Boston brace is used for low curves. All braces are cumbersome, but (d) if well made they need not interfere much with activity.

ble primary curves require operation only if they are greater than 60 degrees and progressing (Kostuik, 1990). Adults may need operation for back pain.

The objectives are (1) to reduce the rotational deformity and lateral deviation, and (2) to arthrodese the entire primary curve. For mobile curves, this is achieved by a posterior operation using either Harrington instrumenta-

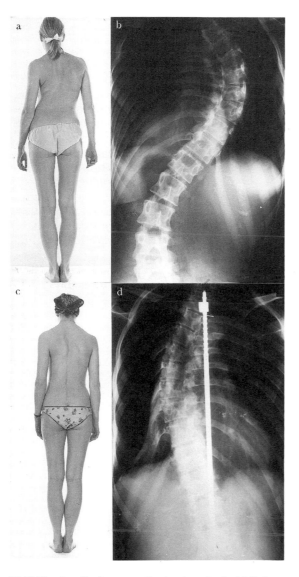

18.10 Fixed scoliosis – operative treatment　(a, b) Before, and (c, d) after correction and fusion using a Harrington rod.

tion combined with sublaminar wiring, but strictly avoiding distraction of the spine (Dickson, 1989), or – the preferred option nowadays – Cotrel–Dubousset instrumentation (Cotrel, Dubousset and Guillaumot, 1988; Kostuik, 1990). These methods provide very secure fixation and postoperative spinal bracing is unnecessary. However, they carry a significant risk of neurological complications, and intra-operative monitoring of somatosensory evoked potentials is recommended.

For rigid curves, and for thoracolumbar curves associated with lumbar lordosis, anterior instrumentation is preferred (Moe, Purcell and Bradford, 1983).

Juvenile idiopathic scoliosis (aged 4–9)

This is uncommon. The characteristics of this group are similar to those of the adolescent group, but the prognosis is worse and fusion may be necessary before puberty. However, if the child is very young, a brace may hold the curve stationary until he is about 10 years old, when fusion is more likely to succeed.

Infantile idiopathic scoliosis (aged 3 or under)

This variety is rare in North America and is becoming uncommon elsewhere, perhaps because most babies nowadays are allowed to sleep prone. Boys predominate and most curves are thoracic with convexity to the left. Although 90% of infantile curves resolve spontaneously, progressive curves can become very severe; those in which the rib–vertebra angle at the apex of the curve differs on the two sides by more than 20 degrees are likely to deteriorate (Mehta, 1972). And because this also influences the development of the lungs, there is a high incidence of cardiopulmonary dysfunction.

Progressive curves should be treated by applying serial elongation derotation flexion (**EDF**) plaster casts under general anaesthesia, until the child is big enough to manage in a brace. Sometimes the curve reaches a certain point and then remains stationary. If it deteriorates after 4 years, it is treated as a juvenile scoliosis (see above).

Osteopathic (congenital) scoliosis

Although fractures and bone softening (as in rickets or osteogenesis imperfecta) may lead to scoliosis, the commonest bony cause is congenital. The anomalies include *hemivertebrae, wedged vertebrae, fused vertebrae* and *absent or fused ribs*; the overlying tissues often show angiomas, naevi, excess hair, dimples or a pad of fat; spina bifida may be associated. Although congenital scoliosis may remain mild, some cases progress to severe deformity, particularly those with unilateral fusion of vertebrae (unilateral unsegmented bar). Before operation is undertaken myelography is essential, to exclude diastematomyelia (in which the cord is bisected by bone projecting backwards from the vertebral body).

If the curve is very severe or progressive, posterior fusion should be carried out as early as possible.

Neuropathic and myopathic scoliosis

Neuromuscular conditions associated with scoliosis include poliomyelitis, cerebral palsy, syringomyelia, Friedreich's ataxia and the rarer lower motor neuron disorders and muscle dystrophies; the curve may take some years to develop. The typical paralytic curve is long, convex towards the side with weaker muscles (spinal, abdominal or intercostal), and at first is mobile. X-ray with traction applied shows the extent to which the deformity is correctible. There is also a strong association of scoliosis with neurofibromatosis; these curves are often short, sharp and difficult to correct.

In severe cases the greatest problem is loss of stability and balance, which may make even sitting difficult or impossible. Additional problems are generalized muscle weakness and loss of sensibility with the attendant risk of pressure ulceration.

Treatment depends upon the degree of functional disability. Mild curves may require no treatment at all. Moderate curves with spinal stability are managed as for idiopathic scoliosis. Severe curves, associated with loss of sitting balance, can often be managed by fitting a suitable sitting support. If this does not suffice, operative treatment may be indicated.

Operation for paralytic curves involves stabilization of the entire paralysed segment – sometimes extending from the second thoracic vertebra to the sacrum. This normally requires combined anterior and posterior instrumentation and fusion. Through an anterior approach, the intervertebral discs are excised and replaced by bone grafts. A steel cable (in Dwyer's operation) or threaded rod (Zielke's instrumentation) is then attached to each vertebral body along the convex side of the curve; by tightening the apparatus, the spine is pulled into correction (Moe, Purcell and Bradford,

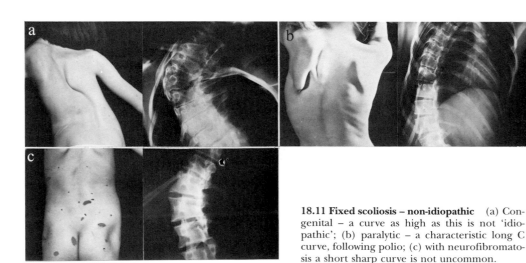

18.11 Fixed scoliosis – non-idiopathic   (a) Congenital – a curve as high as this is not 'idiopathic'; (b) paralytic – a characteristic long C curve, following polio; (c) with neurofibromatosis a short sharp curve is not uncommon.

1983). Two weeks later, posterior instrumentation and fusion is performed, using parallel rods and laminar wiring at each level.

Kyphosis

Rather confusingly, the term 'kyphosis' is used to describe both the normal (the gentle rounding of the dorsal spine) and the abnormal (excessive dorsal curvature or straightening out of the cervical or lumbar lordotic curves). An excessive dorsal curvature is a well-recognized deformity which may be progressive and disabling.

Postural kyphosis is common ('round back' or 'drooping shoulders') and may be associated with other postural defects such as flat feet. It is voluntarily correctible. If treatment is needed, this consists of posture training and exercises.

Compensatory kyphosis is secondary to some other deformity, such as fixed flexion of the hip or increased lumbosacral lordosis. This deformity, too, is correctible.

Structural kyphosis is fixed and associated with changes in the shape of the vertebrae. The most common cause is osteoporosis of the spine, but other causes include congenital abnormalities, Scheuermann's disease (adolescent kyphosis), ankylosing spondylitis, tuberculous spondylitis, and fracture or fracture-dislocation of the spine.

Kyphos, or gibbus, is a sharp posterior angulation due to localized collapse or wedging of one or more vertebrae. This may be the result of a congenital defect, a fracture (sometimes pathological) or spinal tuberculosis.

In *congenital kyphos* vertebral bodies are partly missing or fused anteriorly. Progressive deformity is inevitable, and may result in paraplegia; early operative correction (from the front or the back, or both) is needed (Winter, Moe and Wang, 1973).

In Calvé's disease, a rare condition which is probably the sequel to an eosinophilic granuloma, one vertebral body becomes flattened but the disc spaces remain. A child develops back pain and an angular kyphos. Clinical recovery occurs after a few months' rest.

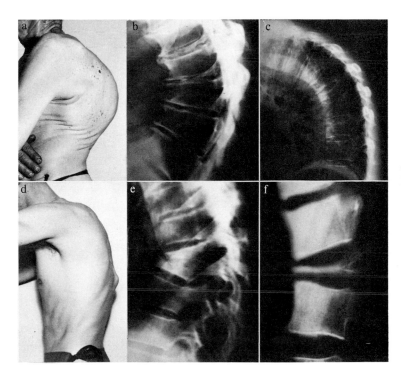

18.12 Kyphosis and kyphos (a, b) Old Scheuermann's disease; (c) senile kyphosis.

(d, e) Small kyphos (gibbus) due to tuberculosis; (f) Calvé's disease.

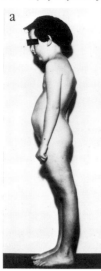
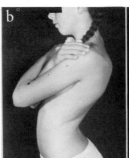
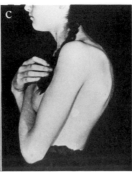
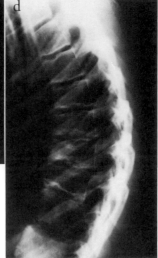

18.13 Kyphosis (continued) (a) Postural kyphosis and (b) kyphosis compensatory to a lumbar 'sway-back'. Unlike these two varieties, the deformity in Scheuermann's disease (c, d) is fixed.

Age at onset

In children, a congenital cause is likely; in adolescents, kyphosis is usually postural or due to Scheuermann's disease; in young adults, ankylosing spondylitis is an important cause; in the elderly, senile kyphosis, pathological fractures and Paget's disease must be considered; at all ages, tuberculosis must be excluded.

Adolescent kyphosis (Scheuermann's disease)

This is a growth disorder of the spine in which the vertebrae become slightly wedge shaped. If this happens in the thoracic spine – and especially if several vertebrae are involved – the normal kyphosis is exaggerated.

The cause of the condition is unknown. Scheuermann used the term 'osteochondritis' because the vertebral epiphyseal end-plates are irregularly ossified. Schmorl drew attention to the function of the cartilage plates in transmitting pressure evenly and suggested that a defect in them threw undue strain on the anterior portion of the vertebral bodies. More recently it has been postulated that a traumatic infraction of the epiphyseal plates occurs in children who

outgrow their bone strength during the pubertal growth spurt; there may also be vertebral osteoporosis and the discs may herniate into the fragile bone.

Clinical features

The condition starts at puberty and is twice as common in girls as in boys. The parents notice that the child, an otherwise fit teenager, is becoming increasingly round-shouldered. The patient may complain of backache and fatigue; this sometimes increases after the end of growth and may become severe.

A smooth thoracic kyphosis is seen; it may produce a distinct hump. Below it is a compensatory lumbar lordosis. The deformity cannot be corrected by changes in posture. Movements are normal but tight hamstrings often limit straight leg raising. Rare complications are spastic paresis of the lower limbs and – with severe deformity of the thorax – cardiopulmonary dysfunction.

X-RAY In lateral radiographs of the spine the vertebral end-plates of several adjacent vertebrae (usually T6–10) appear irregular or fragmented. The changes are more marked anteriorly and one or more vertebral bodies may become wedge shaped. There may also be small

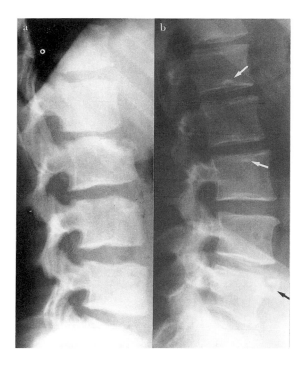

18.14 Scheuermann's disease (a) The x-ray appearances of lumbar Scheuermann's disease are often mistaken for a fracture (or worse). The 'fragmentation' anteriorly is due to abnormal ossification of the ring epiphysis. (b) Schmorl's nodes may also be seen.

translucent defects in the subchondral bone (Schmorl's nodes). Sometimes the lumbar vertebrae are affected and this can cause backache.

The angle of deformity is measured in the same way as for scoliosis (see p. 354), except that here the lateral x-ray is used and the lines mark the uppermost and lowermost affected vertebrae. Wedging of more than 5 degrees in an individual vertebra and an overall kyphosis angle of more than 40 degrees are abnormal.

Differential diagnosis

Postural kyphosis is common in adolescence. It is painless, and the deformity is correctible by the patient's own effort if properly instructed. The curve is a long one and other postural defects are common. The x-ray appearance is normal.

Tuberculosis produces an angular kyphos. X-rays show destruction of at least two adjacent vertebrae with narrowing of the intervening disc and often a paravertebral abscess.

Treatment

Curves of 40 degrees or less require only back-strengthening exercises and postural training. More severe curvature in a child who still has some years of growth ahead responds well to a period of 12–24 months in a brace that holds the lumbar spine flat and the thoracic spine in 'extension' (decreased kyphosis).

The older adolescent or young adult with a rigid curve of more than 60 degrees may, very rarely, need operative correction and fusion using Harrington compression rods. In severe cases this can be a massive undertaking with combined anterior and posterior surgery (Bradford et al., 1980). Indications are a painful severe kyphosis in a skeletally mature patient, or impending spastic paresis.

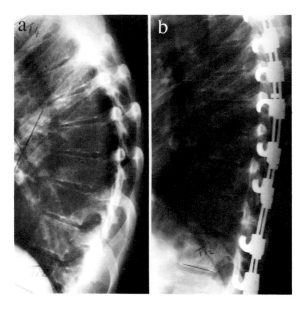

18.15 Scheuermann's disease – operative treatment A severe curve may need operation especially if, as in this girl (a), it is associated with chronic pain. (b) The same girl after operative correction and fixation with Harrington rods; bone grafts were added and can be expected to produce fusion after a year or two.

Kyphosis in the elderly

Degeneration of intervertebral discs probably produces the gradually increasing stoop characteristic of the aged. The disc spaces become narrowed and the vertebrae slightly wedged. There is little pain unless osteoarthritis of the facet joints is also present.

Osteoporotic kyphosis

Postmenopausal osteoporosis may result in one or more compression fractures of the thoracic spine. Patients are usually in their 60s or 70s and may complain of pain. Kyphosis is seldom marked. Often the main complaint is of lumbosacral pain, which results from the compensatory lumbar lordosis in an ageing, osteoarthritic spine. Treatment is directed at the underlying condition and may include hormone replacement therapy.

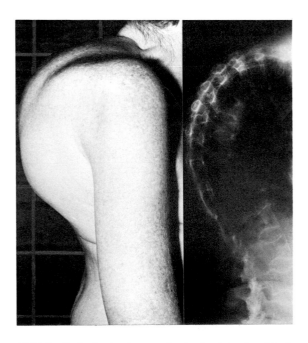

18.16 Senile kyphosis Progressive kyphosis in the elderly can occur because of collapse and wedging of osteoporotic vertebrae. Typically the x-ray shows only faint bony outlines. In a case as severe as this, some pre-existing deformity or long-standing metabolic bone disease was probably present.

Senile osteoporosis affects both men and women. Patients are usually over 75 years of age, often incapacitated by some other illness, and lacking exercise. They complain of back pain, and spinal deformity may be marked. X-rays reveal multiple vertebral fractures. It is important to exclude other conditions such as metastatic disease or multiple myeloma. Treatment is symptomatic. Bed rest and spinal bracing merely aggravate the osteoporosis.

Tuberculosis (see also Chapter 2)

The spine is the most common site of skeletal tuberculosis, and the most dangerous. It is thought that there may be as many as 2 million people with active spinal tuberculosis in the world today.

Pathology

Blood-borne infection usually settles in a vertebral body adjacent to the intervertebral disc. Bone destruction and caseation follow, with infection spreading to the disc space and to the adjacent vertebrae. As the vertebral bodies collapse into each other, a sharp angulation (or kyphos) develops. Caseation and cold abscess formation may extend to neighbouring vertebrae or escape into the paravertebral soft tissues. There is a major risk of cord damage due to pressure by the abscess or displaced bone, or ischaemia from spinal artery thrombosis.

With healing, the vertebrae recalcify and bony fusion may occur between them. Nevertheless, if there has been much forward angulation, the spine is usually 'unsound', and flares are common, with further illness and further collapse. With progressive kyphosis there is again a risk of cord compression.

Clinical features

There is usually a long history of ill-health and backache. In some cases deformity is the dominant feature. Occasionally the patient

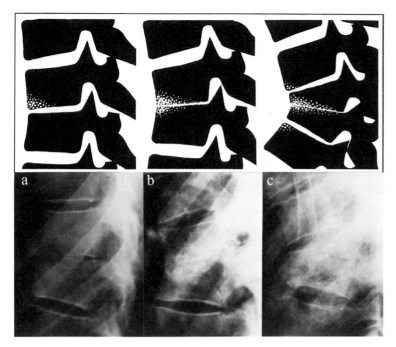

18.17 Spine tuberculosis – pathology (a, b, c) Progressively increasing destruction of the front of the vertebral bodies leads to forward collapse.

presents with a cold abscess pointing in the groin, or with paraesthesia and weakness of the legs.

In the active stage the local signs are as follows.

● LOOK

A characteristic feature in the thoracic spine is an angular kyphos, best seen from the side. In advanced cases the patient is a hunchback. In the lumbar spine the kyphos is scarcely visible but an abscess in the loin or groin may be obvious. If the cervical spine is affected the neck may be stiff.

● FEEL

The fingers can detect a kyphos, however slight; one need only run the hand down the spinous processes. Abscesses are fluctuant and the skin over them is slightly warm (the term 'cold abscess' is merely a reminder that they lack the heat of a pyogenic abscess).

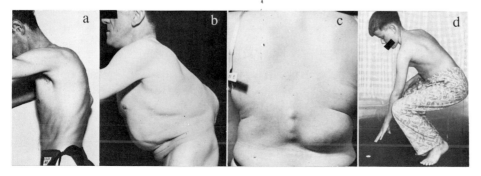

18.18 Spine tuberculosis – clinical features (a) This kyphos is slight but diagnostic. If collapse continues (b), kyphos becomes severe. (c) Large lumbar abscess. (d) The coin test – he bends his hips and knees rather than bending his back.

● MOVE

Diminished movement is undetectable in the thoracic region but easy to observe in the lumbar spine; the back should be carefully watched while movements are attempted. Usually all are limited and the attempt provokes muscle spasm. Formerly the 'coin test' was used; a child with lumbar spasm prefers bending at the hips and knees rather than at the spine when picking a coin up from the floor.

The legs also must be examined for neurological deficit, which may be very slight.

In the healing stage pain vanishes and the patient is fit again, though he may be left with a permanent deformity and the risk of recurrent flares of infection.

Imaging

X-ray The entire spine should be x-rayed, because vertebrae distant from the obvious site may also be affected. The earliest signs of infection are local osteoporosis of two adjacent vertebrae and narrowing of the intervertebral disc space, sometimes with fuzziness of the end-plates. Later there are more obvious signs of bone destruction, and collapse of adjacent vertebral bodies into each other, producing an angular deformity of the spine. Paraspinal soft-tissue shadows may be due either to oedema and swelling or to a paravertebral abscess. This is a characteristic feature of thoracic disease. With healing, bone density increases and the ragged appearance disappears; paravertebral abscesses may calcify.

CT and MRI are useful in the investigation of cord compression.

Investigations

The Mantoux test is positive and in the acute stage the ESR is raised.

If there is serious doubt about the diagnosis, a needle biopsy is performed and material is obtained for histological and bacteriological examination.

Pott's paraplegia

Paraplegia is the most feared complication of spinal tuberculosis.

Early-onset paresis is due to pressure by an abscess, caseous material or a bony sequestrum. The patient presents with lower limb weakness, upper motor neuron signs and sensory dysfunction, together with vertebral disease. CT and MRI may reveal cord compression and myelography demonstrates a block.

Late-onset paresis is due to increasing deformity, or reactivation of disease or vascular in-

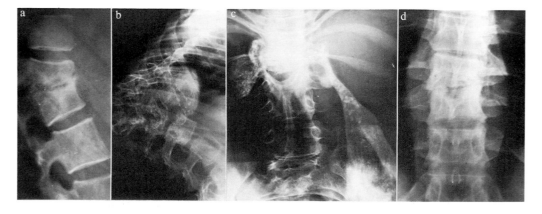

18.19 Spine tuberculosis – x-rays   (a) Early disease with loss of the disc space. (b) If several vertebrae are involved, forward collapse is severe – this patient did not, however, have any signs of paraplegia. (c) Psoas abscesses often calcify during the healing stage. (d) A paravertebral abscess is a fairly constant finding with thoracic disease.

sufficiency of the cord. Imaging and blood investigations may establish the precise diagnosis.

Differential diagnosis

Spinal tuberculosis must be distinguished from other causes of vertebral destruction and kyphosis, particularly pyogenic infection and malignant disease. Metastases may cause vertebral body collapse but, in contrast to tuberculous spondylitis, the disc space is usually preserved.

If the patient presents with paraplegia, other causes of cord compression have to be excluded (see p.205).

Treatment

The objectives are (1) to eradicate or at least arrest the disease, (2) to prevent or correct deformity and (3) to prevent or treat the major complication – paraplegia.

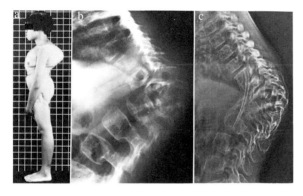

18.20 Spine tuberculosis – operative treatment A severe kyphos (a) may benefit from operation. This curve (b) has been partially corrected and held (c) by both anterior strut grafts and posterior fusion (this film is a xerographic tomograph – the best way of showing these grafts).

Clinical trials conducted by the (British) Medical Research Council (1978) have shown that antituberculous chemotherapy alone is as effective as any other method (including surgical debridement) in stemming the disease; however, during the 10-year follow-up period, kyphosis in the conservatively treated group increased by an average of over 17 degrees. The 'radical school', on the other hand, argue that anterior resection of diseased tissue and anterior spinal fusion with a strut graft offers the double advantage of early and complete eradication of the infection and prevention of spinal deformity (Leong, 1990).

With modern antituberculous drugs, a reasonable compromise would be the following.

Ambulant chemotherapy alone is appropriate for early or limited disease with no abscess formation. Treatment is continued for 6–12 months, or until the x-ray shows resolution of the bone changes. Compliance is sometimes a problem.

Continuous bed rest and chemotherapy may be used for more advanced disease when the necessary skills and facilities for radical anterior spinal surgery are not available, or where the technical problems are too daunting (e.g. in lumbosacral tuberculosis) – provided there is no abscess that needs draining.

Operative treatment is indicated (1) when there is an abscess that can readily be drained and (2) for advanced disease with marked bone destruction and threatened or actual severe kyphosis or paraparesis. Through an anterior approach, all infected and necrotic material is evacuated or excised and the gap is filled with rib grafts that act as a strut. Antituberculous chemotherapy is still necessary, of course.

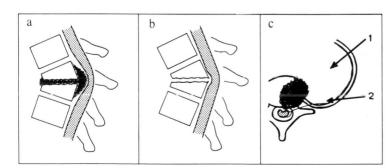

18.21 Spine tuberculosis – paraplegia In Pott's paraplegia the cord may be compressed by an abscess (a) which may resolve with effective conservative treatment; or (b) by a hard knuckle of bone which clearly needs operation. (c) The routes most often used for decompressing the cord: 1, transthoracic; 2 anterolateral.

Pyogenic infection

Pyogenic organisms – usually staphylococci – may infect the vertebral body (pyogenic spondylitis) or the intervertebral disc (discitis).

Pyogenic spondylitis

Vertebral infection is uncommon. Although the usual cause is *Staphylococcus*, unusual organisms such as *E. coli, Salmonella* and *Brucella* may be involved.

PATHOLOGY The infection – usually blood-borne and often from the urinary tract – starts in the intervertebral disc or the bone immediately adjacent to it. Local destruction may be followed by abscess formation. In patients with diminished resistance, infection may spread to involve the cord.

CLINICAL FEATURES   Pain is the chief complaint. It may be localized to the spine and associated with acute muscle spasm, or it may be more vague and radiating into the chest or abdomen. Spinal movements are restricted. Occasionally there are signs of nerve root compression. General examination may reveal some underlying debilitating disease or evidence of drug addiction.

X-rays may reveal narrowing of the disc space and destruction of the adjacent bone. Even before these signs appear, *radioscintigraphy* will almost always show increased activity. In late cases, new bone formation and patchy sclerosis are common – a point of distinction from tuberculous spondylitis. With healing, there may be fusion of adjacent vertebrae.

INVESTIGATIONS   The ESR is usually raised. A positive blood culture is unusual. Antistaphylococcal antibodies may be present in high titres. Agglutination tests for salmonella and brucella should always be performed. A needle biopsy may be required to discover the offending organism.

TREATMENT   Treatment consists of bed rest and intravenous antibiotics for 4–6 weeks; with a positive blood culture or biopsy sample, the most suitable drug can be selected. Once the

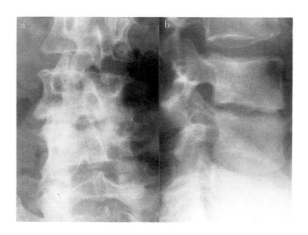

18.22 Pyogenic infection   (a) The intervertebral narrowing and tilt are evidence of bone destruction. (b) The lateral film shows disc narrowing and slight fuzziness of the adjacent vertebral margins. Both films were taken about 6 weeks after the onset of symptoms.

acute infection has subsided, the patient is allowed up in a spinal brace for a further 6 weeks or until x-rays and blood tests show that healing has occurred.

Discitis

Organisms may be blood-borne, and in some cases there is a known source of infection. However, direct infection is probably more common, in many cases introduced iatrogenically during the course of some procedure such as discography, chemonucleolysis or discectomy. As in other types of spinal infection, the vertebral end-plates are rapidly attacked and from there infection spreads into the vertebral body.

CLINICAL FEATURES   With blood-borne infections the patient is often a child; there may be a history of a flu-like illness followed by back pain, local tenderness, muscle spasm and severe limitation of movement.

With direct infection there is always a history of some invasive procedure. Acute back pain and muscle spasm following an injection into the disc should never be attributed merely to the irritant effect of the injection.

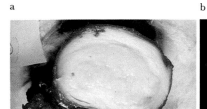

a

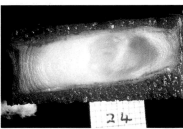

b

18.23 Disc lesions – pathology (1) (a, b) Transverse and sagittal sections through a young (teenage) intervertebral disc. The nucleus is soft, homogenous and almost translucent. The annulus is composed of regular lamellae of fibrocartilage.

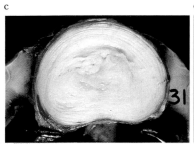

c

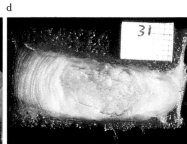

d

(c, d) Mature (50-year-old) normal disc. The nucleus is more fibrous and less homogenous. The annulus is thickened and the vertebral body end-plates are intact.

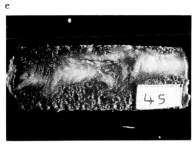

e

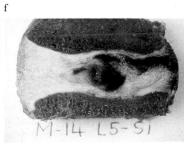

f

(e) Degenerating disc, which is markedly flattened with break-up of the nucleus and disruption of the vertebral body end-plates. (f) Young disc stained with analine blue dye to demonstrate a fissure extending posteriorly through the annulus fibrosus.

Normal disc

Increased nuclear pres-
sure causes bulging

Ruptured annulus and
ligament

Degeneration + joint
displacement

18.24 Disc pathology (2) From above, downwards: an abnormal increase in pressure within the nucleus causes splitting and bulging of the annulus; the posterior ligament may rupture, allowing disc material to extrude into the spinal canal; with chronic degeneration (lowest level) the disc space narrows and the posterior facet joints are displaced, giving rise to osteoarthritis.

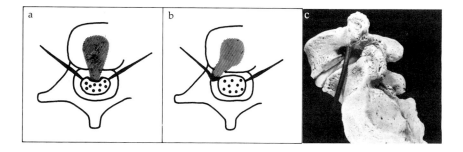

18.25 Disc pathology (3) (a, b) The bulging disc may press on the dura or on a nerve root. (c) The nerve is particularly vulnerable near the entrance to the intervertebral foramen.

Systemic features are usually mild, but the ESR is increased.

X-rays and *radioscintigraphy* show the same features as in pyogenic spondylitis.

TREATMENT Prevention is always better than cure. With injections into the disc, a broad spectrum antibiotic should be given, either locally or intravenously.

Non-iatrogenic discitis is usually self-limiting, and symptoms and signs gradually settle down over a period of a few months. During the acute stage bed rest is prescribed, together with analgesics if necessary. If symptoms do not resolve rapidly, systemic antibiotics are given. Only if there are signs of abscess formation, or cord or nerve root pressure, is surgical evacuation necessary.

Disc degeneration and prolapse

Lumbar backache is one of the most common causes of chronic disability in Western societies, and in the majority of cases the backache is associated with some abnormality of the intervertebral discs at the lowest two levels of the spine (L4/5 and L5/S1).

Pathology

With normal ageing the disc gradually dries out: the nucleus pulposus changes from a turgid, gelatinous bulb to a brownish, desiccated structure, and the annulus fibrosus develops fissures parallel to the vertebral end-plates running mainly posteriorly. Small herniations of nuclear material squeeze through the annulus in all directions and frequently perforate the vertebral end-plates to produce the Schmorl's nodes that are found in over 75% of autopsies.

Disc degeneration is therefore a common expression of senescence. Chronic herniation causes reactive bone formation around the Schmorl's nodes and where the discs protrude at the vertebral margins. The flattening of the disc and the marginal osteophytes are readily seen on x-ray and are referred to as *spondylosis*.

Displacement of the facet joints is an inevitable consequence of disc space collapse, and this in turn leads to *osteoarthritis*; if this is severe, osteophytes may narrow the lateral recesses of the spinal canal and the intervertebral foramina. Encroachment on the spinal canal leads to *spinal stenosis*.

Acute disc herniation* is less common, but more dramatic. Physical stress (a combination of flexion and compression) is the proximate cause but, even at L4/5 or L5/S1 (where stress is most severe), it seems unlikely that a disc would rupture unless there were also some disturbance of the hydrophilic properties of the nucleus. When rupture does occur, fibrocartilaginous material is extruded posteriorly and the annulus usually bulges to one side of the posterior longitudinal ligament. With a complete rupture, part of the nucleus may sequestrate and lie free in the spinal canal or work its way into the intervertebral foramen. A large central rupture may cause compression of the cauda equina. A posterolateral rupture presses on the nerve root proximal to its point of exit through the intervertebral foramen; thus a herniation at L4/5 will compress the fifth lumbar nerve root, and a herniation at L5/S1 the first sacral root. Sometimes a local inflammatory response with oedema aggravates the symptoms.

The pain of acute disc herniation Pressure on the posterior longitudinal ligament and irritation of the dura cause widespread backache but fairly localized tenderness at the affected level; irritation of a nerve root (or, rather, its dural sleeve) causes pain and muscle tenderness in the buttock, thigh and calf (sciatica). Nerve pressure causes paraesthesia, loss of sensation, weakness and depressed reflexes.

Repeated disc rupture leads to rapid degeneration with the features of spondylosis appearing at a younger age than usual.

Symptoms of chronic disc degeneration Radiographic narrowing of the disc space, with osteophyte formation and vertebral sclerosis, is often seen in patients complaining of backache; and almost as often in uncomplaining people!

---

* The terms 'rupture', 'prolapse', 'protrusion' and 'herniation' are used interchangeably.

Does disc degeneration cause pain? And, if so, how? These questions have no ready answer. One can merely speculate that 'disc degeneration' implies the presence of other changes, some of which can cause pain; these are: facet joint malalignment, facet joint arthritis, vertebral instability, and root canal or spinal stenosis. All of these may also cause referred pain or 'sciatica'. And some may cause root irritation and symptoms of 'radiculitis'.

Acute disc rupture (prolapse)

Acute disc prolapse may occur at any age, but is uncommon in the very young and the very old.

Clinical features

The patient is usually a fit adult of 20–45 years. Typically, while lifting or stooping he has severe back pain and is unable to straighten up. Either

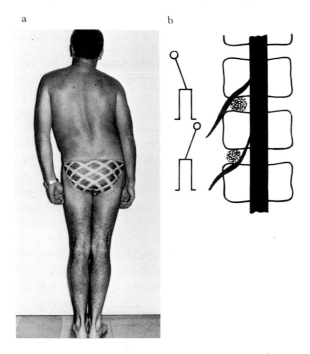

18.26 Lumbar disc – signs (a) The patient has a sideways list or tilt. (b) If the disc protrudes medial to the nerve root the tilt is towards the painful side (to relieve pressure on the root); with a far lateral prolapse (lower level) the tilt is away from the painful side.

then or a day or two later pain is felt in the buttock and lower limb (sciatica). Both backache and sciatica are made worse by coughing or straining. Later there may be paraesthesia or numbness in the leg or foot, and occasionally muscle weakness. Cauda equina compression is rare but may cause urinary retention.

The patient usually stands with a slight list to one side ('sciatic scoliosis'). Sometimes the knee on the painful side is held bent to relax tension on the sciatic nerve; straightening the knee makes the list more obvious. All back movements are severely limited, and during forward flexion the list may increase.

There is often tenderness in the midline of the low back, and paravertebral muscle spasm. Straight leg raising is restricted and painful on the affected side; dorsiflexion of the foot and bowstringing of the lateral popliteal nerve may accentuate the pain. Sometimes raising the unaffected leg causes acute sciatic tension on the painful side ('crossed sciatic tension'). With a high or mid-lumbar prolapse the femoral stretch test may be positive.

NEUROLOGICAL EXAMINATION may show muscle weakness (and, later, wasting), diminished reflexes and sensory loss corresponding to the affected level. L5 impairment causes weakness of big toe extension and knee flexion, sometimes an increased knee jerk (because of the weak antagonists) and sensory loss on the outer side of the leg and the dorsum of the foot. S1 impairment causes weak plantarflexion and eversion of the foot, a depressed ankle jerk and sensory loss along the lateral border of the foot. Occasionally an L4/5 disc prolapse compresses both L5 and S1. Cauda equina compression causes urinary retention and sensory loss over the sacrum.

Imaging

X-rays are helpful, not to show an abnormal disc space but to exclude bone disease. After several attacks the disc space may be narrowed and small osteophytes appear.

Myelography (radiculography) using iopamidol (Niopam) is a reliable method of confirming the disc protrusion, localizing it and excluding

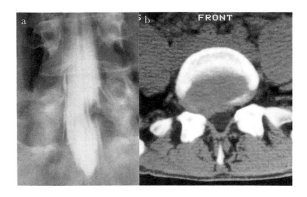

18.27 Lumbar disc – imaging (a) Radiculogram in which absence of the contrast medium shows where a disc has protruded. (b) CT scan showing how disc protrusion can obstruct the intervertebral foramen.

intrathecal tumours; however, it carries a significant risk of unpleasant side effects, such as headache (in over 30%), nausea and dizziness.

Computed tomography has none of the disadvantages of myelography and is now the preferred method of spinal imaging. It is usually performed only when surgery is contemplated.

Magnetic resonance imaging provides sectional images in both the transverse and the longitudinal planes; it can also provide information about disc physiology.

Differential diagnosis

The full-blown syndrome is unlikely to be misdiagnosed, but with repeated attacks and with lumbar spondylosis gradually supervening the features often become atypical. Diagnostically there are three guidelines, three warnings and three major disorders to exclude.

THE GUIDELINES (1) Very young and very old people seldom sustain acute ruptures. In adolescents, look for infection, a benign tumour or spondylolisthesis. In the elderly, look for a compression fracture or malignant disease. (2) An ill patient probably has a more serious disorder. (3) In disc rupture the episodes of pain are punctuated by intervals of normality.

THE WARNINGS (1) Sciatica is referred pain and occurs also in disorders of the facet joints, the sacroiliac joints or with vertebral infections. (2) Disc rupture affects at most two neurological levels; if multiple levels are involved, suspect a neurological disorder. (3) Severe, unrelenting pain is not characteristic of a ruptured disc; suspect a tumour or infection.

THE DIFFERENTIAL DIAGNOSIS (1) Inflammatory disorders, such as infection or ankylosing spondylitis, cause severe stiffness, a raised ESR and erosive changes on x-ray. (2) Vertebral tumours cause severe pain and marked spasm. With metastases the patient is ill, the ESR raised and the x-rays show bone destruction or sclerosis. (3) Nerve tumours, such as neurofibromata of the cauda equina, may cause 'sciatica' but pain is continuous, and myelography may show the defects.

Treatment

Heat and analgesics soothe, and exercises strengthen muscles; but there are only three ways of treating the prolapse itself – *rest, reduction* or *removal;* followed by *rehabilitation.*

REST With an acute attack the patient should be kept in bed, with hips and knees slightly flexed and 10 kg traction to the pelvis. An anti-inflammatory drug such as indomethacin is useful. For mild attacks a spinal corset and reduced activity may suffice.

REDUCTION Continuous bed rest and traction for 2 weeks will reduce the herniation in over 90% of cases. If the symptoms and signs have not improved significantly by then, an epidural injection of corticosteroid and local anaesthetic may help.

Chemonucleolysis – dissolution of the nucleus pulposus by percutaneous injection of a proteolytic enzyme (chymopapain) – is in theory an excellent way of reducing a disc prolapse (McCulloch, 1980). However, properly controlled studies have shown that it is less effective (and potentially more dangerous) than surgical removal of the disc material (Ejeskär et al., 1982).

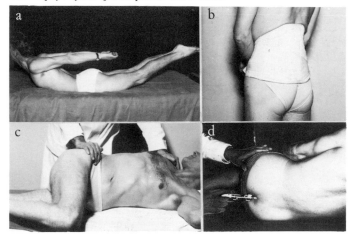

18.28 Lumbar disc – treatment   (a) Exercises; (b) corset; (c) manipulation; (d) epidural injection.

REMOVAL   The indications for operative removal of a disc are: (1) a cauda equina compression syndrome that does not clear up within 6 hours of starting bed rest and traction – this is an emergency; (2) neurological deterioration while under conservative treatment; and (3) persistent pain and signs of sciatic tension (especially crossed sciatic tension) after 3 weeks of conservative treatment. The presence of a prolapsed disc, and the level, must be confirmed by CT, MRI or myelography before operating. Surgery in the absence of a clear preoperative diagnosis is usually unrewarding.

Three types of operation (one of them still experimental) are in use: partial laminectomy and discectomy; microdiscectomy; and percutaneous discectomy.

Partial laminectomy   The lamina and ligamentum flavum on one side are removed, taking great care not to damage the facet joint. The dura and nerve root are then gently retracted towards the midline and the pea-like bulge is displayed. This is incised and the mushy disc material plucked out piecemeal with pituitary forceps. The nerve is traced to its point of exit in order to exclude other pathology.

The main intraoperative complication is bleeding from epidural veins. This is less likely to occur if the patient is placed on his side or in the kneeling position, thus minimizing the rise in venous pressure. The major postoperative complication is disc space infection, but fortunately this is rare.

Microdiscectomy   This is essentially similar to the standard posterior operation, except that the exposure is very limited and the procedure is carried out with the aid of an operating microscope. Morbidity and length of hospitalization are certainly less than with open surgery, but there are drawbacks: careful x-ray control is needed to ensure that the correct level is entered; intraoperative bleeding may be difficult to control; there is a considerable 'learning curve' and the inexperienced operator risks injuring the dura or a stretched nerve root, or missing essential pathology; there is a slightly increased risk of disc space infection, and prophylactic antibiotics are advisable (Wilson and Harbaugh, 1981).

Percutaneous discectomy   In this procedure the herniated material is aspirated through a special suction-probe introduced percutaneously under x-ray control (Onik et al., 1985). The method is still 'on trial'.

REHABILITATION   After recovery from an acute disc rupture, or disc removal, the patient is taught isometric exercises and how to lie, sit, bend and lift with the least strain. Ideally this should be done as part of an education programme in a 'back school' (Zachrisson, 1981).

Persistent postoperative backache and sciatica

Persistent symptoms after operation may be due to: (1) residual disc material in the spinal canal; (2) disc prolapse at another level; or (3) nerve root pressure by a hypertrophic facet joint or a narrow lateral recess ('root canal stenosis'). After careful investigation, any of these may call for reoperation; but second procedures do not have a high success rate – third and fourth procedures still less.

Arachnoiditis

Diffuse back pain and vague lower limb symptoms such as 'cramps', 'burning' or 'irritability' sometimes appear after myelography, epidural injections or disc operations. There may also be sphincter dysfunction and male impotence. Patients complain bitterly and many are labelled neurotic. However, in some cases there are electromyographic abnormalities, and dural scarring with obliteration of the subarachnoid space can be demonstrated at operation.

Treatment is generally unrewarding. Corticosteroid injections at best give only temporary relief, and surgical 'neurolysis' may actually make matters worse. Sympathetic management in a pain clinic, psychological support and a graduated activity programme are the best that can be offered.

Facet joint dysfunction and segmental instability (lumbar spondylosis)

With disc degeneration, and especially after recurrent prolapse, there may be gradual flattening of the disc and displacement of the posterior facet joints. The disturbed movement in flexion and extension constitutes a type of motion segment instability which, despite the paucity of morphological changes, often produces disabling symptoms (Kirkaldy-Willis and Farfan, 1982).

This may continue until the disc has completely collapsed, but the marginal osteophytes

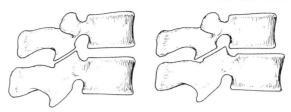

18.29 Facet joint dysfunction Diagrams showing how the sloping facet joints must inevitably be displaced if the disc space collapses.

and progressive osteoarthritis of the facet joints sometimes stabilize that level and the symptom pattern changes.

A less common disorder is softening of the facet articular cartilage in the absence of any obvious preceding abnormality, a condition that has been likened to chondromalacia of the patella (Eisenstein and Parry, 1987).

Clinical features

The patient with lumbar instability often gives a history of acute disc rupture and recurrent attacks of pain over several years. Backache may be intermittent and related to spells of hard work, standing or walking a lot, or sitting in one position during a long journey; it is usually relieved by lying down, though some patients (those with 'chondromalacia'?) prefer to be up and moving about. Pain is often referred to the buttock and the back of the greater trochanter; sometimes it extends down the leg like sciatica. There may be acute incidents of 'locking' or 'giving way'.

As the condition modulates from instability to osteoarthritis of the facet joints, pain is more constant but can sometimes be temporarily relieved by manipulation, local warmth and anti-inflammatory drugs.

The patient is usually over 40 years of age and otherwise fit. Often tender areas are felt in the back and buttocks. Lumbar movements are limited and may be painful at their extremes. With instability there may be a typical 'heave' or 'catch' as the patient straightens up after bending forward. Neurological examination may show residual signs of an old disc prolapse (e.g. an absent ankle jerk). In the very late

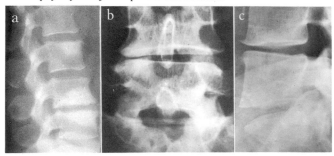

18.30 Segmental instability (a) One of the earliest signs of segmental instability is a wedge of sclerosis adjacent to the disc space – evidence of abnormal loading. Other features are (b, c) vertebral tilting and small anterior traction spurs.

stages, symptoms and signs of spinal stenosis or of unilateral root canal stenosis may supervene.

X-rays

Early signs are slight narrowing of the disc space and retrolisthesis (posterior displacement of the upper vertebra) at L4/5 or L5/S1 in the lateral radiograph (flexion and extension views may show this better). Another telltale feature is localized sclerosis of the vertebral bodies in the unstable segment, a sign of bone reaction to abnormal loading.

Later there is more marked flattening of the disc and bony spurs near the anterior 'corners' of the vertebral bodies. MacNab (1977) has referred to these as 'traction spurs' and they are said to be characteristic of instability.

With advanced degeneration the disc space may show increased radiolucency (the 'vacuum sign'), and oblique views reveal facet joint malalignment and osteoarthritis. Sometimes the vertebral column is tilted or mildly scoliotic, or the patient may develop degenerative spondylolisthesis at L4/5.

Radioscintigraphy shows 'hot spots' over the facet joints at affected levels.

Discography and *facet joint arthrography* are sometimes performed in an attempt to confirm the diagnosis. In the presence of degeneration the contrast medium leaks into the surrounding tissues and its injection may reproduce the symptoms. Whether this proves that disc or facet degeneration is the cause of the patient's symptoms remains in doubt, but it does provide some evidence of pathological change in a fairly well-defined clinical syndrome (Mooney and Robertson, 1976).

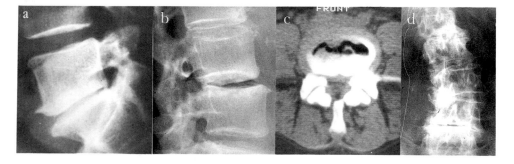

18.31 Spondylosis and osteoarthritis Typical x-ray features are (a) narrowing of the intervertebral space and anterior traction spurs, and (b) retrolisthesis and a vacant area in the disc space – the 'vacuum sign'. (c) CT showing the vacuum sign and hypertrophic osteoarthritis of the facet joints. (d) In advanced cases several levels are involved, with deformity of the spine.

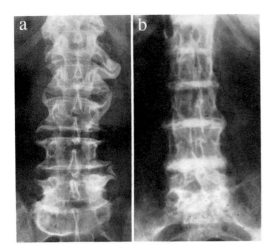

18.32 Other causes of 'spondylosis' (a) In Forestier's disease (see p. 86) there are large spurs at multiple levels, often worse on the right side; (b) in ochronosis (see p. 77) intervertebral calcification is characteristic.

PHYSIOTHERAPY Weight control and strengthening of the vertebral and abdominal muscles may help, and manipulative 'spinal mobilization' often relieves pain dramatically – at least for a while.

CORSETS A soft lumbar support may give relief in some cases; obese patients benefit from having their centre of gravity pulled in close to the spine.

FACET INJECTIONS If clinical and x-ray signs point consistently to one or two facet levels, injection of local anaesthetic and corticosteroids may be carried out under fluoroscopic control. Over 60% of patients can be expected to obtain short-term benefit and about 20% are relieved of symptoms for periods of more than a year (Lippitt, 1984; Lynch and Taylor, 1986).

Facet injection

Another way of showing whether a particular facet joint is responsible for the patient's pain is to inject (under fluoroscopic control) the facet joint and the area around it with local anaesthetic and see if this abolishes the pain (Lippitt, 1984). Unfortunately, there is a significant placebo response to spinal injections and a 'positive' finding does not predict an equally satisfying outcome following arthrodesis at that level.

Treatment

As the disability is seldom severe, and may even decrease with time (as the spine stabilizes itself), conservative measures are encouraged for as long as possible.

GENERAL CARE AND ATTENTION Perhaps the most important thing is to let the patient feel that every effort is being made to clarify the diagnosis. As Nachemson reminds us: 'Thorough examination is half the treatment'.

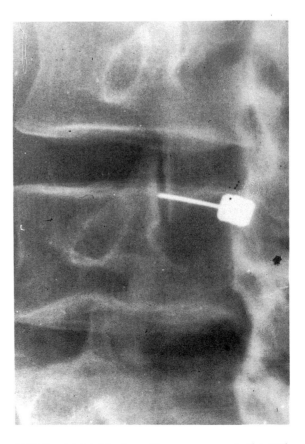

18.33 Facet joint injection Fluoroscopy reveals the position of the needle; injection of local anaesthetic and corticosteroids often gives pain relief.

The technique is as follows. The patient lies prone on the fluoroscopy table. Under local anaesthesia, long 20-gauge needles are introduced perpendicular to the skin 2–3 cm from the midline at the level of the spinous processes (usually both L4/5 and L5/S1 are injected). Each needle is advanced until it strikes bone; the tip will then be close to the facet joint, but the position is checked by rolling the patient into the oblique position (affected joint uppermost) and adjusting the needle under fluoroscopy. About 2 ml is injected at each site.

MODIFICATION OF ACTIVITIES One of the most important aspects of treatment is modification of daily activities (bending, lifting, climbing, etc.) and specific activities relating to work. The patient may need retraining for a different job. The co-operation of employers is essential.

DRUG TREATMENT Mild analgesics may be needed for pain control. However, beware the patient who becomes dependent on increasing doses of medication.

PSYCHOLOGICAL SUPPORT Chronic back pain can be psychologically as well as physically debilitating. Counselling and support are often welcomed by the patient.

SURGERY Only after all the above measures have been tried and found to be ineffectual should a spinal fusion be considered. Even then very strict guidelines should be followed if one is to avoid embarking on a road already crowded with patients labelled 'failed back surgery'. (1) Repeated examination should ensure that there is no other treatable pathology. (2) There should have been at least some response to conservative treatment; patients who 'benefit from nothing' will not benefit from spinal fusion either. (3) There should be unequivocal evidence of facet joint instability or osteoarthritis at a specific level. (4) The patient should be emotionally stable and should not exaggerate his symptoms nor display inappropriate physical signs (see below). And (5) the patient should be warned that: (a) a 'fusion' doesn't always fuse (there is a 10–20% failure rate); and (b) a fusion at one level does not preclude further pathology developing at another level; indeed, Lehmann et al. (1987), in a long-term follow-up of patients who had undergone spinal fusion, found that after 10 years 40% had developed signs of instability elsewhere.

Spinal stenosis

One of the long-term consequences of disc degeneration and osteoarthritis is narrowing of the spinal canal due to hypertrophy at the posterior disc margin and the facet joints. This is more likely if the canal was always small, or if a spondylolisthesis decreases its anteroposterior diameter.

The following classification (based on that of Arnoldi et al., 1976) may be useful.

Congenital stenosis This occurs in achondroplasia and hypochondroplasia, but usually is a developmental variant.

Postdegenerative stenosis As described above, this is more likely if spondylosis is superimposed on developmental narrowing.

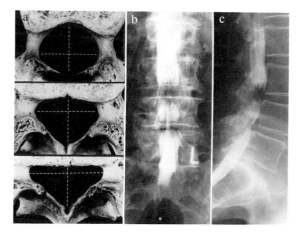

18.34 Spinal stenosis (a) The shape of the lumbar spinal canal varies from oval (with a large capacity) to trefoil (with narrow lateral recesses); further encroachment on an already narrow canal can cause an ischaemic neuropathy and 'spinal claudication'. (b, c) Myelogram showing marked narrowing of the radio-opaque column at the level of stenosis.

Postspondylolisthetic stenosis A degenerative spondylolisthesis at L4/5 quite often produces stenosis and is the commonest cause in elderly patients.

Miscellaneous Paget's disease, a spinal tumour or tuberculosis may present with features of spinal stenosis. Rarely, the condition follows trauma or operation.

Clinical features

The patient, usually a man aged over 50, complains of aching, heaviness, numbness and paraesthesia in the thighs and legs; it comes on only after standing upright or walking for 5–10 minutes, and is consistently relieved by sitting, squatting or leaning against a wall to flex the spine (hence the confusing term 'spinal claudication'). The patient may prefer walking uphill, which flexes the spine, to downhill, which extends it. Symptoms are often unilateral, suggesting an asymmetrical stenosis ('root canal stenosis'). There may be a previous history of disc prolapse or chronic backache.

Examination, especially after getting the patient to reproduce the symptoms by walking, may show neurological deficit in the lower limbs. Electromyography may be helpful if the clinical findings are equivocal.

IMAGING X-rays usually show degenerative spondylolisthesis or advanced disc degeneration and osteoarthritis. Measurement of the spinal canal may be carried out on plain films, but more reliable information is obtained from computed tomography. *Myelography* and/or *MRI* may be performed if operation is planned; these give a better idea of the longitudinal relationships in the spine and of the effect of spinal extension and flexion.

Treatment

Conservative measures, including instruction in spinal posture, may suffice. Most patients are prepared to put up with their symptoms and simply avoid uncomfortable postures. If discomfort is marked and activities are severely restricted, operative decompression is almost always successful. A wide laminectomy is performed, if necessary extending over several levels and outwards to clear the nerve root canals. This relieves the leg pain, but not the back pain, and occasionally it actually increases instability; consequently in patients under 60 the operation is sometimes combined with spinal fusion.

Spondylolisthesis

'Spondylolisthesis' means forward shift of the spine. The shift is nearly always between L4 and L5, or between L5 and the sacrum. Normal laminae and facets constitute a locking mechanism which prevents each vertebra from moving forwards on the one below. Forward shift (or slip) occurs only when this mechanism has failed.

Classification

Various classifications have been suggested. Basically there are six types of spondylolisthesis.

DYSPLASTIC (20%) The superior sacral facets are congenitally defective; slow but inexorable forward slip leads to severe displacement. Associated anomalies (usually spina bifida occulta) are common.

LYTIC OR ISTHMIC (50%) In this, the commonest variety, there are defects in the pars

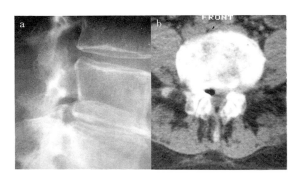

18.35 Spinal stenosis (a) A lateral film shows marked narrowing of the spinal canal, but (b) a CT scan provides even more convincing and dramatic evidence.

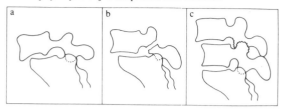

18.36 Spondylolisthesis – varieties (a) The pars inter-articularis is long and attenuated, with forward shift of the upper vertebra on the lower. (b) There is a break in the pars interarticularis – this is a kind of stress fracture. (c) Degeneration of the facet joints (usually at L4/5) has allowed forward slipping to occur.

interarticularis (spondylolysis); or repeated breaking and healing may lead to elongation of the pars. The defect (which occurs in about 5% of people) is usually present by the age of 7, but the slip may only appear some years later (Fredrickson et al., 1984). It is difficult to exclude a genetic factor because spondylolisthesis often runs in families, and is more common in certain races, notably Eskimos; but the incidence increases with age, so an acquired factor probably supervenes to produce what is essentially a stress fracture. The condition is more common than usual in those whose spines are subjected to extraordinary stresses (e.g. competitive gymnasts).

DEGENERATIVE 25% Degenerative changes in the facet joints and the discs permit forward slip (nearly always at L4/5) despite intact laminae. These patients have a high incidence of generalized osteoarthritis and pyrophosphate crystal arthropathy.

POST-TRAUMATIC Unusual fractures may result in destabilization of the lumbar spine.

PATHOLOGICAL Bone destruction (e.g. due to tuberculosis or neoplasm) may lead to vertebral slipping.

POSTOPERATIVE Occasionally, operative removal of bone results in progressive instability.

Pathology

In the common lytic type of spondylolisthesis the pars interarticularis is in two pieces (spondylolysis) and the gap is occupied by fibrous tissue; behind the gap the spinous process, laminae and inferior articular facets remain as an isolated segment. With stress, the vertebral body and superior facets in front of the gap may subluxate or dislocate forwards, carrying the superimposed vertebral column; the isolated segment of neural arch maintains its normal relationship to the sacral facets. When there is no gap, the pars interarticularis is elongated or the facets are defective.

The degree of slip is measured by the amount of overlap of adjacent vertebral bodies and is usually expressed as a percentage.

With forward slipping there may be pressure on the dura mater and cauda equina, or on the emerging nerve roots; these roots may also be compressed in the narrowed intervertebral foramina. Disc prolapse is liable to occur.

Clinical features

Spondylolysis, and even a well-marked spondylolisthesis, may be discovered incidentally during routine x-ray examination.

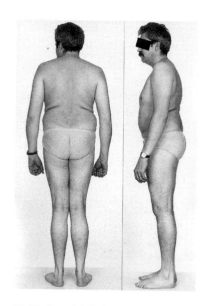

18.37 Spondylolisthesis – clinical appearance The transverse loin creases, forward tilting of the pelvis and flattening of the lumbar spine are characteristic.

In children the condition is painless but the mother may notice the unduly protruding abdomen and peculiar stance.

In adolescents and *adults* backache is the usual presenting symptom; it is often intermittent, coming on after exercise or strain. Sciatica may occur in one or both legs.

Patients aged over 50 are usually women with degenerative spondylolisthesis. They always have backache; some have sciatica; and some present because of pseudoclaudication due to spinal stenosis.

On examination the buttocks look curiously flat, the sacrum appears to extend to the waist and transverse loin creases are seen. The lumbar spine is on a plane in front of the sacrum and looks too short. Sometimes there is a scoliosis.

A 'step' can often be felt when the fingers are run down the spine. Movements are usually normal in the younger patients but there may be 'hamstring tightness'; in the degenerative group the spine is often stiff.

X-RAYS show the forward shift of the upper part of the spinal column on the stable vertebra below; elongation of the arch or defective facets may be seen. The gap in the pars inter-articularis is best seen in the oblique views. In doubtful cases, *CT* may be helpful.

Prognosis

Congenital spondylolisthesis appears at an early age, often goes on to a severe slip and carries a significant risk of neurological complications.

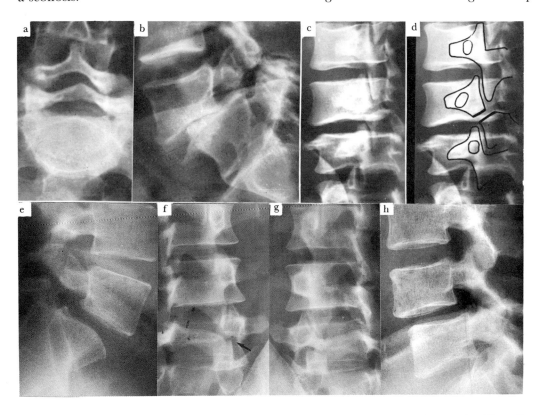

18.38 Spondylolisthesis – x-rays (a) In the anteroposterior x-ray the superior surface of the 'slipped' vertebral body may be seen almost end-on. In the lateral x-ray (b) the slip may be obvious, but the defect in the pars interarticularis is better seen in the oblique view (c, d) where it is likened to a 'collar' around the 'neck' of an illusory 'dog'. (e, f, g) In this case the break in the pars is seen in the lateral x-ray. Oblique views show that on one side there is a defect (arrow) but on the other the break has healed with elongation of the pars. In degenerative spondylolisthesis (h) there is no pars defect; the unstable facet joints permit slipping, usually at L4/5.

Lytic (isthmic) spondylolisthesis with less than 10% displacement is usually asymptomatic, does not progress after adulthood, does not predispose the patient to later back problems and is not a contraindication to strenuous work (Wiltse et al., 1990). With slips of more than 25% there is an increased risk of backache in later life.

Degenerative spondylolisthesis is rare before the age of 50, progresses slowly and seldom exceeds 30%.

Treatment

Conservative treatment, similar to that for segmental instability (facet joint dysfunction) is suitable for most patients.

Operative treatment is indicated: (1) if the symptoms are disabling and interfere significantly with work and recreational activities; (2) if the slip is more than 50% and progressing; and (3) if neurological compression is significant.

For children, posterior intertransverse fusion *in situ* is almost always successful; if neurological signs appear, decompression can be done later. For adults, either posterior or anterior fusion is suitable. However, in the 'degenerative' group, where neurological symptoms predominate, decompression without fusion may suffice.

Note on post-traumatic spondylolisthesis The patient found to have spondylolysis or spondylolis-

thesis after recent back injury (usually hyperextension) may have fractured the pars, or merely have strained the fibrous tissue of a preexisting lesion. If doubt exists (and it usually does) a plaster jacket is worn for 3 months; the recent fracture may join spontaneously. If union does not occur the assumption is that spondylolisthesis was present before injury and treatment is along the lines already indicated.

The backache problem

Chronic backache is such a frequent cause of disability in the community that it has become almost a disease in itself, calling for special skills in its assessment and management.

Diagnosis

Careful history taking and examination will uncover one of five pain patterns.

TRANSIENT BACKACHE FOLLOWING MUSCULAR ACTIVITY This suggests a simple back strain, which will respond to a short period of rest followed by gradually increasing exercise. People with thoracic kyphosis (of whatever origin), or fixed flexion of the hip, are particularly prone to back strain because they tend to compensate for the deformity by holding the lumbosacral spine in hyperlordosis.

SUDDEN, ACUTE PAIN AND SCIATICA In young people (those under 20) it is important to exclude infection and spondylolisthesis; both produce recognizable x-ray changes. Patients aged 20–40 years are more likely to have an acute disc prolapse: diagnostic features are (1) a history of a lifting strain, (2) unequivocal sciatic tension and (3) neurological symptoms and signs. Elderly patients may have osteoporotic compression fractures.

CHRONIC LOW BACK PAIN, WITH OR WITHOUT 'SCIATICA' If the patient is over 40, gives a history suggesting disc prolapse some years previously, with recurrent episodes of increased pain, the most likely diagnosis is facet joint dysfunction, segmental instability or osteoarthritis. Typically, symptoms are aggravated by

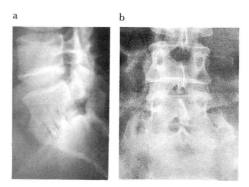

a   b

18.39 Spondylolisthesis – treatment Stability may be restored by (a) an anterior body fusion with bone grafts or (b) by a lateral mass fusion which is simpler and after which the patient can become active more rapidly.

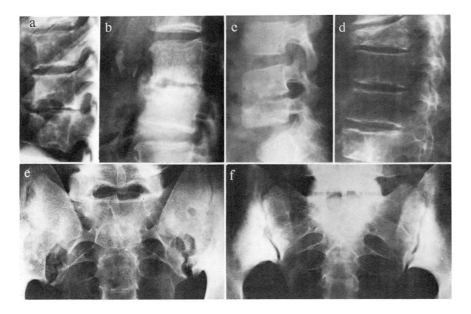

18.40 Some causes of chronic backache   (a) Tuberculosis; (b) acute osteomyelitis – note the sclerosis which developed within a few weeks; (c) discitis. (d) Here, unlike the previous three, the disc spaces are normal – the bodies are not – these are secondary deposits. (e) Bilateral sacroiliac tuberculosis; (f) osteitis condensans ilii, which is probably not the cause of the backache.

activity and relieved by rest. X-rays show characteristic signs of 'spondylosis'. These are the most difficult patients. They need painstaking examination (1) to uncover the features of segmental instability or facet joint osteoarthritis and (2) to determine whether those features account for the symptoms. In the process, disorders such as ankylosing spondylitis, chronic infecton or other bone disease must be excluded by appropriate imaging and blood investigations. Treatment is almost always conservative (see p. 373).

BACK PAIN PLUS PSEUDOCLAUDICATION   These patients are usually aged over 50 and may give a history of previous, long-standing, back trouble. The diagnosis of spinal stenosis should be confirmed by suitable imaging studies.

SEVERE AND CONSTANT PAIN LOCALIZED TO A PARTICULAR SITE   This suggests local bone pathology, such as a compression fracture, Paget's disease, a tumour or infection. Spinal osteoporosis in middle-aged men is pathological and calls for a full battery of tests to exclude primary disorders such as myelomatosis, carcinomatosis, hyperthyroidism, gonadal insufficiency, alcoholism or corticosteroid usage.

The 'chronic back pain syndrome'

Patients with chronic backache may despair of finding a cure for their trouble (or, indeed, even a diagnosis that everyone agrees on), and they often develop affective and psychosomatic ailments which subsequently become the chief focus of their attention. This is not conscious malingering; it is a form of illness behaviour (Waddell et al., 1984) which is both self-perpetuating and self-justifying. It is usually accompanied by recognizable '*non-organic*' (*inappropriate*) *physical signs* (Waddell et al., 1980), such as: (1) pain and tenderness of bizarre degree or distribution; (2) pain on performing impressive but non-stressful manoeuvres such as pressing vertically on the spine or passively rotating the entire trunk; (3) variations in response to tests such as straight leg raising while distracting the patient's attention; (4) sensory diminution or loss affecting an entire lower limb; and (5) overdetermined behaviour during physical examination (trembling, sweating, hyperventilating, inability to move, a tendency to fall and exaggerated withdrawal) – usually accompanied by loud groaning and exclamations of discomfort. Patients with these features are unlikely to respond to surgery and they may require prolonged support and management in a special pain clinic – but only after every effort has been made to exclude organic pathology.

Notes on applied anatomy

THE SPINE AS A WHOLE   The spine has to move, to transmit weight and to protect the spinal cord. In upright man the lumbar segment is lordotic and the column acts like a crane; the paravertebral muscles are the cables that counterbalance any weight carried anteriorly. The resultant force, which passes through the nucleus pulposus of the lowest lumbar disc, is therefore much greater than if the column were loaded directly over its centre; even at rest, tonic contraction of the posterior muscles balances the trunk, so the lumbar spine is always loaded. Nachemson and Morris (1964) measured the intradiscal pressure in volunteers during various activities and found it as high as $10–15 \, kg/cm^2$ while sitting, about 30% less on standing upright and 50% less on lying down. Leaning forward or carrying a weight produces much higher pressures, though when a heavy weight is lifted breathing stops and the abdominal muscles contract, turning the trunk into a tightly inflated bag which cushions the force anteriorly against the pelvis. (Could it be that champion weight-lifters benefit in this way from having voluminous bodies?)

Seen from the side, the dorsal spine is concave forwards (kyphosis); the cervical and lumbar regions are concave backwards (lordosis). In forward flexion the lordotic curves straighten out. Lying supine with the legs straight tilts the pelvic brim forwards; the lumbar spine compensates by increasing its lordosis. If the hips are unable to extend fully (fixed flexion deformity), the lumbar lordosis increases still more until the lower limbs lie flat and the flexion deformity is masked.

THE VERTEBRAL COMPONENTS   Each segment of the vertebral column transmits weight through the vertebral body anteriorly and the facet joints posteriorly. Between adjacent bodies (and firmly attached to them) lie the intervertebral discs. These compressible 'cushions', and the surrounding ligaments and muscles, act as shock-absorbers; if they are degenerate or weak their ability to absorb some of the force is diminished and the bones and joints suffer the consequences.

The vertebral body is cancellous, but the upper and lower surfaces are condensed to form sclerotic end-plates. In childhood these are covered by cartilage, which contributes to vertebral growth. Later the peripheral rim ossifies and fuses with the body, but the central area remains as a thin layer of cartilage adherent to the intervertebral disc. The epiphyseal end-plates may be damaged by disc pressure during childhood, giving rise to irregular ossification and abnormal vertebral growth (Scheuermann's disease).

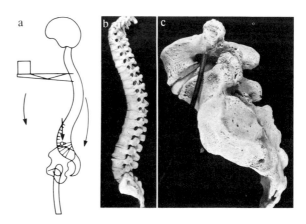

18.41 Anatomy   (a, b) The vertebral column has a series of gentle curves which produce lordosis in the cervical and lumbar regions and kyphosis in the dorsal segment. The column functions like a crane, the weight in front of the spine being counterbalanced by contraction of the posterior muscles. (c) Relationship of nerve root to disc and facet joint.

THE INTERVERTEBRAL DISC The disc consists of a central avascular *nucleus pulposus* – a hydrophilic gel made of protein-polysaccharide, collagen fibres, sparse chondroid cells and water (88%) – surrounded by concentric layers of fibrous tissue, the *annulus fibrosus*. If the physicochemical state of the nucleus pulposus is normal, the disc can withstand almost any load that the muscles can support; if it is abnormal, even small increases in force can produce sufficient stress to rupture the annulus.

MOVEMENTS The axis of movements in the thoracolumbar spine is the nucleus pulposus; the disposition of the facet joints determines which movements occur. In the lumbar spine these joints are in the anteroposterior plane, so flexion, extension and sideways tilting are free but there is virtually no rotation. In the thoracic spine the facet joints face backwards and laterally, so rotation is relatively free; flexion, extension and tilting are possible but are grossly restricted by the ribs. The costovertebral joints are involved in respiration and their limitation is an early feature of ankylosing spondylitis.

THE SPINAL CANAL The shape of the canal changes from ovoid in the upper part of the spine to triangular in the lower. Variations are common and include the trefoil canal whose shape is mainly due to thickening of the laminae posteriorly (Eisenstein, 1980). This shape is harmless in itself, but further encroachment on the canal (e.g. by a bulging disc or hypertrophic facet joints) may cause compression of the spinal contents (spinal stenosis).

THE SPINAL CORD The spinal cord ends at about L1 in the conus medullaris, but lumbosacral nerve roots continue in the spinal canal as the cauda equina and leave at appropriate levels lower down. The dural sac continues as far as S2, and whenever a nerve root leaves the spine it takes with it a dural sleeve as far as the exit from the intervertebral foramen. These dural sleeves can be outlined by contrast medium radiography (radiculography).

THE INTERVERTEBRAL FORAMINA AND NERVE ROOTS Each intervertebral foramen is bounded anteriorly by the disc and adjoining vertebral bodies, posteriorly by the facet joint, and superiorly and inferiorly by the pedicles of adjacent vertebrae. It can therefore be narrowed by a bulging disc or by joint osteophytes. The segmental nerve roots leave the spinal canal through the intervertebral foramina, each pair below the vertebra of the same number (thus, the fourth lumbar root runs between L4 and L5). The segmental blood vessels to and from the cord also pass through the intervertebral foramen. Occlusion of this little passage may occasionally compress the nerve root directly or may cause nerve root ischaemia (especially when the spine is held in extension).

NERVE SUPPLY OF THE SPINE The spine and its contents (including the dural sleeves of the nerve roots themselves) are supplied by small branches from the anterior and posterior primary rami of the segmental nerve roots. Lesions of different structures (e.g. the posterior longitudinal ligament, the dural sleeve or the facet joint) may therefore cause pain of similar distribution. *Pain down the thigh and leg ('sciatica') does not necessarily signify root pressure; it may equally well be referred from a facet joint.*

BLOOD SUPPLY In addition to the spinal arteries, which run the length of the cord, segmental arteries from the aorta send branches through the intervertebral foramina at each level. Accompanying veins drain into the azygos system and inferior vena cava, and anastomose profusely with the extradural plexus which extends throughout the length of the spinal canal (Batson's plexus).

References and further reading

Archer, I.A. and Dickson, R.A. (1989) Spinal deformities. 1. Basic principles. *Current Orthopaedics* **3**, 72–76

Arnoldi, C.C. and Brodsky, A.E., Cauchoix, J. et. al. (1976) Lumbar spinal stenosis and nerve root entrapment. *Clinical Orthopaedics and Related Research* **115**, 4–5

Bradford, D.S., Khalid, B.A., Moe, J.H., Winter, R.B. and Lonstein, J.E. (1980) The surgical management of patients with Scheuermann's disease. *Journal of Bone and Joint Surgery* **62A**, 705–712

Cotrel, Y., Dubousset, J. and Guillamet, M. (1988) New universal instrumentation in spinal surgery. *Clinical Orthopaedics and Related Research* **227**, 10–23

Dickson, R.A. (1989) Idiopathic spinal deformities. *Current Orthopaedics* **3**, 77–85

Dickson, R.A., Lawton, J.D., Archer, I.A. and Butt, W.P. (1984) The pathogenesis of idiopathic scoliosis. *Journal of Bone and Joint Surgery* **66B**, 8–15

Eisenstein, S. (1980) The trefoil configuration of the lumbar vertebral canal. *Journal of Bone and Joint Surgery* **62B**, 73–77

Eisenstein, S.M. and Parry, C.R. (1987) The lumbar facet arthrosis syndrome. *Journal of Bone and Joint Surgery* **69B**, 3–7

Ejeskär, A, Nachemson, A., Herberts, P. et al. (1982) Surgery versus chemonucleolysis for herniated lumbar discs. *Clinical Orthopaedics and Related Research* **171**, 252–259

Fredrickson, B.E., Baker, D.R., McHolick, W.J. et al. (1984) The natural history of spondylolysis and spondylolisthesis. *Journal of Bone and Joint Surgery* **66A**, 699–700

Kellgren, J.H. (1977) The anatomical source of back pain. *Rheumatology and Rehabilitation* **16**, 3–14

Kirkaldy-Willis, W.H. and Farfan, H.F. (1982) Instability of the lumbar spine. *Clinical Orthopaedics and Related Research* **165**, 110–123

Kostuik, J.P. (1990) Operative treatment of idiopathic scoliosis. *Journal of Bone and Joint Surgery* **72A**, 1108–1113

Lehmann, T.R., Spratt, K.F., Tozzi, J.E. et al. (1987) Long-term follow-up of lower lumbar fusion patients. *Spine* **12**, 97–104

Leong, J.C.Y. (1990) Spinal infections. Pyogenic and tuberculous infections. In *The Lumbar Spine* (eds. J.N. Weinstein and S.W. Weisel), W.B. Saunders, Philadelphia, pp. 699–723

Lippitt, A.B. (1984) The facet joint and its role in spinal pain: management with facet joint injections. *Spine* **9**, 746–750

Lonstein, J.E. and Carlson, J.M. (1984) The prediction of curve progression in untreated idiopathic scoliosis during growth. *Journal of Bone and Joint Surgery* **66A**, 1061–1071

Lynch, M.C. and Taylor, J.F. (1986) Facet joint injection for low back pain. *Journal of Bone and Joint Surgery* **68B**, 138–141

McCulloch, J.A. (1980) Chemonucleolysis: experience with 2000 cases. *Clinical Orthopaedics and Related Research* **146**, 128–135

MacNab, I. (1977) *Backache*, Williams & Wilkins, Baltimore

Medical Research Council Working Party on Tuberculosis of the Spine (1978) Sixth Report. *Journal of Bone and Joint Surgery* **60B**, 163–177

Mehta, M.H. (1972) The rib–vertebra angle in the early diagnosis between resolving and progressive infantile scoliosis. *Journal of Bone and Joint Surgery* **54B**, 230–243

Moe, J.H., Purcell, G.A. and Bradford, D.S. (1983) Zielke instrumentation (VDS) for the correction of spinal curvature. *Clinical Orthopaedics and Related Research* **180**, 133–153

Mooney, V. and Robertson, J. (1976) The facet syndrome. *Clinical Orthopaedics and Related Research* **115**, 149–156

Nachemson, A. and Morris, J.M. (1964) In vivo measurements of intradiscal pressure. *Journal of Bone and Joint Surgery* **46A**, 1077–1092

Onik, G., Helms, C.A., Ginsburg, L. et al. (1985) Percutaneous lumbar discectomy using a new aspiration probe. *American Journal of Roentgenology* **144**, 1137–1140

Waddell, G., McCulloch, J.A., Kummel, E. and Venner, R.M. (1980) Nonorganic physical signs in low-back pain. *Spine* **5**, 117–125

Waddell, G., Bircher, M., Finlayson, D. and Main, C.J. (1984) Symptoms and signs: physical disease or illness behaviour. *British Medical Journal* **289**, 739–741

Wilson, D. and Harbaugh, R. (1981) Microsurgical and standard removal of protruded lumbar disc. A comparative study. *Neurosurgery* **8**, 422–427

Wiltse, L.L., Rothman, S.L.G., Milanowska, K., Hanley, E.N. and Bradford, D.S. (1990) Lumbar and lumbosacral spondylolisthesis. In *The Lumbar Spine* (eds. J.N. Weinstein and S.W. Weisel), W.B. Saunders, Philadelphia, pp. 471–545

Winter, R.B., Moe, J.H. and Wang, J.D. (1973) Congenital kyphosis. *Journal of Bone and Joint Surgery* **55A**, 223–256

Zachrisson, M. (1981) The back school. *Spine* **6**, 104–106

The hip
19

Examination

Symptoms

Pain arising in the hip joint is felt in the groin, down the front of the thigh and, sometimes, in the knee; occasionally knee pain is the only symptom! Pain at the back of the hip is seldom from the joint; it usually derives from the lumbar spine.

Stiffness may cause difficulty with putting on socks or sitting in a low chair.

Limp is common and may be associated with either pain or 'weakness'.

Deformity is seldom obvious; instead the patient notices that the leg 'is getting shorter' – or sometimes 'longer'.

Walking distance may be curtailed; or, reluctantly, the patient starts using a walking stick.

Signs with the patient upright

The *gait* is noted, and also whether the patient uses any form of support. If there is a *limp* it may be due to pain (the antalgic gait), to shortening (the short-leg limp) or to abductor weakness (the Trendelenburg lurch).

The *Trendelenburg test* is used to assess stability. The patient is asked to stand, unassisted, on each leg in turn; the other leg is lifted by bending the knee (but not the hip). Normally the weightbearing hip is held stable by the abductors and the pelvis rises on the unsupported side; if the hip is unstable or very

painful, the pelvis drops on the unsupported side. Another way of testing for Trendelenburg's sign is as follows. The examiner faces the patient, placing one hand against the shoulder on the side being tested (the 'test side') and using his other hand to give support on the opposite side (the 'support side'). The patient is now asked to lift one leg and stand on the test side. If he has a positive Trendelenburg he tries to move his body over towards the test side; if he is prevented from doing this (by the examiner's hand on his shoulder) he can support himself only by pressing down hard on the support side. A positive Trendelenburg test is found in: (1) dislocation or subluxation of the hip; (2)

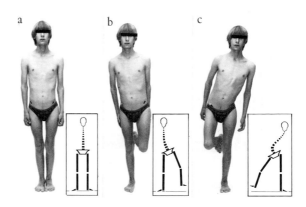

19.1 Trendelenburg's sign (a) Standing normally on two legs. (b) Standing on the right leg which has a normal hip whose abductor muscles ensure correct weight transference. (c) Standing on the left leg whose hip is faulty, and so abduction cannot be achieved; the pelvis drops on the unsupported side and the shoulder swings over to the left.

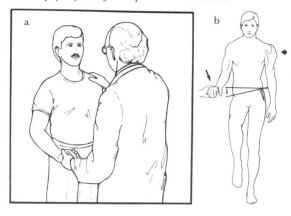

19.2 Trendelenburg's sign An easy way of doing the test is to feel the alteration in load support. (a) The position adopted. The patient's left hip is unstable; the examiner's right hand prevents lateral movement of the body towards that side. (b) Positive Trendelenburg. When the patient takes weight on the abnormal hip, he keeps his balance by pushing down hard with his right hand. The hand positions are then reversed and the test is repeated on the normal hip; the difference is obvious.

weakness of the abductors; (3) shortening of the femoral neck; or (4) any painful disorder of the hip.

The lumbar spine is examined for deformity or limitation of movement.

Signs with the patient lying supine

● LOOK

Skin Scars or sinuses may be seen (or they may be at the back of the hip). In babies, asymmetry of skin creases may be important.

Shape Swelling or wasting is noted.

Position The limb may lie in an abnormal position; excessive rotation is easy to detect but other deformities are often masked by tilting of the pelvis.

Limb length can usually be gauged by looking at the ankles or heels; but first it is necessary to

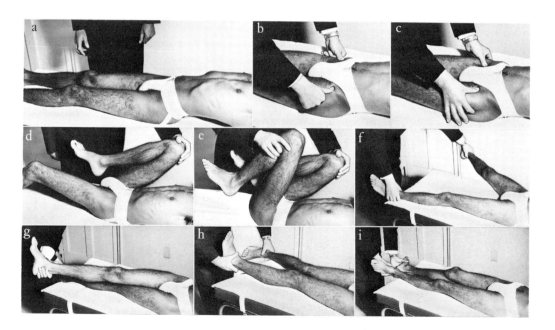

19.3 Signs with patient supine (a) Looking at the patient: his legs and pelvis are square with the couch; the lordosis indicates fixed flexion of the hip. (b) Feeling the anterior superior iliac spines. (c) Locating the top of the greater trochanter. (d) Flexing the right hip causes the left to lift off the couch (fixed flexion). The left hip also has limitation of (e) flexion, (f) abduction, (g) adduction, (h) internal rotation and (i) external rotation.

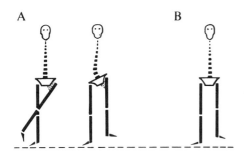

A   B

19.4 Shortening (1) – real or apparent? A leg may look short without actually being short. Thus A, with adduction of his left hip, has to hitch up his pelvis in order to uncross his legs; this makes the leg *appear* short.

B has no hip deformity; unlike A he is able to stand (or lie) with his legs at right angles to his pelvis. His leg really *is* short.

position the pelvis so that the anterior superior iliac spines are at the same level. Provided the pelvis is truly at right angles to the trunk and lower limbs, any visible discrepancy in limb length is probably real. This can be checked by placing the two lower limbs in identical positions in relation to the pelvis and then *measuring* the distance from the anterior superior iliac spine to the medial malleolus on each side.

Sometimes the *real length*, as determined by measuring between two bony points, is quite different from the *apparent length* with the patient lying in repose. This happens when the pelvis is tilted and one limb is hitched upwards. Almost invariably this is due to an uncorrectible

deformity at the hip: with fixed adduction on one side, the limbs would tend to be crossed; when the legs are placed side by side the pelvis has to tilt upwards on the affected side, giving the impression of a shortened limb. The exact opposite occurs when there is fixed abduction, and the limb seems to be longer on the affected side.

If real shortening is present it is usually possible to establish where the fault lies. With the knees flexed and the heels together, it can be seen whether the discrepancy is below or above the knee. If it is above, the next question is whether the abnormality lies above the greater trochanter. The thumbs are pressed firmly against the anterior superior iliac spines and the middle fingers grope for the tops of the greater trochanters; any elevation of the trochanter on one side is readily appreciated.

● FEEL

Skin temperature and *soft tissue* contours can be felt, but are unhelpful unless the patient is very thin.

Bone contours are felt when levelling the pelvis and judging the height of the greater trochanters. *Tenderness* may be elicited in and around the joint.

● MOVE

The assessment of hip movements is difficult because any limitation can easily be obscured by movement of the pelvis. Thus, even a gross limitation of extension, causing a *fixed flexion deformity*, can be completely masked simply by arching the back into excessive lordosis. For-

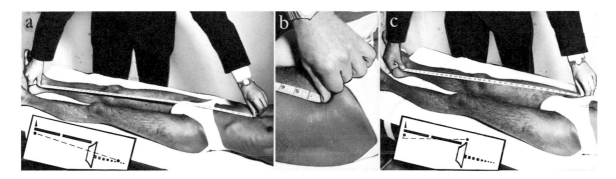

19.5 Shortening (2) – measurements Apparent length (a) is measured from a fixed point in the midline (e.g. the xiphisternum) to the bottom of the medial malleolus. Real length is measured from the anterior superior iliac spine; note how the thumb is pressed hard up against it (b) – also to the medial malleolus (c).

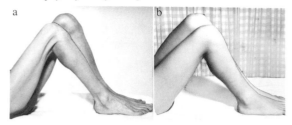

19.6 Shortening (3) Provided the backs of both heels are exactly level, bending the knees immediately shows whether the shortening is (a) above the knee or (b) below it.

tunately it can be just as easily unmasked by performing *Thomas' test*: both hips are flexed simultaneously to their limit, thus completely obliterating the lumbar lordosis; holding the 'sound' hip firmly in position (and thus keeping the pelvis still), the other limb is lowered gently; with any flexion deformity the knee will not rest on the couch. Meanwhile the full range of *flexion* will also have been noted; the normal range is about 130 degrees.

Similarly, when testing *abduction* the pelvis must be prevented from tilting sideways. This is achieved by placing the 'sound' hip (the hip opposite to the one being examined) in full abduction and keeping it there. A hand is placed on one iliac crest to detect the slightest movement of the pelvis. Then after checking that the anterior superior iliac spines are level, the affected joint is moved gently into abduction. The normal range is about 40 degrees.

Adduction is tested by crossing one limb over the other; the pelvis must be watched and felt to determine the point at which it starts to tilt. The normal range of adduction is about 30 degrees.

To test *rotation* both legs, lifted by the ankles, are rotated first internally and then externally; the patellae are watched to estimate the amount of rotation. Rotation in flexion is tested with the hip and knee each flexed 90 degrees.

If internal rotation is full with the hip extended, but restricted in flexion, this suggests pathology in the anterosuperior portion of the femoral head, probably avascular necrosis (the so-called 'sectoral sign'). But in a young person pain on internal rotation with the hip flexed may indicate a torn acetabular labrum.

Abnormal movement Telescoping may be elicited by alternately pulling and pushing the limb in its longest axis; this is a sign of marked instability.

Signs with the patient lying prone

- LOOK   Scars, sinuses or wasting are noted.
- FEEL   Muscle bulk and tautness are most easily assessed when the patient is prone.
- MOVE   Extension of the two hips is most accurately compared with the patient lying prone. Rotation also can be assessed by flexing both knees and then moving the legs (like two handles) first away from each other and then crossing each other.

Imaging

The minimum required is an anteroposterior x-ray of the pelvis showing both hips and a lateral view of each hip separately. The two sides can be compared: any difference in the size, shape or position of the femoral heads is important. With a normal hip Shenton's line,

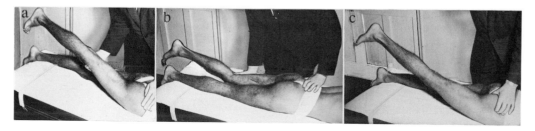

19.7 Signs with patient prone (a) Extension of the good hip is full; (b) in the affected leg it is limited. (c) Testing power in the glutei.

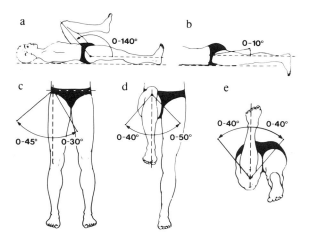

19.8 Normal range of movements (a) The hip should flex until the thigh meets the abdomen, but (b) extends only a few degrees. (c) Abduction is usually greater than adduction. The relative amounts of internal and external rotation vary according to whether the hip is in (d) flexion or (e) extension; in flexion the unwary may confuse internal with external rotation, but a hand on the thigh resolves the difficulty.

Table 19.1 The diagnostic calendar

Age at onset (years)	Probable diagnosis
0 (birth)	Congenital dislocation
0–5	Perthes' disease
10–20	Slipped epiphysis
Adult	Osteoarthritis Avascular necrosis Rheumatoid arthritis

are exceptions to this rule, it is sufficiently true to allow the age at onset to serve as a guide to the probable diagnosis.

which continues from the inferior border of the femoral neck to the inferior border of the pubic ramus, looks continuous; any interruption in the line suggests an abnormal position of the femoral head. Narrowing of the joint 'space' is a sure sign of arthritis.

A lateral view is obligatory for assessing the shape, position and architecture of the femoral head; for example, when a slipped epiphysis or avascular necrosis is suspected.

Arthrography may be used to show the outline of the cartilaginous femoral head in young children. It may also reveal loose bodies, a loose flap of articular cartilage or a tear of the acetabular labrum.

CT is essential in the assessment of fracture dislocations of the hip.

Radioscintigraphy is helpful in the assessment of femoral head blood supply.

MRI is the best method of diagnosing early avascular necrosis, when the changes are predominantly in the marrow.

The diagnostic calendar

Hip disorders are characteristically seen in certain well-defined age groups. Whilst there

Congenital dislocation of the hip

Congenital dislocation is one phase of a spectrum of hip instability in newborn infants. Normally at birth the hips are completely stable and held partially flexed. Occasionally, however, the joint is 'unstable' in the sense that it is either dislocated or is dislocatable – that is, though usually in place, it can easily be made to . dislocate by gentle manipulation.

The reported incidence of instability is 5–20 per 1000 live births (Palmen, 1961; Barlow, 1962; Wilkinson, 1972); however, most of these hips stabilize spontaneously, and on re-examination 3 weeks after birth the incidence of instability is only 1 or 2 per 1000 infants. Girls are much more commonly affected than boys, the ratio being about 7 : 1. The left hip is more often affected than the right; in 1 in 5 cases the condition is bilateral.

Aetiology and pathogenesis

Genetic factors must play a part in the aetiology, for congenital dislocation tends to run in families and even in entire populations (e.g. northern Italians). Wynne-Davies (1970) identified two heritable features which could predispose to hip instability: generalized joint laxity, a dominant trait, and acetabular dysplasia, a polygenic trait which is seen in the smaller group (mainly girls) with persistent instability. However, this cannot be the whole story because in 4 out of 5 cases only one hip is dislocated.

Hormonal factors (e.g. high levels of maternal oestrogen, progesterone and relaxin in the last few weeks of pregnancy) may aggravate ligamentous laxity in the infant. This could account for the rarity of instability in premature babies, born before the hormones reach their peak.

Intrauterine malposition (especially a breech position with extended legs) favours dislocation; this is linked with the higher incidence in firstborn babies, among whom spontaneous version is less likely.

Unilateral dislocation usually affects the left hip; this fits with the usual vertex presentation (left occiput anterior) in which the left hip is somewhat adducted.

Postnatal factors may contribute to persistence of neonatal instability and acetabular maldevelopment. Dislocation is very common in Lapps and North American Indians who swaddle their babies and carry them with legs together, hips and knees fully extended, and is rare in southern Chinese and African Negroes who carry their babies astride their backs with legs widely abducted. There is also experimental evidence that simultaneous hip and knee extension leads to hip dislocation during early development (Yamamuro and Ishida, 1984).

Pathology

At birth the hip, though unstable, is probably normal in shape (McKibbin, 1970), but the capsule is often stretched and redundant.

During infancy a number of changes develop, some of them perhaps reflecting a primary dysplasia of the acetabulum and/or the proximal femur, but most of them from adaptation to persistent instability and abnormal joint loading.

The femoral head dislocates posteriorly but, with extension of the hips, it comes to lie first posterolateral and then superolateral to the acetabulum. The cartilaginous socket is shallow and anteverted. The cartilaginous femoral head is normal in size but the bony nucleus appears late and its ossification is delayed throughout infancy.

The capsule is stretched and the ligamentum teres becomes elongated and hypertrophied. Superiorly the acetabular labrum and its capsular edge may be pushed into the socket by the dislocated femoral head; this fibrocartilaginous limbus may obstruct any attempt at closed reduction of the femoral head.

After weightbearing commences, these changes are intensified. Both the acetabulum and the femoral neck remain anteverted and the pressure of the femoral head induces a false socket to form above the shallow acetabulum. The capsule, squeezed between the edge of the acetabulum and the psoas muscle, develops an hourglass appearance. In time the surrounding muscles become adaptively shortened.

Clinical features

The ideal, still unrealized, is to diagnose every case at birth. For this reason, every newborn child should be examined for signs of hip instability. Where there is a family history of congenital dislocation, and with breech presentations, extra care is taken and the infant may have to be examined more than once.

IN THE NEONATE there are several ways of testing for instability. In *Ortolani's test,* the baby's thighs are held with the thumbs medially and the fingers resting on the greater trochanters; the hips are flexed to 90 degrees and gently abducted. Normally there is smooth abduction to almost 90 degrees. In congenital dislocation the movement is usually impeded, but if pressure is applied to the greater trochanter there is a soft 'clunk' as the dislocation reduces, and then the hip abducts fully (the 'jerk of entry'). If abduction stops half-way and there is no jerk of entry, there may be an irreducible dislocation.

Barlow's test is performed in a similar manner, but here the examiner's thumb is placed in the groin and, by grasping the upper thigh, an attempt is made to lever the femoral head in and out of the acetabulum during abduction and adduction. If the femoral head is normally in the reduced position, but can be made to slip

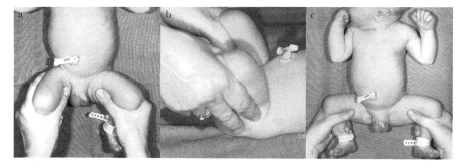

19.9 Congenital hip dislocation – early signs (a, b) Position of the hands for performing Ortolani's test. (c) The test has been performed – the right hip has not abducted fully; with a little more pressure there was a 'jerk of entry'.

out of the socket and back in again, the hip is classed as 'dislocatable' (i.e. unstable).

Every hip with signs of instability – however slight – is examined by *ultrasonography*. This shows the shape of the cartilaginous socket and the position of the femoral head. If there is any abnormality, the infant is placed in a splint with the hips flexed and abducted (see under 'Management') and is recalled for re-examination 6 weeks later. By then it should be possible to assess whether the hip is reduced and stable, reduced but unstable, subluxated or dislocated.

In experienced hands, neonatal screening is highly effective in reducing the incidence of late-presenting dislocation (Hadlow, 1988).

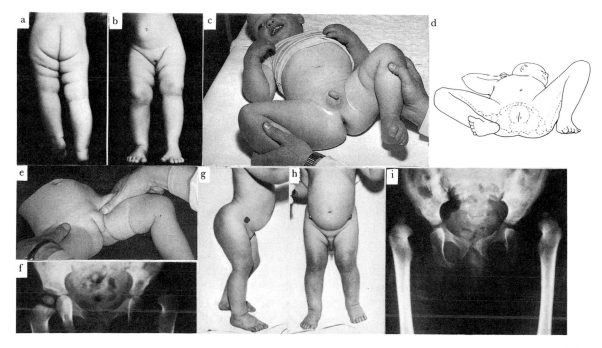

19.10 Congenital hip dislocation – late signs (a, b) Unilateral dislocation of the left hip. (c) The left hip does not abduct more than half way, and (d) the drawing shows why – the femoral head is caught up on the rim of the acetabulum. (e) The thumb sinks in too far on the left hip, because (f) the head is not in the socket. (g–i) The clinical appearance and x-rays of a bilateral dislocation.

APPROACH TO THE LIMPING CHILD

1. *Measure limb length*

2. *Check the foot*
   Splinter? Injury?
   Swollen ankle: Infection? Arthritis?

3. *Examine the knee*
   Swelling: Infection? Arthritis? Tumour?
   Tenderness: Injury? Infection?
   Instability: Patellar subluxation?

4. *Examine the hip*
   Septic arthritis?
   Dislocation? Subluxation? Coxa vara?
   Transient synovitis? Perthes' disease?
   Arthritis? Tumour?

5. *General assessment*
   Exclude non-accidental injury

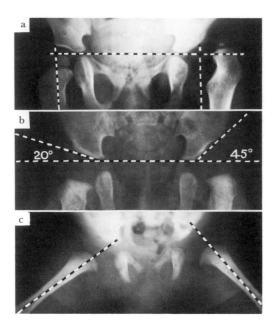

19.11 Congenital hip dislocation – x-rays (a) Perkin's lines: the epiphysis should lie medial to the vertical and below the horizontal line. (b) The acetabular roof angle should be about 20 degrees. (c) Von Rosen's lines: with the hips abducted 45 degrees, the femoral shafts should point into the acetabulum.

LATE FEATURES An observant mother may spot asymmetry, a clicking hip, or difficulty in applying the napkin because of limited abduction.

With unilateral dislocation the skin creases look asymmetrical and the leg is slightly short and externally rotated; a thumb in the groin may feel that the femoral head is missing. With bilateral dislocation there is an abnormally wide perineal gap. Abduction is decreased.

Contrary to popular belief, late walking is not a marked feature; nevertheless, in children who do not walk by 18 months dislocation must be excluded. Likewise, a limp or Trendelenburg gait, or a waddling gait could be a sign of missed dislocation.

Imaging

Ultrasonography has largely replaced radiography for imaging hips in the newborn. At birth the acetabulum and femoral head are cartilaginous and therefore invisible on plain x-rays. Real-time ultrasound gives an accurate picture of their relationship to each other.

Plain x-rays are more useful after the first 6 months, though even then their assessment requires the projection of various 'lines' and 'indices' based on bone outlines rather than the (cartilaginous) anatomical articulation.

Management

THE FIRST 3–6 MONTHS
The simplest policy is to regard all infants with a high-risk background (a family history or extended breech delivery), or a positive Ortolani or Barlow test, as 'suspect' and to nurse them in double napkins or an abduction pillow for the first 6 weeks. At that stage they are re-examined: those with stable hips are left free but kept under observation for at least 6 months; those with persistent instability are treated by more formal abduction splintage (see below) until the hip is stable and x-ray shows that the acetabular roof is developing satisfactorily (usually 3–6 months).

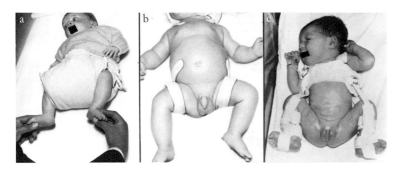

19.12 Congenital hip dislocation – treatment before weightbearing   Reduction is usually easy and can be held by (a) an abduction pillow, (b) Von Rosen's malleable splint, or – best of all – (c) the Pavlik harness. The hips should not be more than about 60 degrees abducted, though flexion sometimes needs to be well beyond a right angle.

However, since 80–90% of hips that are unstable at birth will stabilize spontaneously in 2–3 weeks, it seems more sensible not to start splintage immediately unless the hip is already dislocated. This reduces the small (but significant) risk of epiphyseal necrosis that attends any form of restrictive splintage in the neonate. Thus: if a hip is dislocatable but not habitually dislocated, the baby is left untreated but re-examined weekly; if at 3 weeks the hip is still unstable, abduction splintage is applied (see below). If the hip is already dislocated at the first examination, it is gently placed in the reduced position and abduction splintage is applied from the outset. Reduction is maintained until the hip is stable; this may take only a few weeks, but the safest policy is to retain some sort of splintage until x-ray shows a good acetabular roof.

Where facilities for ultrasound scanning are available, a more refined protocol can be applied. All newborn infants with a high-risk background or a suggestion of hip instability are examined by ultrasonography. If this shows that the hip is reduced and has a normal cartilaginous outline, no treatment is required but the child is kept under observation for 3–6 months. If the anatomy is less than perfect, the hip is splinted in abduction and at 6 weeks ultrasound scanning is repeated. Some hips will now appear normal and these need no further treatment, apart from routine observation for 3–6 months. A few will show persistent abnormality and for these splintage in abduction is continued until a further scan at 3 months or an x-ray at 6 months shows a well-formed acetabular roof.

Splintage   The object of splintage is to hold the hips somewhat flexed and abducted; extreme positions are avoided and the joints should be allowed some movement in the splint. For the newborn, double napkins or a soft abduction pillow may suffice. Von Rosen's splint is an H-shaped malleable splint that has the merit of being easy to apply (and the demerit of being equally easy to take off!). The Pavlik harness is more difficult to apply but gives the child more freedom while still maintaining position. The least complicated – and most resistant to the mother's attentions – is the application of 'knee plasters' with a cross-bar holding the hips in 90 degrees of flexion and about 45 degrees of abduction, or 10 degrees more than the angle at which the 'jerk of entry' is felt (McKibbin et al., 1988). The three golden rules of splintage are: (1) the hip must be properly reduced before it is splinted; (2) extreme positions must be avoided; (3) the hips should be able to move.

Follow-up   Whatever policy is adopted, follow-up is continued until the child is walking. Sometimes, even with the most careful treatment, the hip may later show some degree of acetabular dysplasia.

PERSISTENT DISLOCATION: 6–18 MONTHS
If, after early treatment, the hip is still incompletely reduced, or if the child presents late with a 'missed' dislocation, the hip must be

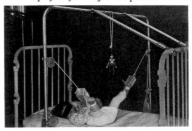

19.13 Congenital hip dislocation – treatment after weightbearing Vertical traction with abduction gradually increased.

reduced – preferably by closed methods but if necessary by operation – and held reduced until acetabular development is satisfactory.

Closed reduction This is the ideal but risks damaging the blood supply to the femoral head and causing necrosis. To minimize this risk reduction must be gradual; traction is applied to both legs, preferably on a vertical frame, and abduction is gradually increased until, by 3 weeks, the legs are widely separated. This manoeuvre alone (aided if necessary by *adductor tenotomy*) may achieve stable concentric reduction. This should be checked by an examination under anaesthesia, x-ray and *arthrography*.

Splintage The concentrically reduced hip is held in a plaster spica at 60 degrees of flexion, 40 degrees of abduction and 20 degrees of internal rotation. After 6 weeks the spica is replaced by a splint which prevents adduction but allows movement – a Pavlik harness or 'knee plasters' with a cross-bar. This is retained for another 3–6 months, checking by x-ray to ensure that the femoral head is concentrically reduced and the acetabular roof is developing normally. Splintage is then gradually abandoned by allowing the child longer and longer periods of freedom.

Operation If, at any stage, concentric reduction has not been achieved, open operation is needed. Any obstruction is dealt with and the hip is reduced. It is usually stable in 60 degrees of flexion, 40 degrees of abduction and 20 degrees of internal rotation. A spica is applied and the hip is splinted as described above.

If stability can be achieved only by markedly internally rotating the hip, a corrective subtrochanteric osteotomy of the femur is carried out, either at the time of open reduction or 6 weeks later. In young children this usually gives a good result (Gibson and Benson, 1982).

PERSISTENT DISLOCATION: 18 MONTHS – THE 'AGE LIMIT'
In the older child, closed reduction is less likely to succeed; many surgeons would proceed straight to arthrography and open reduction.

Traction Even if closed reduction is unsuccessful, a period of traction (if necessary combined with psoas and adductor tenotomy) will help to loosen the tissues and bring the femoral head down opposite the acetabulum.

Arthrography An arthrogram at this stage will clarify the anatomy of the hip and show whether there is an inturned limbus or any marked degree of acetabular dysplasia.

Operation The joint capsule is opened anteriorly, any inturned limbus is removed and the femoral head is seated in the acetabulum. Usually a derotation osteotomy held by a plate and screws will be required. At the same time a small segment can be removed from the proximal femur to reduce pressure on the hip (Klisic and Jankovic, 1976). If there is marked acetabular dysplasia, some form of acetabuloplasty will also be needed – either a pericapsular reconstruction of the acetabular roof (Pemberton, 1965) or an innominate osteotomy which repositions the entire innominate bone and acetabulum (Salter, 1961).

Splintage After operation, the hip is held in a plaster spica for 3 months and then in a splint which permits some hip movement for a further 1–3 months, checking by x-ray to ensure that the hip is reduced and developing satisfactorily.

DISLOCATION ABOVE THE 'AGE LIMIT'
The term 'age limit' implies that above a certain age reduction of the dislocation is unwise. The force needed for reduction may damage the hip, and the risk of avascular necrosis is greatly increased.

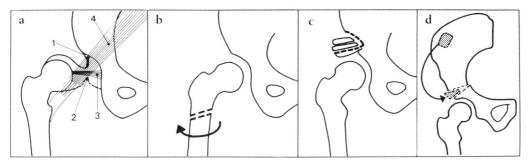

19.14 Congenital hip dislocation – operative treatment (1)   (a) Obstructions to closed reduction: 1, inverted limbus; 2, hourglass constriction of capsule; 3, thick ligamentum teres; 4, tight psoas. (b) Derotation osteotomy. (c) Shelf operation. (d) Innominate osteotomy.

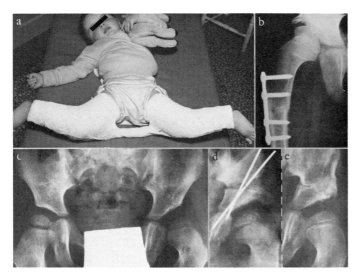

19.15 Congenital hip dislocation – operative treatment (2)   (a) Reduced open, but stable only in medial rotation – 6 weeks later (b) derotation osteotomy.

(c) Reduced open, but head poorly covered; (d, e) innominate osteotomy.

19.16 Congenital hip dislocation – above the age limit   (a) Unilateral dislocation in a young adult. (b) Bilateral dislocation – this patient had no symptoms till aged 40 when she presented with backache.

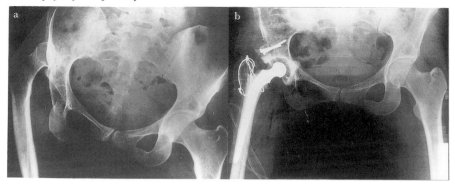

19.17 Congenital hip dislocation – hip replacement   (a) This patient, aged 35, had a very short leg, a severe limp and back pain; she could walk only a few hundred yards. (b) Hip replacement restored her to near normality – clearly the risk was worth taking.

With *unilateral dislocation* the age limit is about 10 years. The untreated hip is mobile; the patient limps but has little pain until middle life. This is the justification for non-intervention. However, persistent *subluxation* may be improved – even in young adults – by a Chiari osteotomy which displaces the acetabulum medially, leaving the femoral head partially covered by the innominate bone (Chiari, 1974).

With *bilateral dislocation* the deformity – and the waddling gait – is symmetrical and therefore not so noticeable; the risk of operative intervention is also greater because failure on one or other side turns this into an asymmetrical deformity. Therefore, in these cases, most surgeons avoid operation above the age of 6 years unless there is pain or deformity is unusually severe. The untreated patient waddles through life and may be surprisingly uncomplaining.

PERSISTENT DISLOCATION IN ADULTS

Adults who appear to have managed quite well for many years may present in their 30s or 40s with increasing discomfort due to an unreduced congenital dislocation. Walking becomes more and more tiring and backache is common. With bilateral dislocation the loss of abduction may seriously hamper sexual intercourse in women. Disability may be severe enough to justify total joint replacement. It should, however, be remembered that the operation is particularly difficult in this group of patients and it should never be undertaken lightly.

Acetabular dysplasia and subluxation of the hips

Acetabular dysplasia may be genetically determined or may follow incomplete reduction of a congenital dislocation, damage to the lateral acetabular epiphysis or maldevelopment of the femoral head. The socket is unusually shallow, the roof is sloping and the femoral head may subluxate; if this occurs, faulty load transmission leads to secondary osteoarthritis.

Clinical features

During infancy, limited abduction of the hip is suspicious and ultrasonography may reveal a deficient acetabulum.

In children the condition is usually asymptomatic and discovered only when the pelvis is x-rayed for some other reason. Sometimes, however, the hip is painful – especially after strenuous activity – and the child may develop a limp. If there is subluxation the Trendelenburg sign is positive, leg length may be asymmetrical and the femoral head may be felt as a lump in the groin. Movement – especially abduction in flexion – may be restricted.

X-rays should be taken lying and standing (the latter may show minor degrees of incongruity). The acetabulum looks shallow, the roof is sloping and the femoral head is uncovered. Subtle abnormalities are revealed by measuring the depth of the socket and the relationship

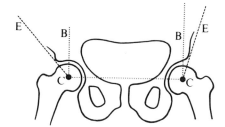

19.18 The centre–edge (CE) angle The line C–C joins the centre of each femoral head; CB is perpendicular to this, and CE cuts the superior edge of the acetabulum. The angle BCE is normally 30 degrees or more, as in the right hip; an angle of less than 20 degrees, as in the left hip, indicates dysplasia.

between the centre of the femoral head and the edge of the acetabulum – Wiberg's centre–edge (CE) angle. With subluxation, Shenton's line is broken.

Congruity and stability of the hip may be best assessed by examination and arthrography under anaesthesia (Catterall, 1992).

Adults may present with secondary osteoarthritis, sometimes confined to the posterior part of the joint and difficult to detect by conventional x-rays. Three-dimensional imaging is helpful in planning operative treatment (Murphy et al, 1990).

Diagnosis

It is often difficult to be sure that the patient's symptoms are due to the dysplastic acetabulum; other conditions causing pain and limp must be excluded (see p. 390).

Bilateral dysplasia is a feature of developmental disorders, such as multiple epiphyseal dysplasia.

Treatment

Infants with subluxation are treated as for dislocation: the hip is splinted in abduction until the acetabular roof looks normal.

Older children may need an operation to restore joint congruity: either a varus osteotomy of the femur or an osteotomy of the pelvis to reposition the acetabular roof.

In adolescents and young adults the indications for operation are pain, weakness, instability and subluxation of the hip.

If the hip is reducible and congruent, simple measures such as muscle strengthening exercises may suffice. If symptoms persist, a realignment operation (innominate or femoral osteotomy, or both) may be necessary.

If the hip is not fully reducible or if congruity cannot be achieved by repositioning the joint, acetabular augmentation is needed. This means either a displacement osteotomy (such as the Chiari procedure) or a lateral shelf reconstruction.

If the acetabulum and femoral head are severely distorted, more complex types of pelvic and/or femoral osteotomy will be required. However, if the patient can be tided over into his 40s, hip replacement may be a better option.

In older adults, the treatment is that of secondary osteoarthritis (see below).

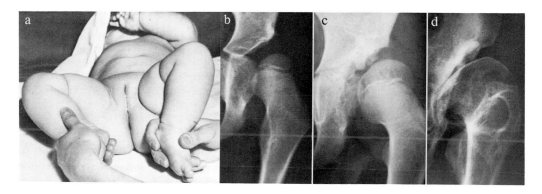

19.19 Congenital subluxation (a) The cardinal physical sign; (b) x-ray in childhood; (c) in adolescence; (d) degeneration in early adult life.

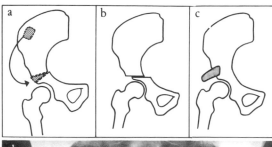

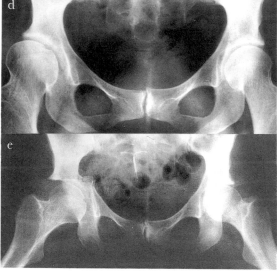

19.20 Congenital subluxation – treatment (a) Salter's innominate osteotomy; (b) Chiari's pelvic osteotomy; (c) shelf. (d, e) Before and after Chiari osteotomy.

Acquired dislocation of the hip

Dislocation occurring after the first year of life is usually due to one of three causes: pyogenic arthritis, muscle imbalance or trauma. Rare causes of acquired dislocation include tuberculosis and Charcot's disease.

Dislocation following sepsis

In infancy the femur may be infected via the umbilicus or via femoral vein puncture; at this age the growth disc is no barrier and infection readily involves the femoral head and the joint. In older children acute osteomyelitis usually affects the metaphysis; but as this is intracapsular again the joint is readily attacked. If the infection is unchecked the head and neck of the femur may be destroyed and a pathological dislocation result. The pus may escape and, when the child recovers, the sinus heals. The hip signs then resemble those of a congenital dislocation, but the telltale scar remains. On x-ray the femoral head appears to be completely absent; however, some part of it often survives, although it is too osteoporotic to be seen.

The dislocation should be treated by traction, followed, if necessary, by open reduction. In the absence of a femoral head, the greater trochanter can be placed in the acetabulum; varus osteotomy of the upper femur helps to achieve stability.

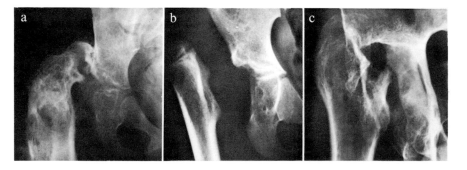

19.21 Acquired dislocation (non-traumatic) (a) Acute suppurative arthritis following osteomyelitis of the femoral neck in a child. (b) Acute suppurative arthritis in infancy has resulted in complete disappearance of the femoral head and neck. (c) Pathological dislocation in tuberculosis.

Dislocation due to muscle imbalance

Unbalanced paralysis in childhood may result in the hip abductors being weaker than the adductors. This is seen in cerebral palsy, in myclomeningocele and after poliomyelitis (see Chapter 10). The greater trochanter fails to develop properly, the femoral neck becomes valgus and the hip may subluxate or dislocate. Treatment is similar to that of congenital dislocation, but in addition some muscle re-balancing operation is essential.

Traumatic dislocation

Occasionally dislocation of the hip is missed while attention is focused on some more distal (and more obvious) injury. Reduction is essential, if necessary by open operation; even if avascular necrosis or hip stiffness supervenes, a hip in the anatomical position presents an easier prospect for reconstructive surgery than one that remains persistently dislocated.

Femoral anteversion (intoe gait)

A familiar sight at every paediatric orthopaedic clinic is the child brought because of the intoe gait. The child walks awkwardly and trips over his feet when running. The cause is rarely serious but a bland assurance that 'he will grow out of it' may fail to convince the parents and certainly won't satisfy the grandparents.

Below the age of 3 years intoeing is usually due to forefoot adduction or tibial torsion, both of which may correct spontaneously as the child grows.

Above the age of 3 years the commonest cause of intoe gait is excessive anteversion (persistent fetal alignment) of the femoral neck, so that internal rotation of the hip is increased and external rotation diminished. The gait may look clumsy but is no bar to athletic prowess and usually improves with growth. These children often sit on the floor in the 'television position' with the knees facing each other. With the child standing, the patellae are turned inwards ('squinting patellae') and there may be compensatory external torsion of the tibiae.

Femoral neck anteversion can be assessed by ultrasonography or by obtaining CT scans across the hips and the knees and measuring the angle between the axis of the femoral neck and the transverse axis across the femoral condyles.

Correction by femoral osteotomy is feasible but seldom indicated, and certainly not before the age of 8 years.

Other causes of intoe gait include femoral shaft torsion, tibial torsion and forefoot adduction. To differentiate these the child is examined first with hips and knees extended, then with both flexed to a right angle; finally the position of the foot is inspected.

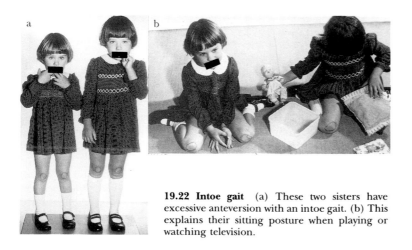

19.22 Intoe gait (a) These two sisters have excessive anteversion with an intoe gait. (b) This explains their sitting posture when playing or watching television.

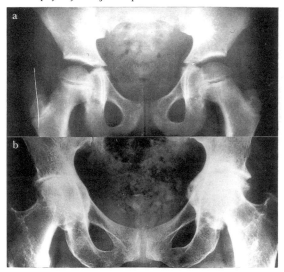

19.23 Protrusio acetabuli   (a) The early stage in a child. (b) In this adult with protrusio, degenerative changes have developed in both hips.

Protrusio acetabuli (Otto pelvis)

In this condition the socket is too deep and bulges into the cavity of the pelvis. The 'primary' form shows a slight familial tendency. It affects females much more often than males and develops soon after puberty; at this stage there are usually no symptoms although movements are limited. X-rays show the sunken acetabulum, with the inner wall bulging beyond the iliopectineal line. Secondary osteoarthritis may develop in later life, but until then the condition does not require treatment.

Protrusio may occur in later life secondary to bone 'softening' disorders, such as osteomalacia or Paget's disease, and in long-standing cases of rheumatoid arthritis. If pain is severe, or movements are markedly restricted, joint replacement is indicated.

Coxa vara

The normal femoral neck-shaft angle is 160 degrees at birth, decreasing to 125 degrees in adult life. An angle of less than 120 degrees is called coxa vara. The deformity may be either congenital or acquired.

Congenital coxa vara

This is a rare disorder of infancy and early childhood. It is due to a defect of endochondral ossification in the medial part of the femoral neck. When the child starts to crawl or stand, the femoral neck bends or develops a stress fracture; with continued weightbearing it collapses increasingly into varus. Sometimes there is also shortening or bowing of the femoral shaft.

CLINICAL FEATURES   The condition is diagnosed when the child starts to walk. The leg is short and the thigh may be bowed. X-ray shows that the physeal line is too vertical; typically, in the infant, there is a separate triangle of bone in the inferior portion of the metaphysis (Fairbank's triangle).

With bilateral coxa vara the patient may not be seen until he presents as a young adult with osteoarthritis.

TREATMENT   If shortening is progressive, the deformity should be corrected by a subtrochanteric valgus osteotomy. Varus does not recur, but there may be some permanent shortening.

Acquired coxa vara

Coxa vara can develop if the femoral neck bends (because it is soft) or if it breaks.

BONE SOFTENING   Bone softening may produce coxa vara in children (rickets, bone dystrophies and possibly Perthes' disease), in adults (osteomalacia) and in the elderly (osteoporosis and Paget's disease).

At any age, tuberculosis or pyogenic infection may soften bone and lead to coxa vara, but the deformity is overshadowed by the causal condition.

FRACTURE   Fracture may produce coxa vara in children (through a solitary cyst), in adolescents (slipped epiphysis) and in the elderly (malunion of a trochanteric fracture).

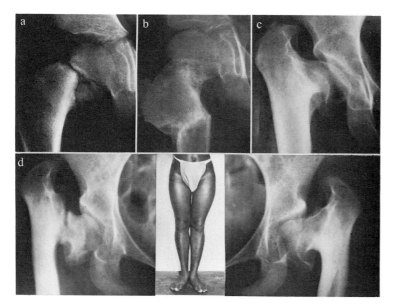

19.24 Infantile coxa vara (a) Growth disc too vertical and triangle of bone on undersurface of neck; (b) abduction osteotomy should be performed early; otherwise (c) the shaft migrates upwards. (d) Bilateral infantile coxa vara – untreated; only some 30 cm of ankle separation was possible.

The irritable hip

This vague term is attached to a well-recognized syndrome of transient hip pain and restriction of movement in an otherwise healthy child. With an incidence of 3% (Landin, Danielsson and Wattsgard, 1987) it is the commonest cause of hip pain in children. Boys are affected twice as often as girls.

Clinical features

The patient – typically between 6 and 12 years of age – presents with pain and a limp, often intermittent and following activity. Pain is felt in the groin or front of the thigh, sometimes reaching as far as the knee. Slight wasting may be detectable but the cardinal sign is that the extremes of all movements are limited, and the attempt to produce them is painful. General examination, blood investigations and x-rays are normal, but ultrasonography may reveal a small joint effusion. Scintigraphy is usually normal during the acute phase.

Characteristically, symptoms last for 1–2 weeks and then subside spontaneously; hence the synonym 'transient synovitis'. The child may have more than one episode, with an interval of months between attacks of pain.

Diagnosis

The condition is important largely because it resembles a number of serious disorders which have to be excluded.

Perthes' disease is the main worry. Symptoms usually last longer than 2 weeks and x-rays may show an increased 'joint space'.

Tuberculous synovitis produces a raised ESR and the Heaf test is positive.

Juvenile chronic arthritis and ankylosing spondylitis may start with synovitis of one hip. There may be a raised ESR.

Slipped epiphysis may present as an 'irritable hip'. Age and build are characteristic and the x-ray appearance is diagnostic, provided a lateral view is also taken.

Treatment

If the child is otherwise completely healthy, the symptoms and signs are mild and the joint effusion is slight, the child can be treated by simple bed rest at home. In more severe cases – and particularly if the diagnosis is in doubt – the child should be admitted for continuous bed rest and traction. The hip should be kept flexed and in some external rotation, as extension and internal rotation increase the intra-articular pressure and may predispose to ischaemia (Vegter, 1987).

Ultrasonography is repeated at intervals and weightbearing is allowed only when the symptoms disappear and the effusion resolves.

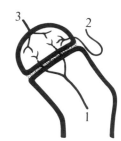

19.25 Perthes' disease – the background 1, Metaphyseal vessels; 2, lateral epiphyseal vessels; 3, vessels in the ligamentum teres.

Perthes' disease

Perthes' disease – or rather Legg–Calvé–Perthes' disease, for in 1910 the condition was described independently by three different people – is a painful disorder of childhood characterized by avascular necrosis of the femoral head. It is uncommon in any community – the quoted incidence is about 1 in 10 000 (Barker and Hall, 1986) – but particularly rare in African Negroes. Patients are usually 4–8 years old and boys are affected four times as often as girls.

The condition may be part of a general disorder of growth. Epidemiological studies in the UK have shown that there is a higher than usual incidence in underprivileged communities. Affected children have retarded growth of the trunk and limbs, with notably small feet; their siblings, too, have retarded trunk growth (Hall et al., 1988).

Pathogenesis

The precipitating cause of Perthes' disease is unknown but the cardinal step in the pathogenesis is ischaemia of the femoral head. Up to the age of 4 months, the femoral head is supplied by: (1) metaphyseal vessels which penetrate the growth disc; (2) lateral epiphyseal vessels running in the retinacula; and (3) scanty vessels in the ligamentum teres. The metaphyseal supply

gradually declines until, by the age of 4 years, it has virtually disappeared; by the age of 7, however, the vessels in the ligamentum teres have developed. Between 4 and 7 years of age the femoral head may depend for its blood supply and venous drainage almost entirely on the lateral epiphyseal vessels whose situation in the retinacula makes them susceptible to stretching and to pressure from an effusion. Although such pressure may be insufficient to block off the arterial flow, it could easily cause venous stasis resulting in a rise in intraosseous pressure and consequent ischaemia. There is both clinical and experimental evidence that this can occur in Perthes' disease (Lin and Ho, 1991).

The immediate cause of capsular tamponade is probably an effusion following trauma (of which there is a history in over half the cases) or a non-specific synovitis. Two or more such incidents may be needed to produce the typical bone changes.

Pathology

The pathological process takes 2–4 years to complete, passing through three stages.

STAGE 1: ISCHAEMIA AND BONE DEATH   All or part of the bony nucleus of the femoral head is dead; it still looks normal on plain x-ray but stops enlarging. The cartilaginous part of the femoral head, being nourished by synovial fluid, remains viable and becomes thicker than normal. There may also be thickening and oedema of the synovium and capsule.

STAGE 2: REVASCULARIZATION AND REPAIR   Within weeks (possibly even days) of infarction, a number of changes begin to appear. Dead marrow is replaced by granulation tissue, which sometimes calcifies. The bone is revascularized and new lamellae are laid down on the dead trabeculae, producing the appearance of increased density on x-ray. Here and there ossification may extend into the epiphyseal cartilage, showing up as flecks of 'calcification' in the x-ray. Beneath the subarticular bone plate, resorption may lead to the appearance of a tangential fracture. Some of the dead trabecular fragments are resorbed and replaced by fibrous tissue. Alternating areas of sclerosis and fibrosis appear on the x-ray as 'fragmentation' of the epiphysis. The metaphysis may become hyperaemic and on x-ray looks rarefied or cystic. Morphological changes may also appear in the acetabulum, particularly in older children and when more than half of the femoral head is involved (Joseph, 1989).

STAGE 3: DISTORTION AND REMODELLING If the repair process is rapid and complete, the bony architecture may be restored before the femoral head loses its shape. If it is tardy, the bony epiphysis may collapse and subsequent growth of the head and neck will be distorted: the head becomes oval or flattened – like the head of a mushroom – and enlarged laterally, while the neck is often short and broad. Slowly the femoral head is displaced laterally in relation to the acetabulum.

Clinical features

The patient – typically a boy of 4–8 years – complains of pain and starts limping. Symptoms continue for weeks on end or may recur intermittently. The child appears to be well, though often somewhat undersized. In 4% there is an associated urogenital anomaly.

The hip looks deceptively normal, though there may be a little wasting. Early on, the joint is irritable so that all movements are diminished and their extremes painful. Often the child is not seen till later, when most movements are full; but abduction (especially in flexion) is nearly always limited and usually internal rotation also.

X-rays

Although the condition may be suspected from the clinical appearances, diagnosis hinges on the x-ray changes.

At first the x-rays may seem normal, though subtle changes such as widening of the 'joint space' and slight asymmetry of the ossific centres are usually present. Radionuclide scanning may show a 'void' in the anterolateral part of the femoral head. The classic feature of increased density of the ossific nucleus occurs somewhat later; this may be accompanied by

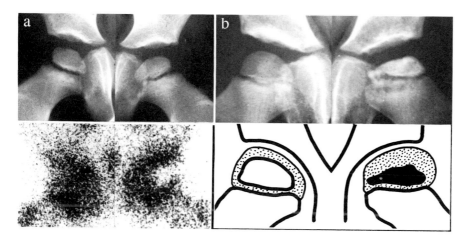

19.26 Perthes' disease – early features (a) This boy had an irritable left hip; his x-ray is virtually normal, but a scan on the same day shows a void in the lateral portion of the femoral head. (b) Later the head became radiologically dense; it stopped growing but the cartilage did not – the diagram shows how this results in an increased 'joint space'.

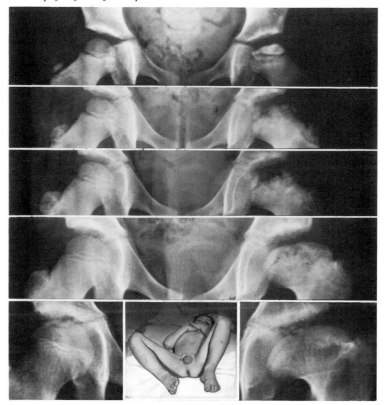

19.27 Perthes' disease Serial x-rays over a period of 5 years. Despite radiological severity the clinical signs are usually slight, but abduction in flexion is nearly always limited (inset).

fragmentation, or a crescentic subarticular fracture often best seen in the lateral view. At this stage scintigraphy shows increased activity.

Later still there is obvious increase in the joint space as well as flattening and lateral displacement of the epiphysis, with rarefaction and widening of the metaphysis.

The picture varies with the age of the child, the stage of the disease and the amount of head that is necrotic. Catterall (1972) described four groups, based on the appearances in both anteroposterior and lateral x-rays. In group 1 the epiphysis has retained its height and less than half the nucleus is sclerotic. In group 2 up to half the nucleus is sclerotic and there may be some collapse of the central portion. In group 3 most of the nucleus is involved, with sclerosis, fragmentation and collapse of the head. Metaphyseal resorption may be present. Group 4 is the worst: the whole head is involved, the ossific nucleus is flat and dense and metaphyseal resorption is marked. Somewhat simpler is the Salter–Thompson classification, into those with

more and those with less than half the head involved (Simmons, Graham and Szalai, 1990).

After healing has occurred the femoral head may appear mushroom shaped, larger than normal and laterally displaced in a dysplastic acetabular socket. A common late finding in the anteroposterior x-ray is a sclerotic line curving across the femoral neck – the 'sagging rope

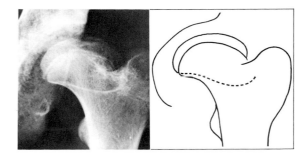

19.28 Perthes' disease The 'sagging rope sign' – the radiological relic of former Perthes' disease.

sign' (Apley and Weintroub, 1981); this may be the result of distortion and remodelling of the femoral head, or it may represent the distal margin of the metaphyseal rarefaction.

Differential diagnosis

The irritable hip of early Perthes' disease must be differentiated from other causes of irritability; the child's fitness, the increased joint space and the patchy bone density are characteristic. In transient synovitis the x-ray is normal.

Morquio's disease, cretinism, multiple. epiphyseal dysplasia, sickle-cell disease and Gaucher's disease may resemble Perthes' disease radiologically, especially if they are bilateral; however, in bilateral Perthes' disease the two sides are always at different stages. Moreover, in the other conditions diagnostic features are usually apparent.

Prognostic features

The greater the degree of femoral head involvement, the worse the outcome (Catterall, 1982). There is a poorer prognosis, too, for girls than for boys. However, age is the biggest prognostic factor: in children under 6 years the outlook is almost always excellent; thereafter, the older the child the less good is the prognosis.

Certain adverse radiological signs presage increasing deformity and displacement or subluxation of the femoral head – the *head at risk*. These are: (1) progressive uncovering of the epiphysis; (2) calcification in the (invisible) cartilage lateral to the ossified epiphysis; (3) a radiolucent area at the lateral edge of the bony epiphysis (Gage's sign); and (4) severe metaphyseal resorption. The recognition of these signs is important, for treatment is based largely on the prediction of progressive femoral head displacement.

Treatment

As long as the hip is irritable the child should be in bed with skin traction applied to the affected leg with the hip in a little flexion and external rotation. Once irritability has subsided, which usually takes about 3 weeks, movement is encouraged – particularly abduction. The clinical and radiographic features are then reassessed, with a choice of further treatment, 'supervised neglect' or 'containment'.

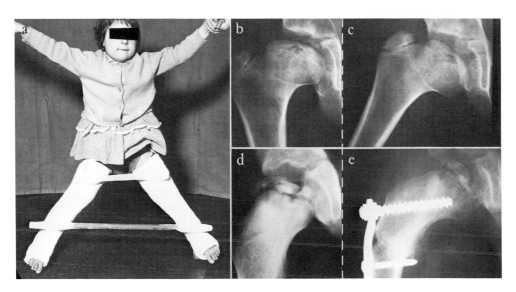

19.29 Perthes' disease – treatment   (a) So-called 'broomstick' plaster; (b) shows this girl's x-ray with her hip in the neutral position; when her hip is abducted (c) containment is achieved. (d, e) Similar containment in another patient, achieved by femoral osteotomy.

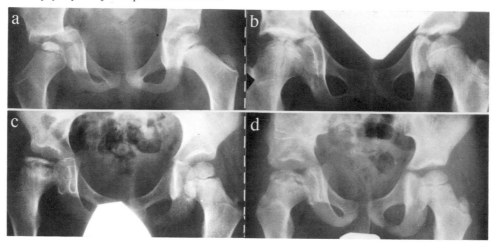

19.30 Perthes' disease – treatment (continued) Pelvic osteotomy also can achieve containment: (a, b) shows the effect of a Chiari osteomy, and (c, d) of an innominate osteotomy.

'SUPERVISED NEGLECT' This somewhat flippant term implies that treatment is abandoned. But not the child; he resumes normal activities and is checked regularly. If symptoms recur or signs increase, treatment by containment is instituted.

'CONTAINMENT' The aim is to counteract lateral displacement and to contain the head within the acetabulum in the hope that it will retain its shape and articular congruence during healing. Containment can be achieved: (1) by holding the hips widely abducted, in plaster or in a removable splint (ambulation, though awkward, is just possible, but the position must be maintained for at least a year); or (2) by operation, either a varus osteotomy of the femur (which always results in a little shortening) or an innominate osteotomy of the pelvis (which usually causes slight lengthening); plaster is worn until the osteotomy has united (6–8 weeks), after which the child is allowed free.

Choice of method

The objectives of treatment are (1) to alleviate symptoms, and (2) to restore or maintain the shape of the femoral head, expecting thereby to postpone or prevent the development of os-

teoarthritis. But once irritability has subsided, the child rarely has any symptoms; and even with considerable radiological deformity, significant symptoms of osteoarthritis are seldom seen before middle life. Consequently, since any form of treatment has disadvantages or dangers, a case can be made out for treating all patients by 'supervised neglect' – except, of course, those in whom symptoms fail to subside with rest or recur when activity is resumed.

Most surgeons, however, believe that the choice between containment and doing nothing should not be decided purely by symptoms and clinical signs; they maintain that it should depend upon the age of onset and the radiological severity of the disease. Patients classified as Catterall group 1 need no treatment. Nor do patients in groups 2 and 3 if they are less than 7 years of age, unless the head is at risk; those aged over 7 or with a head at risk need containment. Group 4 patients of any age also need containment; but if deformity is very severe this may be unattainable, and the attempt to force it is then harmful. Before intervening, plain x-rays and contrast arthrography should be carried out with the hip in varying degrees of abduction and rotation to determine the position of congruence. If the head is too flat, adduction will cause hinging rather than congruent rolling; clearly in that case repositioning offers no advantage.

Even in patients selected for containment, there is still a choice – between splintage and operation. Surgery is not devoid of risk but has the great merit of achieving containment rapidly, so that the child's social development is less affected; the two operations (femoral osteotomy and pelvic osteotomy) give similar results.

Slipped epiphysis

Displacement of the proximal femoral epiphysis – also known as epiphysiolysis – is uncommon and virtually confined to children going through the pubertal growth spurt. Boys (usually between 14 and 16 years old) are affected more often than girls (who are, on average, 2–3 years younger). The left hip is affected more commonly than the right and if one side slips there is a considerable risk of the other side also slipping.

Aetiology

The slip occurs through the hypertrophic zone of the cartilaginous growth plate. Why should the physis give way during a period of accelerated growth? Many of the patients are either fat and sexually immature or excessively tall and thin. It is tempting to formulate a theory of *hormonal imbalance* as the underlying cause of physeal disruption. Normally, pituitary hormone activity, which stimulates rapid growth and increased physeal hypertrophy during puberty, is balanced by increasing gonadal hormone activity, which promotes physeal maturation and epiphyseal fusion. A disparity between these two processes may result in the physis being unable to resist the shearing stresses imposed by the increase in body weight. This occurs most obviously in the hypogonadal 'Fröhlich type' of child, and it may be a factor in cases associated with juvenile hypothyroidism. There are also instances of epiphysiolysis occurring in children with craniopharyngioma after successful treatment and sudden reactivation of pituitary activity.

Trauma plays a part, especially in the 30% of cases with an 'acute' slip. In the other 70% there is a slow, progressive displacement – or a series of slight displacements – sometimes culminating in a major slip after relatively mild mechanical stress (the 'acute-on-chronic' slip).

Pathology

In slipped epiphysis the femoral shaft rolls into external rotation and the femoral neck is displaced forwards while the epiphysis remains seated in the acetabulum. Disruption occurs through the hypertrophic zone of the physis and, relatively speaking, the epiphysis slips posteriorly on the femoral neck. If the slip is severe, the anterior retinacular vessels are torn. At the back of the femoral neck the periosteum is lifted from the bone with the vessels intact; this may be the main – or the only – source of blood supply to the femoral head, and damage to these vessels by manipulation or operation may result in avascular necrosis.

Physeal disruption leads to premature fusion of the epiphysis – usually within 2 years of the onset of symptoms. This is accompanied by considerable bone modelling and, although there may be a permanent external rotation deformity and apparent coxa vara, adaptive changes often ensure good joint function even without treatment.

Clinical features

Slipping usually occurs as a series of minor episodes rather than a sudden, acute event; or there may be a protracted history leading to a severe climax – the 'acute-on-chronic' slip. In over 50% of cases there is a history of injury.

The patient is usually a child around puberty, typically overweight or very tall and thin. Pain, sometimes in the groin, but often only in the thigh or knee, is the presenting symptom. It may be called a 'sprain'; often, and unfortunately, it is disregarded. It soon disappears only to recur with further exercise. Limp also occurs early and is more constant. Sometimes the child becomes aware that the leg is 'turning out'.

On examination the leg is externally rotated and is 1–2 cm short. Characteristically there is

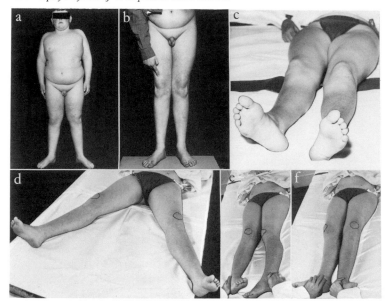

19.31 Slipped epiphysis – clinical features (a) The build is unmistakable; (b) this boy complained of pain only in the knee; (c) the leg lies in external rotation.

Another patient, showing (d) diminished abduction of the right hip; (e) diminished internal rotation; and (f) increased external rotation.

limitation of flexion. abduction and medial rotation. A classic sign is the tendency to increasing external rotation as the hip is flexed.

Following an acute slip, the hip is irritable and all movements are accompanied by pain.

X-ray

Even when slipping is trivial, changes can be seen. In the anteroposterior view the epiphyseal plate seems to be too wide and too 'woolly'. A line drawn along the superior surface of the neck remains superior to the head instead of

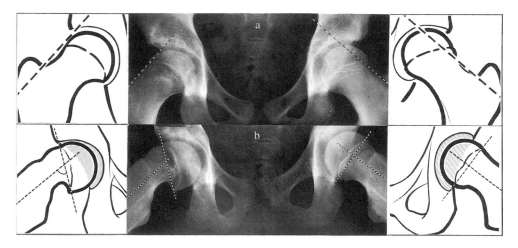

19.32 Slipped epiphysis – x-rays (a) Anteroposterior and (b) lateral views of early slipped epiphysis of the right hip. The upper diagrams show Trethowan's line passing just above the head on the affected side, but cutting through it on the normal side. The lateral view is diagnostically more reliable; even minor degrees of slip can be shown by drawing lines through the base of the epiphysis and up the middle of the femoral neck – if the angle indicated is less than 90 degreees, the epiphysis has slipped posteriorly.

passing through it (Trethowan's sign). In the lateral view the femoral epiphysis is tilted backwards; this is the most reliable x-ray sign and minor abnormalities can be detected by measuring the angle of the epiphyseal base to the femoral neck; this is normally a right angle and anything less than 87 degrees means that the epiphysis is tilted posteriorly (Billing and Severin, 1959).

Complications

SLIPPING AT THE OPPOSITE HIP   In at least 20% of cases slipping occurs at the other hip – sometimes while the patient is still in bed. Forewarned is forearmed: the asymptomatic hip should be checked by x-ray and at the least sign of abnormality the epiphysis should be pinned.

AVASCULAR NECROSIS   Death of the epiphysis used to be common. It is now recognized that it hardly ever occurs in the absence of treatment. This iatrogenic complication is minimized by avoiding forceful manipulation and operations which might damage the posterior retinacular vessels.

ARTICULAR CHONDROLYSIS   Cartilage necrosis probably results from vascular damage (often iatrogenic), but in these cases bone changes are minimal. There is progressive narrowing of the joint space and the hip becomes stiff.

COXA VARA   A slipped epiphysis that goes unnoticed – or is inadequately treated – may result in coxa vara. Except in the most severe cases, this is more apparent than real; the head slips backwards rather than downwards and the deformity is essentially one of *femoral neck retroversion*. Secondary effects are *external rotation deformity* of the hip, possibly *shortening* of

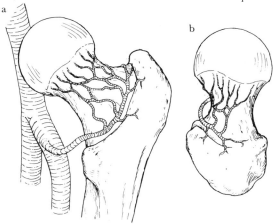

19.34   The femoral neck seen (a) from behind and (b) from above, showing the position of the vessels posterosuperiorly.

the femur and (still a point of contention) *secondary osteoarthritis*.

Treatment

The aims of treatment are (1) to preserve the epiphyseal blood supply, (2) to stabilize the physis and (3) to correct any residual deformity. Manipulative reduction of the slip carries a high risk of avascular necrosis and should be avoided. The choice of treatment depends on the degree of slip.

MINOR SLIPS (less than one-third the width of the epiphysis on the anteroposterior x-ray and less than 20 degrees tilt in the lateral view)   Deformity is minimal and needs no correction. The position is accepted and the physis is stabilized by inserting two or three threaded pins, or a hook-pin (Hansson, 1982), along the femoral neck and into the epiphysis. An alternative is to place a bone graft across the physis, through a window in the anterior femoral neck (Heyman and Herndon, 1954; Weiner, 1989).

MODERATE SLIPS (between one-third and two-thirds of the width of the epiphysis on the anteroposterior x-ray and 20–40 degrees of tilt in the lateral view)   Deformity resulting from this degree of slip, though noticeable, is often tempered by gradual bone modelling and may in the end cause little disability. One can therefore accept the position, fix the epiphysis *in situ* and then wait: if, after a year or two, there

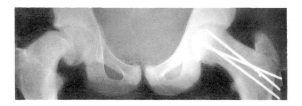

19.33 Slipped epiphysis – sequels   The left side has been pinned, now the right epiphysis has slipped – the patient should be warned of this possibility.

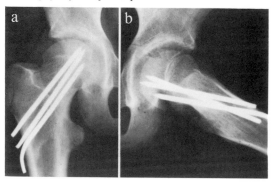

19.35 Slipped epiphysis – treatment Slipping was minimal so no reduction was attempted, but further slipping was prevented by pinning the epiphysis.

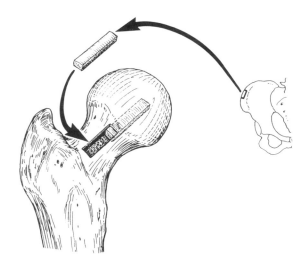

19.36 Slipped epiphysis – treatment The Heyman and Herndon epiphyseodesis.

is a noticeable deformity, a corrective osteotomy is performed below the femoral neck (see below). This approach is safe – but 'fixing' the epiphysis is easier said than done: because the head is tilted backwards, pins driven up the femoral neck will either enter the most anterior segment of the epiphysis (and be very insecure) or will penetrate the posterior cortex of the femoral neck and damage the retinacular vessels. Therefore, short threaded pins are inserted on the anterior femoral neck and directed posteromedially into the centre of the epiphysis. Alternatively – and probably with less risk of complications – fusion can be achieved by bone graft epiphyseodesis (Weiner, 1989). At the same time any protruding bump on the anterosuperior metaphysis can be trimmed to prevent impingement on the lip of the acetabulum.

SEVERE SLIPS (more than two-thirds the width of the epiphysis on the anteroposterior x-ray and 40 degrees of tilt in the lateral view) This, the 'unacceptable slip', causes marked deformity which, untreated, will predispose to secondary osteoarthritis (Boyer, Mickelson and Ponseti, 1981). Closed reduction by manipulation is dangerous. Open reduction by Dunn's method (Dunn and Angel, 1978) gives good results, but should be reserved for the specialist. The greater trochanter is elevated and the femoral neck exposed. By gentle subperiosteal dissection, the posterior retinacular vessels are preserved whilst mobilizing the epiphysis (which is usually stuck down by young callus). A small

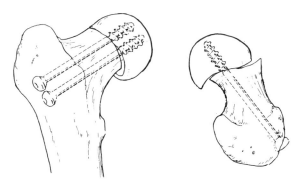

19.37 Slipped epiphysis – treatment A moderate slip can be accepted and fixed internally; it is essential that the threaded pins or screws enter the femur anteriorly so as not to risk damaging the retinacular vessels on the back of the femoral neck.

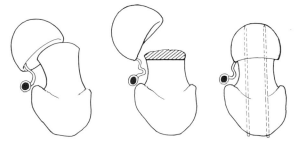

19.38 Slipped epiphysis – treatment Dunn's operation for a severe slip. A small segment of the femoral neck is removed so that the epiphysis can be reduced and pinned without placing tension on the posterior vessels.

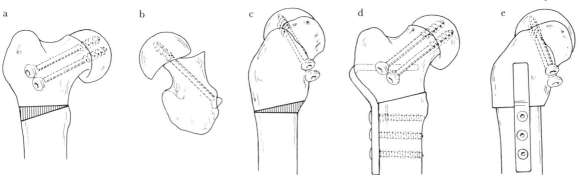

19.39 Slipped epiphysis – treatment (a, b, c) A severe slip can be treated by fixing it and then performing a compensatory osteotomy. Wedges are cut based laterally and anteriorly so as to permit valgus, flexion and rotation at the osteotomy. (d, e) The position after osteotomy and internal fixation.

segment of the femoral neck is then removed, so that the epiphysis can be repositioned without tension on the posterior structures; once reduced, it is held by two or three pins. In all but the most experienced hands, this still carries a 5–10% risk of avascular necrosis or chondrolysis. The alternative – and the method recommended for the less experienced surgeon – is to fix the epiphysis as for a 'moderate slip' and then, as soon as fusion is complete, to perform a compensatory intertrochanteric osteotomy: the easiest is a triplane osteotomy with simultaneous repositioning of the proximal femur in valgus, flexion and medial rotation (Ireland and Newman, 1978); more anatomical is the geometric flexion osteotomy described by Griffith (1976). However, the patient should be told that this may result in 2–3 cm of shortening.

GENERAL NOTE Most of the complications of slipped epiphysis are related to treatment – injudicious attempts at manipulative reduction of the slip, or failure to recognize the hazards of internal fixation (Riley, Weiner and Akron, 1990). The first rule of surgical treatment is 'thou shalt do no harm'.

Pyogenic arthritis (see also Chapter 2)

Pyogenic arthritis of the hip is usually seen in children under 2 years of age. The organism (usually a staphylococcus) reaches the joint either directly from a distant focus or by local spread from osteomyelitis of the femur. Unless the infection is rapidly aborted, the femoral head, which is largely cartilaginous at this age, is liable to be destroyed by the proteolytic enzymes of bacteria and pus.

Clinical features

The child is ill and in pain, but it is often difficult to tell exactly where the pain is! The affected limb may be held absolutely still and all attempts at moving the hip are resisted. With care and patience it may be possible to localize a point of maximum tenderness over the hip; the diagnosis is confirmed by aspirating pus from the joint.

In the acute stage x-rays are of little value but sometimes they show soft-tissue swelling, displacement of the femoral head and a vacuum sign in the joint. Ultrasonography will reveal the joint effusion.

Treatment

Antibiotics should be given as soon as the diagnosis is reasonably certain. The joint is aspirated under general anaesthesia and, if pus is withdrawn, arthrotomy is advisable; antibiotics are instilled locally and the wound is closed without drainage. In the older child with a short history (less than 4 days) aspiration may be sufficient (Wilson and Di Paola, 1986). But

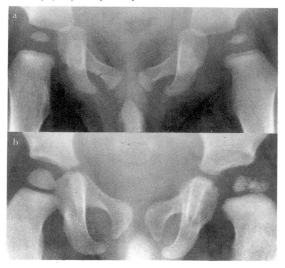

19.40 Pyogenic arthritis in children (a) In this infant, with early pyogenic arthritis, the joint is distended and the head displaced laterally. (b) A later x-ray shows that the epiphysis has been partly destroyed and part of it is avascular. Treatment was delayed too long.

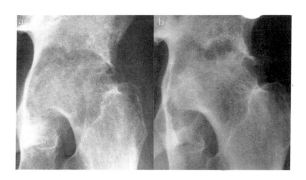

19.41 Pyogenic arthritis in adults Untreated, staphylococcal arthritis may cause rapid bone destruction: (a) 1 month after onset of symptoms; (b) 3 weeks later.

after either arthrotomy or aspiration, systemic antibiotics are essential, and the hip is kept on traction or splinted in abduction until all evidence of disease activity has disappeared.

Complications

If the infection is unchecked the head and neck of the femur may be destroyed and a pathological dislocation result. The pus may escape and, when the child recovers, the sinus heals. The hip signs then resemble those of a congenital dislocation, but the telltale scar remains and on x-ray the femoral head is completely absent.

Tuberculosis (see also Chapter 2)

The disease may start as a synovitis, or as an osteomyelitis in one of the adjacent bones. Once arthritis develops, destruction is rapid and may result in pathological dislocation. Healing usually leaves a fibrous ankylosis with considerable limb shortening and deformity.

Clinical features

The condition starts insidiously with aching in the groin and thigh, and a slight limp; later, pain is more severe and may wake the patient from sleep.

With early disease (synovitis or osteomyelitis) the joint is held slightly flexed and abducted, and extremes of movement are restricted and painful; but until x-ray changes appear the hip is merely 'irritable' and diagnosis is difficult. If arthritis supervenes the hip becomes flexed, adducted and medially rotated, muscle wasting becomes obvious, and all movements are grossly limited by pain and spasm.

X-RAY The earliest change is general rarefaction but with a normal joint space and line; the femoral epiphysis may be enlarged or a bone abscess visible; with arthritis, in addition to the general rarefaction, there is destruction of the acetabular roof (wandering acetabulum) or the femoral head, usually both; the joint may be subluxed or even dislocated. With healing the bones recalcify.

Early disease may heal leaving a normal or almost normal hip; but if there has been arthritis the usual result is an unsound fibrous joint. The leg is scarred and thin; shortening is often severe because many factors contribute – adduction deformity, bone destruction, damage to the upper femoral epiphysis and occasionally premature fusion of the lower femoral epiphysis.

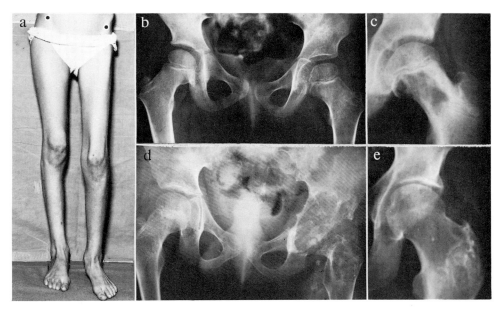

19.42 Hip tuberculosis – active   (a) Apparent lengthening in early disease of the left hip. (b) Synovitis of left hip. (c) Osteomyelitis of the femoral neck. (d) Florid arthritis. (e) Trochanteric infection – this rarely extends to the joint. Note the osteoporosis of the left hip in (b) and (d).

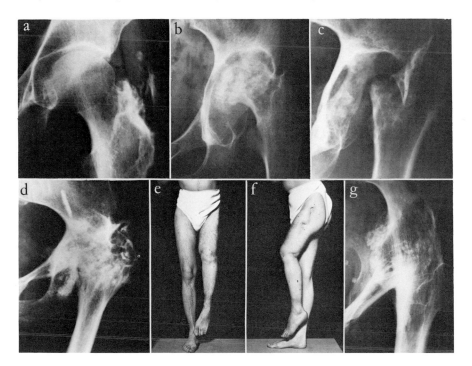

19.43 Hip tuberculosis – healing and aftermath   (a) Healed trochanteric disease with the hip joint still normal. (b) Healing arthritis with gross enlargement of the acetabulum. (c) Healing arthritis with large acetabulum and destruction of the head. (d) Joint destruction with considerable calcification in the aftermath stage; and (e, f) appearance of the hip in this patient – note the gross shortening. (g) A patient in whom secondary infection was followed by bony ankylosis.

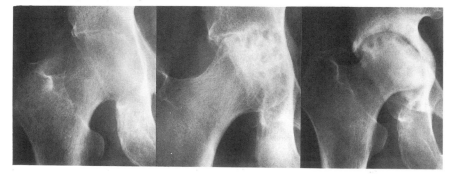

19.44 Hip tuberculosis – drug treatment   In this patient antituberculous drugs alone resulted in healing – though of course hip movements were still limited.

Treatment

Antituberculous drugs are essential, and these alone may result in healing. Skin traction is applied and, for a child, an abduction frame may be used. An abscess in the femoral neck is best evacuated; if the arthritis does not settle, joint 'debridement' is performed. As the disease subsides, traction is discontinued and the patient is got up.

If the joint has been destroyed, arthrodesis may be necessary once all signs of activity have disappeared, but usually not before the age of 14.

In older patients with residual pain and deformity, if the disease has clearly been in-active for a considerable time, total joint replacement is feasible and often successful (Young-Hoo Kim, Dae-Young Han and Byeong-Mun Park, 1989); with antituberculous drugs, which are essential, the chances of recurrence are not great.

Rheumatoid arthritis

(see also Chapter 3)

The hip joint is frequently affected in rheumatoid arthritis; occasionally the disease remains

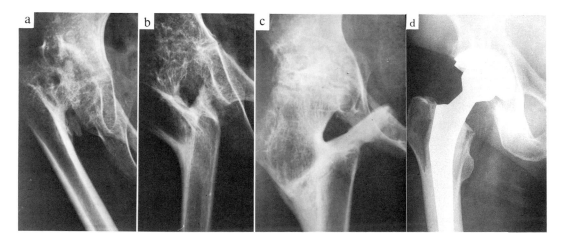

19.45 Hip tuberculosis – operative treatment   (a, b) Before and after osteotomy in the late healing stage. (c) Combined osteotomy and arthrodesis. (d) This patient's disease had been quiescent for 2 years; hip replacement under cover of antituberculous drugs was successful.

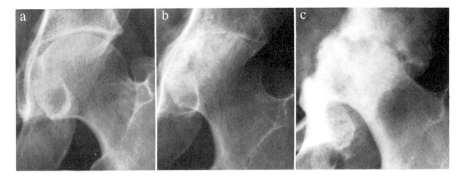

19.46 Rheumatoid arthritis   Three stages in the development of rheumatoid arthritis: (a) loss of joint space; (b) erosion of bone after cartilage has disappeared; (c) perforation of the acetabular floor – such marked destruction is more likely to occur if the patient is having corticosteroids.

monarticular for several years, but eventually other sites are affected. Persistent synovitis in a weightbearing joint soon leads to the destruction of cartilage and bone; the acetabulum is eroded and eventually the femoral head may perforate its floor. The hallmark of the disease is progressive bone destruction on both sides of the joint without any reactive osteophyte formation.

Clinical features

Usually the patient already has rheumatoid disease affecting many joints. Pain in the groin comes on insidiously; limp, though common, may be ascribed to pre-existing arthritis of the foot or knee. With advancing disease the patient has difficulty getting into or out of a chair, and even movements in bed may be painful. Occasionally the slow symptomatic progression is punctuated by acute flares with intense pain in the hip.

Wasting of the buttock and thigh is often marked, and the limb is usually held in external rotation and fixed flexion. All movements are restricted and painful.

X-RAYS   During the early stages there is osteoporosis and diminution of the joint space; later, the acetabulum and femoral head are eroded. Protrusio acetabuli is common. In the worst cases (and especially in patients on corticosteroids) there is gross bone destruction and the floor of the acetabulum may be perforated.

Treatment

If the disease can be arrested by general treatment, hip deterioration may be slowed down. But once cartilage and bone are eroded, no treatment will influence the progression to joint destruction. Total joint replacement is then the best answer. It relieves pain and restores a useful range of movement. It is advocated even in younger patients, because the polyarthritis so limits activity that the implants are not unduly stressed.

Care should be taken during operation to prevent fracture or perforation of the osteoporotic bone.

Children with juvenile chronic arthritis may need custom-made prostheses for their small and often delicate bones.

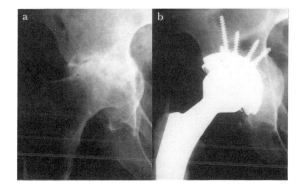

19.47 Rheumatoid arthritis – treatment   Severe erosive arthritis treated by hip replacement with an uncemented socket and bone grafting of the acetabulum.

Postoperative infection poses a greater risk in rheumatoid patients than in others – more particularly if the patient is on corticosteroid therapy. Prophylaxis is even more important than usual.

Osteoarthritis (see also Chapter 5)

The hip joint is one of the commonest sites of osteoarthritis, though in some populations (e.g. African Negroes and southern Chinese) this joint seems peculiarly immune to the disease. This may simply be because certain predisposing conditions (acetabular dysplasia, Perthes' disease, slipped epiphysis) show a similar differential incidence in these populations.

Where there is an obvious underlying cause the term 'secondary osteoarthritis' is applied (Table 19.2); these patients are often in their third or fourth decade and the appearance of the joint reflects the preceding abnormality. Thus in regions where congenital dislocation and acetabular dysplasia are common (e.g. northern Italy), women are more often affected than men, the hips may be the only joints affected and lateral subluxation is common.

When no underlying cause is apparent, the term 'primary osteoarthritis' is used. Patients are somewhat older – usually in their sixth or seventh decade – with a predominance of women, and often other areas (knees or spine) also are affected. There may be evidence of chondrocalcinosis.

Table 19.2 Causes of osteoarthritis of the hip

Abnormal stress	Defective cartilage	Abnormal bone
Subluxation	Infection	Fracture
Coxa magna	Rheumatoid	Necrosis
Coxa vara	Calcinosis	Paget's
Minor deformities	Chondrolysis	Other causes
Protrusio		of sclerosis

Pathology

The articular cartilage becomes soft and fibrillated whilst the underlying bone shows cyst formation and sclerosis. These changes are most marked in the area of maximal loading (chiefly the top of the joint); at the margins of the joint there are the characteristic osteophytes. Synovial hypertrophy is common and capsular fibrosis may account for joint stiffness.

Sometimes – and for no obvious reason – articular destruction progresses very rapidly, with erosion of the femoral head or acetabulum (or both), occasionally going on to perforation of the pelvis.

Clinical features

Pain is felt in the groin but may radiate to the knee. Typically it occurs after periods of activity but later it is more constant and sometimes disturbs sleep. Stiffness at first is noticed chiefly after rest; later it increases progressively until putting on socks and shoes becomes difficult. Limp is often noticed early and the patient may think the leg is getting shorter.

The patient is usually fit and over 50, but secondary osteoarthritis can occur at 30 or even 20 years of age. There may be an obvious limp and, except in early cases, a positive Trendelenburg sign. The affected leg usually lies in external rotation and adduction, so it appears short; there is nearly always some fixed flexion, although this may only be revealed by Thomas' test. Muscle wasting is detectable but rarely severe. Deep pressure may elicit tenderness, and the greater trochanter is somewhat high and posterior. Movements, though often painless within a limited range, are restricted; internal rotation, abduction and extension are usually affected first and most severely.

X-RAY The earliest sign is a decreased joint space, usually maximal in the superior weight-bearing region but sometimes affecting the entire joint. Later signs are subarticular sclerosis, cyst formation and osteophytes. The shape of the femoral head or acetabulum may give a clue to an underlying condition (e.g. old Perthes' disease). Bilateral cases occasionally show features of a generalized dysplasia.

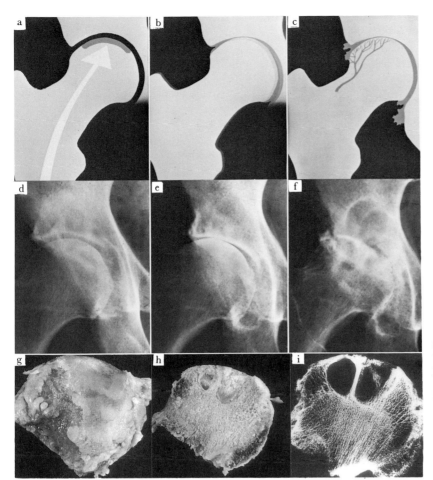

19.48 Osteoarthritis – pathology (a, b, c) Cartilage softening and thinning are greatest in the zone of maximal stress. There is a vascular reaction and new-bone formation in the subchondral bone as well as osteophytic growth at the margins of the joint. These changes, as well as subchondral cyst formation, are reflected in the sequential x-ray appearances (d, e, f) and in the morphology of the excised femoral head (g, h, i).

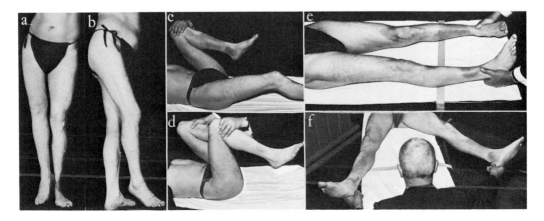

19.49 Osteoarthritis – signs The right hip is osteoarthritic and shows: (a, b) apparent shortening, with adduction and flexion deformity; (c) demonstrating fixed flexion; (d, e, f) limitation of flexion, internal rotation and abduction.

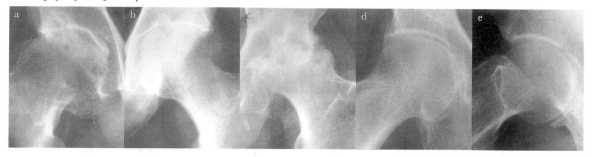

19.50 Osteoarthritis – x-rays   X-ray features of (a) hypertrophic OA, (b) atrophic OA, (c) rapidly destructive OA and (d, e) posterior marginal OA.

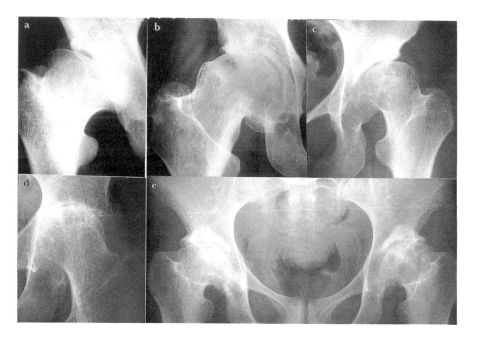

19.51 Secondary osteoarthritis   (a) After Perthes's disease. (b) After slipped upper femoral epiphysis. (c) After congenital subluxation. (d) After rheumatoid disease. (e) Bilateral in a patient with multiple epiphyseal dysplasia.

Treatment

Analgesics and anti-inflammatory drugs may be helpful, and warmth is soothing. The patient is encouraged to use a walking-stick and to try to preserve movement and stability by non-weight-bearing exercises. In early cases physiotherapy (including manipulation) may relieve pain for long periods. Activities are adjusted so as to reduce stress on the hip.

OPERATIVE TREATMENT   The indications for operation are (1) progressive increase in pain, (2) severe restriction of activities, (3) marked deformity and (4) progressive loss of movement (especially abduction), together with (5) x-ray signs of joint destruction.

In the usual case – a patient aged over 60 years with a long history of pain and increasing disability – the preferred operation is *total joint replacement* (see below). In those between 40

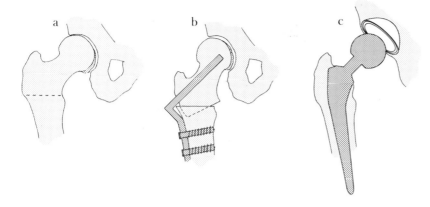

19.52 Osteoarthritis – treatment   (a) When only part of the joint is damaged, a realignment osteotomy may allow redistribution of stress to a less damaged part of the articular surface (b). In older patients, and when articular destruction is marked, joint replacement (c) is indicated.

and 60 years this may still be the best operation if joint destruction is severe.

In younger patients, particularly those with some preservation of articular cartilage, an *intertrochanteric realignment osteotomy* may be considered. If performed early, it can arrest or delay further cartilage destruction, and if the operation is well planned it does not preclude later replacement arthroplasty (Maistelli et al., 1990; Werners, Vincent and Bulstrode, 1990).

Adolescents and young adults with acetabular dysplasia may benefit from a *medial displacement pelvic osteotomy*. A recent 9-year follow-up of Chiari's operation found a good result and arrest of osteoarthritic changes in over 70% of patients, despite the fact that many of them continued to show a positive Trendelenburg sign (Zlatic et al., 1988). An alternative is the 'dial' osteotomy, in which the entire acetabulum is rotated.

Arthrodesis of the hip is a practical solution for young adults with marked destruction of a single joint, and particularly when the conditions for advanced reconstructive surgery are less than ideal. If well executed, the operation guarantees freedom from pain and permanent stability, though it has the disadvantages of restricted mobility and a significant incidence of later deformity and discomfort in other nearby joints (Greiss, Thomas and Freeman, 1980; Roberts and Fetto, 1990).

Osteonecrosis (see also Chapter 6)

The femoral head is the commonest site of symptomatic osteonecrosis – mainly because of its peculiar blood supply which renders it vulnerable to ischaemia from *arterial cut-off* (e.g. following trauma) or *venous stasis* (e.g. from a raised intra-articular or intraosseous pressure in such conditions as septic arthritis, Perthes' disease and Gaucher's disease).

Idiopathic (aseptic) necrosis is usually associated with high dosage corticosteroid therapy, alcohol abuse or a combination of both; the pathogenetic mechanism is disputed.

Pathology

The pathological features, and the stages in the progress of osteonecrosis, are described in Chapter 6.

Clinical features

Post-traumatic necrosis develops soon after a definite and usually severe injury to the hip, but symptoms and signs of the necrosis may take months to appear.

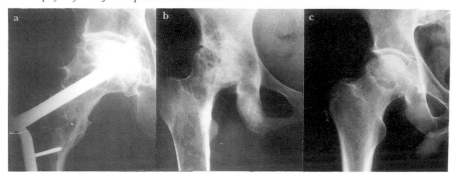

19.53 Osteonecrosis Femoral head necrosis due to (a) femoral neck fracture, (b) Gaucher's disease and (c) chronic alcohol abuse.

Idiopathic necrosis is more insidious. The patient usually a man of 20–50 years who complains of pain in the hip (or, in over 50% of cases, in both hips), which progresses over a period of 2–3 years to become quite severe.

On examination, the patient walks with a limp and may have a positive Trendelenburg sign. The thigh is wasted and the limb may be 1–2 cm short. Movements are restricted, particularly abduction and internal rotation. A characteristic sign is a tendency for the hip to twist into fixed external rotation during passive flexion; this corresponds to the 'sectoral sign' in which, with the hip extended, internal rotation is almost full, but with the hip flexed it is grossly restricted.

X-rays show the classic features of segmental sclerosis, a subchondral fracture line and, eventually, collapse of the femoral head. These are, of course, the late features produced by the competing processes of trabecular collapse and repair. The very earliest stages of ischaemia cause no abnormality on the plain x-ray, but MRI may reveal marked changes even while the patient is asymptomatic (see p. 96).

Diagnosis

There may be a history of trauma, a familial disorder such as sickle-cell disease or Gaucher's disease, an occupational background suggesting dysbaric ischaemia, an underlying disease such as systemic lupus erythematosus, or a known background of corticosteroid administration or alcohol abuse. It is important to recognize that pathogenic factors are cumulative, so a patient with systemic lupus or a moderately severe alcohol habit may develop osteonecrosis following comparatively low doses of cortisone.

Staging (see Chapter 6)

In stage 1 the patient has little or no pain and the plain x-ray shows no abnormality. In stage 2 there are early x-ray signs but the femoral head is structurally intact. Stage 3 is more advanced, with increasing signs of femoral head distortion or fragmentation. Stage 4 is characterized by collapse of the articular surface and secondary osteoarthritis.

Treatment

The treatment of osteonecrosis is discussed on p. 98. A simple protocol for the hip is shown in Table 19.3. However, each case should be

Table 19.3 A suggested guide to management

Stage of osteonecrosis	Traumatic osteonecrosis	Non-traumatic osteonecrosis
I	Reduction and fixation	Decompression
II	Bone grafting	Decompression
III: young	Osteotomy and grafting	Osteotomy and grafting
old	Joint replacement	Joint replacement
IV	Joint replacement	Joint replacement

Reproduced, with permission, from Solomon (1987)

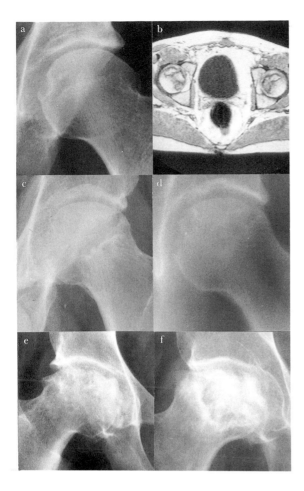

decided on its merits: a young person who is severely disabled, or anyone in severe pain, needs early operative treatment; others – despite advanced x-ray signs – may be uncomplaining and can be treated conservatively (as for osteoarthritis).

OPERATIVE TREATMENT If the femoral head has collapsed completely there are only two options: *arthrodesis* or *total hip replacement* – and few patients will accept arthrodesis. It is the management of early osteonecrosis that is still highly controversial. *Osseous decompression* by drilling is aimed at relieving the venous stasis which is part of the intraosseous compartment syndrome. Clearly it has no place in traumatic necrosis, which is due to arterial interruption. And even in idiopathic necrosis, where high intraosseous pressures can be demonstrated, it can succeed only in the very early stage before bone collapse has occurred. Therefore, patients with stage 1 or 2 idiopathic necrosis, especially if they are beginning to experience pain, may be offered this operation in the hope that it will prevent further bone destruction; that is, provided the underlying cause is also dealt with. Since 50% of cases are bilateral, if the apparently unaffected side has raised intraosseous pressure, it is worth drilling that side also.

Osteotomy is considered in young patients (those under 40) with stage 2 or 3 osteonecrosis limited to a small segment of the femoral head. By suitable realignment (usually a flexion osteotomy) the necrotic zone can be displaced away from the line of maximum stress, thus preserving hip function. Ultimately, if further collapse does occur, they may still qualify for replacement arthroplasty.

19.54 Osteonecrosis (a) This patient in stage 1 had few symptoms and virtually normal x-rays, but (b) the MRI shows osteonecrosis of both femoral heads. (c, d) X-ray and tomogram of stage 2, with increased density but preservation of the spherical shape of the head. (e, f) Stages 3 and 4 – increasing distortion of the femoral head and secondary osteoarthritis.

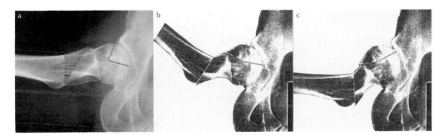

19.55 Osteonecrosis – treatment (a) Flexion osteotomy is planned by marking out the necrotic segment and the proposed anterior wedge excision. (b) After closure of the wedge. (c) When the femur is brought down to the neutral position the necrotic segment rotates out of the line of maximal stress.

Bursitis and tendinitis around the hip

Trochanteric bursitis

Pain over the lateral aspect of the hip and thigh may be due to irritation and inflammation of the trochanteric bursa which lies deep to the tensor fascia lata. There is local tenderness and sometimes crepitus on flexing and extending the hip. X-rays may show evidence of a previous fracture, or a protruding metal implant or trochanteric wires dating from some former operation. There may also be calcification or shadows suggesting swelling of the soft tissues. It is important to exclude underlying disorders such as gout, rheumatoid disease and infection (including tuberculosis).

Other causes of pain and tenderness over the greater trochanter are stress fractures (in athletes and elderly patients), slipped epiphysis (in adolescents) and bone infection (in children). The commonest cause of misdiagnosis is referred pain from the lumbar spine.

The treatment of trochanteric bursitis is rest, administration of non-steroidal anti-inflammatory drugs and (provided infection is excluded) injection of local anaesthetic and corticosteroid.

Gluteus medius tendinitis

Acute tendinitis may cause pain and localized tenderness just behind the greater trochanter. This is seen particularly in dancers and athletes. The clinical and x-ray features are similar to those of trochanteric bursitis, and the differential diagnosis is the same.

Treatment is by rest and injection of corticosteroid and local anaesthetic.

Iliopsoas bursitis

Pain in the groin and anterior thigh may be due to an iliopsoas bursitis. The site of tenderness is difficult to define and there may be guarding of the muscles overlying the lesser trochanter. Hip movements are sometimes restricted; indeed, the condition may arise from synovitis of the hip since there is often a potential communication between the bursa and the joint. The most typical feature is a sharp increase in pain on adduction and internal rotation of the hip.

The differential diagnosis of anterior hip pain includes inguinal lymphadenopathy, hernia, a psoas abscess, fracture of the lesser trochanter, slipped epiphysis, local infection and arthritis.

Treatment is by non-steroidal anti-inflammatory drugs and injection of local anaesthetic and steroid; the injection is best performed under fluoroscopic control.

Snapping hip

'Snapping hip' is a disorder in which the patient – usually a young woman – complains of the hip 'jumping out of place', or 'catching', during walking. The snapping is caused by a thickened band in the gluteus maximus aponeurosis flipping over the greater trochanter. In the swing phase of walking the band moves anteriorly; then, in the stance phase, as the gluteus maximus contracts and pulls the hip into extension, the band flips back across the trochanter, causing an audible 'snap'. This is usually painless but it can be quite distressing, especially if the hip gives way. Sometimes there is tenderness around the hip, and it may be possible to reproduce the peculiar sensation by flexing and extending the hip while abducted.

The condition must be distinguished from other causes of painful clicking, particularly a *tear of the acetabular labrum* or an *osteocartilaginous flap* on the femoral head (similar to osteochondritis dissecans). An arthrogram will exclude these entities.

Treatment of the snapping tendon is usually unnecessary; the patient merely needs an explanation and reassurance. Occasionally, though, if discomfort is marked the band can be either divided or lengthened by a Z-plasty (Brignall and Stainsby, 1991).

Principles of hip operations

Exposure of the hip

Operative approaches to the hip can be broadly divided into anterior, anterolateral, lateral and posterior.

The anterior (Smith-Petersen) approach starts in the plane between sartorius and rectus femoris medially and tensor fascia femoris laterally and remains anterior to the gluteus medius. The hip capsule is exposed by detaching the origins of rectus femoris. This provides adequate exposure for many operations, including open reduction of the dislocated hip in infants and the various types of pelvic osteotomy. However, it is not ideal for major reconstructive surgery in adults.

The anterolateral (Watson-Jones) approach is also anterior to the gluteus medius, but behind the tensor fascia femoris. It provides reasonable exposure of the hip joint, with minimal detachment of muscles, but the gluteus medius is in the way and this makes hip replacement difficult.

Lateral approaches suffer from the fact that the gluteus medius and minimus obstruct the view of the acetabulum. The abductors are dealt with by (1) retracting them posterosuperiorly (a limited solution), or (2) splitting them and raising the anterior portion intact from the greater trochanter (Hardinge's direct lateral approach), or (3) osteotomizing the greater trochanter and retracting it upwards with the attached abductors (as in the Charnley approach for total joint replacement). This provides excellent exposure; however, there may be problems with reattachment of the trochanteric fragment.

The posterior approach is the most direct. By splitting the anterior part of gluteus maximus, the rotators at the back of the hip are exposed and the sciatic nerve is retracted safely beneath the bulk of the posterior portion of gluteus maximus. Once the short rotators are detached, the hip is entered directly. Many surgeons prefer this approach for joint replacement. It has two minor disadvantages: orientation is more difficult, especially for placing the acetabular cup; and it is associated with an increased incidence of postoperative dislocation.

Planning

Reconstructive surgery of the hip needs careful preoperative planning. Ideally this should be based on three-dimensional imaging studies (Murphy et al., 1990). Tracings of plain x-rays are useful for taking measurements and working out repositioning angles in advance.

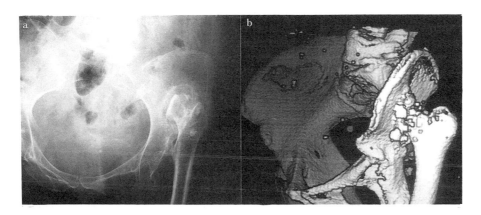

19.56 Planning (a) Plain x-rays showing an old unreduced congenital dislocation. (b) The three-dimensional MRI reveals more clearly the problems of reconstructive surgery.

Intertrochanteric osteotomy

RATIONALE Intertrochanteric osteotomy has three objectives: (1) to change the orientation of the femoral head in the socket so as to reduce mechanical stress in a damaged segment; (2) by realigning the proximal femur, to improve joint congruity; and (3) by transecting the bone, to reduce intraosseous hypertension and relieve pain. An unintentional, and poorly understood, consequence is (4) fibrocartilaginous repair of the articular surface.

INDICATIONS In children osteotomy is used to correct angular or rotational deformities of the proximal femur (e.g. in congenital dislocation, coxa vara or severe slips of the capital epiphysis), or to produce 'containment' of the femoral head in Perthes' disease.

In adults, the main indication is osteoarthritis associated with joint dysplasia, particularly in patients who are younger than 50 years. Pain is often relieved immediately (probably due to reduced vascular congestion) and sometimes the articular space is gradually restored. The other prime indication is in localized avascular necrosis of the femoral head; if only a small segment is involved, realignment can rotate this segment out of the path of maximum stress.

CONTRAINDICATIONS Osteotomy is unsuitable in elderly patients and in those with severe stiffness; movement may be even further decreased afterwards. It is also contraindicated in rheumatoid arthritis, and even in osteoarthritis if there is widespread loss of articular substance; reposi-

tion is useless if other parts of the femoral head are equally damaged.

TECHNICAL CONSIDERATIONS The osteotomy allows repositioning of the femoral head in valgus, varus or different degrees of rotation. Exact placement and angulation can be ensured only by meticulous preoperative planning and painstaking execution of the bone cuts (Müller, 1975). The fragments are fixed with suitably angled plates and screws. Postoperatively the patient is permitted only partial weightbearing for 3–6 months. Müller emphasized that 10–15% of patients require some assistance (a walking stick) for the rest of their lives.

Sugioko (1978) devised a transtrochanteric rotational osteotomy which allows the femoral neck to be rotated on its long axis, thus turning the femoral head through an arc of 90 degrees or more. The operation is used mainly for segmental necrosis of the femoral head.

COMPLICATIONS The main complication is malposition of the bone. Only careful planning can prevent this. Non-union of the osteotomy is rare.

RESULTS Provided the indications are strictly observed, the results are moderately good. In a recent series of 368 osteotomies, survivorship analysis showed that 10 years after osteotomy 47% of patients had required no further surgery (Werners, Vincent and Bulstrode, 1990).

Sugioko's transtrochanteric rotational osteotomy, though evidently successful in the originator's hands, has proved unpredictable in others' (Tooke, Amstutz and Hedley, 1987).

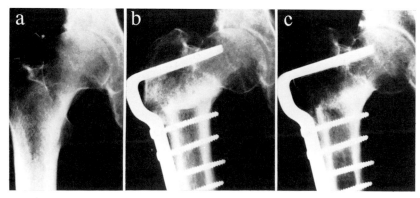

19.57 Osteoarthritis – treatment by osteotomy Following a varus type of osteotomy this patient lost most of her pain, and the x-rays suggest articular cartilage regeneration (would 'rejuvenation' be too strong a word?).

Arthrodesis

RATIONALE Fusion of the hip is guaranteed to relieve pain and provide stability for a lifetime. But at what cost? Surprisingly, though the joint is fused the patient retains a great deal of 'mobility' because lumbosacral tilting and rotation are preserved and often increased. Nevertheless, there are restrictions: for sitting comfortably the hip needs 60 degrees of flexion; for climbing stairs, 45 degrees; and for walking, 20 degrees. In the stance phase of walking the normal hip is in slight abduction, but in the swing phase it is carried in slight adduction. No position of fusion can satisfy all these demands, so one aims at a compromise. And sometimes it is wrong, with the result that function is seriously impaired.

INDICATIONS Arthrodesis should be considered for any destructive condition of the hip when there are serious contraindications to osteotomy or arthroplasty: for example, a patient who is too young, a hip that is already stiff but painful, and previous infection. Young patients adapt well; those aged over 30–40 years respond unpredictably.

CONTRAINDICATIONS Elderly patients, and any patient with a good range of movement, will resent a 'stiff hip'. Other contraindications are lack of bone stock and abnormalities in the 'compensating joints' (lumbar spine, knees and opposite hip).

TECHNICAL CONSIDERATIONS The recommended position for arthrodesis is 20 degrees of flexion, 10 degrees of adduction (unless the leg is short) and neutral or slight external rotation. However, in young people there is a tendency for the 'joint' to drift into further flexion and by the age of 40 this may be as much as 40 degrees. Some form of internal fixation is used to secure the bones in the desired position. It is important to ensure that these implants do not destroy the abductors; though they are not needed while the hip is arthrodesed, they will be essential if ever the fusion is converted to an arthroplasty.

COMPLICATIONS The major complications are (1) failure to fuse and (2) malposition, which hampers function and puts unwanted strain on

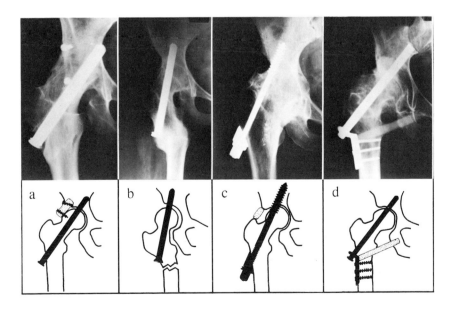

19.58 Arthrodesis (a) Watson-Jones' method. (b) Pyrford arthrodesis – the hip is pinned in its deformed position and the deformity corrected by an osteotomy; the patient is kept on traction for 6 weeks, then in a short hip spica for a further 6 weeks. (c) Compression arthrodesis. (d) Norwich V arthrodesis.

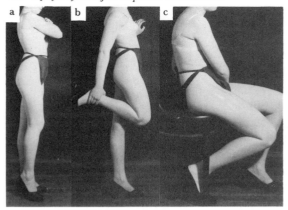

19.59 Arthrodesis Stiffness of the hip is largely disguised by mobility of the spine and knee.

other joints. Late complications are (3) compensatory deformities in other joints (knees and opposite hip) and (4) low backache, which occurs in over 60% of patients 20 years after fusion. Women may complain of (5) difficulty with sexual intercourse. And (6) squatting is, of course, impossible. However, it should be remembered that total replacement is still possible after a hip has been arthrodesed.

RESULTS Provided the 'compensating joints' (lumbar spine, knee and opposite hip) are completely normal, young patients in particular may derive great benefit from arthrodesis, with many years of comfort, a well-disguised limp and the ability to walk long distances and play games. Older patients fare less well: in a 10-year follow-up study. Greiss, Thomas and Freeman (1980) found that over 60% of patients with unilateral arthrodesis had degenerative changes in adjacent joints and all had some degree of backache.

Total hip replacement

RATIONALE Total replacement of the articular surfaces seems the ideal way of treating any disorder causing joint destruction (Charnley, 1979). However, there are several problems to be overcome: (1) the prosthetic implants must be durable; (2) they must permit slippery movement at the articulation; (3) they must be

firmly fixed to the skeleton; and (4) they must be inert and not provoke any unwanted reaction in the tissues. The usual combination is a metal femoral component (stainless steel, titanium or cobalt–chrome alloy) articulating with a polyethylene socket. Ceramic components have better frictional characteristics but are more easily broken. Fixation is either by embedding the implant in methylmethacrylate cement, which acts as a grouting material filling the interstices, or by fitting the implant closely to the bone bed without cement. The 'bond' between bone and the implant surface, or cement, is never perfect. The best that can be hoped for is ingrowth of trabecular bone on the implant or cement (osseointegration). There are various ways of enhancing this process: (1) if cement is used, it is applied under pressure and allowed to cure without movement or extrusion after the implant has been inserted; (2) Ling and his co-workers have shown that a smooth, tapered and collarless femoral prosthesis will continue settling within the cement mantle even after polymerization, thereby maintaining expansile pressure between cement and bone (Fowler et al., 1988); (3) uncemented implants may be covered with a mesh or porous coating

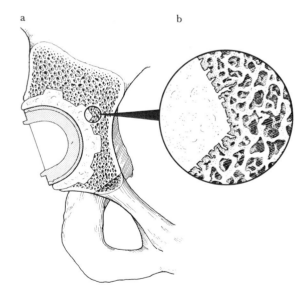

19.60 Prosthetic fixation Fixation between cement and bone is by (a) interlock (interdigitation of large irregularities in cement and bone) and, more completely, by (b) osseointegration (intimate penetration of cement between endosteal trabeculae.

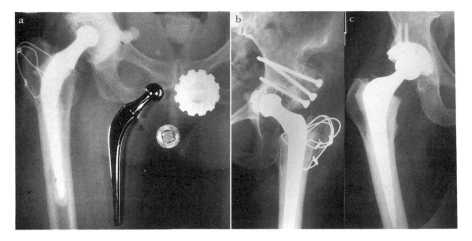

19.61 Total hip replacement (a) The Charnley hip replacement system, forerunner of all the modern methods of total arthroplasty. The small wire-mesh disc is used as a plug to prevent cement extrusion into the pelvis. (b) In this patient with untreated congenital dislocation a small off-set cup has been used, and the dysplastic acetabulum has been augmented with a bone graft. (c) 'Hybrid' arthroplasty, using an uncemented cup and a cemented collarless femoral prosthesis.

that encourages bone ingrowth (Engh, Bobyn and Glassman, 1987); (4) the implant may be coated with hydroxyapatite, an excellent substrate for osteoblastic new-bone formation and osseointegration (Geesink, de Groot and Klein, 1988; Geesink, 1990).

INDICATIONS Because of the tendency for implants to loosen with time, joint replacement is usually reserved for patients over 60 years. However, with improved cementing techniques and rapid advances in the design of uncemented prostheses, the operation is being offered to younger patients with destructive hip disorders, and occasionally even to children severely crippled with rheumatoid disease.

CONTRAINDICATIONS Overt or latent sepsis is the chief contraindication to joint replacement. An infected arthroplasty spells disaster. Patients under 60 years of age are considered only if other operations are unsuitable.

TECHNICAL CONSIDERATIONS The fear of infection dictates a host of prophylactic measures, including the use of special ultra-clean air operating theatres, occlusive theatre clothing and perioperative antibiotic cover (Lidwell et al., 1984; Marotte et al., 1987). In addition, some surgeons routinely use antibiotic-laden cement. A variety of joint exposures is recommended: none has any significant advantages over the others. The choice of implant should depend on sound biomechanical and biological testing, but seems to be determined as much by personal prejudice. The array of over 300 different mechanisms currently on the market represents the triumph of razzle over reason. The argument of 'cemented versus cementless' goes on (Engh, Bobyn and Glassman, 1990; Sarmiento et al., 1990). In the end, sound technique is probably more important than anything else.

Postoperatively the implant should be protected from full loading until osseointegration is advanced; 6–10 weeks on crutches is not unreasonable.

COMPLICATIONS Hip replacements are often performed on patients who are somewhat elderly; some are rheumatoid and may be having steroid therapy. Consequently the general complication rate is by no means trivial; deep vein thrombosis in particular is common.

The remaining complications are more likely to occur with this particular operation, or are peculiar to it. Factors that may contribute to their development include previous hip operations, severe deformity, inadequate 'bone stock', an insufficiently sterile operating environment, and lack of experience or expertise on the part of the surgeon or his team.

Operative complications include perforation or even fracture of the femur. Special care should be taken in patients who are very old or osteoporotic and in those who have had previous hip operations.

Sciatic nerve palsy (usually due to traction but occasionally caused by direct injury) may occur with any type of arthroplasty. If there is reason to suspect nerve damage, the area should be explored. Most cases recover spontaneously.

Postoperative dislocation is rare if the prosthetic components are correctly placed. Reduction is easy and traction in abduction usually allows the hip to stabilize. If malposition of the acetabular component is severe, revision may be needed, or possibly augmentation of the socket.

Heterotopic bone formation around the hip is seen in about 20% of patients 5 years after joint replacement. The cause is unknown, but patients with skeletal hyperostosis (Chapter 5) and ankylosing spondylitis are particularly at risk. In severe cases this is associated with pain and stiffness. Ossification can be prevented in high-risk patients by giving either a course of non-steroidal anti-inflammatory drugs for 3–6 weeks postoperatively (Sodemann, Persson and Nilsson, 1988) or a single dose of irradiation to the hip (Lo et al., 1988).

Aseptic loosening of either the acetabular socket or the femoral stem is the commonest cause of long-term failure. Figures for its incidence vary widely, depending on the criteria used. There is likely to be clinical or radiographic evidence of loosening in about 20% of patients 10 years after operation; at microscopic level many stable implants show cellular reaction and membrane formation at the bone–cement interface (Linder and Carlsson, 1986). Fortunately, only a fraction of these are symptomatic. Pain may be a feature, especially when first taking weight on the leg after sitting or lying, but the diagnosis usually rests on x-ray signs of progressively increasing radiolucency around the implant, fracturing of cement, movement of the implant or bone resorption (Gruen, McNeice and Amstutz,

1979). Radionuclide scanning shows increased activity, and it is claimed that the pattern of ^{99}Tc-MDP and ^{67}Ga uptake can differentiate between aseptic loosening and infection (Taylor et al., 1989). If symptoms are marked, and particularly if there is evidence of progressive bone resorption, the implant and cement should be painstakingly removed and a new prosthesis inserted – either cemented or uncemented, depending on the condition of the bone.

A particularly aggressive form of bone resorption and implant loosening is sometimes seen. It is associated with granuloma formation at the interface between cement (or implant) and bone. This may be due to a severe histiocyte reaction stimulated by cement, polyethylene or metal particles that find their way into the boundary zone. Revision is usually necessary and this should be done using either an uncemented titanium stem (the metal appears to enhance osteoblastic activity) or, if the cavities are very large, morsellized cancellous bone grafts (Eskola et al., 1990).

Infection is the most serious postoperative complication. With adequate prophylaxis the risk should be less than 1%, but it is higher in the very old, in patients with rheumatoid disease or psoriasis, and in those on immunosuppressive therapy (including corticosteroids).

The large bulk of foreign material restricts the access of the body's normal defence mechanism; consequently, even slight wound contamination may be serious (Gristina and Kolkin, 1983). Organisms may multiply in the postoperative haematoma to cause early infection, and, even many years later, haematogenous spread from a distant site may cause late infection.

Early wound infection sometimes responds to antibiotics. Later infection does so less often and may need operative 'debridement' followed by irrigation with antibiotic solution for 3–4 weeks. Once the infection has cleared, a new prosthesis can be inserted, preferably without cement. An alternative, more applicable to 'mild' or 'dubious' infection, is a one-stage exchange arthroplasty using gentamicin-impregnated cement. The results of revision arthroplasty are only moderately good. In a recent series of patients, only 38% of treated

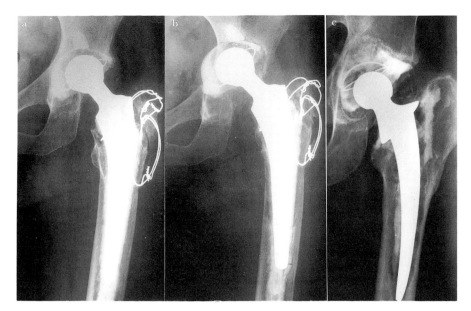

19.62 Hip replacement – loosening   (a) Five years after hip replacement there is a distinct radiolucent line around the femoral implant and resorption of the calcar. (b) A year later the x-ray shows fracturing of the cement mantle, tilting of the femoral prosthesis and migration of the acetabular cup. (c) Another case, showing aggressive osteolysis around a cemented femoral stem.

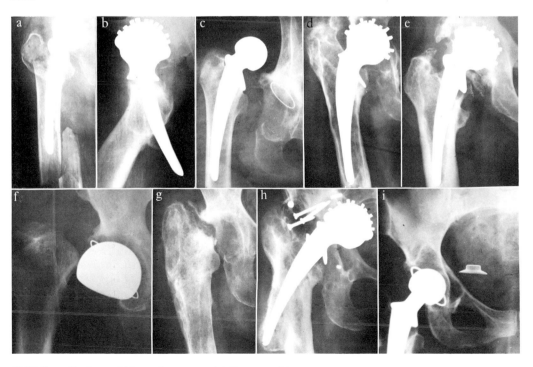

19.63 Complications of hip replacement   (a) Fracture; (b) penetration; (c) dislocation; (d) loosening; (e) infection; (f) fractured femoral neck beneath a double cup. (g) Girdlestone excision – the universal salvage – but salvage is not always needed – this patient (h) requested the same operation to her other hip; and (i) – well, we take our hats off to this one! (With acknowledgements to St Elsewhere's Hospital.)

hips were free of infection at late follow-up (Goodman and Schurman, 1988). If all else fails the prosthesis and cement may have to be removed, leaving an excisional (Girdlestone) arthroplasty.

RESULTS   The success rate of total hip replacement is now so high that only with a prolonged follow-up of a large number of cases can we evaluate the relative merits of different models. Assessment is a complex problem, but standard methods are emerging (Johnston et al., 1990).

Notes on applied anatomy

The ball-and-socket arrangement of the hip combines stability for weightbearing with freedom of movement for locomotion. A deeper acetabulum would confer greater stability but would limit the range of movement. Even with the fibrocartilaginous labrum the socket is not deep enough to accommodate the whole of the femoral head, whose articular surface extends considerably beyond a hemisphere.

The opening of the acetabulum faces downwards and forwards (about 30 degrees in each direction); the neck of the femur points upwards and forwards. Consequently, in the neutral position, the anterior portion of the head is not 'contained'. The amount of forward inclination of the neck relative to the shaft (the angle of anteversion) varies from 10 to 30 degrees in the adult. The upward inclination of the neck is such that the neck–shaft angle is 125 degrees.

A neck–shaft angle of less than 125 degrees is referred to as 'coxa vara' because, were the neck normally aligned relative to the pelvis, the limb would be deviated towards the midline of the body – in varus; a neck–shaft angle greater than 125 degrees (i.e. with the neck unduly vertical) is coxa valga. The angle is mechanically important because the further away the abductor muscles are from the hip, the greater is their leverage and their efficiency.

During standing and walking, the femoral neck acts as a cantilever; the line of body weight passes medial to the hip joint and is balanced

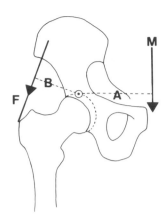

19.64 Forces around the hip When standing on one leg the pelvis is balanced on the femoral head. The vertical force due to the body weight (M) is counterbalanced by contraction of the lateral muscles (F). The force borne by the femoral head at ⊙ is produced by the combined moments M × A and F × B.

laterally by the abductors (especially gluteus medius). The combination of body weight, leverage effect and muscle action means that the resultant force transmitted through the femoral head can be very great – about five times the body weight when walking slowly and much more when running or jumping. It is easy to see why the hip is so liable to suffer from cartilage failure – the essential feature of osteoarthritis.

The ligaments of the hip, though very strong in front, are weak posteriorly; consequently, posterior dislocation is much more common than anterior. When the hip is adducted and medially rotated it is particularly vulnerable, and when this position results from unbalanced paralysis the hip can slip unobtrusively out of position.

During the swing phase of walking not only does the hip flex, it also rotates; this is because the pelvis swivels forwards. As weight comes onto the leg, the abductor muscles contract, causing the pelvis to tilt downwards on the weightbearing side; it is failure of this abductor mechanism which causes the Trendelenburg lurch.

The femoral head receives its arterial blood supply from three sources: (1) intraosseous vessels running up the neck, which are inevitably damaged with a displaced cervical fracture; (2) vessels in the retinacula reflected from capsule to neck, which may be damaged in a fracture or compressed by an effusion; and (3) vessels in the ligamentum teres, which are undeveloped in the early years of life and even later convey only a meagre blood supply. The relative importance of these vessels varies with age, but at all ages avascular necrosis is a potential hazard.

The nerve supply of the hip, unlike the blood supply, is plentiful. Sensory fibres, conveying proprioception as well as pain, abound in the capsule and ligaments. But the venous sinusoids of the bones also are supplied with sensory fibres; a rise in the intraosseous venous pressure accounts for some of the pain in osteoarthritis, and a reduction of this pressure for some of the relief which may follow osteotomy.

The tensor fascia femoris, though a relatively small muscle, has, through its action in tightening the iliotibial tract, a surprisingly large range of functions. This tract is anterior to the axis of knee flexion when the knee is straight, so its tension helps to hold the knee slightly hyperextended while standing. It is also important in getting up from the sitting position, as well as during the phases of walking and running when weight is being taken on the slightly flexed knee.

References and further reading

Apley, A.G. and Weintroub, S. (1981) The sagging rope sign in Perthes' disease and allied disorders. *Journal of Bone and Joint Surgery* **63B**, 43–47

Barker, D.J.P. and Hall, A.J. (1986) The epidemiology of Perthes' disease. *Clinical Orthopaedics and Related Research* **209**, 89–94

Barlow, T.G. (1962) Early diagnosis and treatment of congenital dislocation of the hip. *Journal of Bone and Joint Surgery* **44B**, 292–301

Bickerstaff, D.R., Neal, L.M., Booth, A.J., Brennan, P.D. and Bell, M.J. (1990) Ultrasound examination of the irritable hip. *Journal of Bone and Joint Surgery* **72B**, 549–553

Billing, L. and Severin, E. (1959) Slipping epiphysis of the hip. *Acta Radiologica* suppl. 174

Boyer, D.W., Mickelson, M.R. and Ponseti, I.V. (1981) Slipped capital femoral epiphysis. *Journal of Bone and Joint Surgery* **63A**, 85–95

Brignall, C.G. and Stainsby, G.D. (1991) The snapping hip. Treatment by Z-plasty. *Journal of Bone and Joint Surgery* **73B**, 253–254

Catterall, A. (1972) Coxa vara. In *Modern Trends in Orthopaedics – 6* (ed. A.G. Apley), Butterworths, London

Catterall, A. (1982) *Legg–Calvé–Perthes Disease*, Churchill Livingstone, Edinburgh

Catterall, A. (1992) Assessment of adolescent acetabular dysplasia. In Recent Advances in Orthopaedics – 6 (ed. A. Catterall), Churchill Livingstone, Edinburgh

Charnley, Sir J. (1979) *Low Friction Arthroplasty of the Hip*, Springer, Berlin, Heidelberg, New York

Chiari, K. (1974) Medial displacement osteotomy of the pelvis. *Clinical Orthopaedics and Related Research* **98**, 55–71

Doll, D. (1986) Exposure of the hip by anterior osteotomy of the greater trochanter. *Journal of Bone and Joint Surgery* **68B**, 382–386

Dunn, D.M. and Angel, J.C. (1978) Replacement of the femoral head by open operation in severe adolescent slipping of the upper femoral epiphysis. *Journal of Bone and Joint Surgery* **60B**, 394–403

Engh, C.A., Bobyn, J.D. and Glassman, A.H. (1987) Porous-coated hip replacement: the factors governing bone ingrowth, stress shielding and clinical results. *Journal of Bone and Joint Surgery* **69B**, 45–55

Eskola, A., Santavirka, S., Kouttinen, Y.T., Hoikka, V., Tallroth, K. and Lindholm, T.S. (1990) Cementless revision of aggressive granulomatous lesions in hip replacements. *Journal of Bone and Joint Surgery* **72B**, 212–216

Fowler, J.L., Gil, G.A., Lee, A.J.C. and Ling, R.S.M. (1988) Experience with the Exeter Total Hip since 1970. *Orthopedic Clinics of North America* **19**, 477–489

Geesink, R.G.T. (1990) Hydroxy-apatite-coated total hip prostheses. *Clinical Orthopaedics and Related Research* **261**, 39–58

Geesink, R.G.T., deGroot, K. and Klein, C.P.A.T. (1988) Bonding of bone to apatite-coated implants. *Journal of Bone and Joint Surgery* **70B**, 17–22

Gibson, P.H. and Benson, M.K.D. (1982) Congenital dislocation of the hip: a maturity review. *Journal of Bone and Joint Surgery* **64B**, 164–175

Goodman, S.B. and Schurman, D.J. (1988) Outcome of infected total hip arthroplasty: an inclusive, consecutive series. *Journal of Arthroplasty* **3**, 97–102

Greiss, M.E., Thomas, R.J. and Freeman, M.A.R. (1980) Sequelae of arthrodesis of the hip. *Journal of the Royal Society of Medicine* **73**, 497–500

Griffith, M.J. (1976) Slipping of the capital femoral epiphysis. *Annals of the Royal College of Surgeons of England* **58**, 34–42

Gristina, A.G. and Kolkin, J. (1983) Total joint replacement and sepsis. *Journal of Bone and Joint Surgery* **65A**, 128–134

Gruen, T.A., McNeice, G.M. and Amstutz, H.C. (1979) 'Modes of failure' of cemented stem-type femoral components. *Clinical Orthopaedics and Related Research* **141**, 17–27

Hadlow, V. (1988) Neonatal screening for congenital dislocation of the hip. *Journal of Bone and Joint Surgery* **70B**, 740–743

Hall, A.J., Barker, D.J.P., Dangerfield, P.H., Osmond, C. and

Taylor, J.F. (1988) Small feet and Perthes' disease. *Journal of Bone and Joint Surgery* **70B**, 611–613

Hanson, L.I. (1982) Osteosynthesis with the hook-pin in slipped capital femoral epiphysis. *Acta Orthopaedica Scandinavica* **53**, 87–96

Hardinge, K. (1982) The direct lateral approach to the hip. *Journal of Bone and Joint Surgery* **64B**, 17–19

Heyman, C.H. and Herndon, C.H. (1954) Epiphysiodesis for early slipping of the upper femoral epiphysis. *Journal of Bone and Joint Surgery* **36A**, 539–555

Hogh, J. and MacNicol, M.F. (1987) The Chiari pelvic osteotomy. *Journal of Bone and Joint Surgery* **64B**, 365–373

Ireland, J. and Newman, P.H. (1978) Triplane osteotomy for severely slipped upper femoral epiphysis. *Journal of Bone and Joint Surgery* **60B**, 390–393

Johnston, R.C., Fitzgerald, R.H., Harris, W.H., Poss, R., Müller, M.E. and Sledge, C.B. (1990) Clinical and radiographic evaluation of total hip replacement. *Journal of Bone and Joint Surgery* **72A**, 161–168

Joseph, B. (1989) Morphological changes in the acetabulum in Perthes' disease. *Journal of Bone and Joint Surgery* **71B**, 756–763

Klisic, P. and Jankovic, L. (1976) Combined procedure of open reduction and shortening of the femur in treatment of congenital dislocation of the hip in older children. *Clinical Orthopaedics and Related Research* **119**, 60–69

Landin, L.A., Danielsson, L.G. and Wattsgard, C. (1987) Transient synovitis of the hip. *Journal of Bone and Joint Surgery* **69B**, 238–242

Lidwell, O.M., Lowbury, E.J.L., Whyte, W. et. al. (1984) Infection and sepsis after operations for total hip or knee joint replacement: influence of ultraclean air, prophylactic antibiotics and other factors. *Journal of Hygiene (Camb.)* **83**, 505–529

Lin, S.-L. and Ho. T.-C. (1991) The role of venous hypertension in the pathogenesisi of Legg–Perthes disease. *Journal of Bone and Joint Surgery* **73A**, 194–200

Linder, L. and Carlsson, A.S. (1986) The bone–cement interface in hip arthroplasty: a histologic and enzyme study of stable components. *Acta Orthopaedica Scandinavica* **57**, 495–500

Lo, T.C.M., Healy, W.L., Covall, D.J. et al. (1988) Heterotopic bone formation after hip surgery: prevention with single-dose postoperative hip irradiation. *Radiology* **168**, 851–854

McKibbin, B. (1970) Anatomical factors in the stability of the hip in the newborn. *Journal of Bone and Joint Surgery* **53B**, 148–149

McKibbin, B., Freedman, L., Howard, C. and Williams, L.A. (1988) The management of congenital dislocation of the hip in the newborn. *Journal of Bone and Joint Surgery* **70B**, 423–427

McLauchlan, J. (1984) The Stracathro approach to the hip. *Journal of Bone and Joint Surgery* **66B**, 30–31

Maistrelli, G.L., Gerundini, M., Fusco, U., Bombelli, R., Bombelli, M. and Avai, A. (1990) Valgus-extension osteotomy for osteoarthritis of the hip. *Journal of Bone and Joint Surgery* **72B**, 653–657

Marotte, J.H., Lord, G.A., Blanchard, J.P. et al. (1987) Infection rate in total hip arthroplasty as a function of air cleanliness and antibiotic prophylaxis. *Journal of Arthroplasty* **2**, 77–82

Müller, M.E. (1975) Intertrochanteric osteotomies in adults: planning and operating technique. In *Surgical Management of Degenerative Arthritis of the Lower Limb*. (eds. R.L. Cruess and N.S. Mitchell), Lea and Febiger, Philadelphia, pp. 53–64

Murphy, S.B., Kijewski, P.K., Millis, M.B. and Harless, A. (1990) Acetabular dysplasia in the adolescent and young adult. *Clinical Orthopaedics and Related Research* **261**, 214–223

Olerad, S. and Karlstrom, G. (1985) Recurrent dislocation after total hip replacement. *Journal of Bone and Joint Surgery* **67B**, 402–405

Palmen, K. (1961) Preluxation of the hip joint. *Acta Paediatrica* **50**, suppl. 129

Pemberton, P.A. (1965) Pericapsular osteotomy of the ilium for treatment of congenital subluxation and dislocation of the hip. *Journal of Bone and Joint Surgery* **47A**, 65–86

Riley, P.M., Weiner, D.S. and Akron, R.G. (1990) Hazards of internal fixation in the treatment of slipped capital femoral epiphysis. *Journal of Bone and Joint Surgery* **72A**, 1500–1509

Roberts, C.S. and Fetto, J.F. (1990) Functional outcome of hip fusion in the young patient. *Journal of Arthroplasty* **5**, 89–96

Saito, S., Takaoka, K. and Ono, K. (1986) Tectoplasty for painful dislocation or subluxation of the hip. *Journal of Bone and Joint Surgery* **68B**, 55–60

Salter, R.B. (1961) Innominate osteotomy in the treatment of congenital dislocation and subluxation of the hip. *Journal of Bone and Joint Surgery* **43B**, 518–539

Salter, R.B. (1984) The present status of surgical treatment for Legg–Perthes' disease. *Journal of Bone and Joint Surgery* **66A**, 961–966

Sarmiento, A., Ebramzadeh, E., Gogan, W.J. and McKellop, H.A. (1990) Total hip arthroplasty with cement. *Journal of Bone and Joint Surgery* **72A**, 1470–1476

Simmons, E.D., Graham, H.K. and Szalai, J.P. (1990) Interobserver variability in grading Perthes' disease *Journal of Bone and Joint Surgery* **72B**, 202–204

Sodemann, B., Persson, P.-E. and Nilsson, O.S. (1988) Prevention of heterotopic ossification by nonsteroid antiinflammatory drugs after total hip arthroplasty. *Clinical Orthopaedics and Related Research* **237**, 158–163

Solomon, L. (1987) Avascular necrosis of bone. In *Recent Advances in Orthopaedics* – 5 (ed. A. Catterall), Churchill Livingstone, Edinburgh.

Sugioko, Y. (1978) Transtrochanteric anterior rotational osteostomy of the femoral head in the treatment of osteonecrosis affecting the hip. *Clinical Orthopaedics and Related Research* **130**, 191–201

Taylor, D.N., Maughan, J., Patel, M.P. and Clegg, J. (1989) A simple method of identifying loosening or infection of hip prostheses in nuclear medicine. *Nuclear Medicine Communications* **10**, 551–556

Tooke, S.M.T., Amstutz, H.C. and Hedley, A.K. (1987) Results of transtrochanteric rotational osteotomy for femoral head osteonecrosis. *Clinical Orthopaedics and Related Research* **224**, 150–157

Vegter, J. (1987) The influence of joint posture on intra-articular pressure. *Journal of Bone and Joint Surgery* **69B**, 71–74

Weiner, D.S. (1989) Bone graft epiphysiodesis in the treatment of slipped capital femoral epiphysis. *Instruc-*

tional Course Lectures **38**, 263–272

Werners, R., Vincent, B. and Bulstrode, C. (1990) Osteotomy for osteoarthritis of the hip. *Journal of Bone and Joint Surgery* **72B**, 1010–1013

Wilkinson, J.A. (1972) A post-actual survey for congenital dislocation of the hip. *Journal of Bone and Joint Surgery* **54B**, 40–49

Wilson, N.I.L. and Di Paola, M. (1986) Acute septic arthritis in infancy and childhood. *Journal of Bone and Joint Surgery* **68B**, 584–587

Wynne-Davies, R. (1970) Acetabular dysplasia and familial joint laxity: two aetiological factors in congenital dislocation of the hip. *Journal of Bone and Joint Surgery* **52B**, 704–716

Yamamuro, T. and Ishida, K. (1984) Recent advances in the prevention, early diagnosis and treatment of congenital dislocation of the hip in Japan. *Clinical Orthopaedics and Related Research* **184**, 34–40

Young-Hoo Kim, Dae-Young Han and Byeong-Mun Park (1989) Total hip arthroplasty for tuberculous coxarthrosis. *Journal of Bone and Joint Surgery* **69A**, 718–727

Zlatic, M., Radojevic, B., Lazovic, C. and Lupulovic, I. (1988) Late results of Chiari's pelvic osteotomy. *International Orthopaedics* **12**, 149–154

The knee

20

Examination

Symptoms

Pain is the most common knee symptom. With inflammatory or degenerative disorders it is usually diffuse, but with mechanical disorders and especially after injury it is often localized – the patient can, and should, point to the painful spot. If the patient can describe the mechanism of the injury, this is extremely useful.

Stiffness also is common and, like pain, may result in a limp.

Deformity (knock knees or bandy legs) is common but, in itself, seldom troublesome. Unilateral deformity, especially if it is progressive, is more significant.

Swelling may be localized or diffuse. If there was an injury, it is important to ask whether the swelling appeared immediately (suggesting a haemarthrosis) or only after some hours (typical of a torn meniscus).

Locking is an ambiguous term: patients often use it to describe stiffness. However, the clinical term means that the knee, quite suddenly, could not be straightened fully, although flexion was still possible. This happens when a torn meniscus is caught between the articular surfaces. By wiggling the knee around, the patient may be able to 'unlock' it; sudden unlocking is reliable evidence that something mobile had previously obstructed full extension.

Giving way also suggests a mechanical disorder, although it can result from muscle weakness; when it occurs particularly on stairs, the patellofemoral joint is suspect. Instability sufficient for the patient to fall suggests patellar dislocation.

Signs with the patient upright

Valgus or varus deformity is best seen with the patient standing and bearing weight. Then he should be observed walking: in the stance phase note whether the knee extends fully and if there is any lateral instability; in the swing phase note whether the knee is held rigid or moves freely.

Signs with the patient lying supine

● LOOK

Skin The colour of the skin and any sinuses or scars are noted.

Shape *Wasting* of the quadriceps is a sure sign of joint disorder. The visual impression can be checked by measuring the girth of the thigh at the same level (e.g. a certain distance above the joint line) in each limb.

Swelling of the knee and *lumps* around the joint are observed; the shape of the patella is compared with that of the opposite knee.

Position The knee may lie in valgus or varus, partially flexed or hyperextended. The position of the patella should be noted.

● FEEL

Skin Increased warmth is detected by comparing the two knees. The 'temperature gradient'

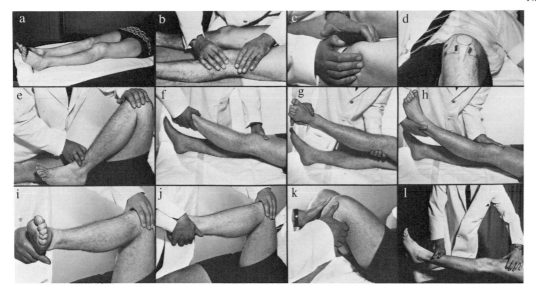

20.1 Examination – supine (a) Looking at both knees – the left is swollen and the thigh wasted; (b) testing for fluid by cross-fluctuation; (c) feeling for synovial thickening; (d) the points which should be palpated for tenderness.

Testing movements: (e) flexion, (f) extension, (g) abduction, (h) adduction. Lateral rotation (i), medial rotation (j) and anteroposterior glide (k) are tested with the knee bent; (l) testing quadriceps power. (Alternative methods are shown in Fig. 20.14 on p. 441, ande Fig 27.33 on p. 681.)

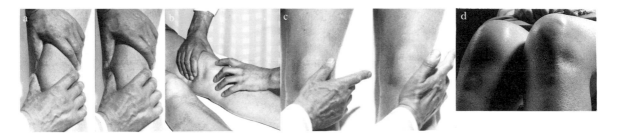

20.2 Tests for fluid (a) Cross-fluctuation, the easiest test for large quantities of fluid. (b) The patellar tap, most likely to be positive with a moderate amount of fluid. (c) The bulge test detects small quantities of fluid. (d) The patellar hollow test – noting at what angle the hollow lateral to the patellar ligament disappears, as compared with the normal side – a very reliable test of even very small quantities of fluid.

is assessed by running a hand down the length of the limb; normally there is a linear decrease in warmth from proximal to distal.

Fluid There are four tests for fluid. (1) Cross-fluctuation: the left hand compresses and empties the suprapatellar pouch while the right hand straddles the front of the joint below the patella; by squeezing with each hand alternately, a fluid impulse is transmitted across the joint. (2) The patellar tap: again the suprapatellar pouch is compressed with the left hand, while the index finger of the right pushes the patella sharply backwards; with a positive test the patella can be felt striking the femur and bouncing off again. (3) The bulge test: this is useful when very little fluid is present. The medial compartment is emptied by pressing on that side of the joint; the hand is then lifted away and the lateral side is sharply compressed;

a distinct ripple is seen on the flattened medial surface. (4) The patellar hollow test: when the normal knee is flexed, a hollow appears lateral to the patellar ligament and disappears with further flexion; with excess fluid the hollow fills and disappears at a lesser angle of flexion (Mann et al., 1991).

The soft tissues and bony outlines are then palpated systematically, feeling for thickening and localized tenderness. This is done first with the knee in extension and then flexed to 90 degrees; in flexion the joint line can be felt more easily. The undersurface of the patella is also accessible if the bone is pushed first to one side and then to the other. Synovial thickening is best appreciated as follows: placing the knee in extension, the examiner grasps the edges of the patella in a pincer made of the thumb and middle finger, and tries to lift the patella forwards; normally the bone can be grasped quite firmly, but if the synovium is thickened the fingers simply slip off the edges of the patella.

● MOVE

Flexion and extension Full extension is assessed by pressing the thigh against the couch and trying to lift the leg. Then flexion is tested. Normally the knee flexes until the calf meets the ham, and extends completely with a snap; even slight loss of extension or 'springiness' on attempting it, is important. The range of flexion is recorded in degrees and any hyper-extension as a minus quantity.

Crepitus during movement may be felt with a hand placed on the front of the knee. It usually signifies patellofemoral roughness.

Movement with stress The medial or lateral compartment of the knee can be loaded sepa-

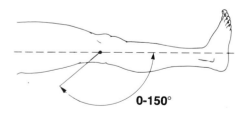

20.3 Normal range of movements Full extension is recorded as 0 degrees. Flexion is usually from 0 to about 150 degrees.

rately during movement by stressing the knee into varus or valgus during flexion. Pain with this manoeuvre signifies cartilage softening in one or other compartment.

Rotation This is tested first with the patient's hip and knee flexed to 90 degrees; one hand steadies and feels the knee, the other rotates the foot. Rotation is then repeated in varying degrees of flexion (see McMurray's test, below).

TESTS FOR STABILITY
In testing for stability it is essential to compare the normal with the abnormal knee.

The medial and lateral ligaments are tested by stressing the knee into valgus and varus: this is best done by tucking the patient's foot under your arm and holding the extended knee firmly with one hand on each side of the joint; the leg is then angulated alternately towards abduction and adduction. The test is performed at full extension and again at 30 degrees of flexion. There is normally some mediolateral move-ment at 30 degrees, but if this is excessive (compared to the normal side) it suggests a torn or stretched collateral ligament. Sideways movement in full extension is always abnormal; it may be due to either (1) torn or stretched ligaments or (2) loss of articular cartilage or bone, which allows the affected compartment to collapse.

The cruciate ligaments are tested by examining for abnormal gliding movements in the antero-posterior plane. With both knees flexed 90 degrees and the feet resting on the couch, the upper tibia is inspected from the side; if its upper end has dropped back, or can be gently pushed back, this indicates a tear of the posterior cruciate ligament (the 'sag sign'). With the knee in the same position, the foot is anchored by the examiner sitting on it (pro-vided this is not painful); then, using both hands, the upper end of the tibia is grasped firmly and rocked backwards and forwards to see if there is any anteroposterior glide (the '*drawer test*'). Excessive anterior movement (a positive anterior drawer sign) denotes anterior cruciate laxity; excessive posterior movements (a positive posterior drawer sign) signifies posterior cruciate laxity. More sensitive is the

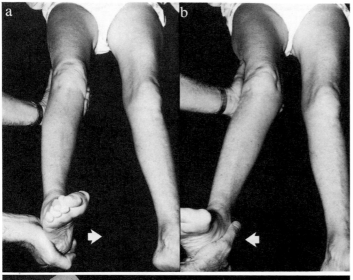

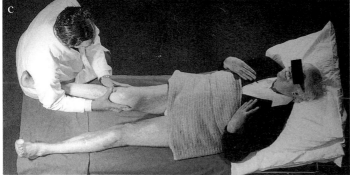

20.4 Tests for instability   Two ways of testing for collateral ligament laxity. (a, b) By stressing first the lateral, then the medial side of the knee, it was easy to see that this patient had medial laxity. (c) If the surgeon holds the leg between his arm and his chest he can impart valgus and varus stresses and, with his hands, detect any knee laxity with precision.

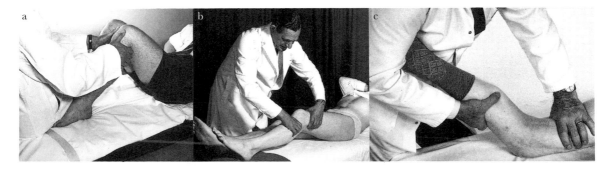

20.5 Testing for instability   Cruciate laxity can be tested with the knee at 90 degrees as shown in (a); the leg can be stabilized by sitting on the patient's foot, and the fingers ensure that the hamstrings are relaxed. The leg is tugged forward and pushed backwards. (b) More reliable is Lachman's test: with the knee at 20–30 degrees the leg and thigh are grasped firmly and moved in opposite directions. (c) The Lachman test is sometimes better performed with the patient prone; one hand stabilizes the thigh, the other moves the tibia.

Lachman test – but this is difficult if the patient has big thighs (or the examiner has small hands). The patient's knee is flexed 20 degrees; with one hand grasping the lower thigh and the other the upper part of the leg, the joint surfaces are shifted backwards and forwards upon each other. If the knee is stable, there should be no gliding.

Other tests for ligamentous stability are described on p. 684).

McMurray's test

This is the classic test for a torn meniscus and is based on the fact that the loose tag can sometimes be trapped between the articular surfaces and then induced to snap free with a palpable and audible click. The knee is flexed as far as possible; one hand steadies the joint and the other rotates the leg medially and laterally while the knee is slowly extended. The test is repeated several times, with the knee stressed in valgus or varus, feeling and listening for the click.

The patellofemoral joint

Lest it be forgotten, the patellofemoral joint is examined separately.

The size, shape and position of the patella are noted. The bone is felt, first on its anterior surface and then along its edges and at the attachments of the quadriceps tendon and the patellar ligament. Much of the posterior surface, too, is accessible to palpation if the patella is pushed first to one side and then to the other; tenderness suggests synovial irritation or articular cartilage softening.

Moving the patella up and down while pressing it lightly against the femur (the 'friction test') causes painful grating if the central portion of the articular cartilage is damaged. Pressing the patella laterally with the thumb while flexing the knee slightly may induce anxiety and resistance to further movement; this, the 'apprehension test', is diagnostic of recurrent patellar subluxation or dislocation.

Signs with the patient lying prone

Scars or lumps in the popliteal fossa are noted. If there is a swelling, is it in the midline (most likely a bulging capsule) or to one side (possibly a bursa)? A semimembranous bursa is usually just above the joint line, a Baker's cyst below it.

The popliteal fossa is carefully palpated. If there is a lump, where does it originate? Does it pulsate? Can it be emptied into the joint?

Apley's test The knee is flexed to 90 degrees and rotated while a compression force is applied; this, the grinding test, reproduces symptoms if a meniscus is torn. Rotation is then repeated while the leg is pulled upwards with the surgeon's knee holding the thigh down; this, the distraction test, produces increased pain only if there is ligament damage (Apley, 1947).

Lachman's test can be readily performed with the patient prone.

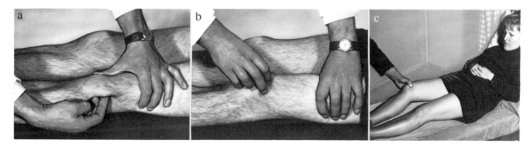

20.6 Examination of patella   (a) Feeling for tenderness behind the patella; (b) the patellar friction test; (c) the apprehension test.

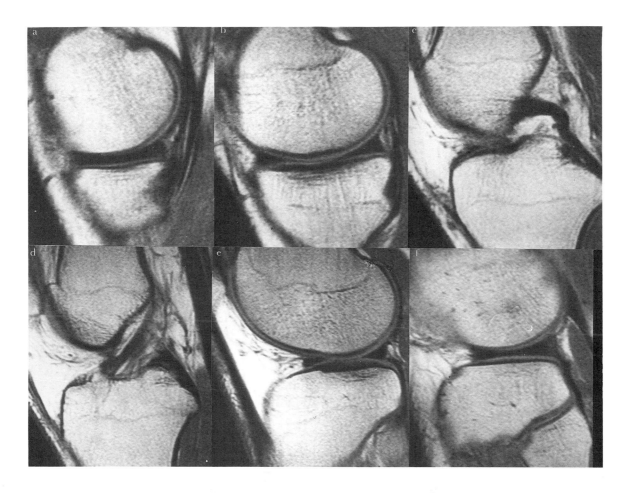

20.7 MRI   A series of sagittal T_1-weighted images proceeding from medial to lateral to show the normal appearances of (a, b) the medial meniscus, (c) the posterior cruciate ligament, (d) the somewhat fan-shaped anterior cruciate ligament and (e, f) the lateral meniscus.

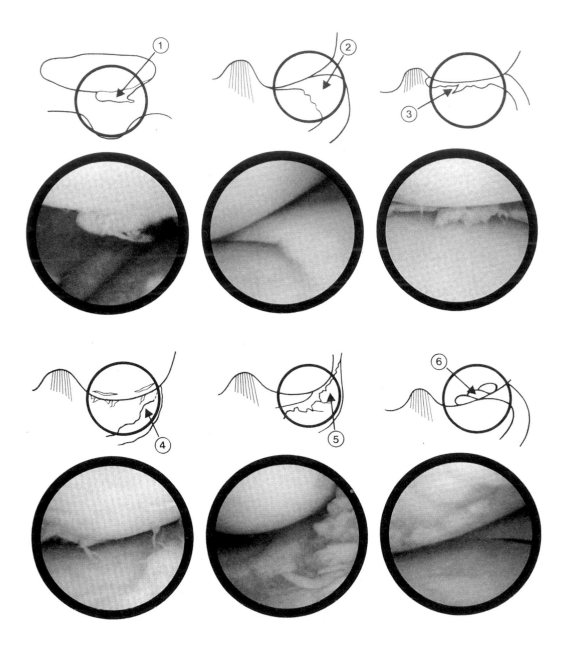

20.8 Arthroscopy   In each case the view is of the right knee from the lateral side. (1) Chondromalacia patellae; (2) normal medial meniscus; (3) torn medial meniscus; (4) degenerate medial meniscus and osteoarthritic femoral condyle; (5) rheumatoid synovium; (6) osteochondritis dissecans medial femoral condyle.

Imaging

Anteroposterior, lateral and sometimes patello-femoral (or skyline) and intercondylar (or tunnel) views are needed. The anteroposterior view should be taken with the patient standing, or better still with the knee stressed into varus and then valgus; unless the femorotibial compartment is loaded, narrowing of the articular space may be missed. Stress films are also essential for diagnosing collateral ligament tears.

When a loose body is seen, its origin should be sought; it should not be confused with a fabella, which lies on the lateral side and behind the line joining the femur to the tibia.

If valgus or varus has to be measured, a long film (from hip to ankle) is needed.

Arthrography and MRI are useful in doubtful meniscal or ligament injuries. Radioisotope scans may show increased activity in the sub-articular bone, an early sign of osteoarthritis.

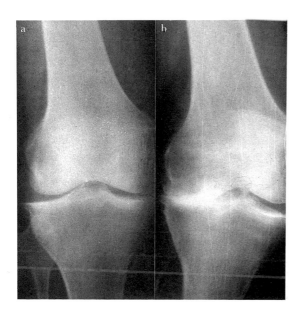

20.9 X-rays These films are of the same knee: (a) with the patient lying on the x-ray table, and (b) with the patient taking weight on the leg. It is easy to see how misleading non-weightbearing films can be.

Arthroscopy

Arthroscopy is useful: (1) to establish or refine the accuracy of diagnosis; (2) to help in deciding whether to operate, or to plan the operative approach with more precision; (3) to record the progress of a knee disorder; and (4) to perform certain operative procedures. Arthroscopy is not a substitute for clinical examination; a detailed history and meticulous assessment of the physical signs are indispensable preliminaries and remain the sheet anchor of diagnosis. However, arthroscopy is especially helpful in diagnosing meniscal injuries – and dealing with them at the same time. *Full asepsis is essential.*

The diagnostic calendar

Depending on the patient's age and the likely diagnosis, different aspects of the examination need to be emphasized.

Adolescents with anterior knee pain are usually found to have chondromalacia patellae, patellar instability, osteochondritis or a plica syndrome. But remember – knee pain may be referred from the hip!

Young adults engaged in sports are the most frequent victims of meniscal tears and ligament injuries. Examination should include a variety of tests for ligamentous instability that would be quite inappropriate in elderly patients.

Patients above middle age with chronic pain and stiffness probably have osteoarthritis. With primary osteoarthritis of the knees, other joints also are often affected; polyarthritis does not necessarily (nor even most commonly) mean rheumatoid arthritis.

Deformities of the knee

In the normal adult the knees are in 5–7 degrees of valgus. Any deviation from this may be regarded as 'deformity', though often it bothers no one – least of all the possessor of the knees. The three common deformities are bow leg (genu varum), knock knee (genu valgum) and hyperextension (genu recurvatum).

Development bow leg and knock knee

Deformity is usually gauged from simple observation. Bilateral bow leg can be recorded by measuring the distance between the knees with the legs held in full extension and the heels touching; it should be less than 6 cm. Similarly, knock knee can be estimated by measuring the distance between the medial malleoli when the knees are held touching with the patellae facing forwards; it is usually less than 8 cm.

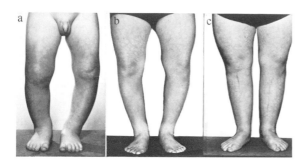

20.10 Bow legs (1)   (a) Infantile, which usually recovers spontaneously. (b) In this older child, deformity persisted and osteotomy was performed (c).

Bow leg in babies and knock knee in 4-year-olds are so common that they are considered to be *normal stages of development*. Other postural abnormalities such as pigeon toes and flat feet may coexist but these children are normal in all other respects. The 'deformity' almost invariably corrects spontaneously by the age of 10–12. Treatment is unnecessary but the parents should be reassured and the child should be seen at intervals of 6 months to record progress. In the occasional case where, by the age of 10, the deformity is still marked (i.e. the intercondylar distance is more than 8 cm or the intermalleolar distance more than 10 cm), operative correction should be advised: either stapling of the medial or lateral side of the knee physis to produce asymmetrical growth (the staples are removed once the knee has overcorrected slightly) or else osteotomy after growth is complete (supracondylar osteotomy for valgus knees and high tibial osteotomy for varus knees).

BLOUNT'S DISEASE   This, a progressive bow-leg deformity associated with abnormal growth of the posteromedial part of the proximal tibial epiphysis, is relatively common in the West

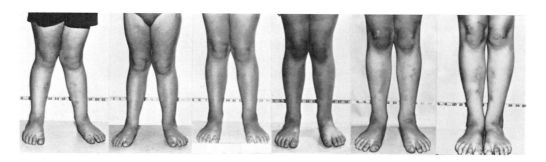

20.11 Genu valgum (1)   Idiopathic knock knee – natural history without treatment. Age: 3 years   3½   4   5   6   7.

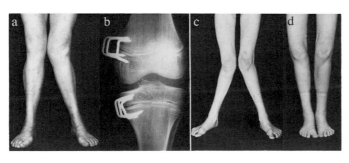

20.12 Genu valgum (2)   Only rarely does knock knee persist: (a, b) an adolescent treated by stapling; (c, d) before and after bilateral osteotomy for severe deformity.

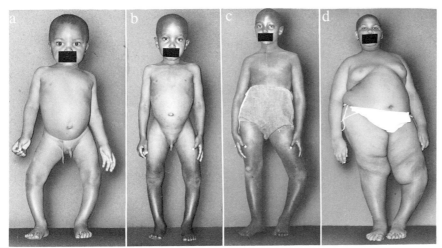

20.13 Bow legs (2) (a) Blount's disease; (b) healed rickets; (c) trauma has damaged the upper tibial epiphysis; (d) this patient has an endocrine disorder and her upper tibial epiphysis has slipped.

Indies and parts of Africa. On x-ray the upper tibial epiphysis is flattened medially and the adjacent metaphysis is somewhat beak-shaped. In the worst cases the epiphysis looks fragmented. Occasionally the femoral epiphysis also is affected. The resulting deformity is nearly always bilateral and is usually associated with internal rotation of the tibia. Spontaneous resolution is rare and, once it is clear that the deformity is progressing, there should be no hesitation in performing a corrective osteotomy, aiming at 6–10 degrees of valgus. Both tibia and fibula need to be osteotomized.

Secondary bow leg and knock knee in children

Disorders that distort physeal growth Genu varum or genu valgum may be seen in disorders that distort physeal growth; for example, dysplasias, rickets and, where the deformity is unilateral, injuries of the growth plate. If angulation is severe, operative correction will be necessary.

'Apparent bow legs' is sometimes seen in children with excessive anteversion of the femoral neck; with the patellae facing forwards the 'varus' deformity disappears. If treatment is needed, it should be a derotation osteotomy of the femur.

Complex deformities – for example, varus of the distal femur together with valgus of the tibia (sometimes with a rotational component also) – may result from either rickets or polyostotic lesions such as multiple exostoses. Corrective osteotomies may be needed above and below the knee. Preoperative planning is crucial.

Genu varum and valgum in adults

Angular deformities are common in adults (usually bow legs in men and knock knees in women). They may be the *sequel to childhood deformity* and if so usually cause no problems. However, if the deformity is associated with the slightest degree of joint instability, this can lead to osteoarthritis – of the medial compartment in varus knees and the lateral compartment in valgus knees. Genu valgum may also cause abnormal tracking of the patella and predispose to patellofemoral osteoarthritis. Even in the absence of overt osteoarthritis, if the patient complains of pain, or if there are clinical or radiological signs of joint damage, a 'prophylactic' osteotomy is justified: above the knee for valgus deformity and below the knee for varus.

Deformity may be *secondary to arthritis* – usually varus in osteoarthritis and valgus in rheumatoid arthritis. In these cases the joint is often unstable and corrective osteotomy less predictable in its effect. Stress x-rays are essential in the assessment of these cases.

Other causes of varus or valgus deformity are *ligament injuries, malunited fractures* and *Paget's disease*. Where possible, the underlying disorder should be dealt with; provided the joint is stable, corrective osteotomy may be all that is necessary.

Hyperextension of the knee (genu recurvatum)

Congenital recurvatum may be due to abnormal intrauterine posture; spontaneous recovery usually occurs. Rarely, gross hyperextension is the precursor of true congenital dislocation of the knee.

Lax ligaments can lead to hyperextension. Normal people with generalized joint laxity tend to stand with their knees back-set.

Prolonged traction, especially on a frame, or holding the knee hyperextended in plaster, may overstretch ligaments, leading to permanent hyperextension deformity. Ligaments may also become overstretched following chronic or recurrent synovitis (especially in rheumatoid arthritis), the hypotonia of rickets, the flailness of poliomyelitis or the insensitivity of Charcot's disease.

Recurvatum of the knee may be secondary to *fixed equinus* of the ankle: in order to set the foot on the ground, the knee is forced into hyperextension. In moderate degrees, this may actually be helpful (e.g. in stabilizing a knee with weak extensors). However, if excessive and prolonged, it may give rise to a permanent deformity. If bony correction is undertaken, the knee should be left with some hyperextension to preserve the stabilizing mechanism. If quadriceps power is poor, the patient may need a caliper. Severe paralytic hyperextension can be treated by fixing the patella into the tibial plateau, where it acts as a bone block (Hong-Xue Men et al., 1991).

Other causes of recurvatum are *growth plate injuries* and *malunited fractures*. These can be safely corrected by osteotomy.

Meniscus lesions

The menisci have an important role in (1) increasing the stability of the knee, (2) controlling the complex rolling and gliding actions of the joint and (3) distributing load during movement.

The medial compartment of the knee carries about 90% of the load during weightbearing (Johnson, Leitl and Waugh, 1980) and the medial meniscus is much less mobile than the lateral. Little wonder that meniscal lesions are much more common on the medial side than on the lateral.

Even in the absence of injury, there is gradual stiffening and degeneration of the menisci with age, so splits and tears are quite common in later life – particularly if there is any associated arthritis or chondrocalcinosis. In young people, meniscal tears are usually the result of trauma.

Tears of the meniscus

The meniscus is split in its length by a force grinding it between the femur and the tibia. In the young this usually occurs when weight is being taken on the flexed knee and there is a twisting strain; hence the frequency in footballers. In middle life, when fibrosis has restricted mobility of the meniscus, tears occur with relatively little force.

Pathology

The medial meniscus is affected far more frequently than the lateral, partly because its attachments to the capsule make it less mobile. Tears of both menisci may occur with severe ligament injuries.

In 75% of cases the split is *vertical* in the length of the meniscus (Dandy, 1990). If the separated fragment remains attached front and back, the lesion is called a *bucket-handle tear*. The torn portion sometimes displaces towards the centre of the joint and becomes jammed between femur and tibia, causing a block to extension ('locking'). If the tear emerges at the free edge of the meniscus, it leaves a tongue

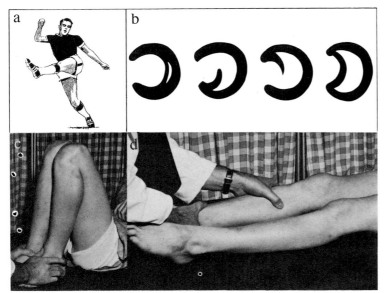

20.14 Torn medial meniscus (a) The meniscus is torn by a twisting force with the knee bent and taking weight; (b) the initial split may extend; (c) a locked knee flexes fully but (d) lacks full extension.

based anteriorly – an *anterior horn tear* – or posteriorly – a *posterior horn tear.*

Horizontal tears are usually 'degenerative' or due to repetitive minor trauma. Some are associated with meniscal cysts (see below).

Most of the meniscus is avascular and spontaneous repair does not occur unless the tear is in the outer third, which is vascularized from the capsule. The loose tag acts as a mechanical irritant, giving rise to recurrent synovial effusion and, in some cases, secondary osteoarthritis.

Clinical features

The patient is usually a young person who sustains a twisting injury to the knee on the sports field. Pain (usually on the medial side) is often severe and further activity is avoided; occasionally the knee is 'locked' in partial flexion. Almost invariably, swelling appears some hours later, or perhaps the following day.

With rest the initial symptoms subside, only to recur periodically after trivial twists or strains. Sometimes the knee gives way spontaneously and this is again followed by pain and swelling.

It is important to remember that in patients aged over 40 the initial injury may be unremarkable and the main complaint is of recurrent 'giving way' or 'locking'.

'Locking' – that is, the sudden inability to extend the knee fully – suggests a bucket-handle tear. The patient sometimes learns to 'unlock' the knee by bending it fully or by twisting it from side to side.

On examination the joint may be held slightly flexed and there is often an effusion. In long-standing cases the quadriceps will be wasted. Tenderness is localized to the joint line, in the vast majority of cases on the medial side. Flexion is usually full but extension is often slightly limited.

Between attacks of pain and effusion there is a disconcerting paucity of signs. The history is helpful, and McMurray's test or Apley's grinding test may be positive.

Plain x-rays are normal but *arthrography*, if properly performed, is a good way of confirming the diagnosis. *MRI* is the most reliable method, and may even reveal tears that are missed by arthroscopy.

Arthroscopy has the advantage that, if a lesion is identified, it can be treated at the same time.

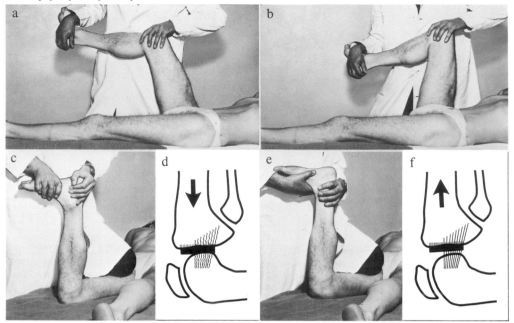

20.15 Torn medial meniscus – tests   (a, b) McMurray's test is performed at varying angles of flexion. (c, d) The grinding test relaxes the ligaments but compresses the meniscus – it causes pain with meniscus lesions. (e, f) The distraction test releases the meniscus but stretches the ligaments and causes pain if these are injured.

Differential diagnosis

Loose bodies   in the joint may cause true locking. The history is much more insidious than with meniscal tears and the attacks are variable in character and intensity. A loose body may be palpable and is often visible on x-ray.

Recurrent dislocation of the patella causes the knee to give way; typically the patient is caught unawares and collapses to the ground. The apprehension test is positive.

Fracture of the tibial spine   may follow an injury. There is tenderness anteriorly and the joint cannot be fully extended. X-ray may show the fracture.

A partial tear of the medial collateral ligament   may heal with adhesions where it is attached to the medial meniscus, so that the meniscus loses mobility. The patient complains of recurrent attacks of pain and giving way, followed by tenderness on the medial side. Sleep may be disturbed if the medial side rests upon the other knee or the bed. As with a meniscus injury, rotation is painful; but unlike a meniscus lesion, the grinding test gives less pain and the distraction test more pain.

A torn anterior cruciate ligament can cause chronic instability, with a sense of the knee 'giving way' or buckling when the patient turns sharply towards the side of the affected knee. Careful examination should reveal signs of rotational instability, a positive Lachman test or a positive anterior drawer sign. MRI or arthroscopy will settle any doubts.

Treatment

DEALING WITH THE LOCKED KNEE   Usually the knee 'unlocks' spontaneously; if not, gentle passive flexion and rotation may do the trick. Forceful manipulation is unwise (it may do more damage) and is usually unnecessary; after a few days' rest the knee may well unlock itself. However, if the knee does not unlock, or if attempts to unlock it cause severe pain, arthro-

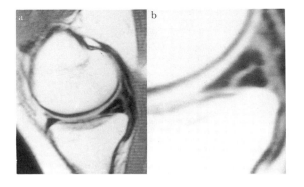

20.16 Torn meniscus – MRI (a) Sagittal proton density sequence showing a horizontal tear of the posterior horn of the medial meniscus. (b) Enlarged image on 'meniscal window' setting. This type of tear is easily missed on arthroscopy.

scopy is indicated: if the tear is confirmed, the offending fragment is removed.

CONSERVATIVE TREATMENT is often acceptable. If the joint is not locked, it is reasonable to hope that the tear is peripheral and can repair. After an acute episode, the joint is held straight in a plaster backslab for 3–4 weeks; the patient uses crutches and quadriceps exercises are encouraged. Operation can be put off as long as attacks are infrequent and not disabling and the patient is willing to abandon those activities that provoke them.

OPERATIVE TREATMENT is indicated (1) if the joint cannot be unlocked and (2) if symptoms are recurrent. For practical purposes, the lesion is usually dealt with as part of the 'diagnostic' arthroscopy. Tears close to the periphery, which have the capacity to heal, can be sutured using the arthroscope and special instruments (Johannsen et al., 1988).

Tears other than those in the peripheral third are dealt with by excising the torn portion (or the bucket handle). Total meniscectomy is thought to cause more instability and so predispose to late secondary osteoarthritis; certainly in the short term it causes greater morbidity than partial meniscectomy and has no obvious advantages (Hede, Hejgaard and Larsen, 1986).

Arthroscopic meniscectomy has distinct advantages over open meniscectomy: shorter hos-pital stay, lower costs and more rapid return to function. However, it is by no means free of complications (Sherman et al., 1986).

After arthroscopic or open meniscectomy a postoperative haemarthrosis may need aspiration. Chronic postoperative pain and swelling may be due to reflex sympathetic dystrophy; the sooner this is recognized the more amenable is it to treatment.

Postoperative pain and stiffness are reduced by prophylactic non-steroidal anti-inflammatory drugs. Quadriceps-strengthening exercises are important.

Outcome

Neither a meniscal tear by itself nor removal of the meniscus necessarily leads to secondary osteoarthritis (Casscells, 1978; Doherty, Watt and Dieppe, 1983). An important factor is the overall state of the knee: if, either because of associated ligament injuries or as a consequence of any operation, the knee becomes unstable, secondary osteoarthritis is likely to follow.

Meniscal degeneration

Patients over 45 years old may present with symptoms and signs of a meniscal tear. Often, though, they can recall no preceding injury. At arthroscopy there may be a horizontal cleavage in the medial meniscus – the characteristic 'degenerative' lesion – or detachment of the anterior or posterior horn without an obvious tear. Associated osteoarthritis or chrondrocalcinosis is common (Noble and Hamblin, 1975).

A detached anterior or posterior horn can be sutured firmly in place. Meniscectomy is indicated only if symptoms are marked or if, at arthroscopy, there is a major tear.

Discoid lateral meniscus

In the fetus the meniscus is not semilunar but disc-like; if this shape persists, symptoms are likely. A young patient complains that, without any history of injury, the knee gives way and 'thuds' loudly. A characteristic clunk may be felt

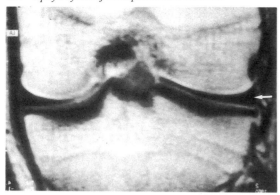

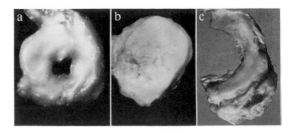

20.18 Other meniscus lesions Whereas tears are much more common on the medial side, discoid meniscus and cysts are much more common on the lateral. (a) Partial and (b) complete discoid lateral meniscus. (c) Cyst of lateral meniscus.

20.17 Discoid meniscus – MRI The discoid lateral meniscus produces a black image across the entire lateral compartment.

at 110 degrees as the knee is bent and at 10 degrees as it is being straightened. The diagnosis is easily confirmed by MRI.

If there is only a clunk, treatment is not essential. If pain is disturbing, the meniscus may be excised, though a more attractive procedure is arthroscopic partial excision leaving a normally shaped meniscus (Dimakopoulos and Patel, 1990).

Meniscal cysts

Cysts of the menisci are probably traumatic in origin, arising from either a small horizontal cleavage tear or repeated squashing of the peripheral part of the meniscus. It is also suggested that synovial cells infiltrate into the vascular area between meniscus and capsule and there multiply (Barrie, 1979). The multilocular cyst contains gelatinous fluid and is surrounded by thick fibrous tissue.

Clinical features

The lateral meniscus is affected much more frequently than the medial. The patient complains of an ache or a small lump at the side of the joint. Symptoms may be intermittent, or worse after activity.

On examination the lump is situated at or slightly below the joint line, usually anterior to the collateral ligament. It is seen most easily with the knee slightly flexed; in some positions

it may disappear altogether. Lateral cysts are often so firm that they are mistaken for a solid swelling. Medial cysts are usually larger and softer.

Differential diagnosis

Apart from cysts, various conditions may present with a small lump along the joint line.

A ganglion is quite superficial, usually not as 'hard' as a cyst, and unconnected with the joint.

Calcific deposits in the collateral ligament usually appear on the medial side, are intensely painful and tender, and often show on the x-ray.

A prolapsed, torn meniscus occasionally presents as a rubbery, irregular lump at the joint line. In some cases the distinction from a 'cyst' is largely academic.

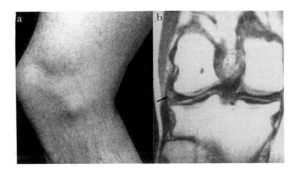

20.19 Meniscal cyst (a) The tense swelling just below the midline. (b) MRI showing the cyst arising from the edge of the lateral meniscus.

Various tumours, both of soft tissue (lipoma, fibroma) and of bone (osteochondroma), may produce a medial or lateral joint lump. Careful examination will show that the lump does not arise from the joint itself.

Treatment

If the symptoms warrant operation, the cyst may be removed. In the past this was usually combined with total meniscectomy, in order to prevent an inevitable recurrence of the cyst. However, it is quite feasible to examine the meniscus by arthroscopy, remove only the torn or damaged portion and then decompress the cyst from within the joint. The recurrence rate following such arthroscopic surgery is negligible (Parisien, 1990).

Chronic ligamentous instability

The knee is a complex hinge which depends heavily on its ligaments for mediolateral, anteroposterior and rotational stability. Ligament injuries, from minor strains through partial ruptures to complete tears, are common in sportsmen, athletes and dancers. Whatever the nature of the acute injury, the victim may be left with chronic instability of the knee – a sense of the joint wanting to give way, or actually giving way, during unguarded activity. Sometimes this is accompanied by pain and recurrent episodes of swelling. There may be a meniscal tear, but meniscectomy is likely to make matters worse; sometimes patients present with meniscectomy scars on both sides of the knee!

Examination should include special tests for ligamentous instability as well as radiological investigation and arthroscopy. It is important not only to establish the nature of the lesion but also to measure the level of functional impairment against the needs and demands of the individual patient before advocating treatment.

The subject is dealt with in detail on p. 683.

Recurrent dislocation of the patella

Recurrent dislocation with minimal stress is seen in the patellofemoral joint, the shoulder and the ankle. When the patella dislocates, it always does so towards the lateral side as the knee is flexed (though medial dislocation may follow an overzealous lateral release operation). A single dislocation occasionally results from an unusual injury; in recurrent dislocation there are other predisposing factors, such as: (1) generalized ligamentous laxity; (2) underdevelopment of the lateral femoral condyle and flattening of the intercondylar groove; (3) maldevelopment of the patella, which may be too high or too small; (4) valgus deformity of the knee; and (5) a primary muscle defect.

During the first episode the capsule on the medial side of the patella is torn and, if it fails to unite properly, lateral laxity persists. Repeated dislocation damages the contiguous surfaces of patella and femoral condyle; this may result in further flattening of the condyle, so facilitating further dislocations. A late complication is secondary osteoarthritis.

Clinical features

Girls are affected more commonly than boys and the condition is often bilateral. Dislocation occurs unexpectedly when the quadriceps muscle is contracted with the knee in flexion. There is acute pain, the knee is stuck in flexion and the patient may fall to the ground.

Although the patella always dislocates laterally, the patient may think it has displaced

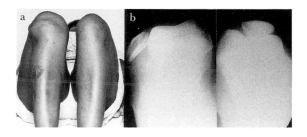

20.20 Dislocated patella (a) Clinical picture and (b) x-ray showing dislocation of the right patella.

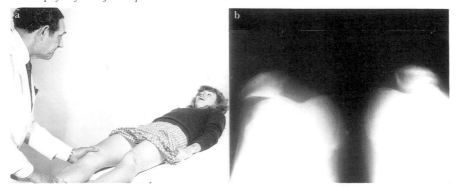

20.21 Patellar instability   (a) The apprehension test – the patient's facial expression shows that she is apprehensive that the patella may dislocate. (b) Subluxation of the patella.

medially because the uncovered medial femoral condyle stands out prominently.

If the knee is seen while the patella is dislocated, the diagnosis is obvious. There is usually tenderness on the medial side of the joint. Later the joint becomes swollen, and aspiration may reveal a blood-stained effusion.

Between attacks the patella may be too high (patella alta) or too small, and there may be signs of generalized joint laxity. One test is

nearly always positive: if the patella is pushed laterally with the knee slightly flexed, the patient resists vigorously. (The term 'apprehension test' has been coined because the patient is apprehensive lest dislocation recur.)

X-rays may show a high-riding patella or, occasionally, other anatomical abnormalities.

Treatment

Only rarely is the patient seen during the first attack, when the ideal treatment would be operative repair of the torn medial structures. Usually the patella has been reduced and a backslab applied. Treatment then should concentrate on strengthening the quadriceps (especially vastus medialis). As the patient grows older the extensor mechanism often becomes more stable.

If conservative measures fail to prevent repeated dislocation, operation is necessary.

The principle of operative treatment is to produce realignment of the extensor mechanism to a mechanically more favourable angle of pull. This can be achieved in several ways (see Fig. 20.24c–f).

SUPRAPATELLAR   REALIGNMENT   (Campbell–Roux)   A strip of the medial retinaculum is detached distally and fashioned into a sling which is passed over and through the quadriceps tendon and reattached firmly on the medial side. A lateral capsular release may be performed at the same time.

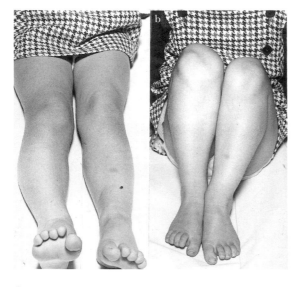

20.22 Habitual dislocation   (a) With the knees extended the patellae are in their normal position, but (b) every time they are flexed the right patella displaces laterally.

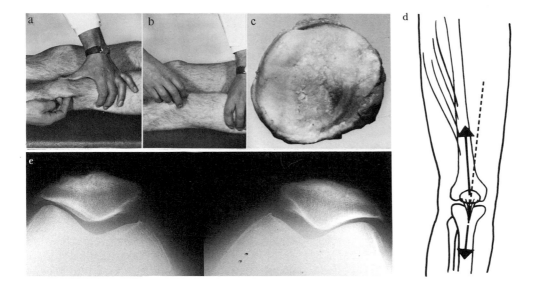

20.23 Patellofemoral overload and chondromalacia (a–c) Chondromalacia, with (a) tenderness of the posterior aspect of the patella, (b) pain on patellar friction and (c) softening and irregulatirty of the articular surface. (d) The Q angle, between the line of the patellar ligament and the line of pull of the quadriceps. (e) The skyline view shows lateral tilting of the patella, worse on the left than the right.

INFRAPATELLAR SOFT-TISSUE REALIGNMENT (Goldthwait) The lateral half of the patellar ligament is detached, threaded under the medial half and reattached more medially and distally. This operation is seldom used by itself but may be combined with suprapatellar realignment.

INFRAPATELLAR BONY REALIGNMENT (Hauser) The patellar ligament with the segment of bone into which it is inserted is freed and reattached more medially and distally. There is a danger that this may tighten the extensor mechanism too much and so limit flexion; careful placement of the transposed bone-block is essential, and this should include slight elevation of the new point of attachment (Noll, Ben-Itzhak and Rossouw, 1988).

PATELLECTOMY Occasionally the patellofemoral cartilage is so damaged that patellectomy is indicated, but this operation should be avoided if possible. There is a small risk that after patellectomy the patellar tendon may continue to dislocate and require realignment by the Hauser technique.

Recurrent subluxation

Recurrent subluxation of the patella is more common than usually supposed. The apprehension test is usually positive and chondromalacia may supervene. Treatment is the same as for recurrent dislocation.

Other types of non-traumatic dislocation

Congenital dislocation, in which the patella is permanently displaced, is fortunately very rare. Reconstructive procedures, such as semitendinosus tenodesis, have been tried but the results are unpredictable.

Habitual dislocation differs from recurrent dislocation in that the patella dislocates every time the knee is bent and reduces each time it is straightened. In long-standing cases the patella may be permanently dislocated.

The probable cause is *contracture of the quadriceps*, which may be congenital or may result from repeated injections (usually antibiotics) into the muscle. The contracture may lead to progressive loss of knee flexion or to habitual dislocation of the patella.

Treatment requires lengthening of the quadriceps. With habitual dislocation, any bands in the vastus lateralis, iliotibial tract and rectus femoris also need to be divided (Bergman and Williams, 1988).

Patellofemoral overload (patellar pain syndrome; chondromalacia of the patella)

The syndrome of anterior knee pain and patellofemoral tenderness is common among active adolescents and young adults. It is often (but not invariably) associated with softening and fibrillation of the articular surface of the patella – *chondromalacia patellae*. Having no other pathological label, orthopaedic surgeons have tended to regard chondromalacia as the cause (rather than one of the effects) of the disorder. Against this are the facts that (1) chondromalacia is commonly found at arthroscopy in young adults who have no anterior knee pain, and (2) some patients with the typical clinical syndrome have no cartilage softening.

CAUSES OF ANTERIOR KNEE PAIN

1. Patellofemoral overload
2. Overuse in athletes
3. 'Jump' knee
4. Patellofemoral subluxation
5. Bipartite patella
6. Patellar cysts or tumours
7. Prepatellar bursitis
8. Plica syndrome
9. Osteochondritis dissecans
10. Discoid meniscus
11. Torn meniscus

Pathogenesis and pathology

The basic disorder is probably mechanical overload of the patellofemoral joint. Rarely, a single injury (sudden impact on the front of the knee) may damage the articular surfaces. Much more common is repetitive overload due to either (1) *malcongruence* of the patellofemoral surfaces because of some abnormal shape of the patella or intercondylar groove or (2) *malalignment* of the extensor mechanism, or weakness of the vastus medialis, which causes the patella to tilt, or subluxate, or bear more heavily on one facet than the other during flexion and extension (Wiberg, 1941; Outerbridge, 1961; Ficat and Hungerford, 1977; Larson, 1979; Annotation, 1981). 'Overload' as used here means either direct stress on a load-bearing facet or sheer stresses in the depths of the articular cartilage at the boundary between high-contact and low-contact areas (Goodfellow et al., 1976).

Patellofemoral overload leads to changes in both the articular cartilage and the subchondral bone, not necessarily of parallel degree. Thus, the cartilage may look normal and show only biochemical changes such as overhydration or loss of proteoglycans, while the underlying bone shows reactive vascular congestion (a potent cause of pain). Or there may be obvious cartilage softening and fibrillation, with or without subarticular intraosseous hypertension. This would account for the variable relationship between (1) malalignment syndrome, (2) cartilage softening, (3) subchondral vascular congestion and (4) anterior knee pain.

Cartilage fibrillation usually occurs on the medial patellar facet or the median ridge, remains confined to the superficial zones and generally heals spontaneously (Bentley, 1985). Thus it is not a precursor of osteoarthritis in later life. Occasionally the lateral facet is involved – Ficat's 'hyperpression zone' syndrome – and this may well be progressive (Ficat and Hungerford, 1977).

Clinical features

The patient, often a teenage girl or an athletic young adult, complains of pain over the front of the knee or 'underneath the knee-cap'. Occasionally there is a history of injury or recurrent

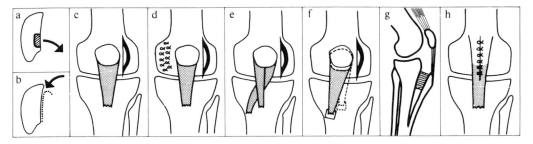

20.24 Chrondromalacia patellae – treatment   (a) Excison of diseased area; (b) 'shaving'; (c) incision of lateral capsule (release); (d) lateral release and medial reefing; (e) release and transfer of part of tendon (Goldthwait); (f) release and transfer of entire extensor insertion (Hauser); (g) tibial tubercle advancement; (h) patellectomy.

displacement. Symptoms are aggravated by activity or climbing stairs, or when standing up after prolonged sitting. The knee may give way and occasionally swells. It sometimes 'catches' but this is not true locking. Often both knees are affected.

At first sight the knee looks normal but careful examination may reveal malalignment or 'squinting' of the patellae. One way of gauging alignment is to measure the quadriceps angle, or Q-angle – the angle subtended by the line of quadriceps pull and the line of the patellar ligament; this should not exceed 20 degrees.

Other signs include quadriceps wasting, fluid in the knee, tenderness under the edge of the patella and crepitus on moving the knee.

Patellofemoral pain is elicited by pressing the patella against the femur and asking the patient to contract the quadriceps – first with central pressure, then compressing the medial facet and then the lateral. If, in addition, the apprehension test is positive, this suggests previous subluxation or dislocation.

Patellar tracking can be observed with the patient seated on the edge of the couch, flexing and extending the knee against resistance; in some cases subluxation is obvious.

Lastly, the structures around the knee are carefully examined for other sources of pain, and the hip is examined to exclude referred pain.

X-RAYS should include skyline views of the patella, which may show abnormal tilting or subluxation, and a lateral view with the knee half-flexed to see if the patella is high or small. The most accurate way of showing and measuring patellofemoral malposition is by CT with the knee in full extension but with the thigh muscles relaxed (Inone et al., 1988).

ARTHROSCOPY can be confusing. Cartilage softening is common in asymptomatic knees, and painful knees may show no abnormality. However, it may be useful in excluding other causes of anterior knee pain (e.g. a plica syndrome).

Differential diagnosis

Other causes of anterior knee pain must be excluded before finally accepting the diagnosis of patellofemoral overload (see box 'Causes of anterior knee pain', earlier). Even then, the cause of 'overload' must be established: is it abnormal posture, overuse, patellar malalignment, subluxation or some abnormality in the shape of the bones?

Treatment

CONSERVATIVE MANAGEMENT In the vast majority of cases the patient will be helped by adjustment of stressful activities and physiotherapy, combined with reassurance that most patients recover without physiotherapy. Exercises are directed specifically at strengthening the medial quadriceps so as to counterbalance the tendency to lateral tilting or subluxation of the patella. Some patients respond to simple measures such as providing support for a valgus foot. Aspirin does no more than reduce pain, and corticosteroid injections should be avoided.

OPERATIVE TREATMENT should be considered only if (1) there is a demonstrable abnormality that is correctible by operation, or (2) conservative treatment has been tried for at least 6 months and (3) the patient is genuinely incapacitated. Operation is intended to improve patellar alignment and patellofemoral congruence, and to reduce patellofemoral pressure.

Lateral release may succeed in mild cases. The lateral part of the extensor retinaculum is divided, either open or arthroscopically.

Proximal realignment is achieved by a combined open release of the lateral retinaculum and reefing of the oblique part of the vastus medialis (Insall, Falvo and Wise, 1976).

Distal elevation of the patellar ligament reduces patellofemoral pressure. In Maquet's tibial tubercle advancement operation (1976) the tubercle, with the attached patellar ligament, is hinged forwards and held there with a bone-block. Some patients resent the bump on the front part of the tibia and the operation may substitute a new set of complaints for the old.

Distal realignment by the Hauser operation (see p. 447) may do more harm than good by increasing patellofemoral pressure; if it is done, the bone-block with the attached patellar ligament should be left proud so as to achieve a 'Maquet' effect (Noll, Ben-Itzhak and Rossouw, 1988).

Chondroplasty, or shaving of the patellar articular surface, is usually performed arthroscopically using a power tool. Soft and fibrillated cartilage is removed, in severe cases down to the level of subchondral bone; the hope is that it will be replaced by fibrocartilage. The operation should be followed by lavage and can be combined with any of the realignment procedures (Ogilvie-Harris and Jackson, 1984).

Patellectomy is a last resort, but patients with severe discomfort are grateful for the relief it brings after other operations have failed.

Osteochondritis dissecans

(see also Chapter 16)

A small, well-demarcated, avascular fragment of bone and overlying cartilage sometimes separates from one of the femoral condyles and appears as a loose body in the joint. The most likely cause is trauma, either a single impact with the edge of the patella or repeated microtrauma from contact with an adjacent tibial ridge. The fact that over 80% of lesions occur on the lateral part of the medial femoral condyle, exactly where the patella makes contact in full flexion, supports the first of these. There may also be some general predisposing factor, because several joints can be affected, or several members of one family. Lesions are bilateral in 25% of cases (Aichroth, 1971).

Pathology

The lower or lateral part of the medial femoral condyle is usually affected, rarely the lateral condyle, and still more rarely the patella. An area of subchondral bone becomes avascular and within this area an ovoid osteocartilaginous segment is demarcated from the surrounding bone. At first the overlying cartilage is intact and the fragment is stable; over a period of months the fragment separates but remains in position; finally the fragment breaks free to become a loose body in the joint. The small crater is slowly filled with fibrocartilage, leaving a depression on the articular surface.

Clinical features

The patient, usually a male aged 15–20 years, presents with intermittent ache or swelling. Later, there are attacks of giving way such that the knee feels unreliable, and locking may occur.

The quadriceps muscle is wasted and there may be a small effusion.

Soon after an attack there are two signs that are almost diagnostic: (1) tenderness localized to one femoral condyle; and (2) Wilson's sign – if the knee is flexed to 90 degrees, rotated

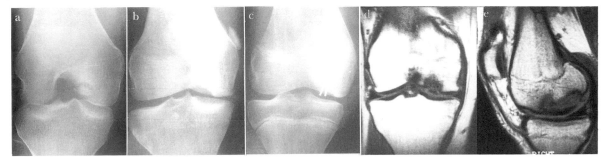

20.25 Osteochondritis dissecans At first the affected area separates ('dissects') but still remains in position. (a) The 'tunnel' view may be the most helpful. (b) The anteroposterior view shows the loose fragment and the crater on the medial femoral condyle from which it came. (c) Pinning the fragment back is one method of treatment. (d, e) MRI shows that the surrounding bone, too, is abnormal.

medially and then gradually straightened, pain is felt which is relieved by lateral rotation.

IMAGING Plain x-rays may show a line of demarcation around a lesion *in situ*, usually in the lateral part of the medial femoral condyle. This site is best displayed in special intercondylar (tunnel) views, but even then a small lesion or one situated far back may be missed. Once the fragment has become detached, the empty hollow may be seen – and possibly a loose body elsewhere in the joint.

Radionuclide scans show increased activity around the lesion, and *MRI* consistently shows an area of low signal intensity in the T1-weighted images; the adjacent bone may also appear abnormal, probably due to oedema. These investigations usually indicate whether the fragment is 'stable' or 'loose' (Mesgarzadeh et al., 1987).

ARTHROSCOPY With early lesions the articular surface looks intact, but probing may reveal that the cartilage is soft. Loose segments are easily visualized.

Differential diagnosis

Avascular necrosis of the femoral condyle – usually associated with corticosteroid therapy or alcohol abuse – may result in separation of a localized osteocartilaginous fragment. However, on x-ray the lesion is always on the dome of the femoral condyle, and this distinguishes it clearly from osteochondritis dissecans.

Treatment

For the purposes of management, it is useful to 'stage' the lesion; hence the importance of radionuclide scanning, MRI and arthroscopy.

In the earliest stage, when the cartilage is intact and the lesion 'stable', *no* treatment is needed but activities are curtailed for 6–12 months. Small lesions often heal spontaneously.

If the fragment is 'unstable' – i.e. surrounded by a clear boundary with sclerosis of the underlying bone, or showing MRI features of separation – treatment depends on the size of the lesion: a small fragment should be removed by arthroscopy and the base drilled; the bed will eventually be covered by fibrocartilage, leaving only a small defect. A large fragment (say more than 1 cm in diameter) should be fixed *in situ* with pins or Herbert screws. In addition, it may help to drill the underlying sclerotic bone to promote union of the necrotic fragment. For drilling, the area is approached from a point some distance away, beyond the articular cartilage.

If the fragment is completely detached but in one piece and shown to fit nicely in its bed, the crater is cleaned and the floor drilled before replacing the loose fragment and fixing it with Herbert screws. If the fragment is in pieces or ill-shaped, it is best discarded; the crater is drilled and allowed to fill with fibrocartilage.

Recent reports show that the osteochondral defect can be resurfaced with a woven carbon fibre pad (Muckle and Minns, 1990).

After any of the above operations the knee is held in a cast for 6 weeks; thereafter movement is encouraged but weightbearing is deferred until x-rays show signs of healing.

Loose bodies

The knee – relatively capacious, with large synovial folds – is a common haven for loose bodies. These may be produced by: (1) injury (a chip of bone or cartilage); (2) osteochondritis dissecans (which may produce one or two fragments); (3) osteoarthritis (pieces of cartilage or osteophyte); (4) Charcot's disease (large osteocartilaginous bodies); and (5) synovial chondromatosis (cartilage metaplasia in the synovium, sometimes producing hundreds of loose bodies).

Clinical features

Loose bodies may be symptomless. The usual complaint is attacks of sudden locking without injury. The joint gets stuck in a position which varies from one attack to another. Sometimes the locking is only momentary and usually the patient can wriggle the knee until it suddenly unlocks. The patient may be aware of something 'popping in and out of the joint'.

In adolescents, a loose body is usually due to osteochondritis dissecans, rarely to injury. In adults osteoarthritis is the most frequent cause.

Only rarely is the patient seen with the knee still locked. Sometimes, especially after the first attack, there is synovitis or there may be evidence of the underlying cause. A pedunculated loose body may be felt; one that is truly loose tends to slip away during palpation (the well-named 'joint mouse').

X-RAY Most loose bodies are radio-opaque. The films also show an underlying joint abnormality.

Treatment

A loose body causing symptoms should be removed unless the joint is severely osteoarthritic. This can usually be done through the arthroscope, but finding the loose body may be difficult; it may be concealed in a synovial pouch or sulcus and a small body may even slip under the edge of one of the menisci.

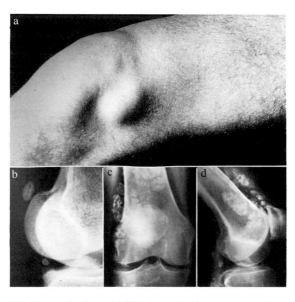

20.26 Loose bodies   (a) This loose body slipped away from the fingers when touched; the term 'joint mouse' seems appropriate. (b) Which is the loose body here? – not the large one (which is a fabella), but the small lower one opposite the joint line. (c, d) Synovial chondromatosis – the multiple loose bodies are characteristic.

Synovial chondromatosis

This is a rare disorder in which the joint comes to contain multiple loose bodies, often in pearly clumps resembling sago ('snowstorm knee'). The usual explanation is that myriad tiny fronds undergo cartilage metaplasia at their tips; these tips break free and may ossify. It has, however, been suggested that chondrocytes may be cultured in the synovial fluid and that some of the products are then deposited onto previously normal synovium, so producing the familiar appearance (Kay, Freemont and Davies, 1989). X-rays reveal multiple loose bodies; on arthrography they show as negative defects.

TREATMENT The loose bodies should be removed. At the same time any patch of abnormal synovium should be carefully excised.

The plica syndrome

A plica is the remnant of an embryonic synovial partition which persists into adult life. During development of the embryo, the knee is divided into three cavities – a large suprapatellar pouch and beneath this the medial and lateral compartments – separated from each other by membranous septa. Later these partitions disappear, leaving a single cavity. But part of a septum may persist as a synovial pleat or plica (from the Latin *plicare* = fold). This is found in over 20% of people, usually as a *median infrapatellar fold* (the ligamentum mucosum), less often as a *suprapatellar curtain* draped across the opening of the suprapatellar pouch or a *mediopatellar plica* sweeping down the medial wall of the joint.

Pathology

The plica in itself is not pathological. But if acute trauma, repetitive strain or some underlying disorder (e.g. a meniscal tear) causes inflammation, the plica may become oedematous, thickened and eventually fibrosed; it then acts as a tight bowstring impinging on other structures in the joint and causing further synovial irritation.

Clinical features

An adolescent or young adult complains of an ache in the front of the knee (occasionally both knees), with intermittent episodes of clicking or 'giving way'. There may be a history of trauma or markedly increased activity. Symptoms are aggravated by exercise or climbing stairs, especially if this follows a long period of sitting.

On examination there may be muscle wasting and a small effusion. The most characteristic feature is tenderness near the upper pole of the patella and over the femoral condyle. Occasionally the thickened band can be felt. Movement of the knee may cause catching or snapping.

ARTHROSCOPY is the definitive way of showing the lesion and dealing with it at the same time.

Diagnosis

The plica syndrome is one cause of anterior knee pain. It may closely resemble other conditions such as patellar overload or subluxation; indeed, the plica may become troublesome only when those other conditions are present, or it may itself predispose to patellar malalignment and chondromalacia (Hardaker, Whipple and Bassett, 1980).

Treatment

The first line of treatment is rest, anti-inflammatory drugs and adjustment of activities. If symptoms persist, the plica can be divided or excised by arthroscopy.

Swelling of the knee – acute

Swelling *of* the knee must be distinguished from swellings *around* the knee (enlarged bursae, soft-tissue tumours, cysts or tumours of the bones). If the joint is swollen, the following disorders must be considered.

Haemarthrosis

Swelling immediately after injury means blood in the joint. The knee is very painful and it feels warm, tense and tender. Later there may be a 'doughy' feel. Movements are restricted. X-rays are essential to see if there is a fracture.

TREATMENT The joint should be aspirated under aseptic conditions. If a ligament injury is suspected, examination under anaesthesia is helpful and may indicate the need for operation; otherwise a crepe bandage is applied and the leg cradled in a back-splint. Quadriceps exercises are practised from the start. The patient may get up when comfortable, retaining the back-splint until muscle control returns.

Bleeding disorders The knee is the most common site for acute bleeds. The patient usually knows when this has happened. If the appropriate clotting factor is available, the knee should be aspirated and treated as for a traumatic haemarthrosis. If the factor is not available, aspiration is best avoided; the knee is splinted in slight flexion until the swelling subsides.

Acute septic arthritis

Acute pyogenic infection of the knee is not uncommon. The organism is usually *Staphylococcus aureus*, but in adults gonococcal infection is almost as .common. The joint is swollen, painful and inflamed; the white cell count and ESR are elevated. Aspiration reveals pus in the joint; fluid should be sent for bacteriological investigation, including anaerobic culture. Treatment consists of systemic antibiotics and drainage of the joint – either open or by arthroscopy and irrigation; if fluid reaccumulates, it can be aspirated through a wide-bore needle. As the inflammation subsides, movement is begun, but weightbearing is deferred for 4–6 weeks.

Traumatic synovitis

Injury stimulates a reactive synovitis; typically the swelling appears only after some hours, and subsides spontaneously over a period of days. There is inhibition of quadriceps action and the thigh wastes. The knee may need to be splinted for several days but movement should be encouraged and quadriceps exercise is essential. If the amount of fluid is considerable, its aspiration hastens muscle recovery. In addition, any internal injury will need treatment.

Aseptic non-traumatic synovitis

Acute swelling, without a history of trauma or signs of infection, suggests gout or pseudogout. Aspiration will provide fluid which may look turbid, resembling pus, but it is sterile and microscopy (using polarized light) reveals the crystals. Treatment with anti-inflammatory drugs is normally effective.

Swelling of the knee – chronic

Chronic swelling is usually due to tuberculosis, rheumatoid arthritis or osteoarthritis; less common causes are pigmented villondular synovitis (see p. 188) and Charcot's disease.

Tuberculosis (see also Chapter 2)

Tuberculosis of the knee may appear at any age, but it is more common in children than in adults.

Clinical features

Pain and limp are early symptoms; or the child may present with a swollen joint. The thigh muscles are wasted, thus accentuating the joint swelling. The knee feels warm and there is synovial thickening. Movements are restricted and often painful. The Mantoux test is positive and the erythrocyte sedimentation rate may be increased.

X-rays show marked osteoporosis and, in children, enlargement of the bony epiphyses. In late cases the joint surfaces are eroded.

Diagnosis Monarticular rheumatoid synovitis, or juvenile chronic arthritis, may closely resemble tuberculosis. A synovial biopsy may be necessary to establish the diagnosis.

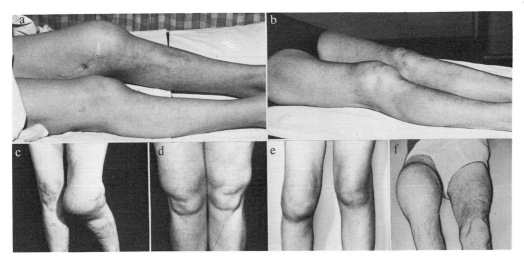

20.27 Swollen knees   Some causes of chronic swelling in the absence of trauma: (a) tuberculous arthritis; (b) rheumatoid arthritis; (c) Charcot's disease; (d) villous synovitis; (e) haemophilia; (f) malignant synovioma.

Treatment

General antituberculous chemotherapy should be given for 3–6 months (see p. 49).

In the active stage the knee is rested in a Thomas' bed knee splint. The synovitis usually subsides, but if it does not the diseased tissue may have to be excised. Bone abscesses should be evacuated.

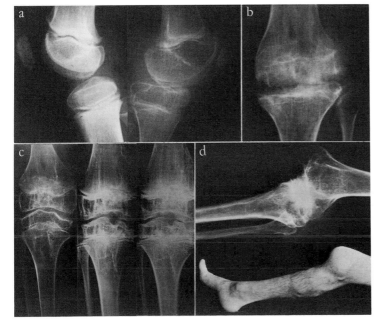

20.28 Tuberculosis – clinical and x-ray   In synovitis (a) the bones are rare and the epiphyses enlarged compared with the normal side; (b) arthritis.

(c) Series showing healing with recalcification, but with joint destruction. (d) The aftermath of arthritis.

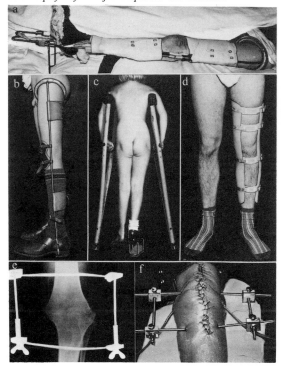

20.29 Tuberculosis – treatment (a) Active disease – traction on a Thomas' splint.
Healing disease: (b) weight-relieving caliper; (c) patten and crutches; (d) removable polythene splint.
(e, f) Arthrodesis in the aftermath stage (Charnley's method).

IN THE HEALING STAGE   the patient is allowed up wearing a weight-relieving caliper. Gradually this is left off, but the patient is kept under observation for any sign of recurrent inflammation. If the articular cartilage has been spared, movement can be encouraged and weight-bearing is slowly resumed. However, if the articular surface is destroyed, immobilization is continued until the joint stiffens.

In the aftermath   the joint may be painful; it is then best arthrodesed, but in children this is usually postponed until growth is almost completed. In some cases, once it is certain that the disease is quiescent, joint replacement may be feasible (Eskola et al., 1988).

Rheumatoid arthritis

(see also Chapter 3)

Occasionally, rheumatoid arthritis starts in the knee as a chronic monarticular synovitis. Sooner or later, however, other joints become involved.

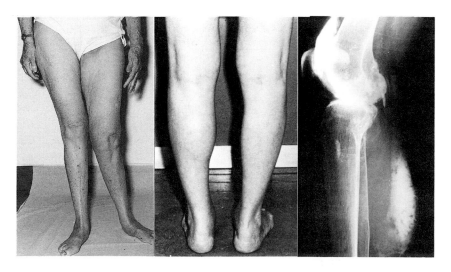

20.30 Rheumatoid arthritis   (a) The typical deformity: slight flexion, valgus and external rotation. (b, c) Sometimes the patient presents with pain and swelling in the calf ('pseudothrombosis'); the arthrogram shows that the capsule has ruptured and fluid has extruded into the calf.

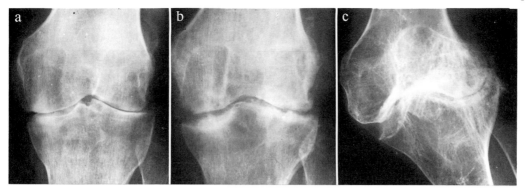

20.31 Rheumatoid arthritis (a) Early changes are cartilage erosion (giving a narrow joint space) and osteoporosis. (b) Later, joint destruction becomes more obvious, and (c) in severe cases gross deformity may result.

Clinical features

DURING STAGE 1 (SYNOVITIS) the patient complains of pain and chronic swelling. There is some wasting, there may be a large effusion and the thickened synovium is easily palpable. At this stage, while the joint is still stable and the muscles are reasonably strong, there is a danger of rupturing the posterior capsule; the joint contents are extruded into a large posterior bursa or between the muscle planes of the calf, causing sudden pain and swelling which closely mimic the features of calf vein thrombosis.

IN STAGE 2 there is increasing instability of the joint, muscle wasting is marked and there is some loss of flexion and extension. X-rays may show loss of joint space and marginal erosions; the condition is easily distinguishable from osteoarthritis by the complete absence of osteophytes, but in the monarticular variety biopsy may be needed to exclude tuberculosis.

IN STAGE 3 pain and disability are usually severe. In some patients stiffness is so marked that the patient has to be helped to stand and the joint has only a jog of painful movement. In others, cartilage and bone destruction predominate and the joint becomes increasingly unstable and deformed. The commonest deformities are fixed flexion and valgus; abnormal mobility (increased anteroposterior glide and lateral wobble) is present. X-rays reveal the bone destruction characteristic of advanced disease.

Treatment

In addition to general treatment, local splintage and injection of methylprednisolone and nitrogen mustard usually reduce the synovitis promptly; a more prolonged effect may be obtained by injecting radiocolloids such as yttrium-90 (^{90}Y). The majority of patients can be managed by conservative measures.

OPERATIVE TREATMENT

SYNOVECTOMY Only if other measures fail to control the synovitis (which nowadays is rare) is synovectomy indicated. This can be done very effectively by arthroscopy. Postoperatively, any haematoma must be drained and movements are commenced as soon as pain has subsided.

SUPRACONDYLAR OSTEOTOMY Marked valgus deformity in a reasonably stable knee is best dealt with by supracondylar osteotomy (an associated flexion deformity can be corrected at the same time). The bones are held by internal fixation, fortified by external plaster splintage for 4–6 weeks; thereafter, movement is encouraged but full weightbearing is allowed only when union is secure.

ARTHROPLASTY Total joint replacement is useful when joint destruction is advanced. However, it is less successful if the knee has been allowed to become very unstable or very stiff; consequently, timing of the operation is most important.

Osteoarthritis (see also Chapter 5)

The knee is the commonest of the large joints to be affected by osteoarthritis. Often there is a predisposing factor: injury to the articular surface, a torn meniscus, ligamentous instability or pre-existing deformity of the hip or knee, to mention a few. However, in many cases no obvious cause can be found.

Osteoarthritis is often bilateral and there is a strong association with Heberden's nodes.

Pathology

Cartilage breakdown usually starts in an area of excessive loading. Thus, with long-standing varus the changes are most marked in the medial compartment. The characteristic features of cartilage fibrillation, sclerosis of the subchondral bone and peripheral osteophyte formation are usually present; in advanced cases the articular surface may be denuded of cartilage and underlying bone may eventually crumble.

Chondrocalcinosis is common, but whether this is cause or effect – or quite unrelated – remains unknown.

Clinical features

Patients are usually over 50 years old; they tend to be overweight and may have long-standing bow-leg deformity.

Pain is the leading symptom, worse after use, or (if the patellofemoral joint is affected) on stairs. After rest, the joint feels stiff and it hurts to 'get going' after sitting for any length of time. Swelling is common, and giving way or locking may occur.

On examination there may be an obvious deformity or the scar of a previous operation. The quadriceps muscle is usually wasted.

Except during an exacerbation, there is little fluid and no warmth; nor is the synovial membrane thickened. Movement is somewhat limited and is often accompanied by patello-femoral crepitus.

It is useful to test movement applying first a varus and then a valgus force to the knee; pain indicates which tibiofemoral compartment is involved. Pressure on the patella may elicit pain.

X-RAY The tibiofemoral joint space is diminished (often only in one compartment) and there is subchondral sclerosis. The true extent of tibiofemoral narrowing can be demonstrated only by an anteroposterior x-ray with the patient bearing weight. Osteophytes are usually present and sometimes there is soft-tissue calcification in the suprapatellar region or in the joint itself (chrondrocalcinosis).

If only the patellofemoral joint is affected, suspect a pyrophosphate arthropathy.

Treatment

If symptoms are not severe, treatment is conservative. Quadriceps exercises are important.

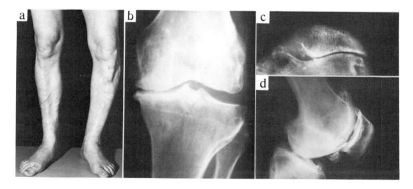

20.32 Osteoarthritis of the knee   (a, b) Varus deformity and degeneration on the medial side. (c, d) Sometimes it is the patellofemoral joint that is mainly affected.

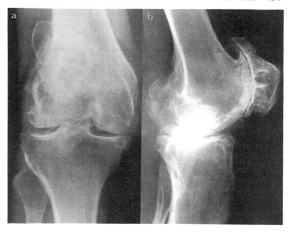

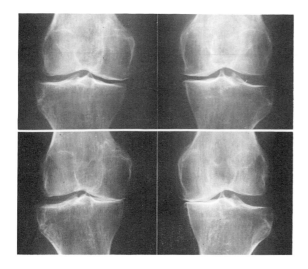

20.33 Osteoarthritis – x-rays The upper films, taken with the patient lying on the x-ray couch, show only slight narrowing of the medial joint space; but with weightbearing, as in the lower films, it is clear that the changes are considerable.

20.34 Patellofemoral osteoarthritis Osteoarthritis mainly in the patellofemoral joint suggests pyrophosphate arthropathy. This patient had other characteristic features: (a) chondrocalcinosis and periarticular ossification; and (b) large trailing osteophytes around the patella.

Analgesics are prescribed for pain, and warmth (e.g. radiant heat or shortwave diathermy) is soothing., A simple elastic support may do wonders, probably by improving proprioception in an unstable knee.

Intra-articular corticosteroid injections will often relieve pain, but this is a stopgap – and not a very good one, because repeated injections may permit (or even predispose to) progressive cartilage and bone destruction.

OPERATIVE TREATMENT Persistent pain, progressive deformity and instability are the usual indications for operative treatment.

Arthroscopic washouts, with trimming of degenerate meniscal tissue and osteophytes, may give temporary relief; this is a useful measure when there are contraindications to reconstructive surgery.

Patellectomy is indicated only in those rare

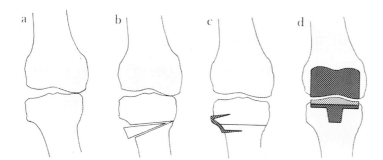

20.35 Osteoarthritis – treatment (a) Medial compartment damage can be treated by wedge osteotomy of the tibia (b, c), which produces a redistribution of stress on the articular surfaces. In more advanced cases, joint replacement of one or both compartments (d) may be more appropriate.

cases where osteoarthritis is strictly confined to the patellofemoral joint. If the tibiofemoral joint is stable, the results are gratifying.

Realignment osteotomy is often successful in relieving symptoms and staving off the need for 'end-stage' surgery. The ideal indication is a 'young' patient (under 50 years) with a varus knee and osteoarthritis confined to the medial compartment: a high tibial valgus osteotomy will redistribute weight to the lateral side of the joint.

Replacement arthroplasty is indicated in older patients with progressive joint destruction. This is usually a 'resurfacing' procedure, with a metal femoral condylar component and a metal-backed polyethylene table on the tibial side. If the disease is largely confined to one compartment, a unicompartmental replacement can be done as an alternative to osteotomy. With modern techniques, and meticulous attention to anatomical alignment of the knee, the results of replacement arthroplasty are excellent.

Arthrodesis is indicated only if there is a strong contraindication to arthroplasty (e.g. previous sepsis) or to salvage a failed arthroplasty.

Osteonecrosis (see also Chapter 6)

'Idiopathic' osteonecrosis of the knee, though not as common as femoral head necrosis, has the same aetiological and pathogenetic background (see p. 92). The usual site is one of the femoral condyles, but occasionally the medial tibial condyle is affected. Corticosteroid therapy and alcohol abuse are the commonest precipitating agents, but sometimes (especially in elderly people) the condition seems to occur 'spontaneously' (Ahlback, Bauer and Bohnc, 1968; Muheim and Bohne, 1970).

Clinical features

Patients are usually over 60 years old and women are affected twice as often as men.

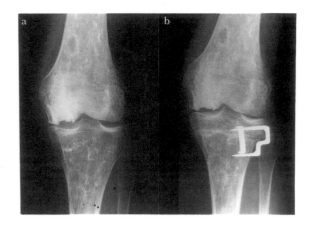

20.36 Osteonecrosis (a) The necrotic segment is always on the highest part of the femoral condyle. (b) The medial femoral condyle can be unloaded by a high tibial valgus osteotomy.

Typically they give a history of sudden, acute pain on the medial side of the joint. Pain at rest also is common.

On examination there is often an effusion; the classic feature is tenderness on pressure upon the medial femoral or tibial condyle rather than along the joint line proper.

X-RAY is often unimpressive at the beginning, but a radionuclide scan will usually show increased activity on the medial side of the joint. Later the classic radiographic features of osteonecrosis appear (see p. 96). On the femoral side, it is always the dome of the condyle that is affected, unlike the picture in osteochondritis dissecans.

Progress is variable. Symptoms and signs may stabilize and the patient be left with no more than slight distortion of the articular surface; or one of the condyles may collapse, leading to osteoarthritis of the affected compartment.

Treatment

Treatment is conservative in the first instance and consists of measures to reduce loading of the joint and analgesics for pain. If symptoms or signs increase, operative treatment may be considered: if only one compartment is involved, a realignment osteotomy may redistribute load from this area to an intact part of the joint (e.g. a valgus tibial osteotomy for medial femoral condyle necrosis). With advanced bone collapse, replacement arthroplasty (uni- or bicompartmental) will be required.

Charcot's disease (see also Chapter 5)

Charcot's disease (neuropathic arthritis) is a rare cause of joint destruction. Because of loss of pain sensibility and proprioception, the articular surface breaks down and the underlying bone crumbles. Fragments of bone and cartilage are deposited in the hypertrophic synovium and may grow into large masses. The capsule is stretched and lax, and the joint becomes progressively unstable.

Clinical features

The patient chiefly complains of instability; pain (other than tabetic lightning pains) is unusual. The joint is swollen and often grossly deformed. It feels like a bag of bones and fluid but is neither warm nor tender. Movements beyond the normal limits, without pain, are a notable feature. Radiologically the joint is subluxated, bone destruction is obvious and irregular calcified masses can be seen.

Treatment

Patients often seem to manage quite well despite the bizarre appearances. However, marked instability may demand treatment – usually a moulded splint or caliper will do – and occasionally pain becomes intolerable. Arthrodesis is feasible but fixation is difficult and fusion is very slow.

Haemophilic arthritis

(see also Chapter 5)

The knee is the joint most commonly involved in bleeding disorders. Repeated haemorrhage leads to chronic synovitis and articular cartilage erosion. Movement is progressively restricted and the joint may end up deformed and stiff.

Clinical features

Fresh bleeds cause pain and swelling of the knee, with the typical clinical signs of a haemarthrosis (see p. 89). Between episodes of bleeding the knee often continues to be painful and somewhat swollen, with restricted mobility. There is a tendency to hold the knee in flexion and this may become a fixed deformity.

X-RAYS may show little abnormality, apart from local osteoporosis. In more advanced cases the joint space is narrowed and large 'cysts' or erosions may appear in the subchondral bone.

Treatment

Both the haematologist and the orthopaedic surgeon should participate in treatment. The acute bleed may need aspiration, but only if this can be 'covered' by giving the appropriate clotting factor; otherwise it is better treated by splintage until the acute symptoms settle down.

Flexion deformity must be prevented by gentle physiotherapy and intermittent splintage. If the joint is painful and eroded, operative treatment may be considered. However, although replacement arthroplasty is feasible, this should be done only after the most searching discussion with the patient, where all the risks are considered, and only if a full haematological service is available.

Injuries of the extensor apparatus

Resisted extension of the knee may tear the extensor mechanism. The patient stumbles on a stair, catches his foot while walking or running, or may only be kicking a muddy football. In all these incidents, active knee extension is pre-

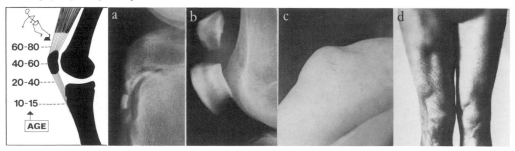

20.37 Extensor mechanism lesions   These follow resisted action of the quadriceps; they usually occur at a progressively higher level with increasing age (diagram). (a) Schlatter's disease – the only one that usually does not follow a definite accident; (b) gap fracture of patella; (c) ruptured quadriceps tendon (note the suprapatellar depression); (d) ruptured rectus femoris causing a lump with a hollow below.

vented by an obstacle. The precise location of the lesion varies with the patient's age. In the elderly the injury is usually above the patella; in middle life the patella fractures; in young adults the patellar ligament can rupture. In adolescents the upper tibial apophysis is occasionally avulsed; much more often it is merely 'strained'.

Rupture above the patella

Rupture may occur in the belly of the rectus femoris. The patient is usually elderly, or on long-term corticosteroid treatment. The torn muscle retracts and forms a characteristic lump in the thigh. Function is usually good, so no treatment is required.

Occasionally a similar injury, but at the musculotendinous junction, occurs in young athletes. If it is diagnosed early, suture is probably advisable, or athletic prowess is likely to be reduced.

Avulsion of the quadriceps tendon from the upper pole of the patella is seen in elderly people and in patients with connective tissue disorders on corticosteroid therapy. Sometimes it is bilateral. Operative repair is essential.

Fracture of the patella

Transverse fracture of the patella occurs in middle life. The patella should be repaired, but the essential is reconstruction of the extensor mechanism, including suture of the torn quadriceps expansion.

Rupture below the patella

This occurs mainly in young people. The ligament may rupture or may be avulsed from the lower pole of the patella. Operative repair is necessary. Pain and tenderness in the middle portion of the patellar ligament may occur in athletes; CT or ultrasonography will reveal an abnormal area. If rest fails to provide relief the paratenon should be stripped (King et al., 1990).

In Johansson–Larsen's disease   the patellar ligament is partially avulsed from the lower pole of the patella; a traction tendinitis develops, usually with calcification. The condition is comparable to Osgood–Schlatter's disease (see below) and usually recovers with rest. A similar condition has been described at the proximal pole of the patella.

Osgood–Schlatter's disease ('apophysitis' of the tibial tubercle)

In this common disorder of adolescence the tibial tubercle becomes painful and 'swollen'. Although often called osteochondritis or apophysitis, it is nothing more than a traction injury of the apophysis into which part of the patellar tendon is inserted (the remainder is inserted on each side of the apophysis and prevents complete separation).

There is no history of injury and sometimes the condition is bilateral. A young adolescent complains of pain after activity, and of a lump. The lump is tender and its situation over the tibial tuberosity is diagnostic. Sometimes active extension of the knee against resistance is painful and x-rays may reveal fragmentation of the apophysis.

Spontaneous recovery is usual but takes time, and it is wise to restrict such activities as cycling and soccer. Occasionally, symptoms persist and, if patience or wearing a back-splint during the day are unavailing, a separate ossicle in the tendon is usually responsible; its removal is then worthwhile.

Calcification and ossification around the knee

Calcification in the medial ligament

Acute pain in the medial collateral ligament may be due to a soft calcific deposit among the fibres of the ligament. There may be a small, exquisitely tender lump in the line of the ligament. Pain is dramatically relieved by operative evacuation of the deposit.

Pellegrini–Stieda disease

X-rays sometimes show a plaque of bone lying next to the femoral condyle under the medial collateral ligament. Occasionally this is a source of pain. It is generally ascribed to ossification of a haematoma following a tear of the medial ligament, though a history of injury is not always forthcoming. Treatment is rarely needed.

Bursitis

Prepatellar bursitis (housemaid's knee)

An uninfected bursitis is due not to pressure but to constant friction between skin and patella. It occurs in carpet layers and miners but rarely in housemaids, who use vacuum cleaners. The swelling is circumscribed and fluctuant but the joint itself is normal. Treatment consists of firm bandaging, and kneeling is avoided; occasionally aspiration is needed. In chronic cases the lump is best excised.

Infection (possibly due to foreign body implantation) results in a warm, tender swelling. Treatment is by rest, antibiotics and, if necessary, aspiration or incision.

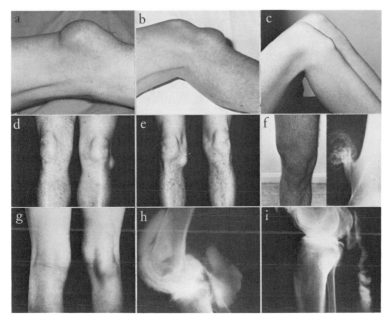

20.38 Lumps around the knee In front: (a) prepatellar bursa; (b) infrapatellar bursa; (c) Schlatter's disease.

On either side: (d) cyst of lateral meniscus; (e) cyst of medial meniscus; (f) cartilage-capped exostosis.

Behind: (g) semimembranosus bursa; (h) arthrogram of popliteal cyst; (i) leaking cyst.

Infrapatellar bursitis (clergyman's knee)

The swelling is superficial to the patellar ligament, being more distally placed than pre-patellar bursitis because one who prays kneels more uprightly than one who scrubs. Treatment is similar to that for prepatellar bursitis. Occasionally the bursa is affected in gout or syphilis.

Semimembranosus bursa

The bursa between the semimembranosus and the medial head of gastrocnemius may become enlarged in children or adults. It presents usually as a painless lump behind the knee, slightly to the medial side of the midline and most conspicuous with the knee straight. The lump is fluctuant but the fluid cannot be pushed into the joint, presumably because the muscles compress and obstruct the normal communication. The knee joint is normal. Occasionally the lump aches, and if so it may be excised through a transverse incision. However, recurrence is common and, as the bursa normally disappears in time, a waiting policy is perhaps wiser.

Two other swellings behind the knee may be confused with an enlarged semimembranosus bursa: a popliteal cyst and a popliteal aneurysm.

Popliteal cyst

This follows synovial rupture or herniation, so the joint itself is abnormal; it may be osteoarthritic (the term 'Baker's cyst' is then used) or, more commonly, rheumatoid. The lump is in the midline of the limb and below the joint line. It fluctuates but is not tender. It may diminish following aspiration and injection of hydrocortisone; excision is not advised, because recurrence is common unless the underlying condition also is treated (e.g. by synovectomy).

The cyst may leak or rupture; fluid then tracks down the calf, which becomes swollen and tender, mimicking a calf vein thrombosis.

POPLITEAL ANEURYSM This is the commonest limb aneurysm and is sometimes bilateral. Pain and stiffness of the knee may precede the symptoms of peripheral arterial disease, so it is essential to examine any lump behind the knee for pulsation. A thrombosed popliteal aneurysm does not pulsate, but it feels almost solid.

Principles of knee operations

Arthroscopy

Arthroscopy is useful: (1) to establish or refine the accuracy of diagnosis; (2) to help in deciding whether to operate, or to plan the operative approach with more precision; (3) to observe and record photographically the progress of a knee disorder; and (4) to perform certain operative procedures. Arthroscopy is not a substitute for clinical examination; a detailed history and meticulous assessment of the physical signs are indispensable preliminaries and remain the sheet anchor of diagnosis.

TECHNIQUE Full asepsis in an operating theatre is essential.

The patient is anaesthetized (though local anaesthesia may suffice for short procedures) and a thigh tourniquet applied. Saline is injected into the joint and, through a tiny incision, a trocar and cannula introduced. Penetration of synovium is recognized by the flow of saline when the trocar is withdrawn. A fibreoptic viewer, light source and irrigation system are attached; a small television camera and monitor make it much easier for the operator to concentrate on manipulating the instruments with both hands ('triangulation'). All compartments of the joint are now systematically inspected; with special instruments and, if necessary, through multiple portals, biopsy, partial meniscectomy, patellar shaving, removal of loose bodies, synovectomy, ligament replacement and many other procedures are possible. Before withdrawing the instrument, saline is squeezed out. A skin stitch is inserted and a firm bandage applied. Postoperative recovery is remarkably rapid.

COMPLICATIONS Intra-articular effusions and small haemarthroses are fairly common but seldom troublesome.

Infection has been reported as a complication in 1–2% of patients, particularly after the use of powered instruments; in such cases it is wise to use prophylactic antibiotics.

Reflex sympathetic dystrophy (which may resemble a low-grade infection during the weeks following arthroscopy) is sometimes troublesome. It usually settles down with physiotherapy and treatment with non-steroidal anti-inflammatory drugs; occasionally it requires more radical treatment (see p. 240).

Osteotomy

Osteotomy may be carried out either above or below the knee. As a general rule, and for sound biomechanical reasons, a valgus osteotomy (i.e. to correct a varus deformity) is best done through the proximal end of the tibia whereas a varus osteotomy (to correct a valgus deformity) is more effective at the femoral supracondylar level (Maquet, 1976).

RATIONALE Osteotomy aims to divide the bone and reposition the fragments, either in order to correct an existing deformity or to alter the load-bearing mechanics of the joint. It may also relieve intraosseous venous congestion.

INDICATIONS Varus or valgus deformity, hyperextension or fixed flexion may result from a variety of conditions; growth defects, epiphyseal injuries, malunited fractures, articular destruction due to arthritis, or stretched ligaments. In these cases the operation is indicated primarily for the correction of deformity, though it may also prevent or delay the development of osteoarthritis.

Osteoarthritis is often associated with varus deformity, and medial compartment overload causes localized pain and progressive destruction of the articular surfaces in one-half of the joint. When this occurs in a relatively young patient, and provided the joint has a reasonable range of movement and is still stable, a high tibial valgus osteotomy offers a reasonable alternative to a hemiarthroplasty. By realigning the joint, load is transferred from the medial compartment to the centre or towards the lateral side. The reduction of pain may, to some extent, be due to decompression of the hypervascular subchondral bone.

TECHNIQUE Angles must be accurately measured and the position of correction carefully calculated before starting the operation. In a high tibial osteotomy the fibula must be released either by dividing it lower down or by disrupting the proximal tibiofibular joint. The tibia is divided and fixed in one of two ways. (1) A wedge of bone, based laterally, is cut out at a level above the attachment of the patellar ligament; the gap is closed and the fragments are fixed with staples in the corrected position; the limb is then immobilized in plaster for 4–6 weeks (Coventry, 1985). (2) Alternatively the tibia is divided in a dome-shaped fashion just above the tibial tubercle, the desired position is obtained and the fragments are held by compression pins until union occurs (Maquet, 1976).

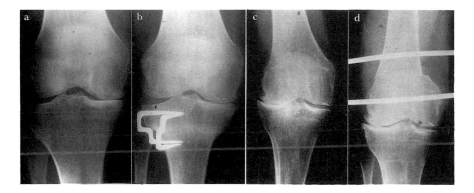

20.39 Osteotomy (a, b) For varus deformity, a high tibial osteotomy is the most effective. (c, d) For valgus deformity, the osteotomy should be on the femoral side of the joint.

RESULTS High tibial valgus osteotomy, when done for osteoarthritis, gives good results provided (1) the disease is confined to the medial compartment and (2) the knee has a good range of movement and is stable. These conditions are seldom strictly observed and in most cases osteotomy is seen as an alternative to a (medial) unicompartmental arthroplasty.

COMPLICATIONS The main complication is failure to correct the deformity, which is really a defect in technique. With medial compartment osteoarthritis, unless a slight valgus position is obtained, the result is liable to be unsatisfactory.

Arthrodesis

A stiff knee is a considerable disability; it makes climbing difficult and sitting in crowded areas distinctly awkward. Consequently, it is not often performed. Nevertheless, it remains the only certain way of relieving pain permanently, and it may particularly be indicated for a failed knee replacement. A short period in plaster before operation enables the patient to decide if the inconvenience is tolerable.

TECHNIQUE A vertical midline incision is used. If the operation is for tuberculosis the diseased synovium is excised; otherwise it is disregarded. The posterior vessels and nerves are protected and the ends of the tibia and femur removed by means of straight saw cuts. Thick Steinmann

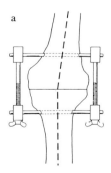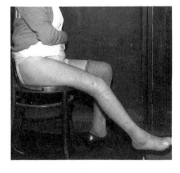

20.40 Arthrodesis (a) Compression arthrodesis with the joint in slight flexion and valgus. (b) The patient with a stiff knee has some difficulty sitting comfortably – and keeping the leg out of the way of passersby.

pins are inserted parallel to each other, through the tibia and femur. The bone ends are apposed and compressed by clamping the pins together (Charnley's method), or by any other method of external fixation. For additional protection a padded plaster is applied. The clamps and pins are removed after 4–6 weeks and a new plaster cylinder is applied; this is worn for a further 6 weeks, after which, provided the x-rays show sufficient union, it is removed.

Knee replacement

INDICATIONS The main indication for knee replacement is pain, especially when combined with deformity and instability. Most replacements are performed for rheumatoid arthritis or osteoarthritis.

TYPES OF OPERATION
Partial replacement Unicompartmental replacement of the medial or lateral portion of the tibiofemoral joint can be used where the disease is appropriately localized. The results are impressive and, to a large extent, the operation has displaced osteotomy as the procedure of choice in this type of case (Broughton, Newman and Bailey, 1986; Goodfellow et al., 1988).

Patellar resurfacing, a kind of partial replacement, is rarely performed alone; usually it is combined with surface replacement of the condyles.

Unconstrained total replacement Most commonly all the articular surfaces are replaced by 'resurfacing' components – metal on the femoral side and polyethylene on the tibial side and patella. It is important to ensure correct placement of the implants so as to reproduce the normal mechanics of the knee as closely as possible. The development of suitable prostheses and instrumentation in recent years has led to vast improvements in technique, so the results are now similar to those of hip replacement.

Constrained joints Joints with fixed hinges are used when there is marked bone loss and severe instability. Their main value nowadays is to provide a mobile joint following resection of tumours at the bone ends. The lack of rotation

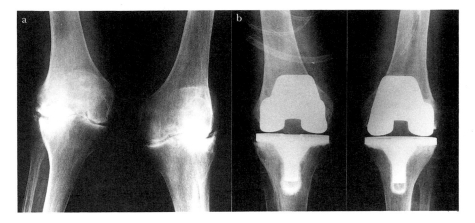

20.41 Total joint replacement X-rays (a) before and (b) after resurfacing of the femur, tibia and patella.

in these implants places severe stresses on the bone/implant interfaces and they are liable to loosen, to break or to erode the tibial or femoral shafts unless inactivity severely limits their use. Moreover, a considerable amount of bone has to be removed, and this makes subsequent arthrodesis difficult.

RESULTS The results of knee replacement have improved greatly in recent years. Thus, Scuderi et al. (1989) report a 10-year 'survival rate' of 97.34% for the cemented posterior stabilized metal femoral prosthesis with a polyethylene tibia. As with hip replacement, there is controversy between the advocates of cemented and uncemented components.

COMPLICATIONS
General As with all knee operations (except arthroscopy) in which a tourniquet is used, there is a high incidence of deep vein thrombosis.

Infection The methods of preventing and treating infection are similar to those used in hip replacement. Treatment by debridement and antibiotics, or by exchange replacement in one or two stages, are obvious possibilities (Rosenberg et al., 1988) though probably the safest salvage operation is arthrodesis.

Loosening This results from faulty prosthetic design or inaccurate bone shaping and placement of the implants. It is important: (1) to

overcome deformity (the knee should finally be about 7 degrees valgus); (2) to promote stability (by tailoring the bone cuts so that the collateral ligaments are reasonably tight in full extension); and (3) to permit rotation (otherwise cemented prostheses are liable to loosen). A loose prosthesis can be recemented, but unless the cause is dealt with loosening will recur.

Patellar problems Though relatively uncommon, these can be very disabling. They include (1) recurrent patellar subluxation or dislocation, which may need realignment, and (2) complications associated with patellar resurfacing, such as loosening of the prosthetic component, fracture of the remaining bony patella, and catching of soft tissues between the patella and the femur.

Notes on applied anatomy

The knee joint combines two articulations – tibiofemoral and patellofemoral. The bones of the tibiofemoral joint have little or no inherent stability; this depends largely upon strong ligaments and muscles. The patellofemoral joint is so shaped that the patella moves in a shallow path (or track) between the femoral condyles; if this track is too shallow the patella readily dislocates, and if its line is faulty the patellar articular cartilage is subject to excessive wear.

One important function of the patella is to increase the power of extension; it lifts the quadriceps forwards, thereby increasing its moment arm.

The patellar tendon is inserted into the upper pole of the patella. It is in line with the shaft of the femur, whereas the patellar ligament is in line with the shaft of the tibia. Because of the angle between them (the Q angle) quadriceps contraction would pull the patella laterally were it not for the fibres of vastus medialis, which are transverse. This muscle is therefore important and it is essential to try to prevent the otherwise rapid wasting that is liable to follow any effusion.

The shaft of the femur is inclined medially, while the tibia is vertical; thus the normal knee is slightly valgus (average 7 degrees). This amount is physiological and the term 'genu valgum' is used only when the angle exceeds 7 degrees; significantly less than this amount is genu varum.

During walking, weight is necessarily taken alternately on each leg. The line of body weight falls medial to the knee and must be counterbalanced by muscle action lateral to the joint (chiefly the tensor fascia femoris). To calculate the force transmitted across the knee, that due to muscle action must be added to that imposed by gravity; moreover, since with each step the knee is braced by the quadriceps, the force that this imposes also must be added.

Clearly the stresses on the articular cartilage are (as they also are at the hip) much greater than consideration only of body weight would lead one to suppose. It is also obvious that a varus deformity can easily overload the medial compartment, leading to cartilage breakdown; similarly, a valgus deformity may overload the lateral compartment.

As the knee bends, the axis of the tibiofemoral 'hinge' moves further and further backwards, so that the rolling movement of the femoral condyles is accompanied by backward gliding of the tibia. As the knee straightens, these are reversed; in addition, during the final stages of extension the tibia rotates laterally (hence the differing shapes of the two femoral condyles). The complex combination of a rolling, gliding and rotating movement is difficult to analyse; it is even more difficult to reproduce in a prosthesis.

Situated as they are between these complexly moving surfaces, the fibrocartilaginous menisci are prone to injury, particularly during unguarded movements of extension and rotation on the weightbearing leg. The medial meniscus is especially vulnerable because, in addition to its loose attachments via the coronary ligaments, it is firmly attached at three widely separated points: the anterior horn, the posterior horn and to the medial collateral ligament. The lateral meniscus more readily escapes damage because it is attached only at its anterior and posterior horns and these are close to each other.

The function of the menisci is not known for certain, but they certainly increase the contact area between femur and tibia. They play a significant part in weight transmission and this applies at all angles of flexion and extension; as the knee bends they glide backwards, and as it straightens they are pushed forwards.

The deep portion of the medial collateral ligament, to which the meniscus is attached, is fan-shaped and blends with the posteromedial capsule. It is, therefore, not surprising that medial ligament tears are often associated with tears of the medial meniscus and of the posteromedial capsule. The lateral collateral ligament is situated more posteriorly and does not blend with the capsule; nor is it attached to the meniscus, from which it is separated by the tendon of popliteus.

The two collateral ligaments resist sideways tilting of the extended knee. In addition, the medial ligament prevents the medial tibial condyle from subluxating forwards. Forward subluxation of the lateral tibial condyle, however, is prevented, not by the lateral collateral ligament but by the anterior cruciate. Only when the medial ligament and the anterior cruciate are both torn can the whole tibia subluxate forwards (giving a marked positive anterior drawer sign). Backward subluxation of the tibia is prevented by the powerful posterior cruciate ligament in combination with the arcuate ligament on its lateral side and the posterior oblique ligament on its medial side.

The cruciate ligaments are crucial, in the sense that they are essential for stability of the knee. The anterior cruciate ligament prevents forward displacement of the tibia on the femur and, in particular, it prevents forward subluxation of the lateral tibial condyle, a movement that tends to occur if a person who is running twists suddenly. The posterior cruciate ligament prevents backward displacement of the tibia on the femur and its integrity is therefore important when progressing downhill.

References and further reading

Ahlback, S., Bauer, G.C.H. and Bohne, W.H. (1968) Spontaneous osteonecrosis of the knee. *Arthritis and Rheumatism* **11**, 705–733

Aichroth, P. (1971) Osteochondritis dissecans of the knee: a clinical survey. *Journal of Bone and Joint Surgery* **53B**, 440–447

Annotation (1981) Biomechanical troubles of the patella. *Lancet* **1**, 1088–1089

Apley, A.G. (1947) The diagnosis of meniscus injuries: some new clinical methods. *Journal of Bone and Joint Surgery* **29**, 78–84

Barrie, H.J. (1979) The pathogenesis and significance of meniscal cysts. *Journal of Bone and Joint Surgery* **61B**, 184–189

Bentley, G. (1985) Articular cartilage changes in chondromalacia patellae. *Journal of Bone and Joint Surgery* **67B**, 769–774

Bergman, N.R. and Williams, P.F. (1988) Habitual dislocation of the patella in flexion. *Journal of Bone and Joint Surgery* **70B**, 415–419

Bose, K. and Chong, K.C. (1976) The clinical manifestations and pathomechanics of contracture of the extensor mechanism of the knee. *Journal of Bone and Joint Surgery* **58B**, 478–484

Broughton, N.S., Newman, J.H. and Bailey, R.A.J. (1986) Unicompartmental replacement and high tibial osteotomy for osteoarthritis of the knee. *Journal of Bone and Joint Surgery* **68B**, 447–452

Casscells, S.W. (1978) The torn or degenerated meniscus and its relationship to degeneration of the weight-bearing areas of the femur and tibia. *Clinical Orthopaedics and Related Research* **132**, 196–200

Coventry, M.B. (1985) Upper tibial osteotomy for osteoarthritis. *Journal of Bone and Joint Surgery* **67A**, 1136–1140

Dandy, D.J. (1985) *Arthroscopy of the Knee: a diagnostic colour index.* Butterworth/Gower Medical, London and New York.

Dandy, D.J. (1990) The arthroscopic anatomy of symptomatic meniscal lesions. *Journal of Bone and Joint Surgery* **72B**, 628–633

Dimakopoulos, P. and Patel, D. (1990) Partial excision of discoid meniscus. *Acta Orthopaedica Scandinavica* **61**, 1–40

Doherty, M., Watt, I. and Dieppe, P. (1983) Influence of primary generalised osteoarthritis on the development of secondary osteoarthritis. *Lancet* **2**, 8–11

Eskola, A., Santavirta, S., Konttinen, Y.T., Tallroth, K. and Lindholm, S.T. (1988) Arthroplasty for old tuberculosis of the knee. *Journal of Bone and Joint Surgery* **70B**, 767–769

Ficat, R.P. and Hungerford, D.S. (1977) *Disorders of the Patello-femoral Joint*, Williams & Wilkins, Baltimore

Goodfellow, J.W., Kershaw, C.J., Benson, M.K.D'A. and O'Connor, J.J. (1988) The Oxford knee for unicompartmental osteoarthritis. *Journal of Bone and Joint Surgery* **70B**, 692–701

Hardaker, W.T., Whipple, T.L. and Bassett, F.H. (1980) Diagnosis and treatment of the plica syndrome of the knee. *Journal of Bone and Joint Surgery* **62A**, 221–225

Heatley, F.W. and Butler-Mannal, A. (1990) Assessment of osteoarthritis of the knee. *Current Orthopaedics* **4**, 79–87

Hede, A., Hejgaard, N. and Larsen, E. (1986) Partial or total open meniscectomy? A prospective randomized study. *International Orthopaedics* **10**, 105–108

Helfet, A.J. (1974) *Disorders of the Knee*, Lippincott, Philadelphia:

Hong-Xue Men, Chan-Hua Bian, Chan-Dou Yang, Zen-Long Zhang, Chi-Chang Wu and Bo-You Pang (1991) Surgical treatment of the flail knee after poliomyelitis. *Journal of Bone and Joint Surgery* **73B**, 195–198

Inone, M., Shino, K., Hirose, H. et al. (1988) Subluxation of the patella. Computed tomography analysis of patellofemoral congruence. *Journal of Bone and Joint Surgery* **70A**, 1331–1337

Insall, J.N., Falvo, K.A. and Wise, D.W. (1976) Chondromalacia patellae. *Journal of Bone and Joint Surgery* **58A**, 1–8

Ireland, J., Trickey, E.L. and Stoker, D.J. (1980) Arthroscopy and arthrography of the knee. *Journal of Bone and Joint Surgery* **62B**, 3–6

Johannsen, H.V., Fruensgaard, S., Holm, A. and Toennesen, P.A. (1988) Arthroscopic suture of peripheral meniscal tears. *International Orthopaedics* **12**, 287–290

Johnson, F., Leitl, S. and Waugh, W. (1980) The distribution of load across the knee. *Journal of Bone and Joint Surgery* **62B**, 346–349

Kay, P.R., Freemont, A.J. and Davies, D.R.A. (1989) The aetiology of multiple loose bodies. *Journal of Bone and Joint Surgery* **71B**, 501–504

King, J.B., Perry, D.J., Mourad, K. and Kumar, S.J. (1990) Lesions of the patellar ligament. *Journal of Bone and Joint Surgery* **72B**, 46–48

Larson, R.L. (1979) Subluxation-dislocation of the patella. In *The Injured Adolescent Knee* (ed. J.C. Kennedy), Williams & Wilkins, Baltimore, pp. 161–204

Mann, G., Finsterbush, A. Frankl, U. et al. (1991) A method of diagnosing small amounts of fluid in the knee. *Journal of Bone and Joint Surgery* **73B**, 346–347

Maquet, P.G.J. (1976) *Biomechanics of the Knee*, Springer, Berlin, Heidelberg, New York

Mesgarzadeh, M., Sapega, A.A., Bonakdarpour, A. et al. (1987) Osteochondritis dissecans: analysis of mechanical stability with radiography, scintigraphy and MR imaging. *Radiology* **165**, 775–780

Muckle, D.S. and Minns, R.J. (1990) Biological response to woven carbon fibre pads in the knee. *Journal of Bone and Joint Surgery* **72B**, 60–62

Muheim, G. and Bohne, W.H. (1970) Prognosis in spontaneous osteonecrosis of the knee. *Journal of Bone and Joint Surgery* **52B**, 605–612

Noble, J. and Hamblin, D.L. (1975) The pathology of the degenerate meniscus lesion. *Journal of Bone and Joint Surgery* **57B**, 180–186

Noll, B.J., Ben-Itzhak, I. and Rossouw, P. (1988) Modified technique for tibial tubercle elevation with realignment for patellofemoral pain. *Clinical Orthopaedics and Related Research* **234**, 174–178

Ogilvie-Harris, D.J. and Jackson, R.W. (1984) The arthroscopic treatment of chondromalacia patellae. *Journal of Bone and Joint Surgery* **66B**, 660–665

Outerbridge, R.E. (1961) The aetiology of chondromalacia patellae. *Journal of Bone and Joint Surgery* **43B**, 752–757

Parisien, J.S. (1990) Arthroscopic treatment of cysts of the menisci. *Clinical Orthopaedics and Related Research* **257**, 154–158

Rosenberg, A.G., Haas, B., Barden, R. et al. (1988) Salvage of infected total knee arthroplasty. *Clinical Orthopaedics and Related Research* **226**, 29–33

Scuderi, G.R., Insall, J.N., Windsor, R.E. and Moran, M.C. (1989) Survivorship of cemented knee replacements. *Journal of Bone and Joint Surgery* **71B**, 798–803

Sherman, O.H., Fox, J.M., Snyder, S.J. et al. (1986) Arthroscopy – no problem surgery: an analysis of complications in two thousand six hundred and forty cases. *Journal of Bone and Joint Surgery* **68B**, 256–265

Smillie, I.S. (1980) *Diseases of the Knee Joint*, 2nd edn, Churchill Livingstone, Edinburgh and London

Wiberg, G. (1941) Roentgenographic and anatomic studies on the femoropatellar joint with special reference to chondromalacia patellae. *Acta Orthopaedica Scandinavica* **12**, 319–410

Wilson, J.N. (1967) A diagnostic sign in osteochondritis dissecans of the knee. *Journal of Bone and Joint Surgery* **49A**, 477–480

The ankle and foot

21

Examination

Symptoms

The most common presenting symptoms are pain, deformity, swelling and sensory change. It is important to know whether standing or walking provokes the symptoms and whether shoe pressure is a factor.

Pain over a bony prominence or a joint is probably due to some local disorder. Pain across the forefoot (metatarsalgia) is less specific and is often associated with muscle fatigue.

Deformity may be in the ankle, the mid-foot or the toes. Parents often worry about their children who are 'flat-footed' or 'pigeon-toed'. Elderly patients may complain chiefly of having difficulty fitting shoes.

Swelling may be diffuse and bilateral, or localized; unilateral swelling nearly always has a surgical cause, bilateral swelling is more often medical in origin. Swelling over the medial side of the first metatarsal head (a bunion) is common in older women.

Corns and callosities Often the main complaint is of shoe pressure on a tender corn over the joints or a callosity on the sole.

Numbness and paraesthesia may be felt in all the toes or in a circumscribed field served by a single nerve.

Signs with the patient standing and walking

The patient, whose lower limbs should be exposed from the knees down, stands first facing the surgeon, then with his back to the surgeon.

● LOOK
The legs, ankles, feet and toes are systematically inspected. Particular points to observe are the colour of the skin and any swelling or deformity.

● FEEL
Palpation is postponed until the patient is sitting.

● MOVE
The patient is asked to stand on tiptoes, then to walk normally and finally to walk on tiptoes. It is important to observe whether the gait is smooth and the foot well balanced or if the patient walks mainly on the inner or the outer border of the foot. Normally the foot relaxes into slight valgus during the stance phase and, as the other leg swings through, the weightbearing ankle moves into dorsiflexion. If the ankle cannot dorsiflex, abnormal stresses are placed on the neighbouring joints and the knee. At push-off, the foot tightens into slight inversion, the metatarsophalangeal joints extend and the intrinsic muscles stabilize the toes; loss of any of these actions causes instability at the moment of maximal weightbearing.

Signs with the patient sitting or lying

The patient is next examined lying on a couch, or it may be more convenient if he sits opposite the examiner and places his feet on the examiner's lap.

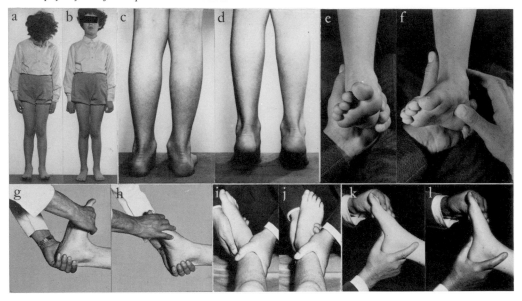

21.1 Examination The patient examined standing, instinctively looks at her feet; this throws her off balance (a); she should look straight ahead (b). Next the feet are examined from behind (c) and on tiptoe (d); then held on the surgeon's lap with the heel square to see if the forefoot is varus (e), and to feel for tenderness (f). Ankle dorsiflexion (g) and plantarflexion (h) are examined; then subtalar inversion (i) and eversion (j). Finally, (k, l) mid-tarsal movements are tested.

● LOOK

The heel is held square so that any foot deformity can be assessed. The toes and sole should be inspected for skin changes. Thickening and keratosis over the proximal toe joints may form corns; similar changes on the sole are called callosities.

● FEEL

The skin temperature is assessed and the pulses are felt. If there is tenderness in the foot it must be precisely localized, for its site is often diagnostic. Any swelling, oedema or lumps must be examined. Sensation may be abnormal; the precise distribution of sensory change is important.

● MOVE

The foot can be regarded as a series of joints which should be examined methodically.

Ankle joint With the heel grasped in the left hand and the mid-foot in the right, dorsiflexion and plantarflexion are tested.

Subtalar joint Grasping the heel alone, inversion and eversion are examined.

Mid-tarsal joint The heel is held still with one hand while the other moves the tarsus up and down and from side to side.

Toes Movement at the metatarsophalangeal and interphalangeal joints is tested.

STABILITY is assessed by moving the joints across the normal physiological planes. With recent ligament injuries, passive stretching causes pain.

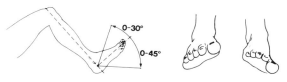

21.2 Normal range of movement All movements are measured from zero with the foot in the 'neutral' or 'anatomical' position: thus, dorsiflexion is 0–30 degrees and plantarflexion 0–45 degrees. Inversion is normally greater than eversion.

MUSCLE POWER is tested by resisting active movement in each direction. Individual tendons may be palpated to establish whether they are intact and functioning.

SHOES should never be neglected because, unless brand new, they may provide valuable evidence of faulty stance or gait.

GENERAL EXAMINATION
If there is any sign of motor weakness or sensory change, a full neurological assessment and examination of the back are imperative.

IMAGING
In the adult, routine anteroposterior and lateral x-rays should be obtained *with the patient standing*. Special views may be required for the calcaneum and the talocalcaneal joint. The best way to visualize the bones in the coronal plane is by *CT. Ultrasonography* is useful for showing tendon lesions and *radioisotope scans* may localize an obscure area of vascular activity or bone reaction.

Babies present special difficulties. The appropriate views and x-ray measurements are described below.

PEDOBAROGRAPHY
Standing or walking on a pressure-sensitive plate produces a graphic display of pressure distribution under the sole. This is particularly useful in planning treatment for neurotrophic ulcers.

Deformities of the foot

Many foot disorders present primarily as 'deformity', which may be due to: (1) congenital defects; (2) muscle imbalance; (3) ligamentous laxity; or (4) joint instability. Any existing deformity is aggravated and perpetuated by abnormal weightbearing and shoe pressure.

Congenital talipes equinovarus (idiopathic club foot)

This relatively common deformity has a polygenic pattern of inheritance. Boys are affected twice as often as girls and the condition is bilateral in one-third of cases. Identical deformities occur with myelomeningocele and in arthrogryposis. In the idiopathic variety there is no obvious neuromuscular defect but the deformity may well be caused by minor degrees of muscle imbalance in the developing fetus.

Pathological anatomy

The talus points downwards (equinus), the neck deviates medially and the body is rotated slightly outwards in relation to the calcaneum; the navicular and the entire forefoot are shifted medially and rotated into supination (the composite varus deformity). The skin and soft tissues of the calf and the medial side of the foot are short and underdeveloped. If the condition is not corrected early, secondary growth changes occur in the bones; these are permanent.

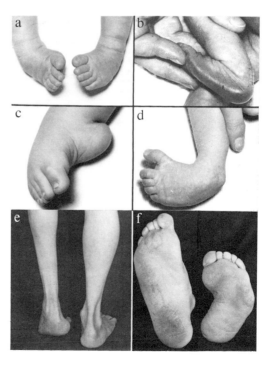

21.3 Talipes equinovarus (club foot) (a) True club foot is a fixed deformity, unlike (b) 'postural' talipes, which is easily correctible by gentle passive movement. (c) With true club foot the poorly developed heel is higher than the forefoot, which is also (d) varus. (e, f) The adult appearance when club foot has not been adequately corrected.

Even with treatment the foot is liable to be short, and the calf may remain thin.

Clinical features

The deformity is usually obvious at birth; the foot is both turned and twisted inwards so that the sole faces posteromedially. More precisely, the ankle is in equinus, the heel is inverted and the forefoot is adducted and supinated; sometimes there is cavus as well, and the talus may protrude on the dorsolateral surface of the foot. The heel is usually small and high, and the calf may be thin.

Gentle attempts at passive correction show the deformity to be fixed; in a normal baby with postural equinovarus the foot can be dorsiflexed and everted until the toes touch the front of the leg.

The infant must always be examined for associated disorders such as spina bifida or arthrogryposis.

In the older child, deformity varies from fairly mild equinus and adductus to the most severe 'club' appearance with weight being taken on the dorsum of the foot.

X-rays

X-rays are used mainly to assess progress after treatment. The *anteroposterior film* is taken with the foot 30 degrees plantarflexed and the tube likewise angled 30 degrees to the perpendicular. Lines are drawn through the long axis of the talus parallel to its medial border and through that of the calcaneum parallel to its lateral border; they normally cross at an angle of 20–40 degrees but in club foot the two lines may be almost parallel.

The *lateral film* is taken with the foot in forced dorsiflexion. Lines drawn through the mid-longitudinal axis of the talus and the lower border of the calcaneum should meet at an angle of about 40 degrees. Anything less than 20 degrees shows that the calcaneum cannot be tilted up into true dorsiflexion; the foot may *seem* to be dorsiflexed but it may actually have 'broken' at the mid-tarsal level, producing the so-called *rocker-bottom deformity*.

Prognosis

Provided treatment is started at birth, the deformity can almost always be largely corrected; however, the condition is not cured and relapse is common, especially in babies with obvious muscle wasting or associated neuromuscular disorders.

Treatment

The objectives are: (1) to correct the deformity early; (2) to correct it fully; and (3) to hold the corrected position until the foot stops growing.

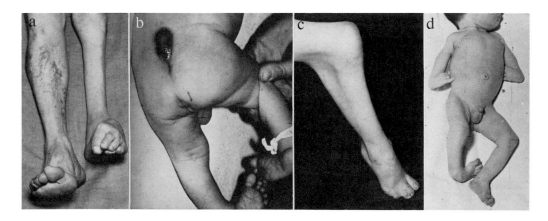

21.4 Other causes of club foot (a) Old polio; (b) spina bifida; (c) arthrogryposis multiplex congenita; (d) multiple deformities in arthrogryposis.

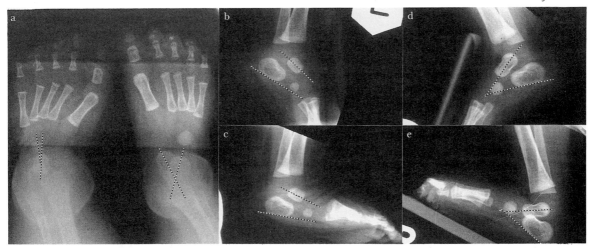

21.5 Talipes equinovarus – x-rays The left foot is abnormal. In the anteroposterior view (a) the talocalcaneal angle is 5 degrees, compared to 42 degrees on the right. In the lateral views, the left talocalcaneal angle is 10 degrees in plantarflexion (b) and 14 degrees in dorsiflexion (c); in the normal foot the angle is unchanged at 44 degrees, whatever the position of the foot (d, e).

There seem to be two varieties of club foot: 'easy' and 'resistant' (Attenborough, 1966). Easy cases respond readily to splinting. Resistant cases respond poorly, relapse quickly and may tempt one to dangerously forceful manipulation; in them, early operative correction is advisable so that manipulation and splintage can be gentle. Resistant cases are recognized by the thin calf and the small, high heel; arthrogrypotic club foot is notoriously resistant.

SPLINTING Treatment begins within 2 or 3 days of birth. Each component of the deformity is corrected in turn, and always in the following order: first the forefoot adduction, then the supination and finally the equinus. Attempts to overcome equinus first may 'break' the foot in the mid-tarsal region, creating a highly refractory 'rocker-bottom' deformity.

Without anaesthesia the foot is gently moulded (but not stretched) towards the desired position and held there by adhesive strapping with felt pads protecting the skin at points of pressure. An alternative method is to apply a light plaster cast over a protective layer of strapping. The process is repeated weekly for 6–8 weeks until the foot is not only corrected but *overcorrected.*

Final correction must be confirmed by x-ray: in the anteroposterior view the longitudinal axes of the talus and calcaneum should be separated by 20 degrees; in the lateral view the calcaneal axis should be at right angles (or less) to the tibia and the talocalcaneal angle should be at least 20 degrees.

OPERATION The resistant case is best operated on by 8 weeks. Through a serpentine medial incision the tendo Achillis and the structures below the medial malleolus are approached without undercutting the skin. The soft-tissue release proceeds stepwise, depending on the amount of correction obtained at each step. It starts with *tendo Achillis elongation;* if some equinus remains, a *posterior release* is obtained by dividing the full width of the posterior ankle capsule and, if necessary, the talocalcaneal capsule. Varus is then corrected by doing a *medial talonavicular release* and *lengthening the tibialis posterior* tendon. The medially displaced talus must be reduced and held with a thin Kirschner wire.

Great care must be taken (1) not to damage articular cartilage and (2) to close the wound without tension. For the less experienced surgeon it may be wise to do the correction in two separate stages (Porter, 1987).

TREATMENT AFTER CORRECTION Whether or not operation was needed, splintage continues; but

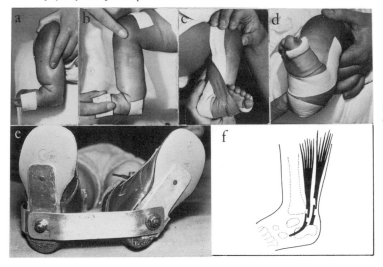

21.6 Treatment of congenital talipes (a–d) Manipulation and strapping.

(e) Denis Browne night shoes. (f) Very early operation.

now the moulding process needs to be repeated only at fortnightly or monthly intervals. This continues until the child starts walking; thereafter, correction can be maintained by Denis Browne night splints and orthoses which permit walking in eversion. Splintage may need to be continued until puberty.

LATE OR RELAPSING CLUB FOOT   Early correction may have been incomplete, or deformity may keep recurring with exasperating persistence. If the child is under 5 years of age, soft-tissue operations can still be successful but an extended *posteromedial release* may be needed. After tendo Achillis lengthening and posterior capsulotomies, the flexor retinaculum is opened, tight invertors and plantarflexors are lengthened, the neurovascular bundle is retracted and the thick fibrous floor of the tunnel is excised to expose the subtalar joint. Talonavicular release is performed, the foot is manipulated into the corrected position and the tarsal bones are held in place with thin Kirschner wires.

In children over the age of 5 years, correction may be impossible without bone reshaping. This may take the form of a dorsolateral wedge-excision of the calcaneocuboid joint (Evans, 1961) or of osteotomy of the calcaneum to correct varus (Dwyer, 1963).

Over the age of 10 the best operation is probably a lateral wedge tarsectomy or, if the foot is mature, a triple arthodesis.

Other varieties of 'talipes'

Sometimes the only deformity is an *adducted forefoot*, which is nearly always correctible by manipulation and splintage. Less than 10% need operation: up to the age of 4 years, dividing the capsules and ligaments of the tarsometatarsal joints permits good realignment; for older children the possibilities are Evans' procedure (see above) or osteotomy of all five metatarsals. Neglected deformities in adults may be severe enough to cause chronic pain. They can be corrected by wedge-excision and arthrodesis of the tarsometatarsal joints.

Talipes calcaneus (the foot dorsiflexed) is common and often associated with valgus de-

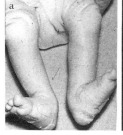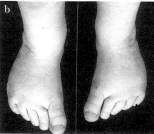

21.7 Other varieties of 'talipes' (a) Bilateral calcaneovalgus (which usually corrects spontaneously). (b) Bilateral forefoot adductus (which may improve, but seldom corrects completely).

formity. The deformity usually disappears spontaneously but, if it is severe or persistent, correction is easily and quickly obtained by weekly manipulation and splintage. With calcaneovalgus deformity it is important to exclude an associated congenital dislocation of the hip.

Flat foot (pes planus; pes valgus)

'Our feet are no more alike than our faces.' This truism from a *British Medical Journal* Editorial (1980) sums up the problem of 'normally abnormal' feet. The medial arch may be normally high or normally low. The term 'flat foot' applies when the apex of the arch has collapsed and the medial border of the foot is in contact (or nearly in contact) with the ground; the heel becomes valgus and the foot pronates at the subtalar–midtarsal complex. The condition is usually asymptomatic but it may cause chronic ache or 'foot strain'.

Causes

Apart from certain rare developmental disorders, flat foot results from excessive ligamentous laxity, loss of stabilizing muscle power, abnormal load distribution or a combination of these factors. The underlying cause is often inherited, hence the common familial incidence.

Pathological varieties

CONGENITAL FLAT FOOT is a rare disorder associated with displacement of the talonavicular joint. It is sometimes associated with muscle imbalance (e.g. in spina bifida) and the foot is usually stiff.

PHYSIOLOGICAL FLAT FOOT is very common in toddlers, especially if they are overweight or have lax joints. It is quite normal for that stage of development and it usually disappears after a few years. Occasionally, however, it persists into adult life as a permanent structural deformity.

JOINT HYPERMOBILITY may manifest as pes valgus. This is seen typically in Marfan's syndrome and the Ehlers–Danlos syndrome.

WEAK FLAT FOOT, due to loss of muscle power, is seen in paralytic disorders, attenuation or rupture of tibialis posterior (e.g. in rheumatoid disease) and following any wasting disease. In old age the combination of obesity and flabby muscles has the same effect.

COMPENSATORY FLAT FOOT may follow some other anatomical defect: (1) fixed ankle equinus or forefoot varus may be accommodated by turning the heel into valgus; (2) with knock knees the body weight is taken medial to the ankles, so the feet collapse into valgus; (3) if the lower limbs are externally rotated the body weight falls anteromedial to the ankle and the foot goes over into valgus – the Charlie Chaplin look.

SPASMODIC FLAT FOOT is produced by spasm or contraction of the peroneal muscles, usually triggered by an inflammatory condition such as Reiter's disease or a congenital tarsal anomaly (see below).

Clinical features

Children seldom complain about their feet – but their parents may do so, either because the feet look flat or because the shoes wear badly. Adults, also, are usually asymptomatic, but they may develop pain because of foot strain, secondary forefoot deformities or osteoarthritis of the tarsal joints.

The foot is examined with the patient standing (when the deformity will be obvious) and then with the patient sitting (to see if there is any tenderness and to test the range of movement). With a tight tendo Achillis, dorsiflexion does not occur without the heel moving into valgus; passively dorsiflexing the hallux normally elevates the arch, but in flat foot it does not (Rose, Welton and Marshall, 1985).

The knees and hips should be examined for associated postural deformities, and general examination may be necessary to exclude any underlying disorder.

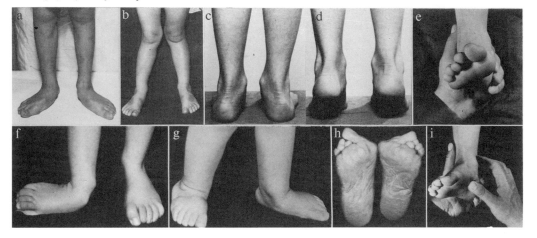

21.8 Flat foot – causal factors   Flat foot may be associated with anatomical faults (upper row), or with physiological faults (lower row). (a) External rotation of the legs; (b) knock knees; (c) a tight tendo Achillis – note that standing on tiptoe (d) restores the arch; (e) a varus forefoot. (f) Paralytic flat foot from old polio; (g) infantile flat foot; (h) middle-aged splay foot; (i) tenderness in temporary flat foot (foot strain).

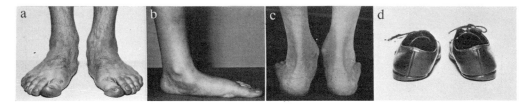

21.9 Flat foot   Clinical features: (a) prominent tuberosity of navicular; (b) flattening of the arch; (c) valgus heels; (d) faulty shoe wear.

Treatment

Small children usually need no treatment; at most, the shoes may be altered to raise the inner side of the heel. Older children and young adults are sometimes helped by heel cups or by placing an arch support inside the shoe. Exercises will strengthen the muscles and reduce the likelihood of foot strain but will do nothing to correct the deformity.

In cases that are clearly due to an underlying disorder (poliomyelitis, rheumatoid arthritis or a ruptured tibialis posterior tendon), operative correction and muscle rebalancing may be needed.

Two types of flat foot – both fortunately rare – may present special problems: congenital flat foot and spasmodic flat foot.

Congenital flat foot

In this condition, sometimes called rigid flat foot or congenital vertical talus, the calcaneum is in equinus, the talus points almost vertically downwards and the talonavicular joint is dislocated. The middle of the sole is the most prominent part (rocker-bottom foot) and the foot feels very stiff.

Treatment demands reduction of the dislocation. If manipulation succeeds (which is unusual) the foot is held in an equinovarus plaster for at least 6 months. If manipulation fails, an anterolateral release is performed, lengthening the anterior tendons and dividing the soft tissues until reduction is achieved. The reduced position is held in an equinovarus plaster for

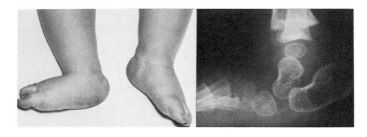

21.10 Flat foot – congenital Note the 'rocker bottom' foot and the vertical talus.

several months and then an extensive posterior release, including lengthening the tendo Achillis, is performed (Walker, Ghali and Silk, 1985). Should open reduction of the dislocation prove impossible the navicular may have to be excised (Colton, 1973).

Spasmodic flat foot

The term is a misnomer: the foot is not flat nor is the disorder spasmodic; but the foot is rigidly everted and the muscles are in spasm.

PATHOLOGY The pathology of spasmodic flat foot has been greatly clarified by the advent of CT (Bower, Keyser and Gilula, 1989). Peroneal muscle spasm is associated with a variety of disorders in the subtalar joint: tarsal coalitions, incomplete coalitions, anatomical abnormalities of the subtalar articular facets, low-grade infection, inflammatory arthritis, fractures and post-traumatic osteoarthritis.

CLINICAL FEATURES The condition usually occurs in adolescents and young adults, is more common in males and is often bilateral. Pain is the presenting symptom. The foot is held everted, and the peroneal and extensor tendons can be seen standing out in spasm under the skin. There may be diffuse tenderness around the tarsus. Ankle movements are normal. Subtalar joint movement is grossly restricted and often painful; even if no spasm was previously visible, attempted movement provokes it. Mid-tarsal movements also are restricted.

X-rays may show an abnormal bar or bridge between adjacent tarsal bones (talonavicular and talocalcaneal in particular) but special views are sometimes needed to demonstrate it.

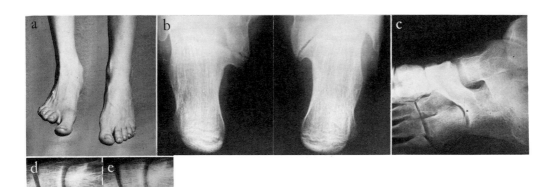

21.11 'Spasmodic' flat foot (a) Evertor spasm, (b) Harris' axial view shows calcaneotalar coalition on the left; this is more difficult to see than (c) a calcaneonavicular bar; (d) before and (e) after excision of a similar bar.

Radioisotope scanning usually reveals a localized area of increased activity. CT scans in the coronal plane are the most helpful for showing talocalcaneal pathology (Bower, Keyser and Gilula, 1989).

TREATMENT is usually conservative. A walking plaster is applied with the foot plantigrade (an anaesthetic may be necessary) and is retained for at least 6 weeks. Even then, splintage with an outside iron and inside T-strap is often necessary for a further 3–6 months. If infection is diagnosed, antibiotics will be required.

Operative treatment is sometimes necessary for removal of an abnormal bar or trimming of bony irregularities or abutting ridges. The space left by excision of a bar can be filled with fat or with a portion of the extensor digitorum brevis muscle. Rarely, triple arthrodesis is offered as a last resort.

Pes cavus

In pes cavus the arch is higher than normal, and often there is also clawing of the toes. The close resemblance to deformities seen in neurological disorders where the intrinsic muscles are weak or paralysed suggests that idiopathic pes cavus is due to a similar type of muscle imbalance.

Pathology

The toes are drawn up into a 'clawed' position, the metatarsal heads are forced down into the sole and the arch at the mid-foot is accentuated. Often the heel is inverted and the soft tissues in the sole are tight. Under the prominent metatarsal heads callosities may form.

Clinical features

Patients usually present at the age of 8–10 years. Deformity may be noticed by the parents or the school doctor before there are any symptoms. There is often a family history, and as a rule both feet are affected. Pain may be felt under the metatarsal heads or over the toes where shoe pressure is most marked. Callosities appear at the same sites.

The deformities are obvious; there is a high instep and the arch stands well clear of the ground. Sometimes the hindfoot is quite normal and the deformity is chiefly one of forefoot equinus (plantaris deformity).

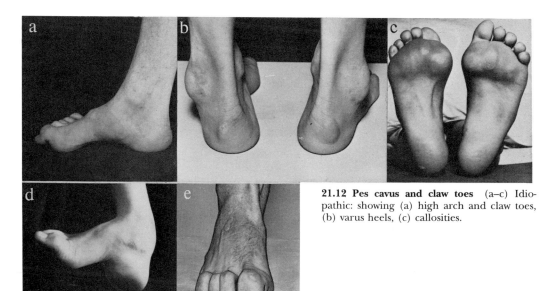

21.12 Pes cavus and claw toes (a–c) Idiopathic: showing (a) high arch and claw toes, (b) varus heels, (c) callosities.

(d) Paralytic cavus. (e) Claw toes with Volkmann's contracture.

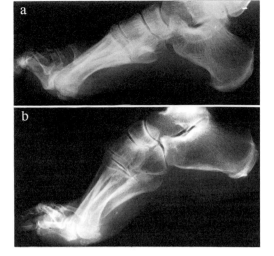

21.13 Pes cavus (a) In pes cavus there is a true elevation of the medial arch when the foot is placed on a flat surface; the x-ray in (b) looks similar, but this is due simply to plantar angulation of the metatarsals – the 'plantaris' deformity.

The toes are held cocked up, with hyperextension at the metatarsophalangeal joints and flexion at the interphalangeal joints. There may be callosities under the metatarsal heads and corns on the toes.

Early on the toe deformities are 'mobile' and can be corrected passively by pressure under the metatarsal heads; as the forefoot lifts, the toes flatten out automatically. Later the deformities become fixed, with the metatarsophalangeal joints permanently dislocated.

Neurological disorders such as peroneal muscular atrophy and Friedreich's ataxia (p. 203) must always be excluded, and the spine should be examined for signs of dysraphism.

Treatment

Often no treatment is required; apart from the difficulty of fitting shoes, the patient has no complaints.

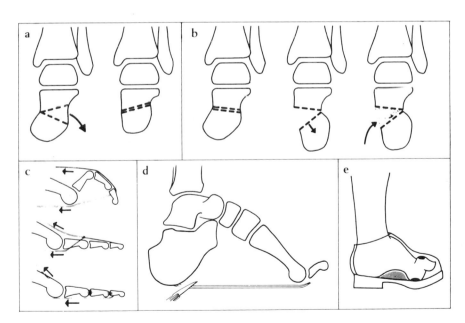

21.14 Treatment of pes cavus and claw toes Correction of the varus heel by (a) excising a laterally based wedge of bone or (b) inserting a medial wedge (Dwyer).
(c) Claw toes due to overaction of the long tendons may be dealt with by transferring flexor to extensor tendons or by arthrodesing the toe joints and reattaching the long extensors more proximally. (d) Division of the plantar fascia (Steindler). (e) Padding and special shoes for the late untreated case.

The patient with symptoms can sometimes be made comfortable by a combination of arch supports and specially made shoes. If not, operation may be necessary. While the forefoot deformities are mobile and passively correctible, a simple rebalancing operation is sufficient: the long flexors are released distally and transferred into the extensor expansions to pull the toes straight; the big toe extensor is transferred to the neck of the first metatarsal and the interphalangeal joint is fused (the Robert Jones procedure). If cavus is pronounced, Steindler's operation may improve matters: the tight tissues spanning the sole are stripped from the calcaneum and the foot is manipulated straight; correction is held by immobilizing the foot in a cast for 6 weeks.

Once the toe deformities have become fixed, they can be corrected only by excising and fusing all the interphalangeal joints.

Bony operations on the arch should be deferred until growth has ceased. For plantaris deformity, wedge excision and arthrodesis of the tarsometatarsal joints provides good correction (Jahss, 1980). If heel varus is marked, calcaneal osteotomy is indicated. In the most severe and neglected deformities, nothing short of a triple arthrodesis with reshaping of the tarsus will suffice; the alternative (often the wiser course) is palliative treatment with specially made shoes.

Hallux valgus

Hallux valgus is the commonest of the foot deformities (and probably of all musculoskeletal deformities). In people who have never worn shoes the big toe is in line with the first metatarsal, retaining the slightly fan shaped appearance of the forefoot. In people who wear shoes the hallux assumes a valgus position; but only if the angulation is excessive is it referred to as 'hallux valgus'.

Splaying of the forefoot, with varus angulation of the first metatarsal, will predispose to lateral angulation of the big toe. Such metatarsus varus may be congenital, or it may result from loss of muscle tone in the forefoot in elderly people. Hallux valgus is also common in rheumatoid arthritis.

Pathological anatomy

The elements of the deformity are: (1) increased width of the forefoot, with the first metatarsal deviated medially (metatarsus primus varus); (2) lateral deviation of the hallux, sometimes causing crowding of the lesser toes; and (3) prominence of the first metatarsal head, due partly to joint angulation, partly to thickening of the bone on the medial side (sometimes amounting to an 'exostosis') and partly to the development of a protective bursa (or bunion) where the shoe rubs. As the deformity increases, the long tendon of the hallux and the sesamoid bones are shifted laterally, the medial capsule is stretched, the great toe rotates so that the nail faces medially, and the abductor hallucis tendon slides under the metatarsal head. Ultimately, malalignment of the metatarsophalangeal joint may lead to osteoarthritis.

Clinical features

Hallux valgus is usually bilateral, and is most common in the sixth decade and in females. There is a variety, strongly familial and by no means uncommon, that presents in adolescents.

Often there are no symptoms apart from the deformity. Pain, if present, may be due to (1) shoe pressure on a large or an inflamed bunion, (2) a hammer toe, (3) an associated wide splay foot with metatarsalgia and pain under the metatarsal heads or (4) secondary osteoarthritis of the first metatarsophalangeal joint.

The deformity is obvious and the bunion is often swollen and inflamed. The forefoot is too wide and the great toe is in valgus and often rotated. The second toe is crowded and hammer toe deformities are common.

The site of tenderness is important and must be accurately localized, for it may influence treatment: it may be (1) over the bunion, (2) in the joint or (3) between the metatarsals.

Unless osteoarthritis has supervened, the metatarsophalangeal joint has a good range of movement.

X-rays should be taken with the patient standing, to show the degree of metatarsal and hallux

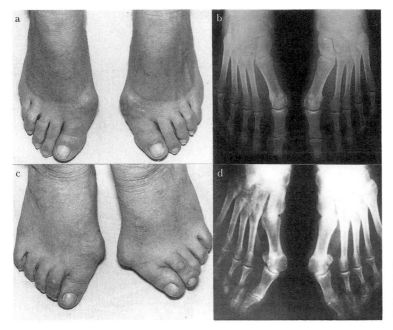

21.15 Hallux valgus (a, b) This girl's feet are well on the way to becoming as deformed as (c, d) those of her mother. Hallux valgus is not uncommonly familial.

angulation. Lines are drawn along the middle of the first and second metatarsals and the proximal phalanx of the great toe; normally the intermetatarsal angle is less than 15 degrees and the hallux angle less than 20 degrees. The first metatarsophalangeal joint may be subluxated, or it may look osteoarthritic.

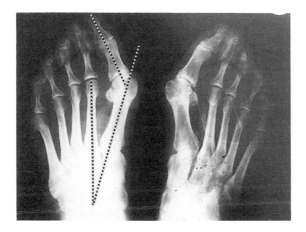

21.16 Hallux valgus – measurements The intermetatarsal angle (between the 1st and 2nd metatarsals) as well as the metatarsophalangeal angle of the hallux are recorded.

Treatment

UNDER 25 YEARS In adolescents and young adults, deformity is usually the only symptom, but the mother is anxious to prevent its becoming as severe as her own. Nothing short of operation can prevent the deformity from increasing. This takes the form of a corrective osteotomy of the first metatarsal and reefing (or tightening) of the medial capsule. It is important that the operation should not shorten the first metatarsal. A *basal osteotomy* with an opening gap is preferred; the metatarsal is realigned laterally and held there with a thick Kirschner wire until union is secure. A *distal osteotomy (Mitchell)* with lateral displacement of the head is also effective, but it does shorten the bone, and care must be taken to prevent dorsal angulation of the distal fragment as this can result in pain under the metatarsal. Some surgeons prefer *Wilson's operation, an oblique osteotomy of the distal shaft,* displacing the distal portion laterally.

25–50 YEARS Provided the metatarsophalangeal joint is well formed (though subluxated), a reconstructive procedure is probably the best. *Exostectomy and capsulorrhaphy* (trimming the

a   b   c   d   e   f

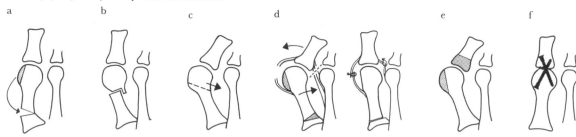

21.17 Hallux valgus – treatment (a) Basal osteotomy with bone graft inserted. (b) Mitchell's osteotomy. (c) Wilson's osteotomy. (d) Before and after basal osteotomy and capsulorrhaphy. (e) Keller's operation. (f) Arthrodesis.

bump and reefing the medial capsule) may suffice for very mild deformity. However, in the usual case this must be combined with *release of the deforming adductor hallucis tendon* from the base of the proximal phalanx and tightening up of the first web space – the Du Vries modification of McBride's operation (Mann, 1986). If the hallux angle is greater than 40 degrees and the first intermetatarsal angle greater than 15 degrees a *basal osteotomy and correction of the first metatarsal* is done as well.

In this age group, and in younger patients, if the metatarsophalangeal joint will not permit congruent alignment, a *chevron osteotomy* of the distal end of the metatarsal will allow the toe to be repositioned without much alteration of the articular relationship.

OVER 50 YEARS Older patients who are still active, with stable big toe joints, are treated as for the previous group. In those who are less active, or less demanding, or where the metatarsophalangeal joint has lost stability, the classic *Keller operation* is the procedure of choice. The proximal third of the proximal phalanx is excised, leaving a gap where the joint once was, and the medial and dorsal exostoses are removed. The toe is unstable but the patient is grateful for the relief of pain. If there is gross varus of the first metatarsal, Keller's operation is combined with a basal metatarsal osteotomy.

Arthrodesis of the first metatarsophalangeal joint, a much under-rated operation, is used by many surgeons instead of Keller's excisional arthroplasty. It is ideal as a salvage operation for failed reconstruction.

Hallux rigidus

The 'rigidity' (joint stiffness) is due to osteoarthritis, the result of local trauma, osteochrondritis dissecans of the first metatarsal head, gout or pseudogout. In marked contrast to hallux valgus, men are more commonly affected than women.

Clinical features

Pain on walking, especially on slopes or rough ground, is the predominant symptom. The hallux is straight and the metatarsophalangeal joint is knobbly. Often there is a callosity under the medial side of the distal phalanx. The outer side of the sole of the shoe may be unduly worn – the result of rolling the foot outwards to avoid pressing on the big toe. The metatarsophalangeal joint feels enlarged and tender. Dorsiflexion is restricted and painful; plantarflexion also is limited, but less so. There may be compensatory hyperextension at the interphalangeal joint.

X-ray The changes are those of osteoarthritis; the joint space is narrowed, there is bone sclerosis and, often, large osteophytes.

Treatment

A rocker-soled shoe may abolish pain by allowing the foot to 'roll' without the necessity for dorsiflexion at the metatarsophalangeal joint.

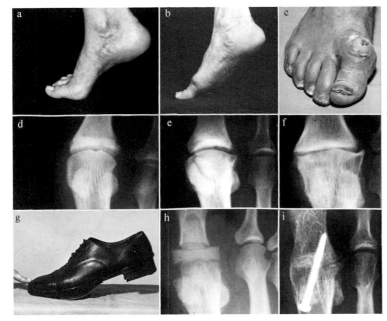

21.18 Hallux rigidus (a) In normal walking the hallux dorsiflexes considerably. With rigidus (b), dorsiflexion is limited; a dorsal callosity (c) may develop.

(d) Splitting osteochondritis or (e) a bipartite sesamoid may be precursors of (f) joint degeneration.

(g) A rocker sole relieves symptoms; operations include joint replacement with a Silastic spacer (h) and arthrodesis (i).

If walking is painful despite this adjustment, an operation is advised. For young patients the best operation is a simple *extension osteotomy* of the proximal phalanx, to mimic dorsiflexion at the interphalangeal joint. In older patients, *cheilectomy* is the procedure of choice: the dorsal osteophytes are removed in an attempt to restore some extension at the metatarsophalangeal joint; even 10 degrees can make a difference to the discomfort that the patient experiences each time the toe is forced into extension at the end of the stance phase in walking.

Joint replacement, using a Silastic prosthesis, may likewise increase movement and relieve pain; Silastic synovitis may develop, but after removing the prosthesis the pain relief and improved movement often remain. *Arthrodesis* of the metatarsophalangeal joint gives a more predictable result, especially in patients engaged in strenuous activities.

Claw toes

Flexion of the interphalangeal joints and hyperextension of the metatarsophalangeal joints constitute claw toes. This 'intrinsic-minus' deformity is seen in neurological disorders (e.g.

peroneal muscular atrophy, poliomyelitis and peripheral neuropathies) and in rheumatoid arthritis. Usually, however, no cause is found and the condition may be associated with idiopathic pes cavus; in such cases there is often a positive family history.

Clinical features

The patient complains of pain in the forefoot (metatarsalgia) and under the metatarsal heads. Usually the condition is bilateral and walking may be severely restricted. At first the joints are mobile and can be passively cor-

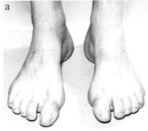
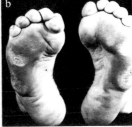

21.19 Claw toes Claw-toe deformity suggests muscle imbalance, with relative weakness of the intrinsics. Only occasionally, however (as in these examples of peroneal muscular atrophy), is a definite neurological defect found.

rected; later the deformities become fixed and the metatarsophalangeal joints subluxed or dislocated. Painful callosities may develop on the dorsum of the toes and under the metatarsal heads. In the most severe cases the skin ulcerates at the pressure sites.

Treatment

So long as the toes can be passively straightened the patient may obtain relief by wearing a metatarsal support or by having a transverse 'metatarsal bar' fitted to the shoe. If this fails, an operation is indicated. 'Dynamic' correction is possible by transferring the long toe flexors to the extensors.

When the deformity is fixed, it may either be accepted and accommodated by special footwear or treated by one of the following operations.

Interphalangeal arthrodesis Even when the toe deformities are fixed, the metatarsophalangeal joints may remain mobile. In these cases (usually young adults) arthrodesis of the toe joints permits active flexion of the metatarsophalangeal joints by the long flexors; this is often combined with transfer of the extensor hallucis longus to the first metatarsal, partly in order to remove a deforming force and partly to provide dynamic 'lift' for the forefoot.

Joint excision If passive toe flexion is not possible, the metatarsal heads can be excised;

the shortened toes fall into reasonable position even though the interphalangeal joints remain flexed, but occasionally they too must be excised and straightened.

Metatarsal osteotomy Oblique osteotomies of the outer four metatarsals (Helal, 1975), allowing the distal segments to slide proximally and dorsally, relax the dorsal structures and take pressure off the metatarsal heads. The theoretical advantages are not always matched by the clinical results unless the surgeon is an expert.

Amputation Toes that are severely contracted, dislocated and ulcerated are worse than none. If the circulation is satisfactory and the patient is willing to accept the appearance, amputation of all ten toes (the 'pobble' procedure) is a useful palliative operation.

Hammer toe

The proximal joint is fixed in flexion, while the distal joint and the metatarsophalangeal joint are extended. The second toe of one or both feet is commonly affected, and hyperextension of the metatarsophalangeal joint may go on to dorsal dislocation. Shoe pressure may produce painful corns or callosities on the dorsum of the toe and under the prominent metatarsal head.

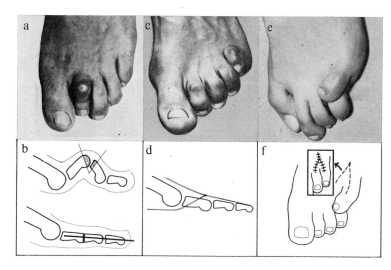

21.20 Toe disorders (a) Hammer toe, and (b) treatment by excision-arthrodesis. (c) Curly toes and (d) treatment by flexor-to-extensor transfer. (e) Overlapping fifth toe, and (f) treatment by V/Y-plasty.

The cause is obscure: the similarity to bou-tonnière deformity of a finger suggests an extensor dysfunction, a view supported by the frequent association with a dropped metatarsal head, flat anterior arch and hallux valgus. A simpler explanation is that the toe was too long or the shoe too short.

Operative correction is indicated for pain or for difficulty with shoes. The toe is shortened and straightened by excising the joint. A large wedge of soft tissue and bone is removed (including the corn if present). When the wound edges are firmly sutured the toe straightens and the excised joint needs no internal fixation. The toe is splinted for 6 weeks using a collodion bandage.

If the metatarsophalangeal joint is dislocated, a dorsal capsulotomy and elongation of the extensor tendon may be necessary; the joint is held in position with a Kirschner wire which is retained for 4 weeks.

Mallet toe

In mallet toe it is the distal interphalangeal joint that is flexed. The toenail or the tip of the toe presses into the shoe, resulting in a painful callosity.

If conservative treatment (chiropody and padding) does not help, operation is indicated. The distal interphalangeal joint is exposed, the articular surfaces excised and the toe straightened. A deep skin suture may suffice to hold the corrected position, but, if not, a thin Kirschner wire is inserted across the joint.

Fifth toe deformities

Overlapping fifth toe

This is a common congenital anomaly. If symptoms warrant, the toe may be straightened by a V/Y-plasty, reinforced by transferring the flexor to the extensor tendon.

Cock-up deformity

The metatarsophalangeal joint is dislocated and the little toe sits on the dorsum of the meta-

tarsal head. Operative treatment is usually successful: through a longitudinal plantar incision, the proximal phalanx is winkled out and removed; the wound is closed transversely, thus pulling the toe out of the hyperextended position.

Tailor's bunion

A bunionette may form over an abnormally prominent fifth metatarsal head. If the shoe cannot be adjusted to fit the bump, the bony prominence can be trimmed, taking care not to sever the tendon of the fifth toe abductor.

Tuberculous arthritis

(see also Chapter 2)

Tuberculous infection of the ankle joint begins as a synovitis or as an osteomyelitis and, because walking is painful, may present before true

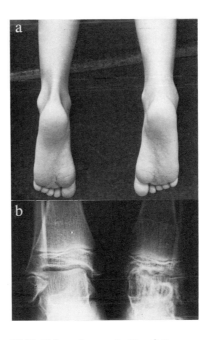

21.21 Tuberculous arthritis of the ankle (a) The swelling is best seen from behind; (b) shows rarefaction and joint destruction.

arthritis supervenes. The ankle is swollen and the calf markedly wasted; the skin feels warm and movements are restricted. Sinus formation occurs early. *X-rays* show generalized rarefaction, sometimes a bone abscess and, with late disease, narrowing and irregularity of the joint space.

TREATMENT In addition to general treatment (Chapter 3) a removable splint is used to rest the foot in neutral position. If the disease is arrested early, the patient is allowed up non-weightbearing in a caliper; gradually he takes more weight, then discards the caliper. Following arthritis, weightbearing is harmless, but stiffness is inevitable and usually arthrodesis is the best treatment.

Rheumatoid arthritis

(see also Chapter 3)

The ankle and foot are affected almost as often as the wrist and hand. During *stage 1* there is synovitis of the metatarsophalangeal, intertarsal and ankle joints, as well as of the sheathed tendons (usually the peronei and tibialis posterior). In *stage 2*, joint erosion and tendon dysfunction prepare the ground for the progressive deformities of *stage 3*.

The ankle and hindfoot

The earliest symptoms are pain and swelling around the ankle. Walking becomes increasingly difficult and, later, deformities appear. On examination, swelling and tenderness are usually localized to the back of the medial malleolus (tenosynovitis of tibialis posterior) or the lateral malleolus (tenosynovitis of the peronei). Less often the ankle swells (joint synovitis) and its movements are restricted. Inversion and eversion may be painful and limited. In the late stages the tibialis posterior may rupture (all

too often this is missed), or become ineffectual due to progressive erosion of the tarsal joints, and the foot gradually drifts into severe valgus deformity. X-rays show osteoporosis and, later, erosion of the tarsal and ankle joints. Soft-tissue swelling may be marked.

Treatment

In the stage of synovitis, splintage is essential (to allow inflammation to subside and to prevent deformity) while waiting for systemic treatment to control the disease. Initially, tendon sheaths and joints may be injected with methylprednisolone, but this should not be repeated more than two or three times. A lightweight below-knee caliper with an inside supporting strap restores stability and may be worn almost indefinitely.

If the synovitis does not subside, operative synovectomy and (if necessary) repair or replacement of the tendon are advisable. For tendon replacement, the common long toe flexor is used as a substitute; it is much thinner than tibialis posterior and the ankle will need to be splinted for at least 3 months after the operation.

In the very late stage, arthrodesis of the ankle and tarsal joints can still restore modest function and abolish pain. Unhappily, replacement of the ankle cannot yet be recommended.

The forefoot

Pain and swelling of the metatarsophalangeal joints are among the earliest features of rheumatoid arthritis. Shoes feel uncomfortable and the patient walks less and less. Tenderness is at first localized to the metatarsophalangeal joints; later the entire forefoot is painful on pressing or squeezing. With increasing weakness of the intrinsic muscles and joint destruction, the characteristic deformities appear: a flattened anterior arch, claw toes and hallux valgus. Subcutaneous nodules are common and may ulcerate. Dorsal corns and plantar callosities also may break down and become infected. In the worst cases the toes are dislocated, inflamed, ulcerated and useless. *X-rays* show

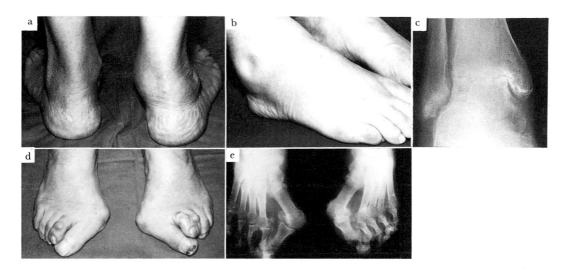

21.22 Rheumatoid arthritis Tenosynovitis of (a) tibialis posterior and (b) of the peronei are both common. (c) Ankle and subtalar arthritis. (d, e) Forefoot deformities due to erosion of metatarsophalangeal joints.

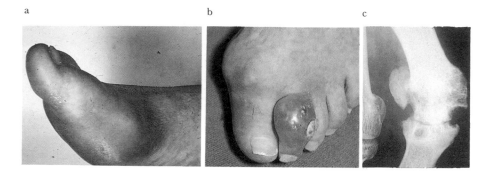

21.23 Gout (a) The classic picture – acute inflammation of the big toe metatarsophalangeal joint. (b) Tophaceous gout of the second toe. (c) X-ray of the first metatarsophalangeal joints; the large excavations are occupied by crystalline tophi.

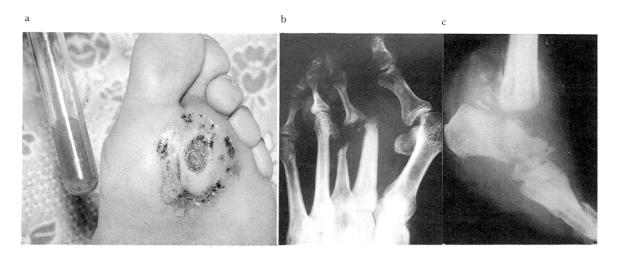

21.24 The diabetic foot (a) Ulceration in a patient with poorly controlled diabetes. (b, c) Despite the severe changes in these two patients with diabetic neuropathy, the feet were relatively painless.

osteoporosis and periarticular erosion at the metatarsophalangeal joints. Curiously – in contrast to the hand – the smaller digits (fourth and fifth toes) are affected first.

Treatment

During the stage of synovitis, anti-inflammatory injections and attention to footwear may relieve symptoms. Once deformity is progressive, treatment is that of the claw toes and hallux valgus. Sometimes a specially made shoe will accommodate the toes in relative comfort. If this does not help, the most effective operation is excision of the metatarsal heads in order to relieve pressure in the sole and to correct the toe deformities. For the hallux, an alternative is metatarsophalangeal fusion. If forefoot surgery is needed and the hindfoot is valgus, this deformity should be corrected by an orthosis (Stockley et al., 1990).

Gout (see also Chapter 4)

Swelling, redness, heat and exquisite tenderness of the metatarsophalangeal joint of the big toe ('podagra') is the epitome of gout. The condition may closely resemble septic arthritis, but the systemic features of infection are absent. The serum uric acid level may be raised.

Sometimes the ankle joint, or one of the toes, may be affected – especially following a minor injury.

Pain under the heel due to plantar fasciitis is another manifestation of gout, though the association may be hard to prove in any particular case.

Treatment with anti-inflammatory drugs will abort the acute attack of gout; until the pain subsides the foot should be rested and protected from injury.

The diabetic foot

Foot disorders are common in diabetes and result from a number of factors: peripheral vascular disease, peripheral neuropathy, osteoporosis and a predisposition to infection.

PERIPHERAL VASCULAR DISEASE   The patient may present with claudication, or continuously painful feet. Trophic changes are common; the skin may feel smooth and cold, and the pulses are weak or absent. Superficial ulceration occurs on the toes, deep ulceration typically under the heel. Small-vessel disease may cause dry gangrene of one or more toes; proximal vascular occlusion can be catastrophic and result in extensive wet gangrene. Treatment is concerned with simple measures such as care of the skin and prevention of infection. Dry gangrene of the toe can be allowed to demarcate before amputation; more severe occlusive disease with wet gangrene may call for immediate amputation.

NEUROPATHY   Sensory impairment may cause numbness, skin blistering, trophic changes and ulceration on the pressure areas under the metatarsal heads. Charcot joints may affect the ankle or the tarsus, giving rise to a swollen, relatively painless foot with typical x-ray changes. Motor loss usually manifests as claw toes; the prominent metatarsal heads are pressure sites for plantar ulceration. 'High spots' can be demonstrated on the pedobarograph and this is helpful in designing weight-relieving orthoses and custom-made shoes. Other forms of treatment include foot care (preferably by a qualified chiropodist), attention to plantar ulcers and the prevention or management of infection. Charcot joints are particularly troublesome and may require stabilizing orthoses or surgical removal of bony prominences that predispose to skin pressure (Newman, 1981).

OSTEOPOROSIS   There is a generalized loss of bone density in diabetes. In the foot the changes may be severe enough to result in insufficiency fractures around the ankle or in the metatarsals. A well-padded cast may relieve pain but it is important not to immobilize the foot for longer than seems essential as this will merely aggravate the osteoporosis.

INFECTION Diabetes (if not controlled) is known to have a deleterious effect on white cell function. This, combined with local ischaemia, insensitivity to skin injury and localized pressure due to deformity, makes sepsis an ever-recurring hazard. Great care is needed with nail trimming; skin cracks should be kept clean and covered; ulcers should be treated with local dressings and antibiotics if necessary. Occasionally, septicaemia calls for admission to hospital and treatment with intravenous antibiotics.

Osteoarthritis (see also Chapter 5)

Osteoarthritis of the ankle is almost always secondary to some underlying disorder: a malunited fracture, recurrent instability, osteochondritis dissecans of the talus, avascular necrosis of the talus or repeated bleeding with haemophilia. Sometimes, however, it is involved in generalized osteoarthritis and pyrophosphate arthropathy.

Symptoms are often quite tolerable, because extremes of range are not required with normal use. *Treatment* is therefore usually conservative – anti-inflammatory drugs and, sometimes, splintage or simply wearing a strong boot. If operation is required, an arthrodesis is performed, even though the complication rate is quite high; however, a reliable prosthetic replacement is not yet available.

Osteochondritis dissecans of the talus

Unexplained pain and slight limitation of movement in the ankle of a young person may be due to a small osteochondral fracture of the upper surface of the talus, though the injury may have been forgotten. X-rays taken at appropriate angles to produce tangential views of the talar surface show the small bony separation (no more than a few millimetres in diameter) at either the anteromedial or the posterolateral part of the superior surface of the talus. The lesion may be visualized directly by arthroscopy.

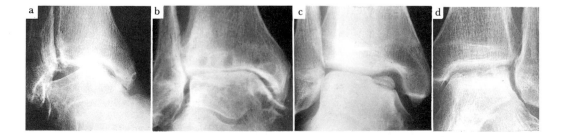

21.25 Osteoarthritis and osteochondritis (a) The obvious malalignment which followed an old injury has led to osteoarthritis. (b) In this ankle the narrowed joint space and subarticular cysts are characteristic of osteoarthritis; the cause is not clear, though it may have been trauma. (c) Osteochondritis dissecans at the common site; this may lead to degeneration. (d) In this unusual example of osteochrondritis a large part of the dome of the talus is affected.

Treatment depends on the degree of cartilage damage. As long as the articular cartilage is intact, it is sufficient to restrict activities. Once it is softened, arthroscopic drilling may be helpful; but if it is also frayed, the affected area should probably be curetted (Pritsch, Horoshovski and Farine, 1986). A loose fragment may need removal, but often the symptoms are insufficient to warrant intervention.

Ruptured tendo Achillis

Probably rupture occurs only if the tendon is degenerate. Consequently most patients are aged over 40. While pushing off (running or jumping), the calf muscle contracts; but the contraction is resisted by body weight and the tendon ruptures. The patient feels as if he has been struck just above the heel, and he is unable to tiptoe. Soon after the tear occurs, a gap can be seen and felt 5 cm above the insertion of the tendon. Plantarflexion of the foot is weak and is not accompanied by tautening of the tendon. Where doubt exists, Simmonds' test is helpful: with the patient prone, the calf is squeezed; if the tendon is intact the foot is seen to plantarflex; if the tendon is ruptured the foot remains still.

Differential diagnosis

INCOMPLETE TEAR   This is uncommon but is frequently diagnosed in error. The mistake arises because, if a complete rupture is not seen within 24 hours, the gap is difficult to feel; moreover, the patient may by then be able to stand on tiptoe (just), by using his long toe flexors.

TEAR OF SOLEUS MUSCLE   A tear at the musculotendinous junction causes pain and tenderness halfway up the calf. This recovers with the aid of physiotherapy and raising the heel of the shoe.

Treatment

If the patient is seen early, the ends of the tendon may approximate when the foot is passively plantarflexed. If so, plaster is applied with the foot in equinus and is worn for 8 weeks. A shoe with a raised heel is worn for a further 6 weeks.

Operative repair is probably safer, but an equinus plaster for 8 weeks and a heel raise for a further 6 weeks are still needed. If repair is performed through a vertical incision, wound breakdown is not uncommon; however, a small transverse incision is probably adequate (Aldam, 1989) and it is even possible to use an entirely percutaneous method (Ma and Griffith, 1977) or not to repair the tendon at all but

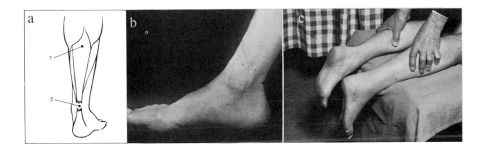

21.26 Tendo Achillis   (a) The soleus may tear at its musculotendinous junction (1) but the tendo Achillis itself ruptures 5 cm above its insertion (2). (b) The depression seen in this picture at the site of rupture later fills with blood. (c) Simmonds' test: both calves are being squeezed but only the left foot plantarflexes – the right tendon is ruptured.

simply approximate the ends with an external fixator and Kirschner wires (Nada, 1985). For ruptures that present late, repair with carbon fibre is a possibility.

Sesamoid chondromalacia

Softening of the articular cartilage on the medial sesamoid may cause pain on walking and localized tenderness. A local injection of methylprednisolone and local anaesthetic often helps; otherwise the sesamoid should be removed.

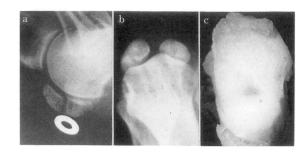

21.27 Sesamoid chondromalacia (a) Bipartite medial sesamoid. This is seldom a cause of symptoms, but it was in this woman; the metal marker indicates the site of her tenderness. (b) Skyline view of the same patient; the appearance resembles that of chondromalacia patellae. (c) The sesamoid had obvious cartilage degeneration; it was removed through a plantar incision, with complete relief of symptoms.

The paralysed foot

Weakness or paralysis of the foot may be symptomless, or may present in one of three characteristic ways: the patient may complain of difficulty in walking; he may 'catch his toe' on climbing stairs (due to weak dorsiflexion); or he may stumble and fall (due to instability).

Clinical features

UPPER MOTOR NEURON LESIONS   Spastic paralysis may occur in children with cerebral palsy or in adults following a stroke. Muscle imbalance usually leads to equinus or equinovarus deformity. The reflexes are brisk but sensation is normal. The entire limb (or both lower limbs) is usually abnormal.

LOWER MOTOR NEURON LESIONS   Poliomyelitis was (and in some parts of the world still is) a common cause of foot paralysis. If all muscle groups are affected, the foot is flail and dangles from the ankle; if knee extension also is weak, the patient cannot walk without a caliper. With unbalanced weakness, the foot develops fixed deformity; it may also be smaller and colder than normal, but sensation is normal. Other lower motor neuron disorders such as spinal cord tumours, peroneal muscular atrophy and severe nerve root compression are rare causes of foot weakness or deformity.

PERIPHERAL NERVE INJURIES   The sciatic, lateral popliteal or peroneal nerve may be affected. The commonest abnormalities are drop foot and weakness of peroneal action. Postoperative or postimmobilization drop foot is due to pressure on the lateral popliteal or on the peroneal nerve as the leg rolls into external rotation. In addition to motor weakness there is an area of sensory loss. Unless the nerve is divided, recovery is possible but may take many months.

Treatment

The weakness may need no treatment at all, or only a splint.

The drop foot following nerve palsy can be treated by transferring the tibialis posterior through the interosseous membrane to the mid-tarsal region.

Spastic paralysis can be treated by tendon release and transfer, but great care is needed to prevent overaction in the new direction. Thus, a spastic equinovarus deformity may be converted to a severe valgus deformity by transferring tibialis anterior to the lateral side; this is avoided if only half the tendon is transferred.

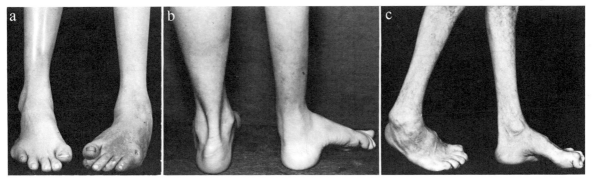

21.28 The paralysed foot   (a) In spina bifida – the small ulcer is an indication of insensitive skin. (b) Poliomyelitis and (c) peroneal muscular atrophy, in both of which sensation is normal.

Fixed deformities must be corrected first before doing tendon transfers. If no adequate tendon is available to permit dynamic correction, the joint may be reshaped and arthrodesed; at the same time muscle rebalancing (even of weak muscles) is necessary, otherwise the deformity will recur.

Painful feet

'My feet are killing me!' The complaint is common but the cause is often elusive. Pain may be due to: (1) mechanical pressure (which is more likely if the foot is deformed); (2) joint inflammation or stiffness; (3) a localized bone lesion; (4) peripheral ischaemia; or (5) muscular strain – usually secondary to some other abnormality. Remember, too, that local disorders may be part of a generalized disease (e.g. diabetes or rheumatoid arthritis), so examination of the entire patient may be indicated.

Specific foot disorders that cause pain are considered below in anatomical sequence.

Painful heel

The common causes of heel pain vary according to age.

CHILDREN

Sever's disease (apophysitis) usually occurs in boys of about 10 years. It is not a 'disease' but a mild traction injury. Pain and tenderness are localized to the tendo Achillis insertion. The x-ray report usually refers to increased density and fragmentation of the apophysis, but often the painless heel looks similar. The heel of the shoe should be raised a little and strenuous activities restricted for a few weeks.

ADOLESCENTS

In girls aged 15–20, a *calcaneal knob* (often bilateral) is common. The posterolateral portion of the calcaneum is too prominent and the shoe rubs on it, causing pain and sometimes blistering. Treatment should be conservative – attention to footwear (open-back shoes are best) and padding of the heel. Operative treatment – removal of the bump or dorsal wedge osteotomy of the calcaneum – is feasible but the results are generally poor (Taylor, 1986).

YOUNG ADULTS

Bursitis just above the insertion of the tendo Achillis may result from ill-fitting footwear, especially in young women and army recruits. Localized pain and tenderness occur. Pain is relieved by removing the stiffener from the heel of the shoe.

Peritendinitis of the tendo Achillis occurs in athletes. The acute form may be relieved by rest, ice-packs, strapping or a hydrocortisone injection (not into the tendon!). The chronic

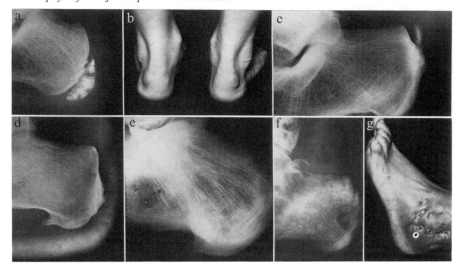

21.29 Heel disorders   (a) Sever's disease – the apophysis is dense and fragmented. (b) Bilateral heel knobs. (c) Achillis bursitis, in this case with calcification. (d) 'Policeman's heel' – both heels had spurs but only one side was painful; were these spurs perhaps associated with gout? (e) Paget's disease. (f, g) Tuberculosis of the calcaneum.

form may need operation. Dividing the investing fascia and freeing adhesions may be adequate but, if there is a necrotic area of the tendon itself, this may need excision.

Acute plantar fasciitis occurs as a 'reactive' disorder associated with gonorrhoea, Reiter's disease and ankylosing spondylitis. Pain and tenderness are localized to the undersurface of the front of the calcaneum. The underlying cause should be treated and the painful area protected from pressure, if necessary with a padded plaster cast.

OLDER ADULTS
'Policeman's heel' affects patients aged 40–60. It is sometimes called *plantar fasciitis* and is thought to be due to traction, followed by an inflammatory reaction, where the plantar fascia is attached to the calcaneum. The only abnormal physical sign is localized tenderness beneath the calcaneum. X-ray sometimes shows a bony spur projecting forwards from the undersurface of the calcaneal tuberosity.

Treatment is conservative: anti-inflammatory drugs or local injection of corticosteroids, and a pad under the heel to off-load the painful area. Pain usually subsides after 6–12 months.

Any *bone disorder in the calcaneum* can present as heel pain: osteomyelitis, osteoid osteoma, cyst-like lesions and Paget's disease are the most likely. X-rays usually provide the diagnosis.

Painful tarsus

In children, pain in the mid-tarsal region is rare: one cause is *Köhler's disease* (osteochondritis of the navicular). The bony nucleus of the navicular becomes dense and fragmented. The child, under the age of 5, has a painful limp, and a tender warm thickening over the navicular. If the foot is strapped and activity restricted for a few weeks, symptoms disappear. The foot eventually becomes normal clinically and radiologically. A comparable condition occasionally affects middle-aged women (Brailsford's disease); the navicular becomes dense, then altered in shape, and later the mid-tarsal joint may degenerate.

In adults, especially if the arch is high, a ridge of bone sometimes develops on the adjacent dorsal surfaces of the medial cuneiform and the first metatarsal (the '*overbone*'). A lump can be seen which feels bony and may become bigger

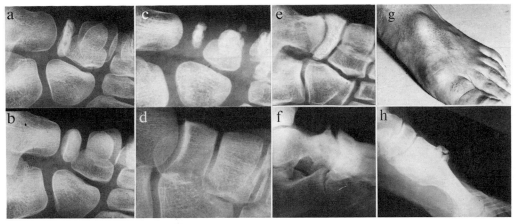

21.30 Painful tarsus (a) Köhler's disease compared with (b) the normal foot. (c) Another example of Köhler's disease, and (d) the same foot fully grown – it has become normal. (e) Brailsford's disease, the adult equivalent of Köhler's disease. (f) Degeneration of the talonavicular joint. (g, h) The 'overbone' at the first cuneiform-metatarsal joint.

and tender if the shoe presses on it. If shoe adjustment fails to provide relief the lump may be bevelled off.

Painful forefoot (metatarsalgia)

Any foot abnormality that results in faulty weight distribution may produce metatarsalgia. The causes are therefore numerous.

THE FOOT AS A WHOLE   A *splay foot* is wide and often associated with *hallux valgus* and *curly toes*. It is commonly seen in middle-aged women who have put on weight. A *cavus foot* with *claw toes* causes pain under the metatarsal heads because weight is taken over too limited an area.

INDIVIDUAL TOES   *Hallux disorders*, including failed operations, are the commonest causes of pain in the metatarsal region, because of faulty weight distribution. If any of the other toes is painful or deformed so that it does not take its proper share of weight, pain under its metatarsal head is liable to occur. Thus, *hammer toe*, *claw toes* and *curly toes* may all produce metatarsalgia.

LOCAL DISORDERS   Three fairly common disorders must be sought.

Freiberg's disease This is a 'crushing' type of osteochondritis of the second metatarsal head (rarely the third). It affects young adults, usually women. A bony lump (the enlarged head) is palpable and tender; the joint is irritable. X-rays show the head to be too wide and flat, the neck thick and the joint space increased. If discomfort is marked, the metatarsal is shortened or the metatarsal head excised.

Stress fracture Stress fracture, usually of the second or third metatarsal, occurs in young adults after unaccustomed activity or in women with postmenopausal osteoporosis. The affected shaft feels thick and tender. The x-ray appearance is at first normal, but later shows fusiform callus around a fine transverse fracture. Long before x-ray signs appear, a radioisotope scan will show increased activity. Treatment is either unneccessary or consists simply of rest.

Morton's metatarsalgia The patient, usually a woman of 40–50 years, complains of sharp pain in the forefoot, radiating to the toes. Tenderness is localized to one of the interdigital spaces – usually the third – and sensation may be diminished in the cleft and adjacent toes. This is essentially an entrapment syndrome affecting

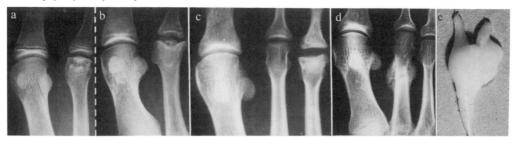

21.31 Metatarsalgia   (a, b) Stages in the development of Freiberg's disease; (c) the comparable disorder in the third metatarsal (Köhler's second disease); (d) stress fracture; (e) 'neuroma' excised from patient with Morton's metatarsalgia.

one of the digital nerves, but secondary thickening of the nerve creates the impression of a 'neuroma'. If symptoms do not respond to protective padding the 'neuroma' is excised.

Tarsal tunnel syndrome

Pain and sensory disturbance in the medial part of the forefoot, unrelated to weightbearing, may be due to compression of the posterior tibial nerve behind and below the medial malleolus. The pain is often worse at night and the patient may seek relief by walking around or stamping his foot. Paraesthesia and numbness may follow the characteristic sensory distribution, but these symptoms are not as well defined as in other entrapment syndromes. The diagnosis is difficult to establish but nerve conduction studies may show slowing of motor or sensory conduction.

Treatment   To decompress the nerve it is exposed behind the medial malleolus and followed into the sole; sometimes it is trapped by the belly of adductor hallucis arising more proximally than usual.

Toenail disorders

The toenail of the hallux may be ingrown, overgrown or undergrown.

INGROWN   The nail burrows into the nail groove; this ulcerates and its wall grows over the nail, so the term 'embedded toenail' would be better. The patient is taught to cut the nail square, to insert pledgets of wool under the ingrowing edges and always to keep the feet clean and dry. If these measure fail, the 'gutter' treatment is worth trying. A small wedge of soft tissue (where the nail digs in) is excised; a fine polythene tube is cut vertically in half and a segment inserted between nail and soft tissue. An alternative is to excise a segment of nail, remove hypertrophied granulation tissue and apply phenol for 3 minutes; this is then carefully wiped off and the toe cleaned with alcohol-soaked gauze (Van der Ham, Hackeng and Tik Ien Yo, 1990). If necessary the entire nail can be removed, taking care to remove the germinal matrix.

OVERGROWN (ONYCHOGRYPOSIS)   The nail is hard, thick and curved. A chiropodist can usually make the patient comfortable, but occasionally the nail may need excision.

UNDERGROWN   A subungual exostosis grows on the dorsum of the terminal phalanx and pushes the nail upwards. The exostosis should be removed.

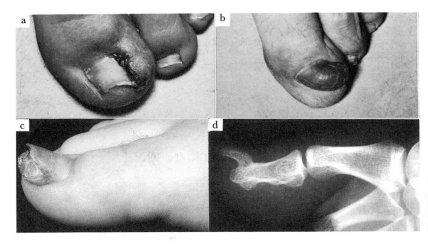

21.32 Toenail disorders (a) In-grown toenail. (b) Overgrown toe-nail (onychogryphosis). (c) Un-dergrown toenail, caused by (d) a subungual exostosis.

Notes on applied anatomy

The ankle and foot function as an integrated unit, and together provide stable support, proprioception, balance and mobility.

THE ANKLE   The ankle fits together like a tenon and mortise; the tibial and fibular parts of the mortise are bound together by the inferior tibiofibular ligament, and stability is augmented by the collateral ligaments. The medial ligament fans out from the tibial malleolus to the talus, the superficial fibres forming the deltoid ligament. The lateral ligament has three thickened bands: the anterior and posterior talofibular ligaments and, between them, the calcaneofibular ligament. Tears of these ligaments may cause tilting of the talus in its mortise. Forced abduction or adduction may disrupt the mortise altogether by (1) forcing the tibia and fibula apart (diastasis of the tibiofibular joint), (2) tearing the collateral ligaments or (3) fracturing the malleoli.

THE FOOT   The footprint gives some idea of the arched structure of the foot. This derives from the tripodial bony framework between the calcaneum posteriorly and the first and fifth metatarsal heads. The medial arch is high, with the navicular as its keystone; the lateral arch is flatter. The anterior arch, formed by the metatarsal bones, thrusts maximally upon the first and fifth metatarsal heads and flattens out (spreading the foot) during weightbearing; it can be pulled up by contraction of the intrinsic muscles, which flex the metatarsophalangeal joints.

MOVEMENTS   The ankle allows movement in the sagittal plane only – plantarflexion and dorsiflexion. Adduction and abduction (turning the toes towards or away from the midline) are produced by rotation of the entire leg below the knee; if either is forced at the ankle, the mortise fractures. Pronation and supination occur at the intertarsal and tarsometatarsal joints; the foot rotates about an axis running through the second metatarsal, the sole turning laterally (pronation) or medially (supination) – movements analogous to those of the forearm. The combination of plantarflexion, adduction and supination is called inversion; the opposite movement of dorsiflexion, abduction and pronation is eversion.

Inversion and eversion are necessary for walking on rough ground or across a slope. If the joints at which they occur are arthrodesed

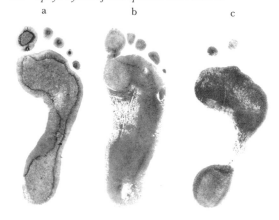

21.33 Footprints   (a) The normal foot, (b) flat foot (the medial arch touches the ground), and (c) cavus foot (even the lateral arch barely makes contact).

in childhood, a compensatory change may occur at the ankle so that it becomes a ball-and-socket joint.

FOOT POSITIONS AND DEFORMITIES   A downward-pointing foot is said to be in equinus; the opposite is calcaneus. If only the forefoot points downwards the term 'plantaris' is used. Supination with adduction produces a varus deformity; pronation with abduction causes pes valgus. An unusually high arch is called pes cavus. Many of these terms are used as if they were definitive diagnoses when, in fact, they are nothing more than Latin translations of descriptive anatomy.

References and further reading

Aldam, C.H. (1989) Repair of calcaneal tendon ruptures. *Journal of Bone and Joint Surgery* **71B**, 486–488

Atar, D., Grant, A.D., Silver, L., Lehman, W.B. and Strongwater, A.M. (1990) The use of a tissue expander in clubfoot surgery. *Journal of Bone and Joint Surgery* **72B**, 574–577

Attenborough, C.G. (1966) Severe congenital talipes equinovarus. *Journal of Bone and Joint Surgery* **48B**, 31–39

Bower, B.L., Keyser, C.K. and Gilula, L.A. (1989) Rigid subtalar joint – a radiographic spectrum. *Skeletal Radiology* **17**, 583–588

Colton, C.L. (1973) The surgical management of congenital vertical talus. *Journal of Bone and Joint Surgery* **55B**, 566–574

Dwyer, F.C. (1963) The treatment of relapsed club foot by the insertion of a wedge into the calcaneum. *Journal of Bone and Joint Surgery* **45B**, 67–75

Editorial (1980) Corrective shoes for children. *British Medical Journal* **280**, 1556–1557

Evans, D. (1961) Relapsed club foot. *Journal of Bone and Joint Surgery* **43B**, 722–733

Helal, B. (1975) Metatarsal osteotomy for metatarsalgia. *Journal of Bone and Joint Surgery* **57B**, 187–192

Jahss, M.H. (1980) Tarsometatarsal truncated-wedge arthrodesis for pes cavus and equinovarus deformity of the fore part of the foot. *Journal of Bone and Joint Surgery* **62A**, 713–722

Ma, G.W.C. and Griffith, T.G. (1977) Percutaneous repair of acute closed ruptured Achilles tendon. *Clinical Orthopaedics and Related Research* **128**, 247–255

Mann, R.A. (1986) *Surgery of the Foot*, C.V. Mosby, St Louis, Toronto, Princeton

Nada, A. (1985) Rupture of the calcaneal tendon. *Journal of Bone and Joint Surgery* **67B**, 449–453

Newman, J.H. (1981) Non-infective disease of the diabetic foot. *Journal of Bone and Joint Surgery* **63B**, 593–596

Perkins, G. (1961) *Orthopaedics*, Athlone Press, London

Phillips, G.E. (1983) A review of elongation of os calcis for flat feet. *Journal of Bone and Joint Surgery* **65B**, 15–18

Porter, R.W. (1987) Congenital talipes equinovarus. II. A staged method of surgical management. *Journal of Bone and Joint Surgery* **69B**, 826–831

Pritsch, M., Horoshovski, H. and Farine, I. (1986) Arthroscopic treatment of osteochondral lesions of the talus. *Journal of Bone and Joint Surgery* **68A**, 862–865

Rose, G.K., Welton, E.A. and Marshall, T. (1985) The diagnosis of flat foot in the child. *Journal of Bone and Joint Surgery* **67B**, 71–78

Stockley, I., Betts, R.P., Rowley, D.I., Getty, C.J.M. and Duckworth, T. (1990) The importance of the valgus hindfoot in forefoot surgery in rheumatoid arthritis. *Journal of Bone and Joint Surgery* **72B**, 705–708

Taylor, G.J. (1986) Prominence of the calcaneus: is operation justified? *Journal of Bone and Joint Surgery* **68B**, 467–470

Van der Ham, A.C., Hackeng, C.A.H. and Tik Ien Yo (1990) The treatment of ingrowing toenails. *Journal of Bone and Joint Surgery* **72B**, 507–509

Walker, A.P., Ghali, N.N. and Silk, F.F. (1985) Congenital vertical talus. *Journal of Bone and Joint Surgery* **67B**, 117–121

Williams, P.F. (1987) Club foot. *Current Orthopaedics* **1**, 404–411

Part 3 — Fractures and Joint Injuries

The management of acute injuries   22

Trauma is the commonest cause of death in people under 40. In the industrial world, road accidents alone claim 1 in 10 000 lives each year. Limb injuries are the commonest, head and visceral injuries the most lethal; this simple observation determines the priorities in management. Most deaths occur within the first hour of injury, before the patient arrives at hospital; the cause of death in these cases is usually severe brain or cardiovascular injury for which countermeasures are of limited value. A second (much lower) peak in trauma deaths occurs between 1 and 4 hours after injury; these usually result from uncompensated blood loss and, with a competent accident service, most are preventable. A third peak in the cumulative mortality rate appears several weeks later when patients die of the late complications of trauma and multiple organ failure.

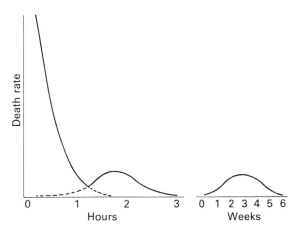

22.1 Death following trauma The trimodal pattern of mortality following severe trauma.

For most severe injuries management proceeds in several well-defined stages: emergency treatment at the scene of the accident and during transit to hospital; resuscitation and evaluation in the accident department; early treatment of visceral injuries and cardiorespiratory complications; provisional fixation followed by definitive treatment of musculoskeletal injuries; and, finally, long-term rehabilitation of the patient.

The scene of the accident

Multiple accidents

The first duty of a doctor arriving at the scene of a major accident is to introduce calm and order into the prevailing chaos. His actions should be swift yet unhurried, cautious yet purposeful. Until the police or other authorities arrive he should assume control and, after rapidly assessing the situation, decide on priorities. If unskilled help is at hand, messages are sent to the emergency services (ambulance, police and fire); the nearest accident centre is alerted and, where mobile operating theatres and surgical teams are available, they may need to be summoned.

The individual patient

Treatment of the individual patient begins as soon as possible. A useful sequence (modified to suit the circumstances) is: obtain access;

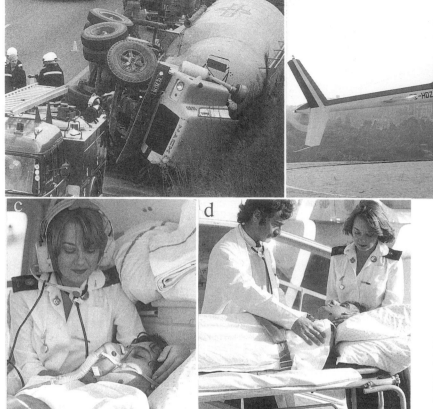

22.2 The major accident (a) Major accidents call for (b) a rapid response, (c) expert care during transport and (d) a 24-hour medical service in the accident centre.

ensure airway and ventilation; examine; extricate; arrest haemorrhage; combat shock; splint fractures; and transport.

ACCESS When a patient is trapped or buried, the objects covering him should be moved, rather than pulling him out from beneath them. Priority is given to freeing the head and trunk. If the patient is conscious he will need immediate reassurance.

AIRWAY AND VENTILATION If the unconscious patient is breathing stertorously the angle of the jaw is pulled forwards and the head extended; should the difficulty persist a finger is inserted into the mouth to ensure that breathing is not being obstructed by the tongue, false teeth or any other foreign body. If, despite clearing the

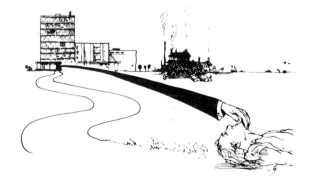

22.3 Severe injuries – danger point This drawing (reproduced by kind permission of Mr R.S. Garden and the Editor of *Injury*) emphasizes the vital (literally) importance of a clear airway, and how it can usually be achieved.

upper airway, the patient still cannot breathe freely, he may have a sucking wound of the chest wall, which should be covered with a dressing strapped firmly in position. If suitable equipment is available, endotracheal intubation can be carried out as an emergency measure and oxygen administered.

EXAMINATION   A detailed examination is neither practicable nor essential, but the pulse is felt, the respirations are observed, and the head, chest, abdomen and limbs, if accessible, are quickly palpated.

EXTRICATION   A patient with fractures should not be dragged forcibly from overlying impedimenta. When obstructions have been lifted he can be gently moved. Twisting and flexion must be avoided if there is the possibility of spinal injury.

HAEMORRHAGE   External bleeding can usually be stopped by pressure with a finger, forceps or a firm pad. Tourniquets are rarely necessary; if one must be used, a label stating the time of its application is attached to the patient in a prominent position.

SHOCK   Morphine is invaluable and, for a severely injured adult, it is probably best to give both 10 mg intravenously and 10 mg intramuscularly; again, adequate labelling is essential. Morphine should not be given to patients with abdominal or head injuries. Where facilities are available, intravenous fluids may be given. *No food or fluids should be given by mouth*; if the patient is unconscious these may enter the trachea, and even if he is conscious their presence in the stomach increases the hazards of anaesthesia during the next few hours.

SPLINTAGE   A broken limb should be gently straightened by traction; it is important to relieve pressure on tented skin so as to avoid turning a closed fracture into an open one. A fractured arm is easily splinted by bandaging it to the trunk, and a leg by tying it to the other leg if this is intact. Ambulances should carry inflatable splints, and only occasionally are improvised splints needed; an umbrella, walking stick, piece of wood or tubular steel is nearly always available. Open wounds are covered with a clean dressing.

TRANSPORT   To move a severely injured patient onto a stretcher at least two, but preferably three, people are required, so that he is transferred 'in one piece' without serious disturbance; this is particularly important with spinal fractures. The unconscious patient is best transported in the semi-prone position. The airway and pulse should be checked once more before the patient leaves in the ambulance.

Ambulances should be equipped with splints, dressings, airways, oxygen and transfusion apparatus. They should be in two-way radio communication with the accident unit. In difficult terrain, helicopter ambulances are almost essential. Ambulance attendants are usually highly trained but every effort should be made by the staff of the accident unit to keep them continually informed, up to date and interested in their work. Their observations on the patient's state of consciousness and general condition are invaluable.

Management in hospital

Patients who arrive in hospital after a major accident are at risk of falling into the second 'mortality peak', with death from hypovolaemic shock. This second period has been dubbed 'the golden hour', during which effective resuscitation can save lives.

There are three stages of care in the emergency room: (1) initial assessment; (2) immediate care and resuscitation; and (3) secondary evaluation and planning of definitive treatment or transfer. Sometimes these steps follow in an orderly sequence; sometimes, however, the situation is so urgent that the first rapid assessment and resuscitation proceed simultaneously, or immediate definitive treatment may be necessary to save a life, or a limb, or to prevent cord damage.

Initial assessment

The patient is stripped and examined rapidly from head to toe. The ABC of initial simultaneous evaluation and treatment is AIRWAY, BREATHING and CIRCULATION. If there are injuries around the head and face, damage to the cervical spine should be assumed and care should be taken not to flex or extend the neck until a cervical spine injury has been definitely excluded.

AIRWAY   The upper airway is cleared of debris, vomitus, false teeth or torn soft tissues; the jaw is pulled forward to dislodge any obstruction by the back of the tongue. If necessary, an oropharyngeal or nasopharyngeal airway is inserted; occasionally, endotracheal intubation or tracheostomy may be called for. During these manoeuvres the neck should be protected from movement.

BREATHING   If, despite a clear airway, ventilation is inadequate the chest should be carefully examined for atelectasis, pneumothorax or a flail segment. Tension pneumothorax is a life-threatening complication and should be treated by immediate decompression: a large-bore needle is inserted into the pleural cavity through the second intercostal space in the mid-clavicular line; once the emergency is over this is replaced by tube thoracostomy through the fifth intercostal space in the mid-axillary line. Sucking chest wounds must be closed and a flail chest requires endotracheal intubation and positive pressure ventilation. It is wise to give all severely injured patients supplemental oxygen and to take a blood sample for measurement of Pco_2 and Po_2.

CIRCULATION   Any major external haemorrhage is controlled by direct pressure. Then the heart is examined, the pulses are felt and the blood pressure is measured (a palpable carotid pulse signifies an arterial pressure of at least 40 mmHg). Wounds – especially small penetrating chest or abdominal wounds – are sought and intravenous infusion is begun. Protruding weapons or other penetrating objects should be left alone and removed only when operative facilities are available and ready.

Cardiac tamponade should be suspected if there is a significant chest injury or penetrating wound, if the blood pressure cannot be maintained by rapid infusion of intravenous fluids, or if there are clinical features such as distended neck veins and a paradoxical pulse. Tamponade is a life-threatening condition and should be treated by immediate decompression with a needle or catheter inserted below the xiphisternum.

FURTHER ASSESSMENT   The abdomen and pelvis are now examined; then the extremities are inspected for wounds or fractures and tested rapidly for muscle activity and sensation. Unless there is pain in the neck or back, the patient is gently rolled onto his side 'in one piece' and the back is inspected and palpated from occiput to natal cleft.

The level of consciousness is assessed on the Glasgow Coma Scale (see later, under 'Head injuries'). All findings are carefully recorded and kept available for comparison with later assessment.

Resuscitation

Resuscitation has begun with the establishment of a clear airway and the restoration of breathing and ventilation. Equally important is to prevent hypovolaemia and treat shock from the earliest moment possible. As a first measure a crystalloid solution such as Ringer's lactate is infused rapidly via one or two large-bore needles or venous cut-down. If the blood pressure does not stabilize after 2 litres of fluid, blood transfusion should be started. Central venous pressure (CVP) is carefully monitored: in hypovolaemic shock the neck veins are collapsed and CVP is low; if the veins are distended and the CVP is increased, tension pneumothorax and cardiac tamponade must be excluded. If the blood pressure cannot be maintained by blood transfusion and cardiac embarrassment has been excluded, the source of continued bleeding must be sought and attended to. In severe shock, pneumatic anti-shock garments are sometimes used. At first only the lower portion of the suit is inflated and the patient's response observed before going any further. Similarly, when the suit is deflated this is done bit by bit so as not to cause a sudden severe fall in blood pressure.

Secondary evaluation

Once the patient has been resuscitated a more careful examination is carried out and the patient sent for x-ray and other investigations. A systematic examination of the head and neck, chest, abdomen and pelvis takes less than 15 minutes. If there is a suspicion of pelvic injury, the perineum should be examined and the penis inspected for bleeding at the meatus; a rectal examination is mandatory. Indeed, a good general adage is 'A finger or a tube in every orifice'.

The extremities are examined in more detail, looking for signs of bone or joint injury. If a vascular injury is suspected, angiography may be necessary. If there are multiple injuries, x-rays of the spine, pelvis and hips may disclose unsuspected fractures or dislocations. In patients with head, spine or pelvic injury, a CT scan may be needed.

Further definitive treatment will be decided by the findings during the secondary review. However, over the next 24–48 hours the patient is still at risk of lethal complications such as shock, respiratory distress syndrome, fat embolism, infection and multiple organ failure. Priority is given at all times to preventive measures such as blood transfusion and oxygenation; there is also evidence that the risk of acute pulmonary dysfunction is lessened by immediate external fixation of unstable fractures.

Shock

Shock is a generalized state of reduced tissue perfusion; if allowed to persist it will result in irreversible damage to the life-supporting organs.

NEUROGENIC SHOCK This occurs with painful injuries, emotional disturbances or both. The blood volume is unchanged but its distribution is faulty, with excess in the non-essential circulation (splanchnic vessels and skeletal muscles) and insufficient in the essential circulation (cerebal and cardiac vessels).

HYPOVOLAEMIC SHOCK This is the result of bleeding, whether internal or external. The blood volume is reduced, but the harmful effects of this reduction are mitigated, again by redistribution; the peripheral and splanchnic vessels contract, so that a higher proportion of the reduced volume becomes available for the heart and brain. In addition, catecholamine release helps to maintain cardiac output. These compensatory mechanisms may fail if the blood loss is great or rapid; the peripheral vessels then become dilated, the cardiac output and blood pressure drop and the circulation fails. This dangerous condition of peripheral vasodilatation is sometimes induced or hastened by heating the patient or giving him alcohol.

Decreased perfusion leads to tissue hypoxia, acidosis and progressive cell damage. Endothelial cell disintegration and capillary leakage contribute further to the cycle of fluid loss, diminished perfusion and irreversible organ failure. Cell membrane disruption and leucocyte/macrophage stimulation result in the release of acute inflammatory mediators such as tumour necrosis factor, interleukins and products of arachidonic acid metabolism.

Clinical features

The bystander who faints at the sight of an accident is suffering from transient neurogenic shock. The injured person also is suffering from neurogenic shock but, because of the blood loss, hypovolaemic shock may supervene. He becomes ill, apathetic and thirsty, his breathing shallow and rapid; the lips and skin are pale and the extremities feel cold and clammy. As compensation fails, the pulse becomes rapid and feeble while the blood pressure drops. Eventually renal function is impaired, urinary output falls and urinary osmolarity increases. Shock must not be diagnosed as purely neurogenic unless careful examination has failed to reveal any serious injury.

Treatment

Neurogenic shock is treated by elevating the legs, relieving pain and dispelling fear. If rapid recovery does not occur, the patient is suffering from hypovolaemic shock or cardiac dysfunction.

The treatment of hypovolaemic shock is urgent: the essentials are to arrest bleeding and to replace lost blood. Morphine (preferably given intravenously) is of great value, but must be withheld if there are head injuries or if abdominal injuries are suspected. Giving oxygen is important, even if the patient is not

a

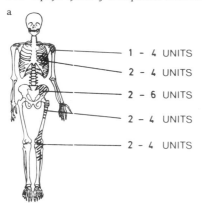

b

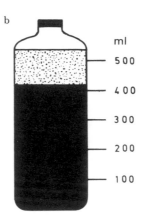

22.4 Severe injuries – danger point   (a) Range of probable blood loss in closed fractures. (b) From a 540-ml container the patient gets only 400–420 ml of actual blood – the rest is anticoagulant and space. *Moral* – The severely injured patient may lose more blood than you think, and get less.

obviously dyspnoeic. Pneumatic antishock garments (military antishock trousers, or 'MAST' suits) are sometimes used; they work by compressing the capillary bed and increasing vascular resistance. They should be applied (and later removed) gradually so as not to cause severe shifts in blood distribution. If there are fractures, early reduction and splintage help to reduce the effects of shock.

The essential feature of treatment, however, is the early restoration of blood volume. A practical routine is to start with the rapid infusion of 2 litres of crystalloid solution such as Ringer's lactate; the patient's response is checked by measuring the heart rate, blood pressure, CVP, urinary output and acid–base balance. If improvement is not sustained and other causes of cardiac embarrassment have been excluded, concealed haemorrhage into the chest or abdomen is probable and should be sought by investigations such as ultrasonography, CT and abdominal paracentesis or lavage.

If the haematocrit (packed cell volume, PCV) is less than 25%, blood transfusion will be necessary and this should be started as soon as possible. In an emergency group O Rh-negative blood may be used until cross-matched blood is available.

It is important not only to give blood but also to give enough blood. Even with closed injuries there is far more bleeding into tissues than is

commonly appreciated: two or three units may be lost with a single major limb fracture and up to 6 units with three major fractures; in trunk fractures with visceral damage, as much as half the blood volume may be lost. Rapid transfusion may be important, for which purpose a pressurized device is valuable. In the previously healthy patient 100 ml/min may be given until the blood pressure reaches 100 mmHg.

Overtransfusion must be guarded against. The CVP is checked repeatedly; however, with severe injuries requiring large amounts of blood, it is better to measure the pulmonary artery wedge pressure directly via a pulmonary artery catheter. Other problems of massive transfusion are hypothermia, hyperkalaemia, acidosis, dilution of endogenous clotting factors and platelets, and an increased risk of intravascular coagulopathy (see below).

Disseminated intravascular coagulation

An insidious complication of severe injury and blood loss is a widespread disorder of coagulation and haemostasis. This is due, at least in part, to the release of tissue thromboplastins into the circulation and the development of endothelial damage and platelet activation. The result is a complex mixture of intravascular coagulation, depletion of clotting factors, fibrinolysis and thrombocytopenia. Microvascular occlusion causes haemorrhagic infarctions and tissue necrosis, while deficient haemostasis leads to abnormal bleeding.

Clinical features

The patient, usually after a period of severe blood loss, shock and transfusion, develops symptoms and signs suggesting diffuse microvascular thrombosis: restlessness, confusion, neurological dysfunction, skin infarcts, oliguria and renal failure. Abnormal haemostasis causes excessive bleeding at operation, oozing drip sites and wounds, spontaneous bruising, gastrointestinal bleeding and haematuria. The diagnosis is confirmed by finding a low haemoglobin concentration, prolonged prothrombin and thrombin times, hypofibrinogenaemia and thrombocytopenia.

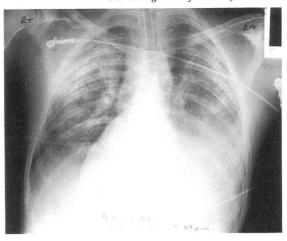

22.5 Adult respiratory distress syndrome X-ray showing diffuse pulmonary infiltrates in both lungs.

Treatment

The best 'treatment' is the prevention or early correction of hypovolaemic shock. If the bleeding is marked, it may help to replace clotting factors and platelets. However, this is a complex problem and it is wise to seek the advice of a haematologist.

Adult respiratory distress syndrome (ARDS)

During the later stages of shock and septicaemia, endothelial cell damage and increased small-vessel permeability lead to the extravasation of haemorrhagic, protein-rich fluid into the pulmonary interstitial tissue and alveoli. Capillary fat emboli and perivascular inflammatory exudates appear; the alveoli become distorted and increasingly awash with fluid, and ventilation is impaired. Over a period of about 10 days the picture changes from a predominantly exudative phase, with pulmonary oedema, to one of pneumocyte proliferation, interstitial fibrosis, microvascular occlusion and alveolar destruction. The early changes are reversible, but once diffuse alveolar damage occurs there is usually an inexorable progression to severe hypoxaemia, multiple organ failure and death.

Clinical features

About 36 hours after injury and (usually) a period of hypovolaemic shock, the patient develops mild dyspnoea. Even before this, if blood gases are measured they may show a diminished Po_2. These changes are common after long-bone fractures, and fat embolism is often suspected. By the second or third day the clinical features are move obvious; the patient is restless, mildly cyanosed and shows signs of respiratory distress. Blood gases remain abnormal, with Po_2 often below 8 kPa (60 mmHg). X-rays may now show diffuse pulmonary infiltrates. Special tests will show features such as reduced lung compliance and tidal volume, increased shunt, increased dead space and increased pulmonary artery pressure. Once the condition reaches this stage the prognosis is poor; deterioration proceeds despite treatment and the outcome is often fatal, due to multiple organ failure and hypoxaemia precipitating cardiac failure and – finally – cardiac arrest.

Treatment

The most important aspect of management is the early and effective treatment of shock. There is also evidence that, in patients with multiple injuries, the incidence of pulmonary dysfunction is reduced by early stabilization of fractures (Phillips and Contreras, 1990).

The treatment of established ARDS is supportive and aims to minimize further lung damage until recovery occurs, whilst optimizing oxygen delivery to the tissues. Oxygen delivery depends upon arterial oxygen saturation, haemoglobin concentration and cardiac output. Careful monitoring is essential, and a pulmonary artery flotation catheter is required to measure the effects of treatment.

Mild ARDS can be managed by continuous positive airway pressure (CPAP) supplied by a close-fitting mask. CPAP increases functional residual volume and reduces shunt, thereby increasing arterial oxygen tension. Usually, however, endotracheal intubation is required, with positive pressure ventilation using minimum airway pressure and the lowest inspired oxygen concentration that will provide adequate arterial oxygenation.

Cardiac output is measured and, if necessary, a cardiac stimulant such as dobutamine may be given. Prostacyclin is sometimes used to improve pulmonary capillary flow and reduce shunt (Holcroft, Vassar and Weber, 1985).

General supportive measures include low-dose dopamine to reduce the risk of renal failure, adequate nutrition – preferably enteral but if necessary parenteral – and selective decontamination of the digestive tract by non-absorbable antibiotics.

Head injuries

Most head injuries result from a blow that causes either direct damage or intracerebral movement due to rapid acceleration or deceleration. Depending on the severity of the injury, damage may consist of: (1) minor neuronal contusion causing transient loss of consciousness or amnesia; (2) severe neuronal contusion or laceration, due either to direct injury or to shearing forces; (3) localized intracranial bleeding with formation of a subdural or an intracerebral haematoma or pressure on the adjacent structures; (4) fractures of the cranium or the base of the skull; (5) localized injury to cranial nerves; (6) diffuse oedema and a rise in intracranial pressure; and (7) intracranial brain shifts resulting in tentorial or tonsillar herniation.

Clinical assessment

The history may give important clues to the type and severity of the injury. Did the patient lose consciousness? If so, for how long? Was there a period of amnesia? Did the patient take drugs or alcohol? Is there a previous history of fits or neurological disorder? What other injuries are present?

There may be obvious swelling and/or bruising of the face. The scalp should be examined for cuts or localized swelling (haematoma); open wounds should be gently explored with a gloved finger to exclude underlying fractures. The nose and ears are examined for CSF leakage; other signs of basal fracture are subconjunctival haemorrhage without a posterior margin, localized periorbital haematomas and retromastoid bruising (Battle's sign).

The bony outlines are felt systematically; in the conscious patient a tender spot may suggest an underlying fracture. The cranial nerves are examined and the eyes are tested for diplopia (which suggests an orbital fracture). If the patient's condition permits, a more complete neurological examination is carried out. In the unconscious patient this can be extremely difficult, but it is important to try to elicit signs of focal intracranial dysfunction that could point to the presence of a haematoma. Motor weakness may be inferred from the response (or asymmetrical lack of response) to painful stimuli such as nail-bed pressure or tendo Achillis squeeze.

The pupils are examined for asymmetrical dilatation and the light reflex is tested on each side. With increased intracranial pressure and tentorial herniation, compression of the IIIrd nerve results in dilatation of the pupil and a failure to react to light.

All patients with a head injury must be x-rayed; CT also may be needed.

Throughout the examination great care must be exercised not to flex or extend the neck unless an associated cervical spine injury has been excluded.

INDICATIONS FOR CT SCANNING FOLLOWING HEAD INJURY

1. Persistent reduction in level of consciousness
2. Focal neurological signs
3. Epileptic fit
4. Depressed skull fracture
5. Penetrating injury
6. Patient on endotracheal intubation and artificial ventilation

The level of consciousness

The most widely accepted system for assessing the level of consciousness is the Glasgow Coma Scale (GCS) (Teasedale and Gennett, 1974). This is based on descending levels of eye opening and verbal and motor responses (Table 22.1). The maximum score, representing normality, is 15; a score of 6 or less implies severe head injury; absence of eye opening, speech and response to commands is indicative of coma. Persistent lack of response to painful stimuli (supraorbital or nail-bed pressure) suggests irrecoverable brain damage.

Management

Most head injuries are fairly trivial and require no more than careful examination and reassurance. The indications for admission to hospital for observation and reassessment are any of the following: (1) a diminished level of consciousness; (2) a history of transient loss of consciousness or amnesia; (3) a skull fracture; and (4) abnormal neurological signs.

In patients who appear to be comatose, drowsy, restless or merely confused it may be difficult to distinguish the effects of a head injury from those of alcohol or drugs. All such patients, as well as those whose cerebral dysfunction may be due to shock or hypoxia,

Table 22.1 Glasgow Coma Scale

	Score
Eye-opening:	
Spontaneous	4
On command	3
On pain	2
Nil	1
Best motor response:	
Obeys	6
Localizes pain	5
Normal flexor	4
Abnormal flexor	3
Extensor	2
Nil	1
Verbal response:	
Orientated	5
Confused	4
Words	3
Sounds	2
Nil	1

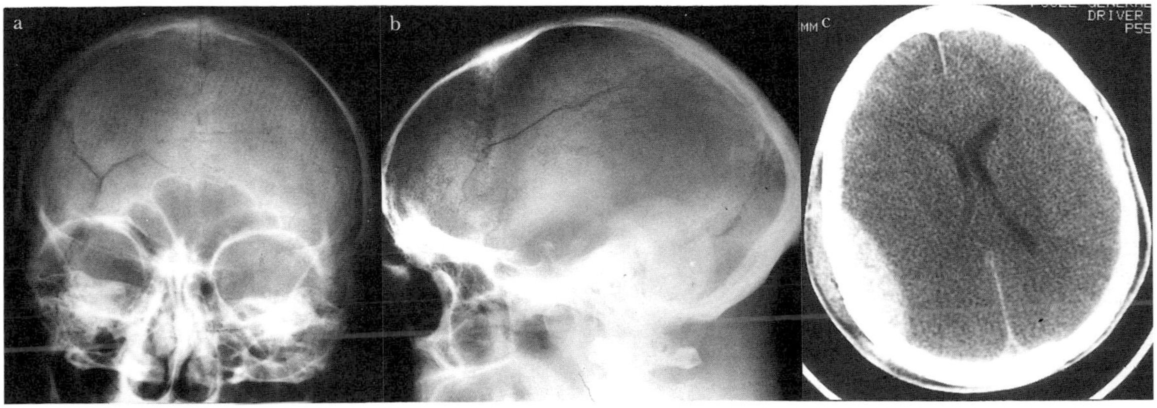

22.6 Head injuries – imaging (a, b) X-rays showing a fracture of the parietal bone. (c) A CT scan shows an extradural haematoma with distortion of the lateral ventricle on that side.

should be graded on the GCS and kept under observation until the diagnosis is clear.

Patients with severe head injuries (a GCS score of 6 or less) should be kept under continuous observation until they recover spontaneously, or develop signs calling for operative treatment, or ultimately show the features of 'brain death'. They are best managed by endotracheal intubation and artificial ventilation. This will, of course, require the use of a general muscle relaxant, which will complicate further neurological assessment. Focal lesions are monitored by testing the pupil reactions and by CT scanning. The main indication for craniotomy is the development of an intracranial haematoma. This aspect of management is best handled by the neurosurgical team.

Other complications that sometimes require surgical treatment are: (1) depressed fractures of the skull; (2) ocular defects (e.g. diplopia) suggesting fractures of the orbit; (3) other cranial nerve defects suggesting localized compression; (4) continuing CSF leakage; (5) deterioration in the level of consciousness.

Chest injuries

Chest injuries may damage the rib cage, the lungs, the heart or the great vessels; precise diagnosis may be vital (literally). Clinical assessment must establish which (if any) of the following is present: (1) a simple fracture of one or two ribs; (2) multiple fractures with a flail segment or stove-in chest; (3) a pneumothorax – open or closed; (4) a haemothorax; (5) cardiac tamponade. Three warnings are important: (1) unconscious patients often have serious chest injuries; (2) small wounds may hide serious complications; and (3) pneumothorax can take many hours to develop, so repeated examination is necessary.

Examination

1. The skin is inspected for open wounds (small ones are the most dangerous) and for bruising (which suggests a crushing injury). The shape of the chest also is noted; a stove-in chest may show obvious asymmetry. The trachea is palpated to see if it is deviated from the midline.
2. Fractured ribs or a stove-in segment can sometimes be palpated.
3. Respiration is observed. Is the patient fighting for breath? During inspiration, if one side of the chest remains still, the lung on that side is probably collapsed; but if one side is sucked in, this paradoxical respiration is diagnostic of a flail segment.
4. Percussion and auscultation may reveal signs of pulmonary collapse, fluid in the chest and mediastinal shift.
5. X-rays are essential; they may reveal fractures, or a pleural effusion, or lung collapse and mediastinal displacement.

Emergency treatment

1. With all severe chest injuries, three measures are important: blood replacement (but not with crystalloid fluids, which aggravate pulmonary congestion); the administration of oxygen; and adequate analgesics (but not respiratory depressants).
2. Open wounds that communicate with the pleural cavity cause a sucking pneumothorax and lung collapse. A moist swab strapped over the hole may suffice temporarily, but the wound should be securely stitched as soon as possible; an intercostal tube connected to an underwater seal allows the lung to expand.
3. A tension pneumothorax occurs when there is no open wound but the injured lung leaks air into the pleural cavity. Increasing respiratory distress follows, with poor chest movements and absent breath sounds. If this lethal condition is even suspected, a large-bore needle should be inserted into the second interspace anteriorly, in the mid-clavicular line. This immediately relieves the tension. It can later be replaced by an intercostal catheter connected to an underwater seal, which is retained until the lung re-expands.
4. Haemothorax (from a torn lung or blood vessel) can be diagnosed by withdrawing blood through a needle. The blood is drained by an intercostal catheter through a low intercostal space. Breathing exercises are encouraged.

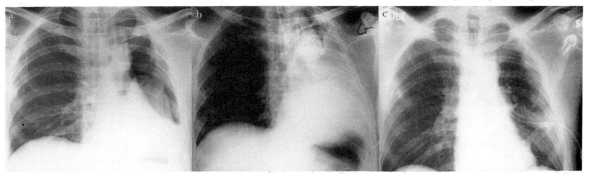

22.7 Tension pneumothorax   A lesson in caution. (a) This young man presented with fractured ribs on the left; soon afterwards he developed respiratory distress and x-rays showed a pneumothorax. This was treated by intercostal drainage and his condition appeared to be satisfactory. However, a few hours later he again became distressed and further x-rays (b) showed complete collapse of the left lung. (c) The situation was quickly rescued by adding tracheal intubation and positive pressure respiration.

5. A stove-in chest with only moderate respiratory difficulty can be treated by strapping a large pack over the mobile segment and administering oxygen. More severe cases need endotracheal intubation and positive pressure ventilation; a chest drain connected to an underwater seal is essential in case there is an associated lung leak. (If ventilation is to be continued for several days a tracheostomy is needed.) The flail segment can be stabilized by rib traction (using wires or towel clips) or by internal fixation.
6. Uncomplicated rib fractures need no treatment other than analgesics. The patient with multiple fractures and extensive bruising should, however, be kept in hospital until complications have been positively excluded.

Abdominal injuries

The most important abdominal injuries are ruptures of viscera and of blood vessels. There is a real danger that abdominal injuries may be overlooked, either because an unconscious patient can give no history or because a conscious but shocked patient may not complain even with serious injury.

Examination

1. The abdomen is inspected for perforating wounds, for bruising and to observe respiratory movements.
2. Palpation may reveal localized tenderness, the boggy fullness of extensive bleeding or board-like rigidity over a ruptured viscus. It must be remembered that considerable bleeding, especially if retroperitoneal, may not be detected on palpation, and rigidity may not develop despite a ruptured viscus if the patient is severely shocked.
3. Auscultation tends to be forgotten but the complete absence of bowel sounds is an important sign of intra-abdominal damage.
4. Percussion may disclose the presence of fluid, or of a decreased area of liver dullness due to gas from a ruptured viscus.
5. Rectal and pelvic examinaton must not be omitted. Injuries to the lower abdomen often damage the bladder and urethra, particularly in men. Blood at the meatus may indicate urethral damage. On rectal examination, upward displacement of the prostate indicates a major urethral disruption. Gross haematuria is an indication for intravenous urography.
6. Intubation of the stomach is often wise; apart from the advantage of aspirating gastric

contents prior to anaesthesia, the with-drawing of blood may suggest gastric injury.

7. Peritoneal lavage is helpful in detectng intra-abdominal haemorrhage, especially when clinical examination is equivocal. It is of particular use in unconscious patients. Prior to insertion of the cannula it is essential to empty the bladder by catheterization.

Emergency treatment

1. An open wound needs to be closed. A temporary dressing is sufficient and formal closure must not be performed if the integrity of the abdominal viscera is in doubt, for laparoscopy or laparotomy is then essential.

2. Continued abdominal bleeding demands emergency transfusion and laparotomy. The patient with hypovolaemic shock who is not responding to transfusion is probably bleeding into his abdomen and, even if the signs are equivocal, exploration is justified. If a retroperitoneal haematoma is found, it should not be explored as this may result in life-threatening haemorrhage.

3. A ruptured viscus must be repaired when the patient has been resuscitated.

Burns

The patient with extensive burns suffers from neurogenic shock because of pain, and from oligaemic shock because (1) fluid exudes copiously from the burnt area, (2) fluid is lost into the tissues and (3) red cells have been damaged. The amount of fluid loss varies with the area of the burn and can be assessed by a special formula (the rule of 9) or from pyrogram charts. Often the depth of the burn cannot be determined until superficial sloughs separate.

Emergency treatment

1. Treatment of shock is urgent. Morphine is given and fluid replacement begun. Every moment of delay in starting the transfusion makes the prognosis worse. For deep burns, whole blood is given; for superficial burns, plasma is used first, though blood usually becomes necessary later.

2. With burns of the face or neck, immediate intubation or tracheostomy may be necessary.

3. With chemical burns, the surface is gently washed. In all other cases the burnt area is not disturbed or treated with topical applications. If the environment is suitable the burn is left exposed, otherwise it is covered with sterile towels.

4. If transfer to a special burns centre is unavoidably delayed, further measures become necessary. Fluid losses must continually be made good with blood, plasma, or plasma and saline solution as required. Antibiotics are started and sedation is continued. Metabolic requirements are met by oral feeding or, in children, intravenously. At least every 4 hours the patient is examined; the skin colour, pulse, blood pressure and urine output are noted. An indwelling catheter is useful in assessing the all-important fluid balance. In severe cases the blood haemoglobin, electrolytes and urea are examined 4-hourly and used as a guide to further treatment.

The metabolic response to trauma

The general effects of trauma are profound and widespread; they involve a host of hormonal and cellular mechanisms designed to counteract the acute effects of tissue damage, blood loss, shock and cardiopulmonary dysfunction, as well as an inflammatory response which initiates the process of repair. Energy requirements for these vital processes are secured at the expense of less dependent tissues such as muscle and fat.

The metabolic adjustments occur in two phases: an early post-traumatic phase, or 'ebb', covering the first 24–48 hours, followed by a more prolonged 'flow' phase which is dominated first by tissue breakdown (the catabolic period) and later by tissue repair (the anabolic period).

The *early response* (or '*ebb*' *phase*) is concerned with the body's defence mechanisms. The fluid shifts that occur during shock trigger a number of humoral mechanisms (mainly increased secretion of renin, aldosterone, cortisol and pituitary antidiuretic hormone) which ensure more effective conservation of sodium and water. At a local level, the inflammatory response to tissue damage is mediated by cytokines such as interleukin 1 (IL-1) and tumour necrosis factor (TNF), arachidonic acid derivatives (prostaglandins), and other vasoactive chemicals.

Ready energy for these processes comes from a number of sources. The classic reaction to stress involves increased hypothalamic–pituitary and sympathetic–adrenal activity. There is increased secretion of ACTH, cortisol, catecholamines (adrenalin, dopamine) and glucagon; among the effects of these hormones are increased glycogenolysis and gluconeogenesis in the liver, reduced glucose utilization by muscle, and stimulation of free fatty acid and glycerol release from the fat stores. Within the first 24 hours after injury the blood sugar rises and there is an increase in metabolic rate, oxygen uptake and body temperature.

As the initial 'fight or flight' reaction subsides, the patient enters the *'flow' phase*. In the early recovery period there is still a need for energy supplies. Blood sugar levels may return to near normal but glucose turnover is increased and gluconeogenesis in the liver continues at an enhanced level. Free fatty acid turnover, likewise, is increased and this is probably the major source of energy in patients who do not receive glucose supplements. One of the most important effects during the catabolic phase is the loss of body protein, resulting in muscle wasting. Amino acids are needed by the liver both for gluconeogenesis and for replenishment of the acute phase proteins required by the inflammatory response. Thus, C-reactive protein levels are at first diminished but, provided the liver is not damaged, the serum levels return to normal or may be increased. These changes are reflected in the continued elevation of the metabolic rate and increased excretion of nitrogen in the urine.

As healing proceeds, the need for increased energy supplies subsides and the patient moves into the anabolic phase of recovery. The metabolic parameters return to normal, body weight increases and muscle bulk is slowly restored.

To supplement or not? With minor or even moderately severe injuries the patient usually adjusts to the metabolic changes quite well, provided blood loss is restored and there is no supervening complication such as sepsis or pulmonary dysfunction. However, in all cases of severe trauma it is important to assess the patient's nutritional status and to ensure that the necessary protein, lipid and energy requirements are being met. If there are major complications such as prolonged bleeding, pulmonary dysfunction or sepsis, enteral or parenteral supplementation will almost certainly be necessary.

Injury severity grading

In a trauma unit, where patients often arrive in clusters, it is useful to have a method of assessing the severity of injury so that priorities can be established and resources allocated on a rational basis. Various attempts have been made to devise 'severity scores' that will correlate reliably with outcome (at least with mortality) and that are easy to apply under a variety of conditions. Some systems are based on measurements that reflect the patient's overall physiological status, for example the Trauma Score (TS) and the Revised Trauma Score (RTS), which combine data from the Glasgow Coma Scale with measurements of cardiovascular and respiratory function (Boyd, Tolson and Copes, 1987; Champion et al., 1989). Diminishing score values indicate a progressively diminishing probability of survival. This type of functional (or 'dynamic') evaluation can be used for pre-hospital and emergency room triage, or for comparative reassessment during and after resuscitation, without the need for accurate diagnosis of structural damage. However, it lacks predictive value in patients with well-compensated physiological reactions whose condition may suddenly deteriorate from one time-point to the next.

An alternative approach is to base the score on the degree of anatomical damage. In the

Abbreviated Injury Scale (AIS) score values range from 1 to 6, with the lower values reflecting minor or moderate injuries and the higher values reflecting increasingly severe tissue damage. The Injury Severity Score (ISS) is similar in principle but allows for assessment of multiple injuries by adding up the squares of the AIS scores for individual injuries (Baker et al., 1974). The main drawback of this system is that it cannot be used for triage or initial emergency room decisions, because at that early stage an accurate anatomical diagnosis may not yet be available.

The preferred approach nowadays is to combine the principles of 'physiological' and 'anatomical' scoring systems. This is the basis of the TRISS method, which uses values from both the Trauma Score and the Injury Severity Score (Boyd, Tolson and Copes, 1987) and a more recent scoring system termed ASCOT (A Severity Characterization Of Trauma) (Champion et al., 1990).

Accident centres and ATLS

Peripheral casualty services (cottage hospitals, health centres and first-aid posts) should deal only with minor injuries. Accident centres are quite different; they must be able to deal with any emergency – medical or surgical. Each

centre should therefore be part of a general hospital; but it also needs the support of a central unit with highly specialized services such as neurosurgery, thoracic surgery and dialysis. It is best designed on an open plan system permitting flexibility of use, and needs to be generously supplied with equipment for communications, patient transport and all forms of emergency care. Of particular importance is equipment for resuscitation, airway management, electrolyte investigations and radiology (portable equipment is inadequate and heavy duty equipment within the centre essential).

Staffing also must be generous, but the leader need not be a surgeon. He must be expert in the diagnosis and management of emergencies, a good organizer, a natural diplomat and a dedicated enthusiast. Recognizing the need for advanced skills in the management of acutely injured patients, the American College of Surgeons in the 1970s introduced special training courses in advanced trauma life support (ATLS); similar schemes are now offered in the UK and other countries throughout the world. Every trainee surgeon and every doctor working in an accident centre should have taken part in at least one of these courses.

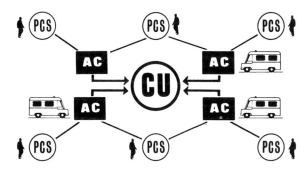

22.8 The organization A three-tier structure is needed: peripheral casualty services (PCS) are for minor injuries and the 'walking wounded'; accident centres (AC) must be able to cope with any emergency, but may need the support of a specialized central unit (CU).

References and further reading

Baker, S.P., O'Neill, B., Haddow, W. et al. (1974) The injury severity score: a method for describing patients with multiple injuries and evaluating emergency care. *Journal of Trauma* **14**, 187–196

Boyd, C.R., Tolson, M.A. and Copes, W.S. (1987) Evaluating trauma care: the TRISS method. *Journal of Trauma* **27**, 370–378

Champion, H.R., Sacco, W.J., Copes, W.S. et al. (1989) A revision of the Trauma Score. *Journal of Trauma* **29**, 623–629

Champion, H.R., Copes, W.R., Sacco, W.J. et al. (1990) A new characterization of injury severity. *Journal of Trauma* **30**, 539–546

Holcroft, J.W., Vassar, M.J. and Weber, C.J. (1985) Prostaglandin E1 and survival in patients with acute respiratory distress syndrome. *Annals of Surgery* **253**, 371–379

Phillips, T.F. and Contreras, D.M. (1990) Timing of operative treatment of fractures in patients who have multiple injuries. *Journal of Bone and Joint Surgery* **72A**, 784–788

Teasedale, G. and Gennett, B. (1974) Assessment of coma and impaired consciousness: a practical scale. *Lancet* **2**, 81–84

Principles of fractures

23

A fracture is a break in the structural continuity of bone. It may be no more than a crack, a crumpling or a splintering of the cortex; more often the break is complete and the bone fragments are displaced. If the overlying skin remains intact it is a *closed* (or *simple*) *fracture*; if the skin or one of the body cavities is breached it is an *open* (or *compound*) *fracture*, liable to contamination and infection.

How fractures happen

Bone is relatively brittle, yet it has sufficient strength and resilience to withstand considerable stress. Fractures result from: (1) a single traumatic incident; (2) repetitive stress; or (3) abnormal weakening of the bone (a 'pathological' fracture).

Fractures due to a traumatic incident

Most fractures are caused by sudden and excessive force, which may be tapping, crushing, bending, twisting or pulling.

With a direct force the bone breaks at the point of impact; the soft tissues also must be damaged. Tapping (a momentary blow) usually causes a transverse fracture and damage to the overlying skin; crushing is more likely to cause a comminuted fracture with extensive soft-tissue damage.

With an indirect force the bone breaks at a distance from where the force is applied; soft-tissue damage at the fracture site is not inevitable.

The force may be: (1) twisting, which causes a spiral fracture; (2) bending, which causes a transverse fracture; (3) bending and compressing, which results in a fracture that is partly transverse but with a separate triangular 'butter-

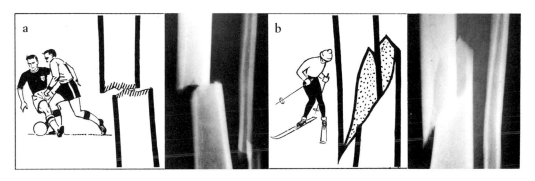

23.1 Mechanisms of injury   (a) A direct blow causes a transverse fracture. (b) A twisting force causes a spiral fracture.

fly' fragment; (4) a combination of twisting, bending and compressing, which causes a short oblique fracture; or (5) pulling, in which a tendon or ligament literally pulls the bone apart.

The above description applies mainly to the long bones. A cancellous bone, such as a vertebra or the calcaneum, when subjected to sufficient force, sustains a comminuted crush fracture. At the knee or elbow resisted extension may cause an avulsion fracture of the patella or olecranon; and in a number of situations resisted muscle action may pull off the bony attachment of the muscle.

Fatigue or stress fractures

Cracks can occur in bone, as in metal and other materials, due to repetitive stress. This is most often seen in the tibia or fibula or metatarsals, especially in athletes, dancers and army recruits who go on long route marches.

Pathological fractures

Fractures may occur even with normal stresses if the bone has been weakened (e.g. by a tumour) or if it is excessively brittle (e.g. in Paget's disease).

Types of fracture

Fractures are infinitely variable in appearance but for practical reasons they are divided into a few well-defined groups.

Complete fractures

The bone is completely broken into two or more fragments. If the fracture is *transverse*, the fragments usually remain in place after reduction; if it is *oblique* or *spiral*, they tend to slip and redisplace even if the bone is splinted. In an *impacted fracture* the fragments are jammed tightly together and the fracture line is indistinct. A *comminuted fracture* is one in which there are more than two fragments; because there is poor interlocking of the fracture surfaces, these lesions are often unstable.

Incomplete fractures

Here the bone is incompletely divided and the periosteum remains in continuity. In a *greenstick fracture* the bone is buckled or bent (like snapping a green twig); this is seen in children, whose bones are more springy than those of adults. Reduction is usually easy and healing is

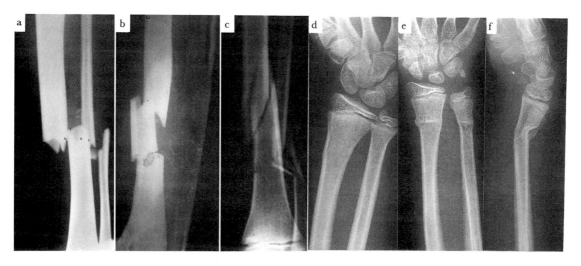

23.2 Varieties of fracture   Complete fractures: (a) transverse; (b) segmental; (c) spiral. Incomplete fractures: (d) buckle or torus; (e, f) greenstick.

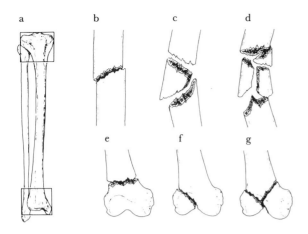

23.3 Müller's classification (a) Each long bone has three segments – proximal, diaphyseal and distal; the proximal and distal segments are each defined by a square based on the widest part of the bone. (b, c, d) Diaphyseal fractures may be simple, wedge or complex. (e, f, g) Proximal and distal fractures may be extra-articular, partial articular or complete articular.

quick. *Compression fractures* occur when cancellous bone is crumpled. This happens in adults, especially in the vertebral bodies. Unless operated upon, reduction is impossible and some residual deformity is inevitable.

Classification of fractures

An alphanumeric classification of fractures, which can be used for computer storage and retrieval, has been developed (Müller et al., 1990). The first digit specifies the bone (1 = humerus, 2 = radius/ulna, 3 = femur, 4 = tibia/fibula) and the second the segment (1 =

proximal, 2 = diaphyseal, 3 = distal, 4 = malleolar). A letter specifies the type of fracture (diaphysis: A = simple, B = wedge, C = complex; proximal and distal: A = extra-articular, B = partial articular, C = complete articular). Two further numbers specify the detailed morphology of the fracture.

How fractures are displaced

After a complete fracture the fragments usually become displaced, partly by the force of the injury, partly by gravity and partly by the pull of muscles attached to them. Displacement is usually described in terms of apposition, alignment, rotation and altered length.

Apposition (shift) The fragments may be shifted sideways, backwards or forwards in relation to each other, such that the fracture surfaces lose contact. The fracture will usually unite even if apposition is imperfect, or indeed even if the bone ends lie side by side with the fracture surfaces making no contact at all.

Alignment (tilt) The fragments may be tilted or angulated in relation to each other. Malalignment, if uncorrected, may lead to deformity of the limb.

Rotation (twist) One of the fragments may be rotated on its longitudinal axis; the bone looks straight but the limb ends up with a rotational deformity.

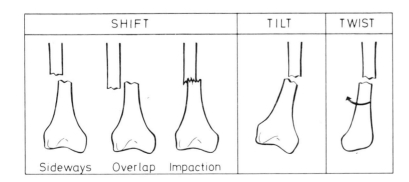

23.4 Fracture displacements

Length The fragments may be distracted and separated, or they may overlap, due to muscle spasm, causing shortening of the bone.

How fractures heal

It is commonly supposed that, in order to unite, a fracture must be immobilized. This cannot be so since, with few exceptions, fractures unite whether they are splinted or not; indeed, without a built-in mechanism for union, land animals could scarcely have evolved. It is, however, naïve to suppose that union would occur if a fracture were kept moving indefinitely; the bone ends must, at some stage, be brought to rest relative to one another. But it is not mandatory for the surgeon to impose this immobility artificially – Nature can do it, with callus; and callus forms in response to movement, not to splintage. *We splint most fractures, not to ensure union but (1) to alleviate pain, (2) to ensure that union takes place in good position and (3) to permit early movement and return of function.*

The process of fracture repair varies according to the type of bone involved and the amount of movement at the fracture site. In a tubular bone, and in the absence of rigid fixation, healing proceeds in five stages.

TISSUE DESTRUCTION AND HAEMATOMA FORMATION Vessels are torn and a haematoma forms around and within the fracture. Bone at the fracture surfaces, deprived of a blood supply, dies back for a millimetre or two.

INFLAMMATION AND CELLULAR PROLIFERATION Within 8 hours of the fracture there is an acute inflammatory reaction with proliferation of cells under the periosteum and within the breached medullary canal. The fragment ends are surrounded by cellular tissue, which bridges the fracture site. The clotted haematoma is slowly absorbed and fine new capillaries grow into the area.

CALLUS FORMATION The proliferating cells are potentially chrondrogenic and osteogenic; given the right conditions, they will start forming bone and, in some cases, also cartilage. The cell population now also includes osteoclasts (probably derived from the new blood vessels) which begin to mop up dead bone. The thick cellular mass, with its islands of immature bone and cartilage, forms the callus or splint on the periosteal and endosteal surfaces. As the immature fibre bone (or 'woven' bone) becomes more densely mineralized, movement at the fracture site decreases progressively and at

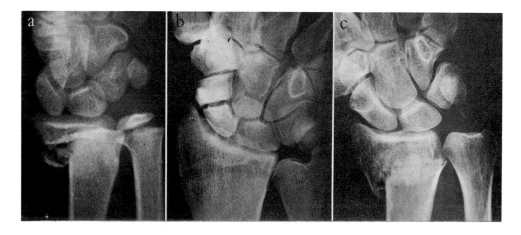

23.5 The patient's age Many fractures have a limited age distribution: each of these patients fell on the outstretched hand. (a) Aged 8 – fracture-separation of lower radial epiphysis; (b) aged 30 – fractured scaphoid; (c) aged 60 – Colles' fracture.

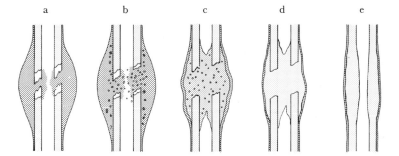

23.6 Fracture healing Five stages of healing. (a) Haematoma: there is tissue damage and bleeding at the fracture site; the bone ends die back for a few millimetres. (b) Inflammation: inflammatory cells appear in the haematoma. (c) Callus: the cell population changes to osteoblasts and osteoclasts: dead bone is mopped up and woven bone appears in the fracture callus. (d) Consolidation: woven bone is replaced by lamellar bone and the fracture is solidly united. (e) Remodelling: the new-formed bone is remodelled to resemble the normal structure.

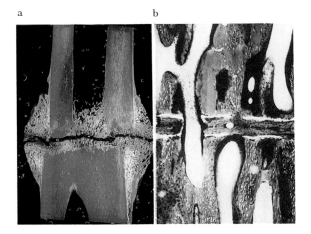

23.7 Fracture healing – histology Experimental fracture healing: (a) by bridging callus and (b) by direct penetration of the fracture gap by a cutting cone.

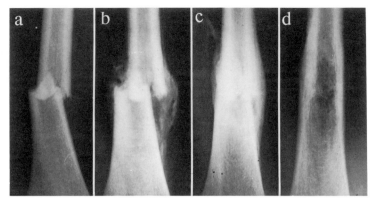

23.8 Fracture repair (a) Fracture; (b) union; (c) consolidation; (d) bone remodelling. The fracture must be protected until consolidated.

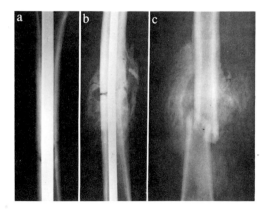

23.9 Callus and movement Three patients with femoral shaft fractures. (a) and (b) are both 6 weeks after fixation – in (a) the Kŭntscher nail fitted tightly, preventing any movement, and there is no callus; in (b) the nail fitted loosely, permitting movement, so there is callus. (c) This patient had cerebral irritation and thrashed around wildly – at 3 weeks callus is excessive.

about 4 weeks after injury the fracture 'unites'.

CONSOLIDATION With continuing osteoclastic and osteoblastic activity the woven bone is transformed into lamellar bone. The system is now rigid enough to allow osteoclasts to burrow through the debris at the fracture line, and close behind them osteoblasts fill in the remaining gaps between the fragments with new bone. This is a slow process and it may be several months before the bone is strong enough to carry normal loads.

REMODELLING The fracture has been bridged by a cuff of solid bone. Over a period of months, or even years, this crude 'weld' is reshaped by a continuous process of alternating bone resorption and formation. Thicker lamellae are laid down where the stresses are high; unwanted buttresses are carved away; the medullary cavity is reformed. Eventually, and especially in children, the bone reassumes something like its normal shape.

Clinical and experimental studies (McKibbin, 1978) have shown that callus is the response to movement at the fracture site. It serves to stabilize the fragments as rapidly as possible – a necessary precondition for bridging by bone. If the fracture site is absolutely immobile – for example, an impacted fracture in cancellous bone, or a fracture rigidly immobilized by a metal plate – there is no need for callus. Instead, osteoblastic new bone formation occurs directly between the fragments. Gaps between the fracture surfaces are invaded by new capillaries and osteoprogenitor cells growing in from the edges and new bone is laid down on the exposed surface (*gap healing*). Where the crevices are very narrow (less than 200 μm), osteogenesis produces lamellar bone; wider gaps are filled first by woven bone which is then remodelled to lamellar bone. By 3–4 weeks the fracture is solid enough to allow penetration and bridging of the area by bone remodelling units – i.e. osteoclastic 'cutting cones' followed by osteoblasts. Where the exposed fracture surfaces are in intimate contact and held rigidly from the outset, internal bridging may occasionally occur without any intermediate stages (*contact healing*).

Healing by callus, though less direct (the term 'indirect' could be used) has distinct advantages: it ensures mechanical strength while the bone ends heal; and, with increasing stress, the callus grows stronger and stronger (an example of Wolff's law). With rigid metal fixation, on the other hand, the absence of callus means that there is a long period during which the bone depends entirely upon the metal implant for its integrity. Moreover, the implant diverts stress away from the bone, which may become osteoporotic and not recover fully until the metal is removed. Flexible implants are now being tried in the hope of overcoming these drawbacks.

Union, consolidation and non-union

Repair of a fracture is a continuous process: any stages into which it is divided are necessarily arbitrary. In this book the terms 'union' and 'consolidation' are used, and they are defined as follows.

UNION
Union is incomplete repair; the ensheathing callus is calcified. Clinically the fracture site is still a little tender and, though the bone moves in one piece (and in that sense is united), attempted angulation is painful. X-rays show the fracture line still clearly visible, with fluffy callus around it. Repair is incomplete and it is not safe to subject the unprotected bone to stress.

CONSOLIDATION
Consolidation is complete repair; the calcified callus is ossified. Clinically the fracture site is not tender, no movement can be obtained and attempted angulation is painless. X-rays show the fracture line to be almost obliterated and crossed by bone trabeculae, with well-defined callus around it. Repair is complete and further protection is unnecessary.

TIMETABLE
How long does a fracture take to unite and to consolidate? No precise answer is possible because age, constitution, blood supply, type of fracture and other factors all influence the time taken.

Approximate prediction is possible and Perkins' timetable is delightfully simple. A spiral fracture in the upper limb unites in 3 weeks; for consolidation multiply by 2; for the lower limb multiply by 2 again; for transverse fractures multiply again by 2. A more sophisticated formula is as follows. A spiral fracture in the upper limb takes 6–8 weeks to consolidate; the lower limb needs twice as long. Add 25% if the fracture is not spiral or if it involves the femur. Children's fractures, of course, join more quickly. These figures are only a rough guide; there must be clinical and radiological evidence of consolidation before full stress is permitted without splintage.

NON-UNION

Sometimes the normal process of fracture repair is thwarted and the bone fails to unite. Causes of non-union are: (1) distraction and separation of the fragments; (2) interposition of soft tissues between the fragments; (3) excessive movement at the fracture line; and (4) poor local blood supply.

Cell proliferation is predominantly fibroblastic; the fracture gap is filled by fibrous tissue and the bone fragments remain mobile, creating a false joint or pseudarthrosis. In some cases periosteal bone formation is active so that, while new bone fails to bridge the fracture gap, the fragment ends are thickened or widened; this *hypertrophic non-union* will ultimately proceed to union provided the bone fragments are placed in contact with each other and held more or less immobile until bridging occurs. In other cases bone formation seems to peter out altogether, resulting in an *atrophic non-union* which will never heal unless the fragments are immobilized and grafted with cancellous bone.

Clinical features

History

There is usually a history of *injury*, followed by *inability to use the injured limb*. But beware! The fracture is not always at the site of the injury: a blow to the knee may fracture the patella, the femoral condyles, the shaft of the femur or even the acetabulum. The patient's age and the mechanism of injury are important. If a fracture occurs with trivial trauma, suspect a pathological lesion. *Pain, bruising* and *swelling* are common symptoms, but they do not distinguish a fracture from a soft-tissue injury. *Deformity* is much more suggestive.

Always enquire about *symptoms of associated injuries*: numbness or loss of movement, skin pallor or cyanosis, blood in the urine, abdominal pain, transient loss of consciousness.

Ask about *previous injuries* that might cause confusion when the x-ray is seen.

Finally, a *general medical history* is important, in preparation for anaesthesia or operation.

General signs

A broken bone is part of a patient. It is important to look for evidence of: (1) shock or haemorrhage; (2) associated damage to brain, spinal cord or viscera; and (3) a predisposing cause (such as Paget's disease).

Local signs

Injured tissues must be handled gently. To elicit crepitus or abnormal movement is unnecessarily painful; x-ray diagnosis is more reliable. Nevertheless the familiar headings of clinical examination should always be considered, or damage to arteries and nerves may be overlooked.

● LOOK Swelling, bruising and deformity may be obvious, but the important point is whether the skin is intact; if the skin is broken and the wound communicates with the fracture, the injury is 'open' ('compound').

● FEEL There is localized tenderness, but it is necessary also to examine distal to the fracture in order to feel the pulse and to test sensation. A vascular injury is a surgical emergency.

● MOVE Crepitus and abnormal movement may be present, but it is more important to ask if the patient can move the joints distal to the injury.

X-ray

X-ray examination is mandatory. Certain pitfalls must be avoided, as follows.

Two views A fracture or a dislocation may not be seen on a single x-ray film, and at least two views (anteroposterior and lateral) must be taken.

Two joints In the forearm or leg, one bone may be fractured and angulated. Angulation, however, is impossible unless the other bone also is broken, or a joint dislocated. The joints above and below the fracture must both be included on the x-ray films.

Two limbs In x-rays of children's bones, normal epiphyses may confuse the diagnosis of a fracture, and films of the uninjured limb are then helpful.

Two injuries Severe force often causes injuries at more than one level. Thus, with fractures of the calcaneum or femur it is important also to x-ray the pelvis and spine.

Two occasions Soon after injury, a fracture (e.g. of the carpal scaphoid) may be difficult to see. If doubt exists, further examination 10–14 days later may, as a result of bone resorption, make diagnosis easier.

Special imaging

Sometimes the fracture – or the full extent of the fracture – is not apparent on the plain x-ray. *Tomography* may be helpful in lesions of the spine or fractures of the tibial condyles; *CT* or *MRI* may be the only way of showing whether a fractured vertebra is threatening to compress

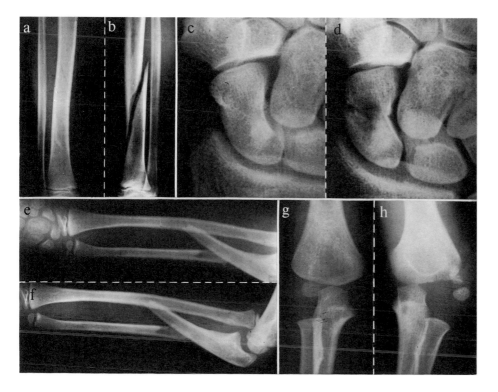

23.10 X-ray examination must be 'adequate' (a, b) Two films of the same tibia: the AP fails to show the fracture. (c) Fractured scaphoid not visible on the day of injury, but clearly seen (d) 2 weeks later. (e, f) Monteggia fracture-dislocation: failure to include both joints in forearm fractures (e) may result in a radioulnar dislocation (f) being missed. (g, h) Fractured lateral condyle (h) – in a child comparison with the uninjured side (g) is useful.

the spinal cord; indeed, transectional images are essential for accurate visualization of fractures in 'difficult' sites such as the calcaneum or acetabulum, and three-dimensional reconstructed images are even better. *Radioisotope scanning* is helpful in diagnosing a suspected stress fracture or other undisplaced fractures.

Description

Diagnosing a fracture is not enough; the surgeon should picture it (and describe it) in all its complexity. (1) Is it open or closed? (2) Which bone is broken, and where? (3) Has it involved a joint surface? (4) What is the shape of the break?

A transverse fracture is slow to join because the area of contact is small; if the broken surfaces are accurately apposed, however, the fracture is stable on compression. A spiral fracture joins more rapidly (because the contact area is large) but is not stable on compression. Short oblique fractures, those with a separate 'butterfly' fragment and comminuted fractures are all slow to join and unstable on compression.

DISPLACEMENT can be resolved into three components:

1. *Shift* (backwards, forwards, sideways, or longitudinally with impaction or overlap).
2. *Tilt or angulation* (sideways, backwards or forwards).
3. *Twist* (rotation in any direction).

A problem often arises in the description of angulation. 'Anterior angulation' could mean that the apex of the angle points anteriorly or that the distal fragment is tilted anteriorly: in this text it is always the latter meaning which is intended.

Secondary injuries

Certain fractures are apt to cause secondary injuries and *these should always be assumed to have occurred until proved otherwise.*

SPINAL CORD INJURY With any fracture of the spine, neurological examination is essential – (1) to establish whether the spinal cord or nerve roots have been damaged and (2) to obtain a baseline for later comparison if neurological signs should change.

PELVIC AND ABDOMINAL INJURIES Fractures of the pelvis may be associated with visceral injury. It is especially important to enquire about urinary function; if a urethral or bladder injury is suspected, diagnostic catheterization may be necessary.

THORACIC INJURIES Fractured ribs or sternum may be associated with injury to the lungs or heart. It is essential to check cardiorespiratory function.

PECTORAL GIRDLE INJURIES Fractures and dislocations around the pectoral girdle may damage the brachial plexus or the large vessels at the base of the neck. Neurological and vascular examination are essential.

Treatment of closed fractures

General treatment is the first consideration: to treat the patient, not simply the part. The sequence is: (1) first aid; (2) transport; and (3) the treatment of shock, haemorrhage and associated injuries. These are discussed in Chapter 21).

In principle the treatment of fractures consists of manipulation to improve the position of the fragments, followed by splintage to hold them together until they unite; meanwhile, joint movement and function must be preserved. Fracture healing is promoted by physiological loading of the bone, so muscle activity and early weightbearing are encouraged. These objectives are covered by three simple injunctions: REDUCE, HOLD, EXERCISE.

The problem is how to hold a fracture adequately and yet use the limb sufficiently: this is a conflict (*Hold* v *Move*) which the surgeon seeks to resolve as rapidly as possible (e.g. by internal fixation); but he also wants to avoid unnecessary risks – here is a second conflict (*Speed* v *Safety*). This dual conflict epitomizes the four factors that dominate fracture management (the term 'fracture quartet' seems appropriate).

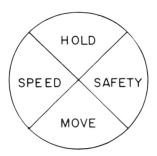

HOLD

SPEED SAFETY

MOVE

The fracture quartet

Treatment is determined not only by the type of fracture but also by the condition of the soft tissues. Tscherne (1984) has provided a helpful classification of closed injuries: grade 0 is a simple fracture with little or no soft-tissue injury; grade 1 is a fracture with superficial abrasion or bruising of the skin and subcutaneous tissue; grade 2 is a more severe fracture with deep soft-tissue contusion and swelling; and grade 3 is a severe injury with marked soft-tissue damage and a threatened compartment syndrome. The more severe grades of injury are more likely to require some form of mechanical fixation.

Reduce

Although general treatment and resuscitation must always take precedence, there should be no undue delay in attending to the fracture; swelling of the soft parts during the first 12 hours makes reduction increasingly difficult. However, there are some situations in which reduction is unnecessary: (1) when there is little or no displacement; (2) when displacement does not matter (e.g. in fractures of the clavicle); and (3) when reduction is unlikely to succeed (e.g. with compression fractures of the vertebrae).

Alignment of the fragments is more important than apposition; provided normal alignment is obtained, overlap of the fracture surfaces may be acceptable. The exception is a fracture involving an articular surface; this should be reduced as near to perfection as possible because any irregularity will predispose to degenerative arthritis.

There are two methods of reduction: closed and open.

CLOSED REDUCTION

Under appropriate anaesthesia and muscle relaxation, the fracture is reduced by a three-fold manoeuvre: (1) the distal part of the limb is pulled in the line of the bone; (2) as the fragments disengage, they are repositioned (by reversing the original direction of force if this can be deduced); and (3) alignment is adjusted in each plane. This is most effective when the periosteum and muscles on one side of the fracture remain intact; the soft-tissue strap prevents over-reduction and stabilizes the fracture after it has been reduced.

Some fractures (e.g. of the femoral shaft) are difficult to reduce by manipulation because of powerful muscle pull and may need prolonged traction.

In general, closed reduction is used for all minimally displaced fractures, for most fractures in children and for fractures that are not unstable after reduction.

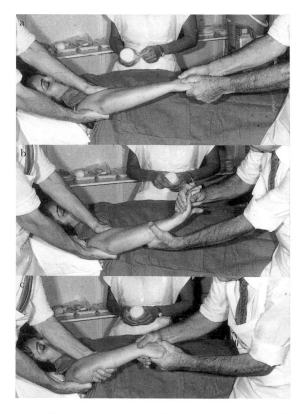

23.11 Closed reduction (a) Traction in the line of the bone. (b) Disimpaction. (c) Pressing fragment into reduced position.

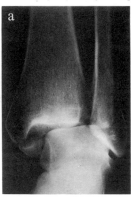
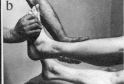
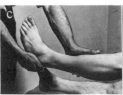
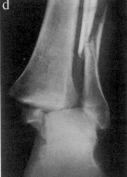

23.12 Closed reduction   These two ankle fractures look somewhat similar but are caused by different forces. The causal force must be reversed to achieve reduction: (a) requires internal rotation (b); an adduction force (c) is needed for (d).

OPEN REDUCTION

Operative reduction of the fracture under direct vision is indicated: (1) when closed reduction fails, either because of difficulty in controlling the fragments or because soft tissues are interposed between them; (2) when there is a large articular fragment that needs accurate positioning; or (3) for traction fractures in which the fragments are held apart. As a rule, however, open reduction is merely the first step to internal fixation.

treatment for fractures with severe soft-tissue damage. Other contraindications to non-operative methods are inherently unstable fractures, multiple fractures and fractures in confused or uncooperative patients. If these constraints are borne in mind, closed methods can be sensibly considered in choosing the most suitable method of fracture splintage. Remember, too, that the objective is to splint the fracture, not the entire limb!

Hold reduction

The word 'immobilization' has been deliberately avoided because the objective is seldom complete immobility; usually it is the prevention of displacement. Nevertheless, some restriction of movement is needed to promote soft-tissue healing and to allow free movement of the unaffected parts.

The available methods of holding reduction are: (1) continuous traction; (2) cast splintage; (3) functional bracing; (4) internal fixation; and (5) external fixation.

In the modern technological age, 'closed' methods are often scorned – an attitude arising from ignorance more than from experience. The muscles surrounding a fracture, if they are intact, act as a fluid compartment; traction or compression creates a hydraulic effect which is capable of splinting the fracture. Therefore closed methods are most suitable for fractures with intact soft tissues, and are liable to fail if they are used as the primary method of

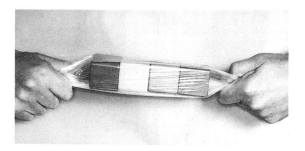

23.13 Hold reduction   Showing how, if the soft tissues around a fracture are intact, traction will align the bony fragments.

CONTINUOUS TRACTION

Traction is applied to the limb distal to the fracture, so as to exert a continuous pull in the long axis of the bone. This is particularly useful for shaft fractures which are oblique or spiral and easily displaced by muscle contraction.

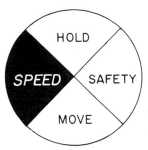

Continuous traction 'Speed' is the weak member of the quartet.

Traction cannot *hold* a fracture still; it can pull a long bone straight and hold it out to length but to maintain accurate reduction is sometimes difficult. And meanwhile the patient can *move* his joints and exercise his muscles.

Traction is *safe* enough, provided it is not excessive and care is taken when inserting the traction pin. The problem is *speed*: not because the fracture unites slowly (it does not) but because lower limb traction keeps the patient in hospital. Consequently, as soon as the fracture is 'sticky' (deformable but not displaceable), traction should be replaced by bracing, if this method is feasible.

TRACTION BY GRAVITY This applies only to upper limb injuries. Thus, with a wrist sling the weight of the arm provides continuous traction to the humerus; for comfort and stability, especially with a transverse fracture, a U-slab of plaster may be bandaged on or, better, a removable plastic sleeve from the axilla to just above the elbow is held on with Velcro.

SKIN TRACTION Skin (or Buck's) traction will sustain a pull of no more than 4 or 5 kg. Holland strapping or one-way-stretch Elastoplast is stuck to the shaved skin and held on with a bandage. The malleoli are protected by Gamgee tissue, and cords or tapes are used for traction.

SKELETAL TRACTION A Kirschner wire, Steinmann pin or Denham pin is inserted, usually behind the tibial tubercle for hip, thigh and knee injuries, lower in the tibia or through the calcaneum for tibial fractures. If a pin is used, hooks that can swivel freely are attached, and cords tied to them for applying traction.

Traction must always be opposed by counteraction; that is, the pull must be exerted against something, or it merely drags the patient down the bed.

Fixed traction The pull is exerted against a fixed point; for example, the tapes are tied to the cross-piece of a Thomas' splint and pull the leg down until the root of the limb abuts against the ring of the splint.

Balanced traction The pull is exerted against an opposing force provided by the weight of the body when the foot of the bed is raised. The cords may be tied to the foot of the bed, or run over pulleys and have weights attached.

Combined traction A Thomas' splint is used. The tapes are tied to the end of the splint and the splint is suspended, or is tied to the end of the bed, which is raised.

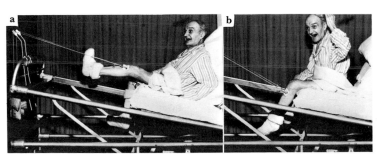

23.14 Continuous traction Balanced skeletal traction – the patient can move his joints while traction holds position; people imagine that without a splint the patient must be uncomfortable – but look at his face!

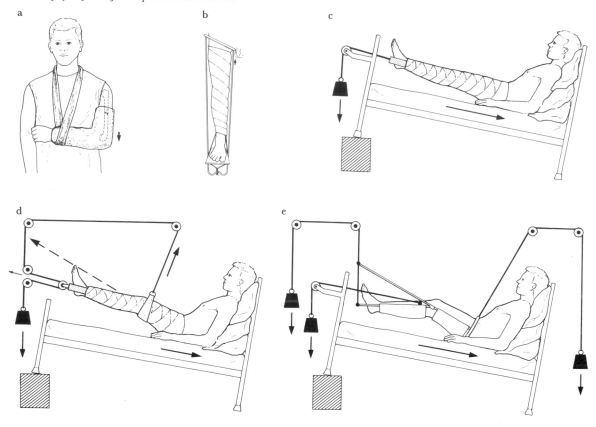

23.15 Methods of traction   (a) Traction by gravity. Skin traction: (b) fixed; (c) balanced; (d) Hamilton Russell; (e) skeletal traction with a splint and a knee-flexion piece.

COMPLICATIONS   There are two important complications of traction which should be guarded against. In children especially, traction tapes and circular bandages *may constrict the circulation*; for this reason 'gallows traction', in which the baby's legs are suspended from an overhead beam, should never be used for children over 12 kg in weight. In older people, leg traction may predispose to *peroneal nerve injury* and a resultant drop foot; the limb should be checked repeatedly to see that it does not roll into external rotation during traction. A very occasional complication is a *compartment syndrome* following excessive traction through a calcaneal pin.

CAST SPLINTAGE
Plaster of Paris is still widely used as a splint, especially for distal limb fractures and for most children's fractures. It is *safe* enough, so long as one is alert to the danger of a tight cast and provided pressure sores are prevented. The *speed* of union is neither greater nor less than with traction, but the patient can go home sooner. *Holding* reduction is usually no problem and patients with tibial fractures can bear weight on the cast. However, joints encased in plaster cannot *move* and are liable to stiffen; stiffness, which has earned the sobriquet 'fracture disease', is the problem with conventional plasters. If the haematoma of a fractured shaft is

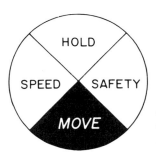

Casts 'Move' is the weak member of the quartet.

are impervious to water, and also lighter) but as long as they are used as full casts the basic drawback is the same.

Stiffness can be minimized by: (1) delayed splintage – that is, by using traction until movement has been regained, and only then applying plaster; or (2) starting with a conventional cast but, after a few days, when the limb can be handled without too much discomfort, replacing the cast by a functional brace which permits joint movement.

not milked away by exercises, adhesions form which bind muscle fibres to each other and to the bone; with articular fractures, plaster perpetuates surface irregularities (closed reduction is seldom perfect) and lack of movement inhibits the healing of cartilage defects. Newer substitutes have some advantages over plaster (they

TECHNIQUE After the fracture has been reduced, stockinette is threaded over the limb and the bony points are protected with wool. Plaster is then applied. While it is setting the surgeon moulds it away from bony prominences; with shaft fractures three-point pres-

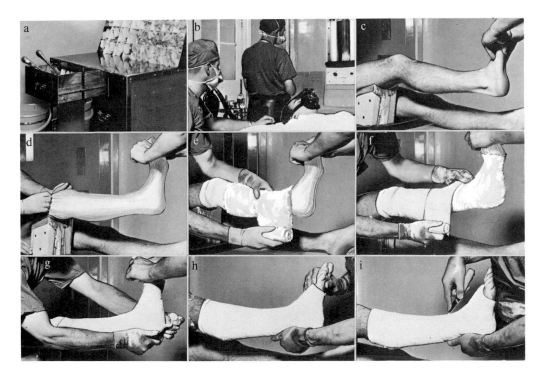

23.16 Plaster technique Applying a well-fitting and effective plaster needs experience and attention to detail. (a) A well-equipped plaster trolley is invaluable. (b) Adequate anaesthesia and careful study of the x-ray films are both indispensable. (c) For a below-knee plaster the thigh is best supported on a padded block. (d) Stockinette is threaded smoothly onto the leg. (e) For a padded plaster the wool is rolled on and it must be even. (f) Plaster is next applied smoothly, taking a tuck with each turn, and (g) smoothing each layer firmly onto the one beneath. (h) While still wet the cast is moulded away from the bony points. (i) With a recent injury the plaster is then split.

sure can be applied to keep the intact periosteal hinge under tension and thereby maintain reduction.

If the fracture is recent, further swelling is likely; the plaster and stockinette are therefore split from top to bottom, exposing the skin. Check x-rays are essential and the plaster may need to be wedged.

With fractures of the shafts of long bones, rotation is controlled only if the plaster includes the joints above and below the fracture. In the lower limb, the knee is usually held slightly flexed, the ankle at a right angle and the tarsus and forefoot neutral (this 'plantigrade' position is essential for normal walking). In the upper limb the position of the splinted joints varies with the fracture. Splintage must not be discontinued (though a functional brace may be substituted) until the fracture is consolidated; if plaster changes are needed, check x-rays are essential.

COMPLICATIONS   Plaster immobilization is safe, but only if care is taken to prevent certain complications. These are tight cast, pressure sores and abrasion or laceration of the skin.

Tight cast   The cast may be put on too tightly, or it may become tight if the limb swells. The patient complains of diffuse pain; only later – sometimes much later – do the signs of vascular compression appear. The limb should be elevated, but if the pain persists the only safe course is to split the cast and ease it open (1) throughout its length and (2) through all the padding down to skin. Whenever swelling is anticipated the cast should be applied over thick padding and the plaster should be split before it sets, so as to provide a firm but not absolutely rigid splint.

Pressure sores   Even a well-fitting cast may press upon the skin over a bony prominence (the patella, the heel, the elbow or the head of the ulna). The patient complains of localized pain precisely over the pressure spot. Such localized pain demands immediate inspection through a window in the cast.

Skin abrasion or laceration   This is really a complication of removing plasters, especially if an electric saw is used. Complaints of nipping

or pinching during plaster removal should never be ignored; a ripped forearm is good reason for litigation.

FUNCTIONAL BRACING
Functional bracing, using either plaster of Paris or one of the lighter materials, is one way of preventing joint stiffness while still permitting fracture splintage and loading. Segments of a cast are applied only over the shafts of the bones, leaving the joints free; the cast segments are connected by metal or plastic hinges which allow movements in one plane. The splints are 'functional' in that joint movements are much less restricted than with conventional casts.

Functional bracing is used most widely for fractures of the femur or tibia, but, since the brace is not very rigid, it is usually applied only when the fracture is beginning to unite, i.e. after 3–6 weeks of traction or conventional plaster. Used in this way, it comes out well on all four of the basic requirements: the fracture can be *held* reasonably well; the joints can be *moved*; the fracture joins at normal *speed* (or perhaps slightly quicker) without keeping the patient in hospital and the method is *safe*. However, except in experienced hands there is a greater risk of fracture malunion than with the use of full-length casts.

TECHNIQUE   Considerable skill is needed to apply an effective brace. First the fracture is 'stabilized': by a few days on traction or in a conventional plaster for tibial fractures; and by a few weeks on traction for femoral fractures (till the fracture is sticky, i.e. deformable but not displaceable). Then a hinged cast or splint is applied which holds the fracture snugly but permits joint movement; functional activity, including weightbearing, is encouraged. Details of technique and applications are given by Sarmiento and Latta (1981).

INTERNAL FIXATION
Bone fragments may be fixed with screws, transfixing pins or nails, a metal plate held by screws, a long intramedullary nail (with or without locking screws), circumferential bands, or a combination of these methods.

Properly applied, internal fixation *holds* a fracture securely so that *movements* can begin at

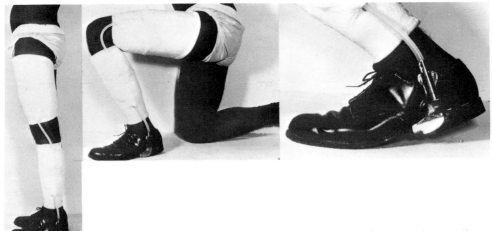

23.17 Functional bracing (cast-bracing) Despite plaster the patient has excellent joint movement (by courtesy of John A. Feagin MD). Note the polypropylene 'hinges' at the knee and ankle.

once; with early movement the 'fracture disease' (stiffness and oedema) is abolished. As far as *speed* is concerned, the patient can leave hospital as soon as the wound is healed, but he must remember that, even though the bone moves in one piece, the fracture is not united – it is merely held by a metal bridge; unprotected weightbearing is, for some time, unsafe. The greatest *danger*, however, is sepsis; if infection supervenes, all the manifest advantages of internal fixation (precise reduction, immediate stability and early movement) may be lost. The risk of infection depends upon: (1) the patient – devitalized tissues, a dirty wound and an unfit patient are all dangerous; (2) the surgeon – thorough training, a high degree of surgical dexterity and adequate assistance are all essential; and (3) the facilities – a guaranteed aseptic routine, a full range of implants and staff familiar with their use are all indispensable.

INDICATIONS Internal fixation is often the most desirable form of treatment. The chief indications are:

1. Fractures that cannot be reduced except by operation.
2. Fractures that are inherently unstable and prone to redisplacement after reduction (e.g. mid-shaft fractures of the forearm and displaced ankle fractures); also, those liable to be pulled apart by muscle action (e.g. transverse fracture of the patella or olecranon).
3. Fractures that unite poorly and slowly, principally fractures of the femoral neck.
4. Pathological fractures, in which bone disease may prevent healing.
5. Multiple fractures, where early fixation (by either internal or external fixation) reduces the risk of general complications and late multisystem organ failure (Phillips and Contreras, 1990).
6. Fractures in patients who present nursing difficulties (paraplegics, those with multiple injuries and the very elderly).

Internal fixation 'Safety' is the weak member of the quartet.

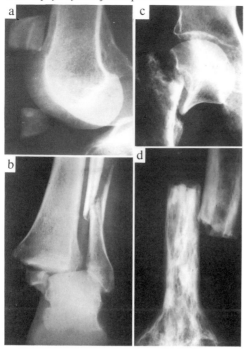

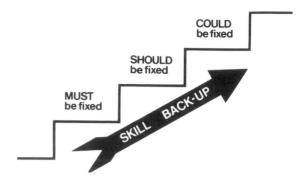

23.20 The indications staircase The indications for fixation are not immutable; thus, if the surgical skill or back-up facilities (staff, sterility and equipment) are of a low order, internal fixation is indicated only when the alternative is unacceptable (e.g. with femoral neck fractures). With average skill and facilities, fixation is indicated when alternative methods are possible but very difficult or unwise (e.g. multiple injuries). With the highest levels of skill and facilities, fixation is reasonable if it saves time, money or beds.

23.18 Indications for internal fixation (a) This patella has been pulled apart and can be held together only by internal fixation. (b) Fracture-dislocation of the ankle is often unstable after reduction and usually requires fixation. (c) This patient was considered to be too ill for operation; her femoral neck fracture has failed to unite without rigid fixation. (d) Pathological fracture in Paget bone; without fixation, union may not occur.

TECHNIQUE Many methods are available, including the use of wires, screws, plates, intramedullary rods and combinations of these. When plates are used they should, if possible, be applied to the tensile surface, which is usually the convex side of the bone. When intramedullary nails are used they may be 'locked' with transverse screws (Muller et al., 1991).

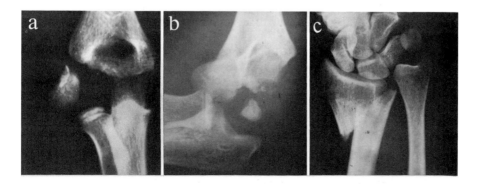

23.19 Further indications for internal fixation (a) The elbow was grossly swollen and this fractured lateral condyle could not be reduced by closed manipulation. (b) Similarly this medial epicondyle could be extricated from the joint only by open operation. (c) The sharp fragment of radius had impaled muscle and could not be freed without operation.

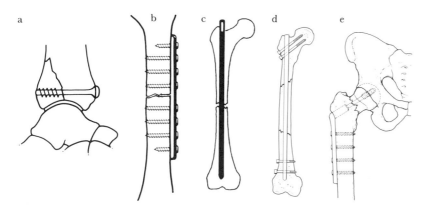

23.21 Internal fixation The method used must be appropriate to the situation: (a) screws – interfragmentary compression; (b) plate and screws – most suitable in the forearm; (c) intramedullary nail – for the larger long bones; (d) interlocking nail and screws – ideal for the femur and tibia; (e) dynamic compression screw and plate – ideal for the proximal and distal ends of the femur.

COMPLICATIONS   Most of the complications of internal fixation are due to poor technique, poor equipment or poor operating conditions.

Infection Iatrogenic infection is now the most common cause of chronic osteitis; the metal does not predispose to infection but the operation does.

Non-union If the bones have been fixed rigidly with the ends apart, the fracture may fail to unite. This is more likely in the leg or the forearm if one bone is fractured and the other remains intact.

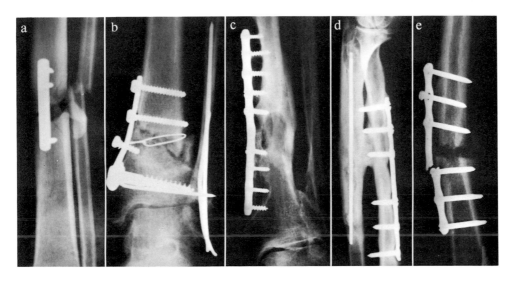

23.22 Bad fixation (how not to do it)   (a) Timidity. (b) Overexuberance. (c) The screws are too short and the bone is infected. (d) Unorthodoxy has resulted in cross-union. (e) Any plate is liable to break unless protected from stress until the fracture has joined.

Implant failure Metal is subject to fatigue, and until some union of the fracture has occurred metal implants are precarious. Stress must therefore be avoided and a patient with a plated tibia should walk with crutches and minimal weightbearing for the first 3 months. Pain at the fracture site is a danger signal and must be investigated.

Refracture It is important not to remove metal implants too soon, or the bone may refracture. A year is the minimum and 18 or 24 months safer; for several weeks after removal the bone is weak, and care or protection is needed.

EXTERNAL FIXATION
A fracture may be held by transfixing screws or tensioned wires which pass through the bone above and below the fracture and are attached to an external frame. This is especially applicable to the tibia and the pelvis, but the method is also used for fractures of the femur, the humerus, the lower radius and even the bones of the hand.

INDICATIONS External fixation is particularly useful for:

1. Fractures associated with severe soft-tissue damage where the wound can be left open for inspection, dressing or skin grafting.
2. Fractures associated with nerve or vessel damage.
3. Severely comminuted and unstable fractures, which can be held out to length until healing commences.

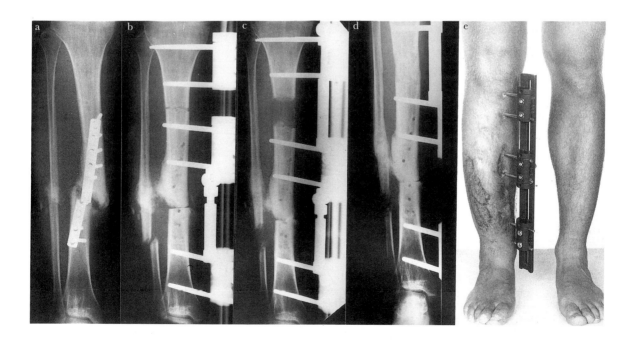

23.23 External fixation This young man broke his leg in a skiing accident. Despite internal fixation, the fracture went on to non-union (a). Osteotomy and callotasis in the proximal half of the bone permitted simultaneous lengthening of the tibia and compression fixation of the ununited fracture (b, c, d). The patient meanwhile was able to get about with his external fixator (e). Three months later the fracture was united and the external fixator could be removed.

4. Ununited fractures, which can be excised and compressed; sometimes this is combined with elongation.
5. Fractures of the pelvis, which often cannot be controlled by any other method.
6. Infected fractures, for which internal fixation might not be suitable.
7. Severe multiple injuries, where early stabilization reduces the risk of serious complications (Phillips and Contreras, 1990).

TECHNIQUE The principle of external fixation is simple: the bone is transfixed above and below the fracture and the proximal and distal transfixing screws or wires are then connected to each other by rigid bars. There are numerous variations in techniques and fixation devices: transfixion by pins, screws or wires; connecting bars on both sides of the bone or on one side only; triangular, quadrangular and circular configurations; fixed connections or adjustable connections; bars and pins of varying rigidity and stability which, together with the specific geometry of the system, provide varying degrees of fracture 'immobilization' (Behrens, 1988). What is essential is that the equipment permits adjustment of length and accurate reduction of the fracture in all three planes. An additional facility (e.g. in the Orthofix appliances) allows 'dynamization'; once stability has been achieved, small amounts of axial movement are permitted – this promotes callus and accelerates union (Kenwright et al., 1991). The system of hoops and tension wires devised by Ilizarov (1992) is particularly versatile; it can be used to immobilize fractures, correct deformities, lengthen bones and transpose segments of bone in almost any part of the peripheral skeleton.

COMPLICATIONS The main complications of external fixation are: (1) overdistraction of the fragments, which are then held rigidly apart; (2) reduced load transmission through the bone, which delays fracture healing and causes osteoporosis (for this reason, external fixators should be dynamized or removed after 6–8 weeks, and replaced by some alternative form of splintage which will allow bone loading); and (3) pin-track infection.

Exercise

More correctly, 'restore function' – not only to the injured parts but also to the patient as a whole. The objectives are to reduce oedema, preserve joint movement, restore muscle power and guide the patient back to normal activity.

Prevention of oedema Swelling is almost inevitable after a fracture and may cause skin stretching and blisters. Persistent oedema is an important cause of joint stiffness, especially in the hand; it should be prevented if possible, and treated energetically if it is already present, by a combination of elevation and exercise. Not every patient needs admission to hospital, and less severe injuries of the upper limb are successfully managed by placing the arm in a sling; but it is then essential to insist on active use, with movement of all the joints that are free. With most closed fractures, all open fractures and all fractures treated by internal fixation it must be assumed that swelling will occur; the limb should be elevated and active exercises begun as soon as the patient will tolerate this. The essence of soft-tissue care may be summed up thus: elevate and exercise; never dangle, never force.

Elevation An injured limb usually needs to be elevated; after reduction of a leg fracture the foot of the bed is raised and exercises are begun. If the leg is in plaster the limb must, at first, be dependent for only short periods; between these periods, the leg is elevated on a chair. The patient is allowed, and encouraged, to exercise the limb actively, but not to let it dangle. When plaster is finally removed, the leg is bandaged and a similar routine of activity punctuated by elevation is practised until circulatory control is fully restored.

Injuries of the upper limb also need elevation. A sling must not be a permanent passive arm-holder; the limb must be elevated intermittently or, if need be, continuously.

Active exercise Active movement helps to pump away oedema fluid, stimulates the circulation, prevents soft-tissue adhesion and promotes fracture healing. A limb encased in plaster is still capable of static muscle contraction and the patient should be taught how to do this. When splintage is removed the joints are mobilized and muscle-building exercises are steadily in-

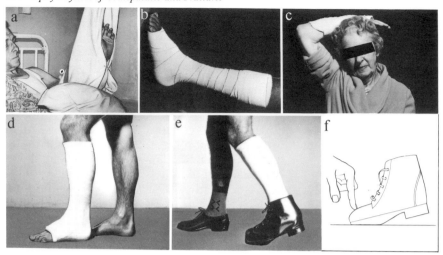

23.24 Some aspects of soft-tissue treatment Swelling is minimized by (a) elevation and (b) firm support. Stiffness is minimized by exercises: this patient (c) with a Colles' fracture is in no danger of a stiff shoulder. To exercise muscles under a plaster is less easy – a walking plaster should be plantigrade (d); an over-boot with rocker action (e, f) facilitates normal walking and muscle activity.

creased. Remember that the unaffected joints need exercising, too; it is all too easy to neglect a stiffening shoulder while caring for an injured wrist or hand.

Assisted movement It has long been taught that passive movement can be deleterious, especially with injuries around the elbow where there is a high risk of developing myositis ossificans. Certainly forced movements should never be permitted, but gentle assistance during active exercises may help to retain function or regain movement after fractures involving the articular surfaces. Nowadays this is done with machines that can be set to provide a specified range and rate of movement ('continuous passive motion').

Functional activity As the patient's mobility improves, an increasing amount of directed activity is included in the programme. He may need to be taught again how to perform everyday tasks such as walking, getting in and out of bed, bathing, dressing or handling eating utensils. Experience is the best teacher and the patient is encouraged to use the injured limb as much as possible. Those with very severe or extensive injuries may benefit from spending time in a special rehabilitation unit. But the best incentive to full recovery is the promise of re-entry into family life, recreational pursuits and meaningful work.

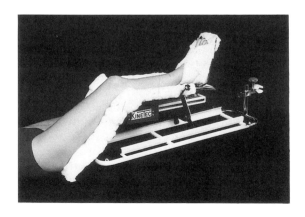

23.25 Continuous passive motion The motorized frame provides continuous flexion and extension to preset limits.

Treatment of open fractures

General considerations

Many patients with open fractures have multiple injuries and severe shock; for them, appropriate treatment at the scene of the accident is essential. The wound should be covered with a sterile dressing or clean material and left undisturbed until the patient reaches the accident department. In hospital a rapid general assessment is the first step, and any life-threatening conditions are addressed. The wound is then inspected; ideally it should be photographed with a Polaroid camera, so that it can again be covered and left undisturbed until the patient is in the operating theatre. Four questions need to be answered: (1) what is the nature of the wound? (2) what is the state of the skin around the wound? (3) is the circulation satisfactory? and (4) are the nerves intact?

All open fractures, no matter how trivial they may seem, must be assumed to be contaminated; it is important to try to prevent them from becoming infected. To this end the four essentials are: (1) immediate wound cover; (2) antibiotic prophylaxis; (3) early wound debridement; and (4) stabilization of the fracture. These are discussed below, but first Gustilo's valuable classification of open fractures is outlined (Gustilo, Merkow and Templeman, 1990).

Classification

Type I The wound is usually a small, clean puncture through which a bone spike has protruded. There is little soft-tissue damage with no crushing and the fracture is not comminuted.

Type II The wound is more than 1 cm long, but there is no skin flap. There is not much soft-tissue damage, and no more than moderate crushing or comminution of the fracture.

Type III There is extensive damage to skin, soft tissue and neurovascular structures, with considerable contamination of the wound. There are three grades of severity. In type III A the fractured bone can be adequately covered by soft tissue; in type III B it cannot and there is also periosteal stripping, as well as severe comminution of the fracture; the fracture is classified as type III C if there is an arterial injury which needs to be repaired, regardless of the amount of other soft-tissue damage. High-velocity injuries are classified as III B or C; although the wound is small, internal damage is severe.

The incidence of wound infection correlates directly with the extent of soft-tissue damage, rising from less than 2% in type I to over 10% in type II fractures.

Early management

The wound should be kept covered until the patient reaches the operating theatre. Antibiotics are given as soon as possible, no matter how small the laceration, and are continued until the danger of infection has passed. In most cases a combination of benzylpenicillin and flucloxacillin given 6-hourly for 48 hours will suffice; if the wound is heavily contaminated, it is prudent to cover also for Gram-negative organisms by adding gentamicin or metronidazole and to continue treatment for 4 or 5 days.

Tetanus prophylaxis is equally important: toxoid for those previously immunized, human antiserum if not.

Debridement

The operation aims to render the wound devoid of foreign material and of dead tissue, leaving a good blood supply throughout. Under general anaesthesia the patient's clothing is removed, while an assistant maintains traction on the injured limb and holds it still. The dressing previously applied to the wound is replaced by a sterile pad and the surrounding skin is cleaned and shaved. The pad is then taken off and the wound is irrigated thoroughly with copious amounts of physiological saline; the final irrigation may be with an antibacterial agent such as bacitracin. A tourniquet is not used because it would endanger the circulation still further and make it difficult to recognize which structures are devitalized. The tissues are then dealt with as follows.

SKIN   Only the merest sliver of skin is excised from the wound edges; as much skin as possible is spared. The wound often needs to be extended by planned incisions to obtain adequate exposure; once it is enlarged clothing and other foreign material may be picked out.

FASCIA   Fascia is divided extensively so that the circulation is not impeded.

MUSCLE   Dead muscle is dangerous; it provides food for bacteria. It can usually be recognized by its purplish discoloration, its mushy consistency, its failure to contract when stimulated and its failure to bleed when cut. All dead and doubtfully viable muscle is excised.

BLOOD VESSELS   Large bleeding vessels are tied meticulously but, to minimize the amount of catgut left in the wound, small vessels are clamped with artery forceps and twisted.

NERVES   It is usually best to leave a cut nerve undisturbed. If, however, the wound is clean and the nerve ends present without dissection, the sheath is sutured using non-absorbable material for ease of later identification.

TENDONS   As a rule, cut tendons are also left alone. As with nerves, suture is permissible only if the wound is clean and dissection unnecessary.

BONE   The fracture surfaces are gently cleaned and replaced in the correct position. Bone, like skin, should be spared, and fragments removed only if they are small and totally detached.

JOINTS   Open joint injuries are best treated by wound toilet, closure of synovium and capsule, and systemic antibiotics; drainage or suction irrigation is used only if contamination is severe.

Wound closure

To close or not to close the skin – this can be a difficult decision. A small, uncontaminated type I wound, operated on within a few hours of injury may, after debridement, be sutured (provided this can be done without tension) or skin grafted. All other wounds must be left open until the dangers of tension and infection have passed. The wound is lightly packed with sterile gauze and is inspected after 5 days: if it is clean, it is sutured or skin grafted (delayed primary closure).

Stabilization of the fracture

It is now recognized that stability of the fracture is important in reducing the likelihood of infection. For a type I or small type II wound with a stable fracture a widely split plaster is permissible or, for the femur, traction on a splint. But more severe wounds (and gunshot wounds) need to have the fracture fixed more securely.

The safest method is external fixation. Intramedullary nailing (with locking if the fracture is comminuted) can be used for the femur or tibia; it is best not to do preliminary reaming which increases the risk of infection. Plates and screws can be used for metaphyseal or articular fractures, but only if the surgeon is experienced in their use and the circumstances are ideal.

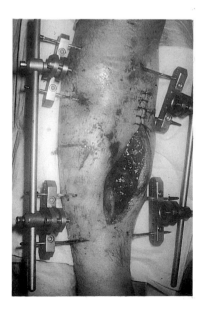

23.26 Open fractures – treatment Stabilization of the fracture is crucial and this is usually best achieved by external fixation.

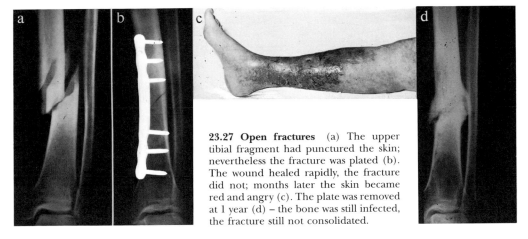

23.27 Open fractures (a) The upper tibial fragment had punctured the skin; nevertheless the fracture was plated (b). The wound healed rapidly, the fracture did not; months later the skin became red and angry (c). The plate was removed at 1 year (d) – the bone was still infected, the fracture still not consolidated.

Aftercare

In the ward, the limb is elevated and its circulation carefully watched. Shock may still require treatment. Chemotherapy is continued; the organism is cultured and, if necessary, a different antibiotic is substituted.

If the wound has been left open, it is inspected at 5–7 days. Delayed primary suture is then often safe, or, if there has been much skin loss, split-skin grafts are applied. If toxaemia or septicaemia persists in spite of chemotherapy, the wound is drained (the only safe treatment if an infected fracture is not seen until 24 hours after injury).

Sequels to open fractures

SKIN   If there has been skin loss or contracture, grafting may be necessary. When reparative or reconstructive surgery to deeper tissues is required, a full-thickness skin graft is highly desirable.

BONE   Infection may lead to sequestra and to sinuses. Small sequestra should be removed early, but large pieces of bone should not be excised.

Delayed union is inevitable after an infected fracture, but union will occur if infection is controlled and treatment continued for sufficient time.

JOINTS   When an infected fracture communicates with a joint, the principles of treatment are the same as with bone infection; namely, drugs, drainage and splintage. The joint should be splinted in the optimum position for ankylosis, lest this occur.

With any open fracture, even if not communicating with a joint, some stiffness is almost inevitable. It can be minimized by slowly increasing active exercises, or by continuous passive motion, once it is certain that infection has been overcome.

Gunshot injuries

Missile wounds are looked upon as a special type of open injury. Tissue damage is produced by: (1) direct injury in the immediate path of the missile; (2) contusion of muscles around the missile track; and (3) bruising and congestion of soft tissues at a greater distance from the primary track. The exit wound (if any) is usually larger than the entry wound.

With high-velocity missiles (bullets, usually from rifles, travelling at speeds above 600 m/s) there is marked cavitation and tissue destruction over a wide area. With low-velocity missiles (bullets from civilian hand-guns travelling at speeds of 300–600 m/s) cavitation is much less, and with smaller weapons tissue damage may be virtually confined to the bullet track. However, with all gunshot injuries debris is sucked into the wound, which is therefore contaminated from the outset.

EMERGENCY MANAGEMENT   As always, the arrest of bleeding and general resuscitation take priority. The wounds should each be covered with a sterile dressing and the area examined for artery or nerve damage. Antibiotics should be given immediately.

DEFINITIVE TREATMENT   Traditionally, all missile injuries were treated as severe open injuries, by exploration of the missile track and formal debridement. However, it has been shown that low-velocity wounds with relatively clean entry and exit wounds can be treated as Gustilo type I injuries, by superficial debridement, splintage of the limb and antibiotic cover; the fracture is then treated as for similar open fractures (Woloszyn, Uitrlugt and Castle, 1986).

High-velocity injuries demand thorough cleansing of the wound and debridement, with excision of deep damaged tissues and, if necessary, splitting of fascial compartments to prevent ischaemia; the wound is left open (covered only with gauze dressings) and the limb is elevated and splinted. The safest plan, if contamination is considerable, and if anatomical considerations permit, is to join the entry and exit wounds and leave the entire track open. If there are comminuted fractures, these are best managed by external fixation. Delayed primary closure is performed after 7 days.

Aphorisms of fracture management

Think before you start   Are you treating the patient? Or merely the x-ray?

Think before you reduce   Have you worked out how to do it? And how to hold your reduction?

Think before you hold   Is your splint necessary? Is it harmful?

Think before you operate   Are your facilities good enough? Are you good enough?

Complications of fractures

General complications

Shock, diffuse coagulopathy and *respiratory dysfunction* occur during the first 24 hours after injury. There is also a late *metabolic response* to trauma which occurs days or weeks after injury; it includes increased catabolism and requires nutritional support (Michelsen and Askanazi, 1986). These are discussed in Chapter 22.

Crush syndrome

The crush syndrome may occur if a large bulk of muscle is crushed, as by fallen masonry, or if a tourniquet has been left on too long. When compression is released, acid myohaematin (cytochrome c), from muscle breakdown, is carried in the circulation to the kidneys and blocks the tubules. An alternative explanation is that renal artery spasm occurs and the anoxic tubule cells necrose.

Shock is profound. The released limb is pulseless and later becomes red, swollen and blistered; sensation and muscle power may be lost. Renal secretion diminishes and a low-output uraemia with acidosis develops. If renal secretion returns within a week the patient survives; most patients, unless treated by renal dialysis, become increasingly drowsy and die within 14 days.

To avert disaster, a limb crushed severely and for several hours should be amputated. Thus, if a tourniquet has been left on for more than 6 hours the limb must be sacrificed. Amputation is carried out above the site of compression and before compression is released.

Once the compression force has been released, amputation is valueless. The limb must be kept cool and the patient's shock treated. If oliguria develops, fluid and protein intake are reduced, carbohydrates given (by mouth or into a large vein), protein catabolism is reduced (by giving neomycin and an anabolic steroid) and the serum electrolyte balance maintained. Renal dialysis should be instituted.

Venous thrombosis and pulmonary embolism

Deep venous thrombosis (DVT) is the commonest complication of trauma and surgery.

The true incidence is unknown but is probably greater than 30% (Hedges and Kakkar, 1988). Thrombosis occurs most frequently in the veins of the calf, and less often in the proximal veins of the thigh and pelvis. It is mainly from the latter sites that fragments of clot are carried to the lungs, the incidence of pulmonary embolism after major orthopaedic operations being about 5% and of fatal embolism about 0.5%.

The primary cause of DVT in surgical patients is hypercoagulability of the blood, due mainly to activation of factor X by thromboplastins released from damaged tissues. Once thrombosis has been initiated, secondary factors become important: stasis may result from a tourniquet or tight bandage, pressure against the operating table or mattress, and prolonged immobility; endothelial damage and an increase in the number and stickiness of platelets may result from trauma or operation.

Those at greatest risk of developing DVT are old people, patients with cardiovascular disease, patients confined to bed after trauma and patients undergoing hip arthroplasty (in whom reaming of the bone and excessive manipulation of the limb may be added predisposing factors).

CLINICAL FEATURES
DVT is, in the main, an occult disease, considerably more common than the signs suggest; the patient with symptoms has already had the condition for several days (Ruckley, 1986).

There may be pain in the calf or thigh; however, following trauma or operation even those who do not complain should be examined regularly for swelling, soft-tissue tenderness and a sudden slight increase in temperature and pulse rate. Typically in calf thrombosis there is increased pain on dorsiflexion of the foot (Homans' sign).

The diagnosis, as well as the exact site of the thrombosis, may be established by ascending venography, which should be done bilaterally. Of the non-invasive methods, B-mode ultrasound scanning is highly accurate for detecting proximal DVT, the most significant prelude to pulmonary embolism. Less reliable methods of detection are measuring radioactive iodine-labelled fibrinogen uptake in the clot or using the Doppler technique to measure blood flow.

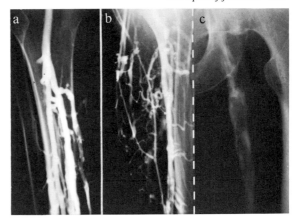

23.28 Deep vein thrombosis – phlebograms This patient's right calf (a) is normal, but his left calf (b) shows thrombosis; his left femoral vein (c) also is thrombosed; the filling defect is surrounded by contrast on all sides so the thrombus is potentially mobile, but it does not look recent so the danger is not great. (By courtesy of Dr N. W. T. Grieve.)

Pulmonary embolism, which almost always originates in the pelvis or thigh rather than the calf, is difficult to diagnose reliably; only a minority of patients have features such as chest pain, dyspnoea or haemoptysis. The occasional patient is seized with sudden chest pain, turns pale and falls dead. All patients with established DVT should be examined for signs of pulmonary consolidation; in suspicious cases, chest x-rays, lung scintigraphy and pulmonary angiography may be necessary to clinch the diagnosis.

Chronic lower limb oedema and leg ulcers (the postphlebitic syndrome) occur in almost all patients with iliofemoral thrombosis and in 10% of those with calf thrombosis.

PREVENTION
The risk of DVT and pulmonary embolism can be significantly reduced by prophylactic treatment (Parker-Williams and Vickers, 1991). Simple physical measures include elevation of the foot of the bed, the use of elastic stockings or graduated compression stockings, and above all the encouragement of exercises and getting the patient out of bed and walking as soon as possible. These are more effective when combined with anticoagulant treatment, which is

now generally advocated in known high-risk patients. The usual regimen is subcutaneous low-dose heparin, 5000 units preoperatively and then three times a day postoperatively until the patient is mobile. Unfortunately, this carries a risk of increased bleeding after operation and it is contraindicated in elderly people. More recently, low molecular weight heparin has been introduced: this is just as effective as unfractionated heparin in preventing DVT but is said to be less likely to cause bleeding; moreover, its main effect is on proximal venous thrombosis, the major cause of pulmonary embolism (Eriksson et al., 1991; Leyvraz et al., 1991).

TREATMENT
Localized DVT in the calf can be treated simply by applying elastic stockings and giving low-dose subcutaneous heparin (5000 units three times a day) until the patient is fully mobile. More extensive DVT, and certainly pelvic or thigh vein thrombosis, or established pulmonary embolism, should be treated immediately by bed rest, the use of elastic stockings and full anticoagulation. A tendency to bleed and peptic ulceration are contraindications.

Heparin is given intravenously, either in a fixed dose of 10 000 units 6-hourly, with protamine as an antidote should bleeding occur, or preferably in variable doses adjusted to maintain the activated partial thromboplastin at 1.5–2.0 times normal. This is continued for 5–7 days; during the last 2 days of this period oral warfarin is introduced and heparin is discontinued. The daily dose of warfarin is adjusted to maintain the prothrombin time at about twice the normal; treatment is continued for approximately 3 months.

Acute, severe pulmonary embolism demands cardiorespiratory resuscitation, vasopressors for shock, oxygen and a large dose (15 000 units) of heparin. Streptokinase is used both to dissolve clots and to prevent more forming. Antibiotics may be given to prevent lung infection.

Tetanus

The tetanus organism flourishes only in dead tissue. It produces an exotoxin which passes to the central nervous system via the blood and the perineural lymphatics from the infected region. The toxin is fixed in the anterior horn cells and therefore cannot be neutralized by antitoxin.

Established tetanus is characterized by tonic, and later clonic, contractions, especially of the muscles of the jaw and face (trismus, risus sardonicus), those near the wound itself, and later of the neck and trunk. Ultimately, the diaphragm and intercostal muscles may be fixed in spasm and the patient dies of asphyxia.

PROPHYLAXIS
Active immunization of the whole population by tetanus toxoid is an attainable ideal. To the patient so immunized, booster doses of toxoid are given after all but trivial skin wounding. In non-immunized patients prompt and thorough wound toilet together with antibiotics may be adequate, but if the wound is contaminated, and particularly with delay before operation, antitoxin is advisable. Horse serum carries a considerable risk of anaphylaxis, and human antitoxin (tetanus immunoglobulin) should be used. The opportunity is taken to initiate active immunization with toxoid at the same time.

TREATMENT
With established tetanus, intravenous antitoxin (again, human for choice) is advisable. Heavy sedation and muscle relaxant drugs may help; tracheal intubation and controlled respiration are employed for the patient with respiratory and swallowing embarrassment.

Gas gangrene

This terrifying condition is produced by clostridial infection (especially *C. welchii*). These are anaerobic organisms that can survive and multiply only in tissues with low oxygen tension; the prime site for infection, therefore, is a dirty wound with dead muscle that has been closed without adequate debridement. Toxins produced by the organisms destroy the cell wall and rapidly lead to tissue necrosis, thus promoting the spread of the disease.

Clinical features appear within 24 hours of the injury: the patient complains of intense pain and swelling around the wound and a brownish discharge may be seen; gas formation is usually not very marked. There little or no pyrexia but the pulse rate is increased and a

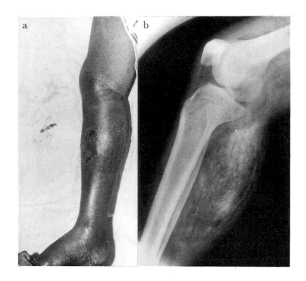

23.29 Gas gangrene (a) Clinical picture of gas gangrene. (b) X-rays show diffuse gas in the muscles of the calf.

characteristic smell becomes evident (once experienced this is never forgotten). Rapidly the patient becomes toxaemic and may lapse into coma and death.

It is essential to distinguish gas gangrene, which is characterized by myonecrosis, from anaerobic cellulitis, in which superficial gas formation is abundant but toxaemia usually slight. Failure to recognize the difference may lead to unnecessary amputation for the non-lethal cellulitis.

PREVENTION
Deep, penetrating wounds in muscular tissue are dangerous; they should be explored, all dead tissue should be completely excised and, if there is the slightest doubt about tissue viability, the wound should be left open. Unhappily there is no effective antitoxin against *C. welchii.*

TREATMENT
The key to life-saving treatment is early diagnosis. General measures, such as fluid replacement and intravenous antibiotics, are started immediately. Hyperbaric oxygen has been used as a means of limiting the spread of gangrene. However, the mainstay of treatment is prompt decompression of the wound and removal of all dead tissue. In advanced cases, amputation may be essential.

Fat embolism

Circulating fat globules larger than 10 µm in diameter, and histological traces of fat emboli in the lungs, occur in most adults after closed fractures of long bones; fortunately only a small percentage of patients develop the fat embolism syndrome, which is now thought to be part of the wider spectrum of post-traumatic respiratory dysfunction (see p. 507).

The source of the fat emboli is probably the bone marrow, and the condition is more common in patients with multiple closed fractures; however, fat embolism has been reported in a variety of disorders other than skeletal trauma (e.g. burns, renal infarction and cardiopulmonary operations); the pathogenesis is still a matter of controversy.

CLINICAL FEATURES
The patient with symptoms is usually a young adult with a lower-limb fracture. Early warning signs (within 72 hours of injury) are a slight rise of temperature and pulse rate. In more pronounced cases there is breathlessness and mild mental confusion or restlessness; petechiae should be sought on the front and back of the chest and in the conjunctival folds. In the most severe cases there may be marked respiratory

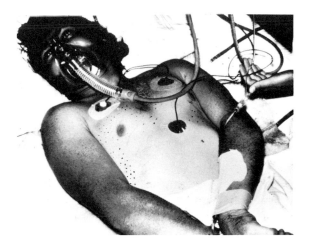

23.30 Fat embolism This man with bilateral femoral shaft fractures (closed) sustained fat embolism. When this photograph was taken he was unconscious, his face was congested and he was on continuous oxygen with cardiac monitoring. The petechiae were smaller and fainter than shown here; they have been accentuated for clarity and to show their distribution.

distress and coma, due partly to hypoxia and partly to cerebral emboli. The features at this stage are essentially those of adult respiratory distress syndrome (see p. 507). Indeed, fat embolism is probably one of the major predisposing factors in the development of ARDS (Alho, 1980). Other important factors are hypovolaemia, inappropriate fluid replacement and sepsis.

SPECIAL INVESTIGATIONS
There is no infallible test for fat embolism but a fairly constant finding is hypoxaemia; the blood Po_2 should always be monitored during the first 72 hours of any major injury, and values below 8 kPa (60 mmHg) must be regarded with grave suspicion.

TREATMENT
In mild cases no treatment is required but accurate monitoring of blood Po_2 and fluid balance is essential. If there are signs of hypoxia, oxygen should be given; patients with severe respiratory distress require intensive care, with sedation, assisted ventilation and Swan–Ganz catheterization for monitoring cardiac function.

Fluid balance must be maintained, and other supportive measures have their advocates; for example, heparin to counteract thromboembolism, steroids to help reduce pulmonary oedema, or aprotinin (Trasylol) which may prevent the aggregation of chylomicrons.

Local complications

Local complications may appear *early* (during the first few weeks following injury) or *late* (anything from a few weeks to several years after the fracture). They can be further subdivided into those affecting the *bone* and those involving the *soft tissues and joints.*

Early complications – bone

Infection

Open fractures may become infected; closed fractures hardly ever do unless they are opened by operation.

Post-traumatic wound infection is now the most common cause of chronic osteitis. This does not necessarily prevent the fracture from uniting, but union will be slow and the chance of refracturing is increased.

CLINICAL FEATURES
The history is of an open fracture or an operation on a closed fracture. The wound becomes inflamed and starts draining sero-purulent fluid, a sample of which may yield a growth of staphylococci or mixed bacteria. Even if the bacteriological examination is negative, if the clinical features are suggestive the patient should be kept under observation continuously and treatment with intravenous antibiotics begun.

LOCAL COMPLICATIONS OF FRACTURES

	Early	*Late*
Bone	Infection	Avascular necrosis Delayed and non-union Malunion
Soft tissues	Blisters and plaster sores Torn muscles and tendons Vascular injuries (including compartment syndrome) Nerve injuries Visceral injury	Bed sores Myositis ossificans Tendinitis and tendon rupture Nerve compression and entrapment Volkmann's contracture
Joints	Haemarthrosis and infection Ligament injury Algodystrophy	Instability Stiffness Algodystrophy

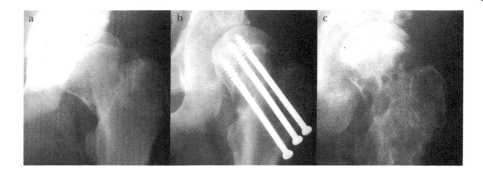

23.31 Infection   (a) This fracture of the femoral neck was treated by internal fixation. (b) Two weeks later the patient was in pain and x-rays showed the femoral head being displaced laterally, probably by fluid or pus in the joint. (c) The outcome was a chronic osteomyelitis with necrosis of the entire femoral head.

TREATMENT

All open fractures should be regarded as potentially infected and treated by giving antibiotics and meticulously excising all devitalized tissue. With acute infection the tissues around the fracture should be opened and drained; the choice of antibiotic is dictated by bacterial sensitivity.

If chronic osteitis supervenes the discharging sinus should be dressed daily and the fracture immobilized in an attempt to achieve union. External fixation is useful in such cases, but if an intramedullary nail has already been inserted this should not be removed; even worse than an infected fracture is one that is both infected and unstable.

The further treatment of chronic osteitis is discussed in Chapter 2.

Early complications – soft tissues

Fracture blisters

These are due to elevation of the superficial layers of skin by oedema, and can sometimes be prevented by firm bandaging. They should be covered with a sterile dry dressing.

Plaster sores

Plaster sores occur where skin presses directly onto bone. They should be prevented by padding the bony points and by moulding the wet plaster so that pressure is distributed to the soft tissues around the bony points. While a plaster sore is developing the patient feels localized burning pain. A window must immediately be cut in the plaster, or warning pain quickly abates and skin necrosis proceeds unnoticed.

Torn muscle fibres

Torn muscle fibres are common with any fracture. Unless the muscle is actively exercised the torn fibres may become adherent to untorn fibres, capsule or bone; if adhesions have been allowed to develop, lengthy rehabilitation will be necessary after the fracture has consolidated. The fracture and the torn muscles both need treatment; it is better to serve two sentences concurrently than consecutively.

Haemarthrosis

Fractures involving a joint may cause acute haemarthrosis. The joint is swollen and tense and the patient resists any attempt at moving it. The blood should be aspirated before dealing with the fracture.

Vascular injury

The fractures most often associated with damage to a major artery are those around the knee

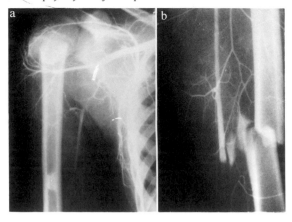

23.32 Gangrene In both these patients the peripheral part of the limb was cold and pulseless; arteriography shows a cut-off of a major artery in association with (a) a fractured neck of humerus, and (b) a fractured shaft of femur.

and elbow, and those of the humeral and femoral shafts. The artery may be cut, torn, compressed or contused, either by the initial injury or subsequently by jagged bone fragments. Even if its outward appearance is normal, the intima may be detached and the vessel blocked by thrombus, or a segment of artery may be in spasm. The effects vary from transient diminution of blood flow to profound ischaemia, tissue death and peripheral gangrene.

CLINICAL FEATURES
The patient may complain of paraesthesia or numbness in the toes or the fingers. The injured limb is cold and pale, or slightly cyanosed, and the pulse is weak or absent. X-rays will probably show one of the 'high-risk' fractures listed above. If a vascular injury is suspected an angiogram should immediately be performed; if it is positive, emergency treatment must be started without further delay.

TREATMENT
All bandages and splints should be removed. The fracture is re-x-rayed and, if the position of the bones suggests that the artery is being compressed or kinked, prompt reduction is necessary. The circulation is then reassessed repeatedly over the next half hour. If there is no improvement, the vessels must be explored by operation – preferably with the benefit of preoperative or peroperative angiography. A torn vessel can be sutured, or a segment may be replaced by a vein graft; if it is thrombosed, endarterectomy may restore the blood flow. Where it is practicable, the fracture should be fixed internally.

Compartment syndrome

Fractures of the arm or leg can give rise to severe ischaemia even if there is no damage to a major vessel. Bleeding, oedema or inflammation (infection) may increase the pressure within one of the osteofascial compartments; there is reduced capillary flow which results in muscle ischaemia, further oedema, still greater pressure and yet more profound ischaemia – a vicious circle that ends, after 12 hours or less, in necrosis of nerve and muscle within the compartment. Nerve is capable of regeneration but muscle, once infarcted, can never recover and is replaced by inelastic fibrous tissue (*Volkmann's ischaemic contracture*). A similar cascade of events may be caused by swelling of a limb inside a tight plaster cast.

CLINICAL FEATURES
'High-risk' injuries are fractures of the elbow, the forearm bones and the proximal third of the tibia. Other precipitating factors are operation (usually for internal fixation) or infection. The classic features of ischaemia are the five Ps: Pain, Paraesthesia, Pallor, Paralysis and Pulselessness. But it is criminal to wait until they are all present; the diagnosis can be made long before that. Ischaemic muscle is highly sensitive

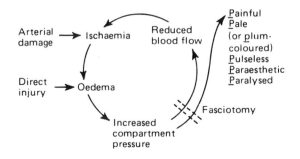

23.33 The vicious circle of Volkmann's ischaemia (Modified from the *Journal of Bone and Joint Surgery*, 1979, **61B**, 298, by kind permission of Mr C. E. Holden and the Editor.)

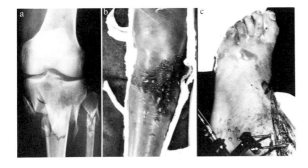

23.34 Compartment syndrome (a) A fracture at this level is always dangerous. This man was treated in plaster. Pain became intense and when the plaster was split (which should have been done immediately after its application), the leg was swollen and blistered (b). A tibial compartment decompression was performed – but too late; 2 days later (c) the foot became gangrenous.

to stretch. If the limb is unduly painful, swollen or tense, the muscles (which may be tender) should be tested by stretching them – when the toes or fingers are passively hyperextended there is increased pain in the calf or forearm. The presence of a pulse does not exclude the diagnosis. In doubtful cases the intracompartmental pressures can be measured directly: if it is higher than 40 mmHg, and the patient has a normal diastolic pressure, urgent treatment is called for. Obviously if the patient is shocked, measurement of the compartment pressure will be unreliable.

TREATMENT

The threatened compartment (or compartments) must be promptly decompressed. Casts, bandages and dressings must be completely removed – merely splitting the plaster is utterly useless. The compartment pressure should be measured; if it is more than 40 mmHg, immediate open fasciotomy is needed. If it is less than 40 mmHg, the limb may be closely observed and re-examined over the next hour; if the condition of the limb improves, repeated clinical evaluation is continued until the danger has passed. If there is no improvement, or if the compartment pressure rises, fasciotomy should be performed. In the case of the leg, 'fasciotomy' may mean opening all four compartments, if necessary by excising a segment of the fibula. The wound should be left open and inspected 5 days later: if there is some muscle

necrosis, debridement can be done; if the tissues are healthy, the wound can be sutured (without tension), or skin-grafted or simply allowed to heal by secondary intention.

Nerve injury

Fractures may be complicated by *nerve injury*. This is particularly common with fractures of the humerus or injuries around the elbow or the knee. The telltale signs should be looked for during the initial examination (see Chapter 11). In closed injuries the nerve is seldom severed, and spontaneous recovery should be awaited. If recovery has not occurred by the expected time, the nerve should be explored; sometimes it is trapped between the fragments and occasionally it is found to be divided. In open fractures a complete lesion (neurotmesis) is more likely; the nerve is explored during wound debridement and repaired, either then or as a 'secondary' procedure 3 weeks later.

Acute nerve compression sometimes occurs with fractures or dislocations around the wrist. Complaints of numbness or paraesthesia in the distribution of the median or ulnar nerve should be taken seriously and the nerve promptly explored and decompressed.

Visceral injury

Fractures around the trunk are often complicated by injuries to underlying viscera, the most important being penetration of the lung with life-threatening pneumothorax following rib fractures and rupture of the bladder or urethra in pelvic fractures. These injuries require emergency treatment, before the fracture is dealt with.

Late complications – bone

Avascular necrosis (see also Chapter 6)

Certain regions are notorious for their propensity to develop ischaemia and bone necrosis after injury. They are: (1) the head of the femur (after fracture of the femoral neck or dislocation of the hip); (2) the proximal part of the scaphoid (after fracture through its waist); (3)

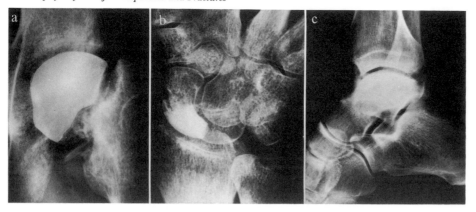

23.35 Avascular necrosis If the fracture cuts off the blood supply to part of the bone, the avascular part becomes dense on x-ray. Three common sites are: (a) head of femur, (b) proximal portion of scaphoid, (c) posterior half of talus.

the lunate (following dislocation); and (4) the body of the talus (after fracture of its neck).

Accurately speaking, this is an early complication of bone injury, because ischaemia occurs during the first few hours following fracture or dislocation. However, the clinical and radiological effects are not seen until weeks or even months later.

CLINICAL FEATURES
There are no symptoms associated with avascular necrosis, but if the fracture fails to unite or if the bone collapses the patient may complain of pain. X-ray shows the characteristic increase in bone density (the consequence of new bone ingrowth in the necrotic segment and disuse osteoporosis in the surrounding parts).

TREATMENT
Treatment usually becomes necessary when joint function is threatened. In old people with necrosis of the femoral head an arthroplasty is the obvious choice; in younger people, realignment osteotomy (or even arthrodesis) may be wiser. Avascular necrosis in the scaphoid or talus may need no more than symptomatic treatment, but arthrodesis of the wrist or ankle is sometimes needed.

Delayed union

The timetable on p. 520 is no more than a rough guide to the period in which a fracture

may be expected to unite and consolidate. It must never be relied upon in deciding when treatment may be discontinued. If the time is unduly prolonged, the term 'delayed union' is used.

CAUSES

Inadequate blood supply Whenever a fracture occurs through bone that is bare of muscle fibres there is the risk of delayed union. The vulnerable bones include those which are liable to avascular necrosis, and also the lower tibia (especially a double fracture).

Infection An open fracture is slow to join, probably because there is little fracture haematoma in which ensheathing callus can form; infection delays union still further.

Incorrect splintage This includes (1) insufficient splintage – thus, a standard below-knee plaster does not hold a fractured shaft of tibia adequately; and (2) excessive traction, which pulls the bones apart.

Intact fellow bone If one bone in the forearm or leg is unbroken, the fractured ends of the other may be held apart, and some delay then follows.

CLINICAL FEATURES
The fracture site is usually tender. The bone may appear to move in one piece; if, however, it is subjected to stress, pain is immediately felt

and the bone may angulate; the fracture is not consolidated.

X-ray The fracture remains visible and there is very little callus formation or periosteal reaction. However, the bone ends are not sclerosed.

TREATMENT

Conservative Delayed union is the signal to continue treatment of the fracture, and to continue it efficiently until consolidation is complete. If plaster is being used, it must be sufficient to prevent movement at the fracture

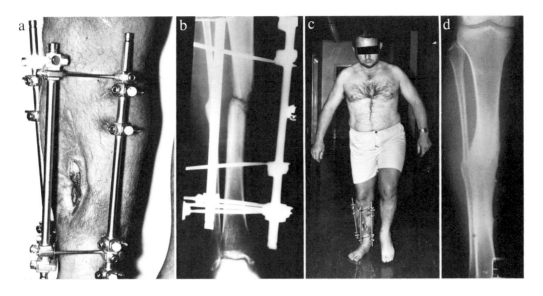

23.36 Infection and delayed union (a) Infected fracture of the tibia treated by wound excision and external fixation; (b) the x-ray after 6 weeks; (c) he was able to walk around with his apparatus, and gradually the wound healed; at 1 year (d) the fracture was completely solid.

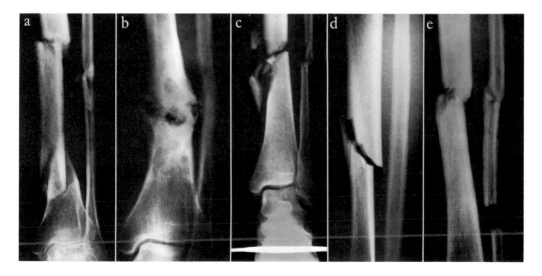

23.37 Delayed union Causes of delay include (a) a double fracture, (b) infection, (c) excessive traction, and (d) an intact fibula. In (e) both bones were fractured but the fibula joined first and splinted the tibia apart; the delayed union is obvious – 2.5 cm of fibula was therefore excised.

CAUSES OF NON-UNION

The injury	*The bone*	*The surgeon*	*The patient*
1. Soft tissue loss	1. Poor blood supply	1. Distraction	1. Immense
2. Bone loss	2. Poor haematoma	2. Poor splintage	2. Immoderate
3. Intact fellow bone	3. Infection	3. Poor fixation	3. Immovable
4. Soft tissue interposition	4. Pathological lesion	4. Impatience	4. Impossible

---

site. If traction is being used it must not be excessive; it is sometimes better replaced by plaster splintage and weightbearing. Functional bracing is an excellent method of promoting bony union. Another approach, though still somewhat controversial, is the application of pulsed electromagnetic fields (Sharrard, 1990).

Operative If a fractured tibia is being held apart by a fibula which was not fractured or which has united quickly, it is worth while excising 2.5 cm of fibula and reapplying plaster.

If union is delayed for more than 6 months and there is no sign of callus formation, internal fixation and bone grafting are indicated.

Non-union

CAUSES
Unless delayed union is recognized, and the fracture adequately treated, non-union is liable to result. Other causes include too large a gap and interposition of tissues.

Too large a gap If the fracture surfaces are too widely separated, union takes a very long time or may never occur. The gap may be due to a gunshot fracture which destroys a large section of bone; to a portion of bone having been expelled during the accident which caused the fracture; to muscle retraction in which the patient's own muscles pull the fragments apart (as in a fractured patella); or to treatment with excessive traction.

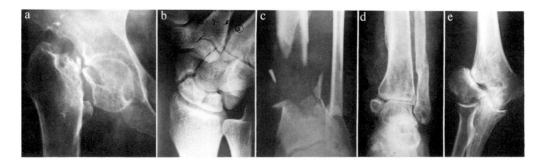

23.38 Non-union The femoral neck (a) and the carpal scaphoid (b) are two common sites of non-union. This tibia (c) could hardly be expected to unite – so much bone had been left at the scene of the accident. (d) This medial malleolus failed to unite, presumably because a flap of periosteum was interposed. (e) This lateral condyle had rotated, and so articular cartilage prevented union.

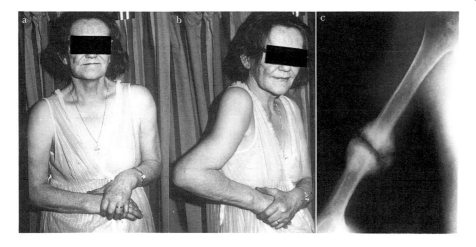

23.39 Non-union (a, b) The amount of movement shown was obviously painless, the cardinal sign of (c) established non-union.

Interposition Non-union may develop when any one of the following tissues is interposed between the bone ends: periosteum (e.g. a flap of periosteum in association with a fractured medial malleolus); muscle (e.g. a fractured femur may spike through the quadriceps muscle); cartilage (e.g. a fractured lateral condyle of humerus may be so rotated that its cartilaginous articular surface faces the shaft).

CLINICAL FEATURES

Movement can be elicited at the fracture site, and this movement (unless excessive) is painless; such painless movement is diagnostic of non-union as distinct from delayed union.

X-ray The fracture is visible and the bone on each side of it may be sclerosed. Two varieties of non-union can be distinguished: (1) hypertrophic with bulbous bone ends, indicating osteogenic activity (as if in the attempt to form bridging callus); and (2) atrophic, with no calcification around the bone ends.

TREATMENT

Conservative Non-union is occasionally symptomless, needing no treatment or, at most, a removable splint. Even if symptoms are present, operation is not the only answer; with hypertrophic non-union, functional bracing may be sufficient to induce union, but treatment often needs to be prolonged. Electrical stimulation promotes osteogenesis and also is sometimes

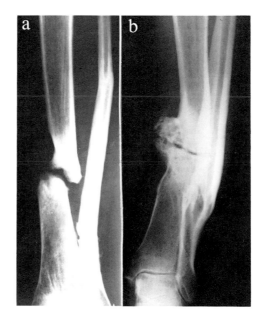

23.40 Non-union (a) Atrophic non-union – bone grafting is needed. (b) Hypertrophic non-union – rigid fixation would probably suffice.

successful; an induced current can be applied through a plaster cast, or electrodes may be implanted.

Operative With hypertrophic non-union and in the absence of deformity, very rigid fixation alone (internal or external) may lead to union.

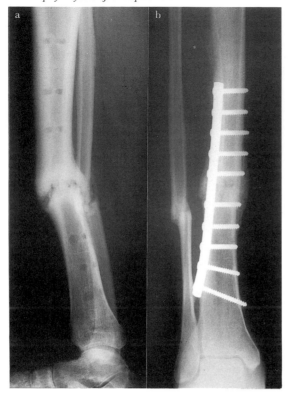

23.41 Non-union – treatment   (a) Hypertrophic non-union after internal fixation. The metal was removed and the intervening fibrous tissue excised. (b) Rigid fixation has resulted in bony union.

With atrophic non-union, fixation alone is not enough and bone grafts should be added; it is wise first to excise any fibrous tissue interposed between the bone ends, and it is important also to correct any deformity.

Malunion

When the fragments join in an unsatisfactory position (unacceptable angulation, rotation or shortening) the fracture is said to be malunited. Causes are failure to reduce a fracture adequately, failure to hold reduction while healing proceeds, or gradual collapse of comminuted or osteoporotic bone.

CLINICAL FEATURES
The deformity is usually obvious, but sometimes the true extent of malunion is apparent only on x-ray. Rotational deformity of the femur, tibia, humerus or forearm may be missed unless the limb is compared with its opposite fellow. Rotational deformity of a metacarpal fracture is detected by asking the patient to flatten the fingers onto the palm and seeing whether the normal regular fan-shaped appearance is reproduced (see p. 609).

X-rays are essential to check the position of the fracture while it is uniting. This is particularly important during the first 3 weeks when

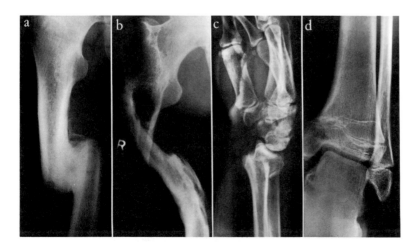

22.42 Malunion   Primary malunion (a) with overlap, (b) with angulation. (c) Secondary malunion – this Colles' fracture was reduced satisfactorily, but displaced in plaster. (d) Secondary malunion following damage to the lower tibial ephiphysis (e).

the situation may change without warning. At this stage it is sometimes difficult to decide what constitutes 'malunion'; acceptable norms differ from one site to another and these are discussed under the individual fractures.

TREATMENT
Incipient malunion may call for treatment even before the fracture has fully united; the decision on the need for remanipulation or correction may be extremely difficult. A few guidelines are offered.

1. In adults, fractures should be reduced as near to the anatomical position as possible. However, apposition is less important than alignment and rotation. Angulation of more than 15 degrees in a long bone, or a noticeable rotational deformity, may need correction by remanipulation, or by osteotomy and internal fixation.
2. In children, angular deformities near the bone ends will usually remodel with time; rotational deformities will not.
3. In the lower limb, shortening of more than 2.5 cm is seldom acceptable to the patient and a limb lengthening procedure may be indicated.
4. The patient's expectations (often prompted by cosmesis) may be quite different from the surgeon's; they are not to be ignored.
5. Early discussion with the patient, and a guided view of the x-rays, will help in deciding on the need for treatment and may prevent later misunderstanding.
6. Very little is known of the long-term effects of small angular deformities on joint function. However, it seems likely that malalignment of more than 15 degrees in any plane may cause asymmetrical loading of the joint above or below and the late development of secondary osteoarthritis; this applies particularly to the large weightbearing joints.

Growth disturbance

In children, damage to the physis may lead to abnormal or arrested growth. A transverse fracture through the growth plate is not disastrous; the fracture runs through the hypertrophic and calcified layers and not through the germinal zone so, provided it is accurately reduced, there is seldom any disturbance of growth. But fractures that split the epiphysis inevitably traverse the growing portion of the physis, and so further growth may be asymmetrical and the bone end characterisically angulated; if the entire physis is damaged, there may be slowing or complete cessation of growth.

The subject is dealt with in more detail on p. 560.

Late complications – soft tissues

Bed sores

Bed sores occur in elderly or paralysed patients. The skin over the sacrum and heels is especially vulnerable. Careful nursing and early activity can usually prevent bed sores; once they have developed, treatment is difficult; it may be necessary to excise the necrotic tissue and apply skin grafts.

Myositis ossificans

Heterotopic ossification in the muscles sometimes occurs after an injury, particularly dislocation of the elbow or a blow to the brachialis, the deltoid or the quadriceps. It is thought to be due to muscle damage, but it also occurs without a local injury in unconscious or paraplegic patients.

CLINICAL FEATURES
Soon after the injury, the patient (usually a fit young man) complains of pain; there is local swelling and soft-tissue tenderness. X-ray is

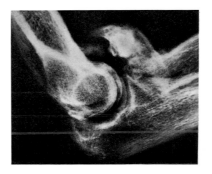

23.43 Myositis ossificans Myositis ossificans following a fractured head of radius.

normal but a bone scan may show increased activity. Over the next 2–3 weeks the pain gradually subsides, but joint movement is limited; x-ray may show fluffy calcificaton in the soft tissues. By 8 weeks the bony mass is easily palpable and is clearly defined in the x-ray.

TREATMENT

The worst treatment is to attack an injured and stiffish elbow with vigorous muscle-stretching exercises; this is liable to precipitate or aggravate the condition. The joint should be rested in the position of function until pain subsides; gentle active movements are then begun.

Months later, when the condition has stabilized, it may be helpful to excise the bony mass.

Tendinitis

Tendinitis may affect the tibialis posterior tendon following medial malleolar fractures. It should be prevented by accurate reduction, if necessary at open operation.

Tendon rupture

Late rupture of the extensor pollicis longus tendon may occur 6–12 weeks after a fracture of the lower radius. Direct suture is seldom possible and the resulting disability is treated by transferring the extensor indicis proprius tendon to the distal stump of the ruptured thumb tendon. Late rupture of the long head of biceps after a fractured neck of humerus usually requires no treatment.

Nerve compression

Nerve compression may damage the lateral popliteal nerve if an elderly or emaciated patient lies with the leg in full external rotation. Radial palsy may follow the faulty use of crutches. Both conditions are due to lack of supervision.

Nerve entrapment

Bone or joint deformity may result in local nerve entrapment with typical features such as numbness or paraesthesia, loss of power and muscle wasting in the distribution of the affected nerve. Common sites are: (1) the ulnar nerve, due to a valgus elbow following an ununited lateral condyle fracture; (2) the median nerve, following injuries around the wrist; (3) the posterior tibial nerve, following fractures around the ankle (p. 496). Treatment is by early decompression of the nerve; in the case of the ulnar nerve this may require anterior transposition.

Volkmann's contracture

Following arterial injury or a compartmental syndrome, the patient may develop ischaemic contractures of the affected muscles. However, nerves injured by ischaemia sometimes recover, at least partially; thus the patient presents with deformity and stiffness, but numbness is inconstant. The sites most commonly affected are the forearm and hand, the leg and the foot.

In a severe case affecting the forearm, there will be wasting of the forearm and hand and clawing of the fingers; if the wrist is passively flexed, the patient can extend the fingers, showing that the deformity is largely due to contracture of the forearm muscles. Detachment of the flexors at their origin and along the interosseous membrane in the forearm may improve the deformity, but function is no better if sensation and active movement are not restored. A pedicle nerve graft, using the proximal segments of the median and ulnar nerves (p. 224) may restore protective sensation in the hand, and tendon transfers (wrist extensors to finger and thumb flexors) will allow active grasp. In less severe cases, median nerve sensibility may be quite good and, with appropriate tendon releases and transfers, the patient regains a considerable degree of function.

Ischaemia of the hand may follow forearm injuries, or swelling of the fingers associated with a tight forearm bandage or plaster. The intrinsic hand muscles fibrose and shorten, pulling the fingers into flexion at the metacarpophalangeal joints, but the interphalangeal joints remain straight. The thumb is adducted across the palm (Bunnell's 'intrinsic-plus' position).

Ischaemia of the calf muscles may follow injuries or operations involving the popliteal

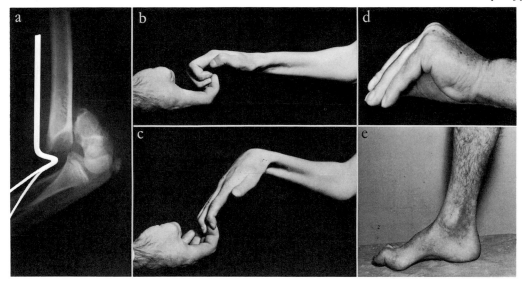

23.44 Volkmann's ischaemia (a) Kinking of the main artery is an important cause. (b, c) Volkmann's contracture of the forearm; the fingers can be straightened only when the wrist is palmarflexed (the constant-length phenomenon). (d) Ischaemic contracture of the small muscles of the hand (Bunnell). (e) Ischaemic contracture of the calf muscles with clawing of the toes.

artery or its divisions. This is more common than is usually supposed. The symptoms, signs and subsequent contracture are similar to those following ischaemia of the forearm. Occasionally, ischaemia may affect the intrinsic muscles of the foot, causing claw toes.

Late complications – joints

Instability

Following injury a joint may give way. Causes include the following.

Ligamentous laxity, especially at the knee, the ankle and the metacarpophalangeal joint of the thumb.

Muscle weakness, especially if splintage has been excessive or prolonged, and exercises have been inadequate (again the knee and ankle are most often affected).

Bone loss, especially after a gunshot fracture or severe compound injury.

Injury may also lead to *recurrent dislocation.* The commonest sites are: (1) the shoulder – if the glenoid labrum has been detached; and (2) the patella – if, after traumatic dislocation, the capsule heals poorly.

A more subtle form of instability is seen after fractures around the wrist. Patients complaining of persistent discomfort or weakness after wrist injury should be fully investigated for *chronic carpal instability* (see pp. 301 and 602).

Joint stiffness

Joint stiffness after a fracture commonly occurs in the knee, the elbow, the shoulder and (worst of all) the small joints of the hand. Sometimes the joint itself has been injured; a haemarthrosis forms and leads to synovial adhesions. More often the stiffness is due to oedema and fibrosis of the capsule, the ligaments and the muscles around the joint, or adhesions of the soft tissues to each other or to the underlying bone. All these conditions are made worse by prolonged immobilization; moreover, if the

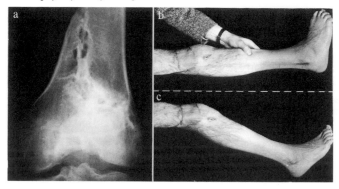

23.45 Joint stiffness (a) This heavily contaminated open fracture resulted in gross knee stiffness (b, c) which was eventually treated by quadriceps-plasty.

joint has been held in a position where the ligaments are at their shortest, no amount of exercise will afterwards succeed in stretching these tissues and restoring the lost movement completely.

In a small percentage of patients with fractures of the forearm or leg, early post-traumatic swelling is accompanied by tenderness and progressive stiffness of the distal joints. These patients are at great risk of developing reflex sympathetic dystrophy (algodystrophy); whether this is an entirely separate entity or merely an extension of the 'normal' post-traumatic soft-tissue reaction is uncertain. What is important is to recognize this type of 'stiffness' when it occurs and to insist on skilled physiotherapy until normal function is restored.

TREATMENT

The best treatment is prevention – by exercises that keep the joints mobile from the outset. If a joint has to be splinted, make sure that it is held in the 'position of safety' (see p. 327). Joints that are already stiff take time to mobilize, but prolonged and patient physiotherapy can work wonders. If the situation is due to intra-articular adhesions, gentle manipulation under anaesthesia may free the joint sufficiently to permit a more pliant response to further exercise.

Occasionally, adherent or contracted tissues need to be released by operation (e.g. when knee flexion is prevented by adhesions in and around the quadriceps).

Algodystrophy (Sudeck's atrophy)

Sudeck, in 1900, described a condition characterized by painful osteoporosis of the hand. The same condition sometimes occurs after fractures of the extremities and it is now recognized that this is the end stage of post-traumatic algodystrophy (see p. 240). It is much more common than originally believed (Atkins, Duckworth and Kanis, 1990) and may follow relatively trivial injury.

The patient complains of continuous, burning pain; at first there is local swelling, redness and warmth, as well as tenderness and moderate stiffness of the nearby joints. As the weeks go by the skin becomes pale and atrophic, movements are increasingly restricted and the patient may develop fixed deformities. X-rays characteristically show patchy rarefaction of the bone.

The earlier the condition is recognized and treatment begun, the better the prognosis. Elevation and active exercises are important after all injuries, but in algodystrophy they are essential. If this does not produce improvement within a few weeks, sympathetic block or sympatholytic drugs such as intravenous guanethidine may help; even then, prolonged and dedicated physiotherapy will be needed.

Osteoarthritis

A fracture involving a joint may severely damage the articular cartilage and give rise to post-

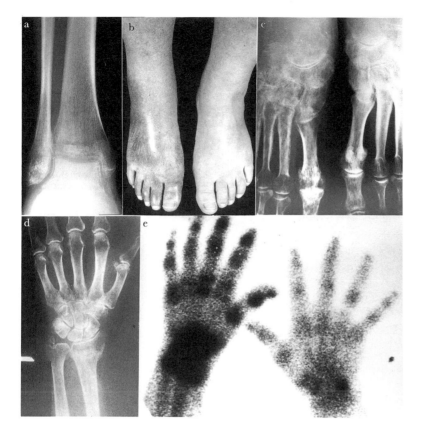

23.46 Sudeck's atrophy (a) Fractures of the tibia frequently lead to 'disuse osteoporosis'. The radiolucent bands seen here are typical. (b) In Sudeck's atrophy the soft tissues also are involved; the right foot is somewhat swollen and the skin has become dusky, smooth and shiny. (c) In the full-blown case, x-rays show a typical patchy osteoporosis. (d) Similar changes may occur in the hand and this is always accompanied by (e) increased activity in the radionuclide scan.

traumatic osteoarthritis within a period of months. Even if the cartilage heals, irregularity of the joint surface may cause localized stress and so predispose to secondary osteoarthritis years later. Little can be done to prevent this once the fracture has united.

Malunion of a shaft fracture may radically alter the mechanics of a nearby joint and this, too, can give rise to secondary osteoarthritis. Residual angulation of more than 15 degrees in a lower limb bone should be carefully assessed for its effect on joint function and, if necessary, corrected by osteotomy.

Stress fractures

A stress or fatigue fracture is one occurring in the normal bone of a healthy patient. It is caused not by a specific traumatic incident but by repetitive stresses, which are of two main kinds – bending and compression.

Bending stress causes breaching of one cortex; healing begins, but with repeated stress the breach may extend across the bone. This variety affects young adults and is probably due to muscular action, which tends to deform bone; the athlete in training builds up muscle power quickly but bone strength only slowly, and a stress fracture may result; this accounts for the high incidence of stress fractures in military recruits.

Compression stress acts on soft cancellous bone; with frequent repetition an impacted fracture may follow.

NOTE It has been suggested that a stress fracture is the initial lesion in some of the osteochondrites; for example, Freiberg's disease.

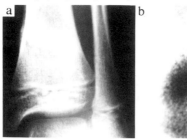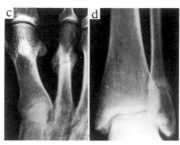

23.47 Stress fractures   (a) The stress fracture of this tibia is only just visible, but it had already been diagnosed 2 weeks earlier when the scan (b) showed a hot spot above the ankle. (c, d) Stress fractures of the second metatarsal and the fibula.

Sites affected

Least rare are the following: shaft of humerus (adolescent cricketers); pars interarticularis of fifth lumbar vertebra (causing spondylolysis); pubic rami (inferior in children, both in adults); femoral neck (at any age); femoral shaft (chiefly lower third); patella (children and young adults); tibial shaft (proximal third in children, middle third in athletes and trainee paratroopers, distal third in the elderly); distal shaft of fibula (the 'runner's fracture'); calcaneum (adults); navicular (athletes); and metatarsals (especially the second – see p. 715).

Clinical features

There may be a history of unaccustomed and repeated activity. A common sequence of events is: pain after exercise – pain during exercise – pain without exercise. Occasionally the patient presents only after the fracture has healed; he may then complain of a lump (the callus).

The patient is usually healthy. The affected site may be swollen or red. It is sometimes warm and usually tender; the callus may be palpable. 'Springing' the bone (attempting to bend it) is often painful.

X-ray

Early on, the fracture is difficult to detect, but a bone scan will show increased activity at the painful spot. A few weeks later one may see a small transverse defect in the cortex and, later still, localized periosteal new-bone formation. These appearances can be mistaken for those of an osteosarcoma, a horrifying trap for the unwary.

Compression stress fractures (especially of the femoral neck and upper tibia) may show as a hazy transverse band of sclerosis with (in the tibia) peripheral callus.

Diagnosis

Many disorders, including osteomyelitis, scurvy and the battered baby syndrome, may be confused with stress fractures. The great danger, however, is a mistaken diagnosis of osteosarcoma; scanning shows increased uptake in both conditions and even biopsy may be misleading.

Treatment

Most stress fractures need no treatment other than an elastic bandage and avoidance of the painful activity until the lesion heals; surprisingly, this can take many months and the forced inactivity is not easily accepted by the hard-driving athlete or dancer.

An important exception is stress fracture of the femoral neck. This should be suspected in all elderly people who complain of pain in the hip for which no obvious cause can be found. If the diagnosis is confirmed by bone scan, the femoral neck should be pinned as a prophylactic measure.

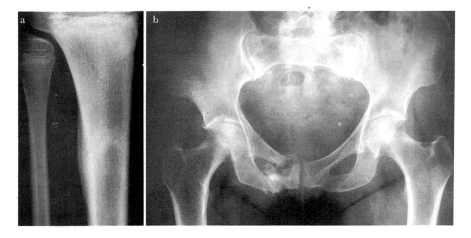

23.48 Stress fractures   Stress fractures are often wrongly diagnosed. (a) This tibial fracture was at first thought to be an osteosarcoma. (b) Stress fractures of the pubic rami in elderly women can be mistaken for metastases.

CAUSES OF PATHOLOGICAL FRACTURE

Generalized bone disease

1. Osteogenesis imperfecta
2. Postmenopausal osteoporosis
3. Metabolic bone disease
4. Myelomatosis
5. Polyostotic fibrous dysplasia
6. Paget's disease

Local benign conditions

1. Chronic infection
2. Solitary bone cyst
3. Fibrous cortical defect
4. Chondromyxoid fibroma
5. Aneurysmal bone cyst
6. Chondroma
7. Monostotic fibrous dysplasia

Primary malignant tumours

1. Chondrosarcoma
2. Osteosarcoma
3. Ewing's tumour

Metastatic tumours

Metastatic carcinoma from breast, lung, kidney, thyroid and prostate

Pathological fractures

When abnormal bone gives way this is referred to as a pathological fracture. The causes are numerous and varied; often the diagnosis is not made until a biopsy is examined (see the boxed summary).

The history

Bone that fractures spontaneously, or after trivial injury, must be regarded as abnormal until proved otherwise. In older patients one should always ask about previous illnesses or operations; a malignant tumour, no matter how long ago it occurred, may be the source of a late metastatic lesion; a history of gastrectomy, intestinal malabsorption, chronic alcoholism or prolonged drug therapy should suggest a metabolic bone disorder.

Symptoms such as loss of weight, pain, a lump, cough or haematuria suggest that the fracture may be through a secondary deposit.

In younger patients, a history of several previous fractures may suggest a diagnosis of osteogenesis imperfecta, even if the patient does not show the classic features of the disorder.

Examination

Local signs of bone disease (an infected sinus, an old scar, swelling or deformity) should not be missed. The site of the fracture may suggest the diagnosis: patients with involutional osteoporosis develop fractures of the vertebral bodies and the corticocancellous junctions of long bones; a fracture through the shaft of the bone in an elderly patient is a pathological fracture until proved otherwise.

General examination may be informative. Congenital dysplasias, fibrous dysplasia, Cushing's syndrome and Paget's disease all produce characteristic appearances. The patient may be wasted (possibly due to malignant disease). The lymph nodes or liver may be enlarged. Is there a mass in the abdomen or pelvis? Old scars should not be overlooked. And rectal and vaginal examinations are mandatory.

Under the age of 20 the common causes of pathological fracture are benign bone tumours and cysts. Over the age of 40 the common causes are myelomatosis, secondary carcinoma and Paget's disease.

X-rays Understandably, the fracture itself attracts most attention. But the surrounding bone must also be examined, and features such as cyst formation, cortical erosion, abnormal trabeculation and periosteal thickening should be sought. The type of fracture, too, is important: vertebral compression fractures may be due to severe osteoporosis or osteomalacia, but they can also be caused by skeletal metastases or myeloma. Middle-aged men, unlike women, do not normally become osteoporotic: x-ray signs of bone loss and vertebral compression in a male under 75 years should be regarded as 'pathological' until proved otherwise.

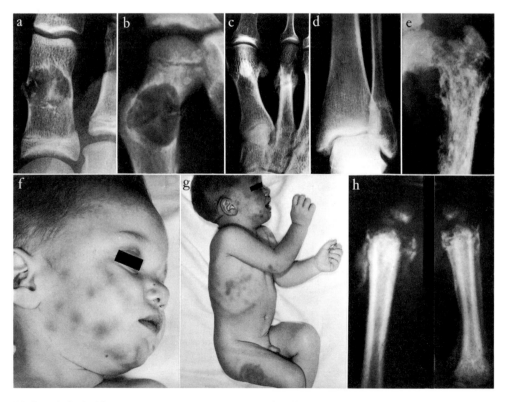

23.49 Pathological fractures – in the young   (a) Through a chondroma of the hallux; (b) through a cyst of the femoral neck; (c) stress fracture of second metatarsal; (d) stress fracture of the fibula – a less common site; (e) fracture through bone weakened by acute osteomyelitis.
(f, g, h) The battered baby syndrome. The fractures are not pathological but the family is; the metaphyseal lesions in each humerus (h) are characteristic.

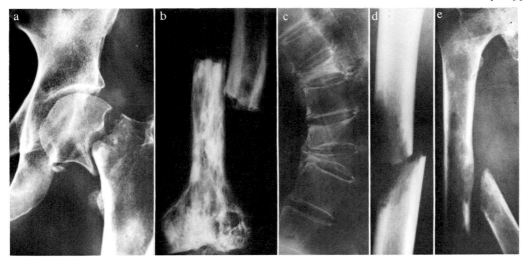

23.50 Pathological fractures – in older people   (a) A fractured femoral neck in an elderly woman with osteoporosis is probably the commonest. Fractures through Paget bone (b) also are usually in old people. Fractures through secondary deposits (c and d) and through myelomatosis (e) may occur somewhat earlier.

Additional investigations

X-RAY EXAMINATION   X-ray of other bones, the lungs and the urogenital tract may be necessary to exclude malignant disease.

BLOOD INVESTIGATION   Investigations should always include a full blood count, ESR, protein electrophoresis, and tests for syphilis and metabolic bone disorders.

URINE EXAMINATION   Urine examination may reveal blood from a tumour, or Bence-Jones protein in myelomatosis.

SCANNING   Local radionuclide imaging may help elucidate the diagnosis, and whole body scanning is important in revealing or excluding other deposits.

Biopsy

Some lesions are so typical that a biopsy is unnecessary (solitary cyst, fibrous cortical defect, Paget's disease). Others are more obscure and a biopsy is essential for diagnosis. If open reduction of the fracture is indicated, the biopsy can be done at the same time; otherwise a definitive procedure should be arranged.

Treatment (see also Chapter 9)

The principles of fracture treatment remain the same: REDUCE, HOLD, EXERCISE. But the choice of method is influenced by the condition of the bone; and the underlying pathological disorder may need treatment in its own right.

GENERALIZED BONE DISEASE   In most of these conditions (including Paget's disease) the bones fracture more easily, but they heal quite well provided the fracture is properly immobilized. Internal fixation is therefore advisable (and for Paget's disease almost essential). Patients with osteomalacia, hyperparathyroidism, renal osteodystrophy and Paget's disease may need systemic treatment as well.

LOCAL BENIGN CONDITIONS   Fractures through benign cyst-like lesions usually heal quite well and they should be allowed to do so before tackling the local lesion. Treatment is therefore the same as for simple fractures in the same area, although in some cases it will be necessary to take a biopsy before immobilizing the fracture. When the bone has healed, the tumour can be dealt with by curettage or local excision.

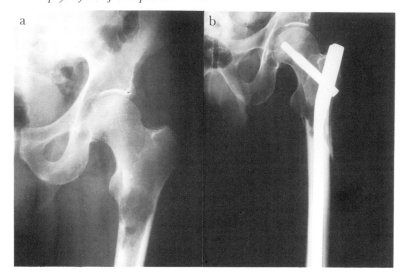

23.51 Pathological fractures – treatment   (a) This patient with a secondary deposit below the lesser trochanter was advised to have prophylactic nailing. While she was being prepared she sustained an undisplaced fracture. This was securely fixed (b) and was followed by radiotherapy.

PRIMARY MALIGNANT TUMOUR   The fracture may need splinting but this is merely a prelude to definitive treatment of the tumour, which by now will have spread to the surrounding soft tissues. The prognosis is almost always very poor.

METASTATIC TUMOURS   Fractures through metastatic lesions heal poorly (and some do not heal at all). If the patient is to be spared the agony of spending the remaining months in bed, and often in pain, internal fixation is the treatment of choice. If there is much bone destruction, metal fixation can be supplemented by packing the area with methylmethacrylate cement. This is followed by local irradiation of the bone.

Usually the primary malignant tumour will have been diagnosed (and treated) before. If not, certain basic investigations should be carried out to exclude myelomatosis and primary carcinomas of the breast, lung, kidney, thyroid and prostate. A bone scan should also be performed, to disclose other skeletal lesions.

A pathological compression fracture of the spine may lead to paraplegia; if a metastasis or myeloma is suspected, the smallest sign of neurological disturbance (e.g. difficulty with micturition) signals an emergency, and local radiotherapy should be started even before investigations are complete. If this fails to halt deterioration, surgical decompression (laminectomy) may still succeed.

PROPHYLACTIC FIXATION   If a metastatic focus is found in an intact long bone and the x-ray shows that it is a destructive lesion, prophylactic internal fixation should be carried out (preferably without exposing the lesion). This is then followed by local irradiation.

Injuries of the physis

In children over 10% of fractures involve injury to the growth plate (or physis). Because the physis is a relatively weak part of the bone, joint strains that might cause ligament injuries in adults are liable to result in separation of the physis in children. The fracture usually runs transversely through the hypertrophic or the calcified layer of the growth plate, often veering off into the metaphysis at one of the edges to include a triangular lip of bone. This has little effect on longitudinal growth, which takes place in the germinal and proliferating layers of the physis. However, if the fracture traverses the cellular 'reproductive' layers of the plate, it may result in premature ossification of the injured part and serious disturbances of bone growth.

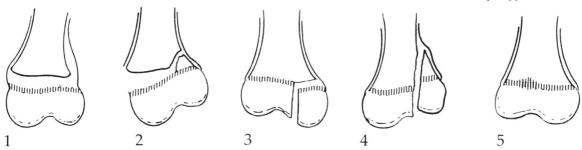

23.52 Physeal injuries Type 1 – separation of the epiphysis – usually occurs in infants but is also seen at puberty as a slipped femoral epiphysis. Type 2 – fracture through the physis and metaphysis – is the commonest; it occurs in older children and seldom results in abnormal growth. Type 3 – an intra-articular fracture of the epiphysis – needs accurate reduction to restore the joint surface. Type 4 – splitting of the physis and epiphysis – damages the articular surface and may also cause abnormal growth; if it is displaced it needs open reduction. Type 5 – crushing of the physis – may look benign but ends in arrested growth.

Classification

The most widely used classification of physeal injuries is that of Salter and Harris (1963), which distinguishes five basic types of injury.

Type 1 A transverse fracture through the hypertrophic or calcified zone of the plate. Even if the fracture is quite alarmingly displaced, the growing zone of the physis is usually not injured and growth disturbance is uncommon.

Type 2 This is essentially similar to type 1, but towards the edge the fracture deviates away from the physis and splits off a triangular metaphyseal fragment of bone.

Type 3 A fracture that splits the epiphysis and then veers off transversely to one or the other side, through the hypertrophic layer of the physis. Inevitably it damages the 'reproductive' layers of the physis and may result in growth disturbance.

Type 4 As with type 3, the fracture splits the epiphysis, but it extends into the metaphysis. These fractures are liable to displacement and a consequent misfit between the separated parts of the physis, resulting in asymmetrical growth.

Type 5 A longitudinal compression injury of the physis. There is no visible fracture but the growth plate is crushed and this may result in growth arrest.

Mechanism of injury

Physeal fractures usually result from falls or traction injuries. They occur mostly in road accidents and during sporting activities or playground tumbles.

Clinical features

These fractures are more common in boys than in girls and are usually seen either in infancy or between the ages of 10 and 12. Deformity is usually minimal, but any injury in a child followed by pain and tenderness near the joint should arouse suspicion, and x-ray examination is essential.

X-rays The physis itself is radiolucent and the epiphysis may be incompletely ossified; this makes it hard to tell whether the bone end is damaged or deformed. The younger the child, the smaller the 'visible' part of the epiphysis and thus the more difficult it is to make the diagnosis; comparison with the normal side is a great help. Telltale features are widening of the physeal 'gap', incongruity of the joint or tilting of the epiphyseal axis. If there is marked displacement the diagnosis is obvious, but even type 4 fracture may at first be so little displaced that the fracture line is hard to see; if there is the faintest suspicion of a physeal fracture, re-x-ray after 4 or 5 days is essential. Type 5 injuries are usually diagnosed only in retrospect.

Treatment

Undisplaced fractures may be treated by splinting the part in a cast or a close-fitting plaster slab for 2–4 weeks (depending on the site of injury and the age of the child). However, with

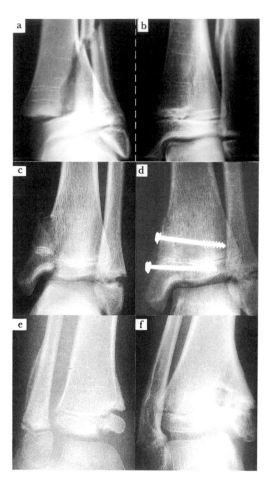

23.53 Physeal injuries (a) Type 2 injury. The fracture does not traverse the width of the physis; after reduction (b) bone growth is not distorted. (c) This type 4 fracture of the tibial physis and separation (type 1) of the fibular physis was treated immediately by open reduction and internal fixation, and (d) a good result was obtained. (e) In this case accurate reduction was not achieved and the physeal fragment remained displaced; (f) the end-result was severe deformity of the ankle.

undisplaced type 3 and 4 fractures, a check x-ray after 4 days and again at about 10 days is mandatory in order not to miss late displacement.

Displaced fractures should be reduced as soon as possible. With types 1 and 2 this can usually be done closed; the part is then splinted securely for 3–6 weeks. Type 3 and 4 fractures demand perfect anatomical reduction. An attempt can be made to achieve this by gentle manipulation under general anaesthesia; if this is successful, the limb is held in a cast for 4–8 weeks (the longer periods for type 4 injuries). If a type 3 or 4 fracture cannot be reduced accurately by closed manipulation, immediate open reduction and internal fixation with smooth Kirschner wires is essential. The limb is then splinted for 4–6 weeks, but it takes that long again before the child is ready to resume unrestricted activities.

Complications

Type 1 and 2 injuries, if properly reduced, have an excellent prognosis and bone growth is not adversely affected. However, complications such as malunion or non-union may occur if the diagnosis is missed and the fracture remains unreduced (e.g. fracture-separation of the medial humeral epicondyle).

Type 3 and 4 injuries may result in premature fusion of part of the growth plate or asymmetrical growth of the bone end. Type 5 fractures cause premature fusion and retardation of growth. The size and position of the bony bridge across the physis can be assessed by tomography or MRI. If the bridge is relatively small (less than half the width of the physis) it can be excised and replaced by a fat graft, with some prospect of preventing or diminishing the growth disturbance (Langenskiold, 1975). However, if the bone bridge is more extensive the operation is contraindicated as it can end up doing more harm than good.

Established deformity, whether from asymmetrical growth or from malunion of a displaced fracture (e.g. a valgus elbow due to proximal displacement of a lateral humeral condylar fracture) should be treated by corrective osteotomy. If further growth is abnormal, the osteotomy may have to be repeated.

Injuries to joints

Joints are usually injured by twisting or tilting forces that stretch the ligaments and capsule. If the force is great enough the ligaments may tear, or the bone to which they are attached may be pulled apart. The articular cartilage, too, may be damaged if the joint surfaces are compressed or if there is a fracture into the joint.

As a general principle, forceful angulation will tear the ligaments rather than crush the bone, but in older people with porotic bone the ligaments may hold and the bone on the opposite side of the joint is crushed instead, while in children there may be a fracture-separation of the physis.

Torn ligaments heal by fibrous scarring. If the separated ends are tightly sutured, scarring will be minimal and the tensile strength of the ligament will approach normality. If the ends are left apart, or are imperfectly sutured, the gap will be filled by fibrous tissue which inevitably stretches under tension.

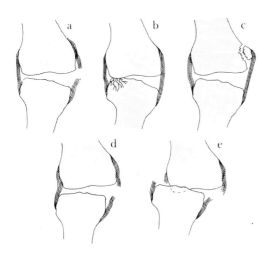

23.54 Joint injuries Severe stress may cause various types of injury. (a) A ligament may rupture, leaving the bone intact. If the soft tissues hold, the bone on the opposite side may be crushed (b), or a fragment may be pulled off by the taut ligament (c). Subluxation (d) means the articular surfaces are partially displaced; dislocation (e) refers to complete displacement of the joint.

Strained ligament

Only some of the fibres in the ligament are torn and the joint remains stable. This follows an injury in which the joint is momentarily twisted or bent into an abnormal position. The joint is painful and swollen, and the tissues may be bruised. Tenderness is localized to the injured ligament and tensing the tissues on that side causes a sharp increase in pain.

Treatment

The joint should be firmly strapped and rested until the acute pain subsides. Thereafter, active movements are encouraged, and exercises practised to strengthen the muscles.

Ruptured ligament

The ligament is completely torn and the joint is unstable. Sometimes the ligament holds and the bone to which it is attached is avulsed; this is effectively the same lesion but easier to deal with because the bone fragment can be securely reattached.

As with a strain, the joint is suddenly forced into an abnormal position; sometimes the patient actually hears a snap. The joints most likely to be affected are the ones that are least well protected by surrounding muscles: the knee, the ankle and the finger joints.

Pain is severe and there may be considerable bleeding under the skin; if the joint is swollen, this is probably due to a haemarthrosis. The patient is unlikely to permit a searching examination, but under general anaesthesia the instability can be demonstrated; it is this that distinguishes the lesion from a strain. X-ray may show a detached flake of bone where the ligament is inserted.

Treatment

A torn ligament will heal spontaneously by fibrosis if it is held without tension for 4–6 weeks. In the past this formed the basis of treatment for most ligament injuries and it is still acceptable (1) when surgical repair is particularly difficult or unrewarding, and (2) when joint instability is not very marked, especially (3) in elderly patients who will make light demands on the joint. After a period of immobilization, movement and exercise are encouraged while avoiding tension on the ligament.

In younger individuals, and in most cases where instability is marked, surgical repair is the treatment of choice – and the sooner the better, for once the tissues retract it may be impossible to appose them by suturing. Postoperatively the joint is immobilized to take tension off the ligament; after 3–4 weeks, movements are begun but the joint is protected for another 4–6 weeks.

Dislocation and subluxation

'Dislocation' means that the joint surfaces are completely displaced and are no longer in contact; 'subluxation' implies a lesser degree of displacement, such that the articular surfaces are still partly apposed.

Clinical features

Following an injury the joint is painful and the patient tries at all costs to avoid moving it. The shape of the joint is abnormal and the bony landmarks may be displaced. The limb is often held in a characteristic position; movement is painful and restricted. X-rays will usually clinch the diagnosis; they will also show whether there is an associated bony injury affecting joint stability – i.e. a fracture-dislocation.

The apprehension test If the dislocation is reduced by the time the patient is seen, the joint can be tested by stressing it as if almost to reproduce the suspected dislocation: the patient develops a sense of impending disaster and violently resists further manipulation.

Recurrent dislocation If the ligaments and joint margins are damaged, repeated dislocation may occur. This is seen especially in the shoulder and the patellofemoral joint.

Habitual (voluntary) dislocation Some patients acquire the knack of dislocating (or subluxating) the joint by voluntary muscle contraction. Ligamentous laxity may make this easier, but the habit often betrays a manipulative and neurotic personality. It is important to recognize this because such patients are seldom helped by operation.

Treatment

The dislocation must be reduced as soon as possible; usually a general anaesthetic is required, and sometimes a muscle relaxant as well. The joint is then rested or immobilized until soft-tissue healing occurs – usually after 3–4 weeks. If ligaments have been torn, they may have to be repaired.

Complications

Many of the complications of fractures are seen also after dislocations: vascular injury, nerve injury, avascular necrosis of bone, heterotopic ossification, joint stiffness and secondary osteoarthritis. The principles of diagnosis and management of these conditions have been discussed above.

References and further reading

Alho, A. (1980) Fat embolism syndrome. Etiology, pathogenesis and treatment. *Acta Chirurgica Scandinavica* suppl. 499, 75–85

Atkins, R.M., Duckworth, T. and Kanis, J.A. (1990) Features of algodystrophy after Colles' fracture. *Journal of Bone and Joint Surgery* **72B**, 105–110

Bassett, C.A.L., Valdes, M.G. and Hernandez, E. (1982) Modification of fracture repair with selected pulsing electromagnetic fields. *Journal of Bone and Joint Surgery* **64A**, 888–895

Behrens, F. (1988) External fixation. *Current Orthopaedics* **2** 9–13

Charnley, J. (1961) *The Closed Treatment of Common Fractures*, 3rd edn, Livingstone, Edinburgh

Coombs, R., Green, S. and Sarmiento, A. (eds) (1989) *External Fixation and Functional Bracing*, Orthotext, London

Devas, M. (1975) *Stress Fractures*, Churchill Livingstone, London, New York

Eriksson, B.I., Kalebo, P., Anthmyr, B.O. et al. (1991)

Prevention of deep-vein thrombosis and pulmonary embolism after total hip replacement. *Journal of Bone and Joint Surgery* **73A**, 484–493

Goodship, A.E. and Kenwright, J. (1985) The influence of induced micromovement upon the healing of experimental tibial fractures. *Journal of Bone and Joint Surgery* **67B**, 650–655

Gustilo, R.B., Merkow, R.L. and Templeman, D. (1990) Current concepts: the managment of open fractures. *Journal of Bone and Joint Surgery* **72A**, 299–304

Hedges, A.R. and Kakkar, V.V. (1988) Prophylaxis of pulmonary embolus and deep vein thrombosis. *Hospital Update* **14**, 1159–1174

Holden, C.E.A. (1979) The pathology and prevention of Volkmann's ischaemic contracture. *Journal of Bone and Joint Surgery* **61B**, 296–300

Ilizarov, G.A. (1992) *Transosseous Osteosynthesis*, Springer, Berlin, Heidelberg, New York

Kenwright, J., Richardson, J.B., Cunningham, J.L. et al. (1991) Axial movement and tibial fractures. *Journal of Bone and Joint Surgery* **73B**, 654–659

Langenskiold, A. (1975) An operation for partial closure of an epiphyseal plate in children and its experimental basis. *Journal of Bone and Joint Surgery* **57B**, 325–330

Leyvraz, P.F., Bachmann, F., Hoek, J. et al. (1991) Prevention of deep vein thrombosis after hip replacement: randomised comparison between unfractionated heparin and low molecular weight heparin. *British Medical Journal* **303**, 543–548

McKibbin, B. (1978) The biology of fracture healing in long bones. *Journal of Bone and Joint Surgery* **60B**, 150–162

Michelsen, C.B. and Askanazi, J. (1986) The metabolic response to injury. *Journal of Bone and Joint Surgery* **68A**, 782–787

Müller, M.E., Nazarian, S., Koch, P. and Schatzker, J. (1990) *The Comprehensive Classification of Long Bones*, Springer, Berlin, Heidelberg, New York

Müller, M.E., Allgöwer, M., Schneider, R. and Willeneger, H. (eds.) (1991) *Manual of Internal Fixation*, 3rd edn, Springer, Heidelberg, Berlin, New York

Parker-Williams, J. and Vickers, R. (1991) Major orthopaedic surgery on the leg and thromboembolism. *British Medical Journal* **303**, 531–532

Perkins, G. (1958) *Fractures and Dislocations*, Athlone Press, London

Phillips, T.F. and Contreras, D.M. (1990) Timing of operative treatment of fractures in patients who have multiple injuries. *Journal of Bone and Joint Surgery* **72A**, 784–788

Roberts, P. and Carnes, S. (1990) The orthopaedic scooter. *Journal of Bone and Joint Surgery* **72B**, 620–621

Ruckley, C.V. (1986) Venous thrombosis and pulmonary embolism. *Current Orthopaedics* **1**, 75–79

Salter, R.B. and Harris, W.R. (1963) Injuries involving the epiphyseal plate. *Journal of Bone and Joint Surgery* **45A**, 587–622

Sarmiento, A. and Latta, L.L. (1981) *Closed Functional Treatment of Fractures*, Springer, Berlin, Heidelberg, New York

Sharrard, W.J.W. (1990) A double-blind trial of pulsed electromagnetic fields for delayed union of tibial fractures. *Journal of Bone and Joint Surgery* **72**, 347–355

Tscherne, H. (1984) The management of open fractures. In *Fractures with Soft Tissue Injuries* (eds. H. Tscherne and L. Gotzen), Springer, Berlin

Watson-Jones, R. (1982) *Fractures and Joint Injuries*, 6th edn (ed. J.N. Wilson), Churchill Livingstone, Edinburgh

Woloszyn, J.T., Uitrlugt, G.M. and Castle, M.E. (1986) Management of civilian gunshot fractures of the extremities. *Clinical Orthopaedics and Related Research* **226**, 247–251

I. *The shoulder and upper arm*

The great bugbear of upper limb injuries is stiffness – particularly of the shoulder but sometimes of the elbow and hand as well. Two points should be constantly borne in mind: (1) in elderly patients it is often best to disregard the fracture and to concentrate on regaining movement; (2) whatever the injury, and however it is treated, the fingers should be exercised from the start.

Fractures of the clavicle

In children the clavicle fractures easily, but it almost invariably unites rapidly and without complications. In adults this is a much more troublesome injury.

Mechanism of injury

A fall on the shoulder or the outstretched hand breaks the clavicle. In the common mid-shaft fracture, the outer fragment is pulled down by the weight of the arm and the inner half is held up by the sternomastoid muscle. In fractures of the outer third, if the ligaments are intact there is little displacement; but if the coracoclavicular ligaments are torn, displacement may be severe and closed reduction impossible.

Clinical features

The arm is clasped to the chest to prevent movement. A subcutaneous lump may be ob-

vious and occasionally a sharp fragment threatens the skin. Though vascular complications are rare, it is prudent to feel the pulse and gently to palpate the root of the neck.

X-RAY
The fracture is usually in the middle third of the bone, and the outer fragment lies below the inner.

A fracture of the outer third may be missed, or the degree of displacement underestimated, unless additional views of the shoulder are obtained.

Treatment

For the common *middle third fracture*, accurate reduction is neither possible nor essential. All that is needed is to support the arm in a sling until the pain subsides (usually 2–3 weeks). Thereafter active shoulder exercises should be encouraged; this is particularly important in older patients.

Severely displaced *outer third fractures* (i.e. those in which the coracoclavicular ligaments are torn) usually cannot be reduced closed. Left untreated, they cause deformity and, in some cases, discomfort and weakness of the shoulder. Operative treatment is therefore indicated: through a supraclavicular incision the fragments are apposed and held with a smooth pin, which is passed laterally through the outer fragment and the acromion, and then back into the clavicular shaft. The arm is held in a sling for 6 weeks and thereafter full movement is encouraged.

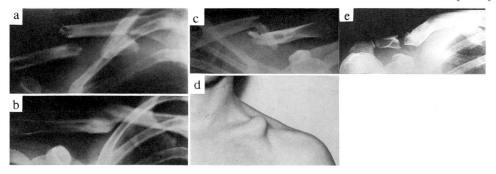

24.1 Fractured clavicle (a) The common site and displacement. (b) Uniting in the usual somewhat faulty position. (c) Comminuted fracture which united leaving (d) a large lump. (e) Fracture near the lateral end, with non-union; this is not uncommon with these far lateral fractures.

Complications

EARLY

Damage to vessels or nerves is very rare.

LATE

Non-union rarely occurs unless a surgeon has been unwise enough to operate on a mid-shaft fracture. It can be treated by secure internal fixation and bone grafting.

Malunion is invariable and leaves a lump; in a child the lump always disappears in time, and in an adult it usually does. Someone anxious to obtain a good cosmetic result quickly may be willing to undergo more drastic treatment: the fracture is manually reduced under anaesthesia and held reduced by a plaster cuirass.

Stiffness of the shoulder is common but temporary; it results from fear of moving a fracture. Unless the fingers are exercised, they also may become stiff and take months to regain movement.

Fractures of the scapula

Mechanisms of injury

The *body of the scapula* is fractured by a crushing force, which usually also fractures ribs and may dislocate the sternoclavicular joint. The *neck of the scapula* may be fractured by a blow or by a fall on the shoulder. The *coracoid process* may fracture across its base or be avulsed at the tip.

Fracture of the acromion is due to direct force. *Fracture of the glenoid rim* may occur with dislocation of the shoulder.

Clinical features

The arm is held immobile and there may be severe bruising over the scapula or the chest wall. Fractures of the body of the scapula are often associated with severe chest injuries.

X-RAY

The films may reveal a comminuted fracture of the body of the scapula, or a fractured scapular neck with the outer fragment pulled downwards by the weight of the arm. Occasionally a crack is seen in the acromion or the coracoid process. CT is useful for demonstrating glenoid fractures.

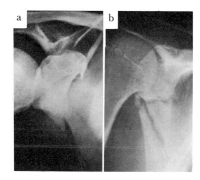

24.2 Scapular fractures (a) Of the neck of the scapula; (b) of the body.

Treatment

Reduction is usually impossible and unnecessary. The patient wears a sling for comfort, and from the start practises active exercises to the shoulder, elbow and fingers.

A large glenoid fragment, due to fracture-dislocation of the shoulder, should be fixed with a screw.

Complications

Fractures of the body are sometimes associated with injuries to the *chest wall* or *lungs* (look for pneumothorax); and with all scapular fractures there may also be injury of the *brachial plexus* (a careful neurological examination is essential).

Acromioclavicular joint injuries

Mechanism of injury

A fall on the shoulder tears the acromioclavicular ligaments, and upward subluxation of the clavicle may occur; more severe injury also tears the coracoclavicular ligaments and results in complete dislocation of the joint.

Clinical features

The patient can usually point to the site of injury and the area may be bruised. If there is tenderness but no deformity, the injury is probably a strain or a subluxation. With dislocation the patient is in severe pain and a prominent 'step' can be seen and felt. Shoulder movements are limited.

X-RAY

The films show either a subluxation with only slight elevation of the clavicle or dislocation with considerable elevation. Not all dislocations are obvious, so stress views are advisable. An anteroposterior x-ray including both shoulders is taken with the patient upright, arms by the side and holding a 5 kg weight in each hand. The distance between the coracoid process and the inferior border of the clavicle is measured on each side; a difference of more than 6 cm is diagnostic of acromioclavicular dislocation.

Treatment

Subluxation does not affect function and does not require any special treatment; the arm is rested in a sling until pain subsides (usually no more than a week) and shoulder exercises are then begun.

Dislocation is poorly controlled by padding and strapping. In patients with physically demanding occupations, operative reduction is preferable; a screw is passed from the clavicle downwards into the base of the coracoid process, drawing the two bones together; the surrounding soft tissues are repaired. The shoulder is rested for 3 weeks and exercises are then encouraged. The screw is removed after 8 weeks.

In elderly patients, and those with sedentary occupations, the injury may be treated as for a subluxation; although the 'bump' persists, disability is usually mild.

Complications

An unreduced subluxation causes no disability. An unreduced dislocation is ugly and some-

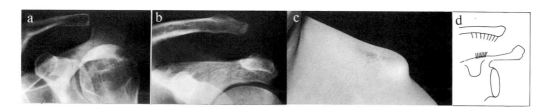

24.3 Acromioclavicular joint   With subluxation (a) deformity is slight. With complete dislocation (b, c) displacement is marked; (d) the conoid and trapezoid ligaments are torn.

times affects function. If necessary, the outer 2.5 cm of the clavicle may be excised, or the clavicle anchored down to the coracoid process. Alternatively, the coracoid process may be detached and, with its muscles, fixed to the clavicle, thus stabilizing the joint.

A late complication is osteoarthritis of the acromioclavicular joint; this can usually be managed conservatively, but if pain is marked the outer end of the clavicle can be excised.

Sternoclavicular dislocations

Mechanism of injury

This uncommon injury is usually caused by lateral compression of the shoulders; for example, when someone is pinned to the ground following a road accident or an underground rock-fall. Rarely, it follows a direct blow to the chest.

Anterior dislocation is much more common than posterior.

Clinical features

Anterior dislocation   is easily diagnosed; the dislocated medial end of the clavicle forms a prominent bump over the sternoclavicular joint. The condition is painful but there are usually no cardiothoracic complications.

Posterior dislocation,   though rare, is much more serious. Discomfort is marked; there may be pressure on the trachea or large vessels; ribs

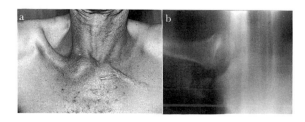

24.4 Sternoclavicular joint   (a) Anterior dislocation is clinically obvious though difficult to demonstrate on plain x-rays. (b) A tomogram shows the displacement well, though a CT would have been even better.

may be fractured and sometimes the patient is shocked and dyspnoeic.

Because of overlapping shadows, plain x-rays are difficult to interpret. CT is the ideal method of diagnosing anterior or posterior dislocation and excluding fractures of the medial end of the clavicle.

Treatment

Anterior dislocation   can usually be reduced by exerting pressure over the clavicle and pulling on the arm with the shoulder abducted. However, the joint usually redislocates. Not that this matters much; full function will be regained, though this may take several months. Internal fixation is unnecessary and dangerous (because of the large vessels behind the sternum).

Posterior dislocation   should be reduced as soon as possible. This can usually be done closed (if necessary under general anaesthesia) by lying the patient supine with a sandbag between the scapulae and then pulling on the arm with the shoulder abducted and extended. The joint reduces with a snap and stays reduced. If this manoeuvre fails, the medial end of the clavicle is grasped with bone forceps and pulled forwards. If this, too, fails (a very rare occurrence) open reduction is justified, but great care must be taken not to damage the mediastinal structures. After reduction, the shoulders are braced back with a figure-of-eight bandage, which is worn for 3 weeks.

Anterior dislocation of the shoulder

Of the large joints, the shoulder is the one that most commonly dislocates. This is due to a number of factors: the shallowness of the glenoid socket; the extraordinary range of movement; underlying conditions such as ligamentous laxity or glenoid dysplasia; and the sheer vulnerability of the joint during stressful activities of the upper limb.

Mechanism of injury

Dislocation is usually caused by a fall on the hand. The humerus is driven forward, tearing the capsule or avulsing the glenoid labrum. Occasionally the posterolateral part of the head is crushed. Rarely, the acromion process levers the head downwards and luxatio erecta (with the hand pointing upwards) results; nearly always the arm then drops, bringing the head to its subcoracoid position.

Clinical features

Pain is severe. The patient supports the arm with the opposite hand and is loath to permit any kind of examination. The lateral outline of the shoulder may be flattened and, if the patient is not too muscular, a bulge may be felt just below the clavicle. The arm must always be examined for nerve and vessel injury.

X-RAY

The anteroposterior x-ray will show the overlapping shadows of the humeral head and glenoid fossa, with the head usually lying below and medial to the socket.

A lateral view aimed along the blade of the scapula will show the humeral head out of line with the socket.

If the joint has dislocated before, routine x-rays may show flattening or an excavation of the posterolateral contour of the humeral head, where it has been indented by the anterior edge of the glenoid socket (Hill and Sachs, 1940).

Treatment

Numerous methods of reduction have been described, some of them now of no more than historical interest.

In a patient who has had previous dislocations, simple traction on the arm may be successful.

For reduction of a 'first-time' dislocation, the patient should be heavily sedated or anaesthetized and in the supine position. Gently increasing traction is applied to the arm with the shoulder in slight abduction, while an assistant applies firm counter-traction to the body (a towel slung around the patient's chest, under the axilla, is helpful). If anaesthesia is contraindicated, the prone position with the arm hanging, may facilitate reduction.

Kocher's method is sometimes used. The elbow is bent to 90 degrees and held close to the body; no traction should be applied. The arm is slowly rotated 75 degrees laterally, then the point of the elbow is lifted forwards, and finally the arm is rotated medially.

An x-ray is taken to confirm reduction and exclude a fracture. When the patient is fully awake, active abduction is gently tested to exclude an axillary nerve injury.

The arm is rested in a sling for a week or two and active movements are then begun, but combined abduction and lateral rotation must be avoided for at least 3 weeks. Throughout this period, elbow and finger movements are practised every day.

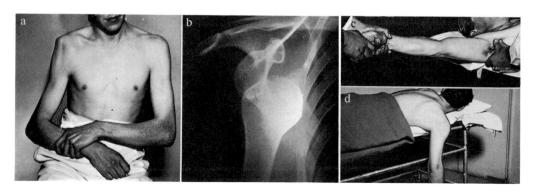

24.5 Shoulder dislocations – anterior   (a, b) Anterior dislocation of the shoulder, (c, d) Two methods of reduction.

Complications

EARLY

Nerve injury The axillary nerve may be injured; the patient is unable to contract the deltoid muscle and there may be a small patch of anaesthesia over the muscle. This is usually a neurapraxia which recovers spontaneously after a few weeks or months.

Occasionally the posterior cord of the brachial plexus is injured. This is somewhat alarming, but fortunately it usually recovers with time.

Vascular injury The axillary artery may be damaged. The limb should always be examined for signs of ischaemia. Management is described on p. 544.

Fracture-dislocation If there is an associated fracture of the proximal humerus, open reduction and internal fixation may be necessary.

The greater tuberosity may be sheared off during dislocation. It usually falls into place during reduction, and no special treatment is then required. If it remains displaced, surgical reattachment is feasible.

LATE

Shoulder stiffness Prolonged immobilization may lead to stiffness of the shoulder, especially in patients over the age of 40. There is loss of lateral rotation, which automatically limits abduction.

Active exercises will usually loosen the joint. They are practised vigorously, bearing in mind that full abduction is not possible until lateral rotation has been regained. Manipulation under anaesthesia is advised only if progress has halted and at least 6 months have elapsed since injury. Lateral rotation should be restored before abduction, and the manipulation should be gentle and repeated rather than forceful.

Unreduced dislocation Surprisingly, a dislocation of the shoulder sometimes remains undiagnosed. This is more likely if the patient is (1) unconscious or (2) very old. Closed reduction is worth attempting up to 6 weeks after injury; manipulation later may fracture the bone or tear vessels or nerves.

Operative reduction is indicated after 6 weeks only in the young, because it is difficult, dangerous and followed by prolonged stiffness. An anterior approach is used, and the vessels and nerves are carefully identified before the dislocation is reduced. 'Active neglect' summarizes the treatment of unreduced dislocation in the elderly. The dislocation is disregarded and gentle active movements are encouraged. Moderately good function is often regained.

Recurrent dislocation If an anterior dislocation tears the shoulder capsule, repair occurs spontaneously and the dislocation does not recur; but if, instead, the glenoid labrum is detached, or the capsule is stripped off the front of the neck of the glenoid, repair is less likely and recurrence common. Bandaging the arm to the side after reducing the acute dislocation does not seem to influence the outcome. Detachment of the labrum occurs particularly in young patients, and, if at injury a bony defect has been gouged out of the posterolateral aspect of the humeral head, recurrence is even more likely.

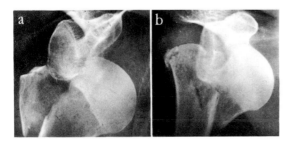

24.6 Anterior fracture – dislocation Anterior dislocation of the shoulder may be complicated by fracture of (a) the greater tuberosity or (b) the neck of the humerus – this often needs open reduction and internal fixation.

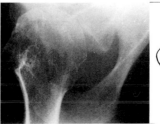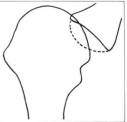

24.7 Recurrent subluxation X-ray showing anterior subluxation; the humeral head is riding on the lip of the glenoid.

The history is diagnostic. The patient complains that the shoulder dislocates with relatively trivial everyday actions. Often he can reduce the dislocation himself. Any doubt as to diagnosis is quickly resolved by the apprehension test: if the patient's arm is passively placed behind the coronal plane in a position of abduction and lateral rotation, his immediate resistance and apprehension are pathognomonic.

Even more common, but less readily diagnosed, is *recurrent subluxation*. The management of both types of instability is dealt with in Chapter 13.

Posterior dislocation of the shoulder

Posterior dislocation is rare, accounting for less than 2% of all dislocations around the shoulder.

Mechanism of injury

Indirect force producing marked internal rotation and adduction must needs be very severe to cause a dislocation. This happens most commonly during a fit or convulsion, or with an electric shock.

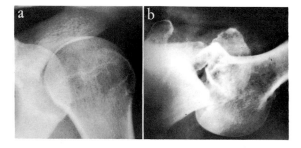

24.8 Shoulder dislocations – posterior   (a) The antero-posterior view may look almost normal, but (b) the lateral view shows obvious subluxation.

Clinical features

The diagnosis is frequently missed – partly because reliance is placed on a single antero-posterior x-ray (which may look almost normal) and partly because those attending to the patient failed to think of it. There are, in fact, several well-marked clinical features. The arm is held in medial rotation and is locked in that position. The front of the shoulder looks flat with a prominent coracoid, but swelling may obscure this deformity; seen from above, however, the posterior displacement is usually apparent.

X-RAY

In the anteroposterior film the humeral head, because it is medially rotated, looks abnormal in shape (like an electric light bulb) and it stands away somewhat from the glenoid fossa (the 'empty glenoid' sign). A lateral film is essential; it shows posterior subluxation or dislocation and sometimes a deep indentation on the anterior aspect of the humeral head. Fractures of the neck of the humerus are sometimes complicated by posterior dislocation.

In difficult cases CT is helpful.

Treatment

The acute dislocation is reduced (usually under general anaesthesia) by pulling on the arm with the shoulder in abduction; a few minutes are allowed for the head of the humerus to disengage and the arm is then gently rotated laterally while the humeral head is pushed forwards. If reduction feels stable the arm is immobilized in a sling; otherwise the shoulder is held widely abducted and laterally rotated in a plaster spica for 3 weeks. Shoulder movement is regained by active exercises.

Complications

Unreduced dislocation   At least half the patients with posterior dislocation have 'unreduced' lesions when first seen. Sometimes weeks or months elapse before the diagnosis is made. Typically the patient holds the arm internally rotated; he cannot abduct the arm more than

70–80 degrees, and if he lifts the extended arm forwards he cannot then turn the palm upwards.

If the patient is young, or is uncomfortable and the dislocation fairly recent (say up to 8 weeks old), open reduction is indicated. Through a posterior approach, capsular repair and reefing are performed.

Late dislocations, especially in the elderly, are best left, but movement is encouraged.

Recurrent dislocation or subluxation Chronic posterior instability of the shoulder is discussed on p. 276.

Special features in children

Traumatic dislocation of the shoulder is exceedingly rare in children. Children who give a history of the shoulder 'slipping out' almost invariably have either voluntary or involuntary (atraumatic) dislocation or subluxation. With *voluntary dislocation,* the child can demonstrate the instability at will. With *involuntary dislocation,* the shoulder slips out unexpectedly during everyday activities. Most of these children have generalized joint laxity and some have glenoid dysplasia. Examination may show that the shoulder subluxates in almost any direction (multidirectional instability). X-rays may confirm the diagnosis.

Treatment Atraumatic dislocation should be viewed with great caution. Some of these children have behavioral problems and this is where treatment should be directed. A pro-

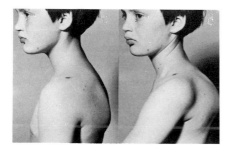

24.9 Habitual (voluntary) dislocation This boy was able (and willing) to dislocate his shoulder posteriorly – and obviously it was painless.

longed exercise programme may also help. Only if the child is genuinely distressed by the disorder, and provided psychological factors have been excluded, should one consider reconstructive surgery – usually a meticulous reefing procedure (Neer and Foster, 1980).

Fractures of the proximal humerus

Fractures of the proximal humerus usually occur after middle age and are most common in osteoporotic, postmenopausal women. In the majority of cases displacement is not marked and treatment presents few problems. However, in about 20% there is considerable displacement of one or more fragments and a significant risk of complications.

Mechanism of injury

Fracture usually follows a fall on the outstretched arm – the type of injury which, in younger people, might cause dislocation of the shoulder. Sometimes, indeed, there is both a fracture and a dislocation.

The most widely accepted classification is that of Neer (1970), who drew attention to the four major segments involved in these injuries: (1) the head, (2) the lesser tuberosity, (3) the greater tuberosity, and (4) the shaft. The classification distinguishes between the number of displaced or separated fragments. Thus, however many fracture lines there are, if the fragments are undisplaced it is regarded as a *one-part fracture*; if one segment is separated from the others, it is a *two-part fracture*; if two fragments are displaced, that is a *three-part fracture*; if all the major parts are displaced, it is a *four-part fracture*. The grading is based on x-ray appearances.

The great value of this classification is that it correlates well with the outcome: minimally displaced fractures cause few problems; two-part fractures can usually be managed by closed reduction; three-part fractures are difficult to

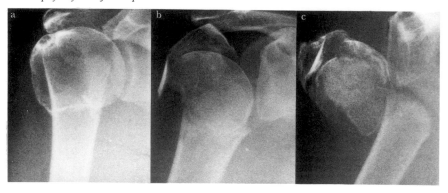

24.10 Fractures of the upper humerus Classification is all very well, but x-rays are more difficult to interpret than line drawings. (a) Two-part fracture. (b) Three-part fracture involving the neck and the greater tuberosity. (c) Four-part fracture.

reduce and may need internal or external fixation; and four-part fractures, which generally have a poor outcome, are best treated by prosthetic replacement.

Clinical features

Because the fracture is often firmly impacted, pain may not be severe. However, the appearance of a large bruise on the upper part of the arm is suspicious. Signs of axillary nerve or brachial plexus injury should be sought.

In elderly patients there often appears to be a single, impacted fracture extending across the surgical neck. However, with good x-rays, several undisplaced fragments may be seen.

In younger patients, the fragments are usually more clearly separated.

In adolescents, fracture-separation of the upper humeral epiphysis occurs; the shaft shifts upwards and forwards, leaving the head in the socket.

An axillary view should always be obtained, to exclude dislocation of the shoulder.

Treatment

Minimally displaced fractures – the vast majority – need no treatment apart from a short period of rest with the arm in a sling until the pain subsides, and then gentle passive movements of the shoulder. Once the fracture has united (usually after 6 weeks), active exercises are encouraged; the hand is, of course, actively exercised from the start.

Two-part fractures – i.e. displacement of one sizeable fragment from the rest – can usually be reduced closed. If the displacement is at the surgical neck, the fragments are gently manipulated into alignment and the arm is immobilized in a Velpeau chest-bandage for 4 weeks. Elbow and hand exercises are encouraged throughout this period; shoulder exercises are commenced at about 4 weeks. The results of conservative treatment are generally satisfactory, considering that most of these patients are over 65 and do not demand perfect function. However, if there is marked displacement with instability, or gross separation of the greater tuberosity, open reduction and internal fixation may be necessary. The rare displaced fracture of the anatomical neck usually results in avascular necrosis of the articular fragment. A large fragment should be screwed back in position – this is essentially an autogenous osteochondral graft.

Three-part fractures – usually with displacement of the surgical neck and the greater tuberosity – are extremely difficult to reduce closed. In active individuals this injury is best managed by open reduction and internal fixation. An alternative method is to use external fixation, holding the humeral head with two threaded pins and the shaft with three; after reduction the connecting bar, which has two ball joints, is attached (Kristiansen and Kofoed, 1987).

Four-part fractures – i.e. with displacement of the surgical neck and both tuberosities – are severe injuries with a high risk of complications such as vascular injury, brachial plexus damage, injuries of the chest wall and (later) avascular necrosis of the humeral head. The x-ray diagnosis is difficult (how many fragments are there, and are they displaced?); a recent study showed poor interobserver agreement on the x-ray assessment (Kristiansen et al., 1988). Often the most one can say is that there are 'multiple displaced fragments', sometimes together with glenohumeral dislocation. Closed treatment and attempts at open reduction and fixation usually result in continuing pain and stiffness; the treatment of choice is prosthetic replacement of the proximal humerus (Stableforth, 1984).

Complications

Shoulder dislocation Fracture-dislocation – either anterior or posterior – is not uncommon. The dislocation can usually be reduced closed and the fracture is then treated in the usual way. However, with three-part fractures, open reduction may be necessary.

Vascular injuries and nerve injuries may occur and should be sought at the initial examination.

Stiffness of the shoulder is common and important, but is minimized by early and persistent exercises. Unlike a frozen shoulder, the stiffness is maximal at the outset.

Malunion is not uncommon. In the elderly it causes little disability; in the young adolescent the bone grows straight.

Special features in children

Fractures of the proximal epiphysis or physis are rare before adolescence. Because of the marked growth and remodelling potential of the proximal humerus, malunion is readily compensated for during the remaining growth

period. These injuries can, therefore, almost always be treated conservatively – by manipulation (if necessary) and immobilization of the arm in a Velpeau bandage for 3 weeks, followed by exercises. Occasionally a severely rotated proximal fragment requires that the arm be held elevated and externally rotated in a spica.

Fractured shaft of humerus

Mechanism of injury

A fall on the hand may twist the humerus, causing a spiral fracture. A fall on the elbow with the arm abducted may hinge the bone, causing an oblique or transverse fracture. A direct blow to the arm causes a fracture which is either transverse or comminuted. A fracture of the shaft in an elderly patient may be due to a metastasis.

With fractures above the deltoid insertion, the proximal fragment is adducted by pectoralis major. With fractures lower down, the proximal fragment is abducted by the deltoid.

Injury to the radial nerve is common, though fortunately recovery is usual.

Clinical features

The arm is painful, bruised and swollen. Active extension of the fingers should be tested because the radial nerve may be damaged.

X-RAY
The site of the fracture, its line (transverse, spiral or comminuted) and any displacement are readily seen. The possibility that the fracture may be pathological should be remembered.

Treatment

Fractures of the humerus heal readily. They require neither perfect reduction nor immobilization; the weight of the arm with an external cast is usually enough to pull the fragments into alignment. A 'hanging cast' is applied from shoulder to wrist with the elbow flexed 90

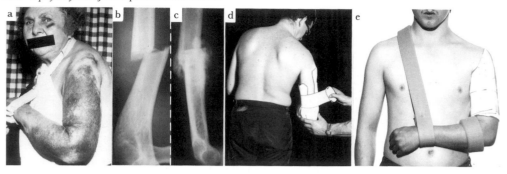

24.11 Fractured shaft of humerus   (a) The telltale bruise. (b, c) Transverse fracture with only moderate displacement. (d) A U-slab of plaster (after a few days in a shoulder-to-wrist hanging cast) is usually adequate, though (e) a ready-made functional brace is simpler and probably better.

degrees and the forearm section suspended by a sling around the patient's neck. This cast may be replaced after 2–3 weeks by a short (shoulder to elbow) cast or a functional polypropylene brace which is worn for a further 6 weeks. The wrist and fingers are exercised from the start. Pendulum exercises of the shoulder are begun within a week, but active abduction is postponed until the fracture has united. Alternatively, the fracture can be held reduced by an external fixator.

If the fracture is very unstable and difficult to control, internal fixation is preferable – either a plate and screws or a long intramedullary nail. Plating needs considerable expertise, and nailing has the disadvantage that the proximal end of the nail may interfere with the action of the supraspinatus.

Spiral fractures unite in about 6 weeks; the other varieties take 4–6 weeks longer. Once united, only a sling is needed until the fracture is consolidated.

Complications

EARLY

Nerve injury   Radial nerve palsy (wrist drop and paralysis of the metacarpophalangeal extensors) may occur with shaft fractures. In closed injuries the nerve is very seldom divided, so there is no hurry to operate. A 'lively' splint is used to support the wrist and hand while recovery is awaited. If there is no sign of this by 6 weeks, the nerve should be explored. In complete lesions (neurotmesis), nerve suture is often unsatisfactory, but function can be largely restored by tendon transfers (see p. 230).

Vascular injury   If there are signs of vascular insufficiency in the limb, brachial artery damage must be excluded. Angiography will show the level of the injury. This is an emergency, requiring exploration and either repair of the vessel or grafting to bypass the damage; in these circumstances, internal fixation is probably advisable.

LATE

Delayed union   may occur in transverse fractures, especially if excessive traction has been used (a hanging cast must not be too heavy) or if the patient has not actively exercised the elbow flexors and extensors.

Non-union   may follow. The dangerous combination is incomplete union and a stiff joint. If elbow or shoulder movements are forced before consolidation, the humerus refractures, and non-union may occur.

The treatment of established non-union is operative. The bone ends are freshened, bone chips packed around them and an intramedullary nail is inserted, a plate screwed on or an external fixator applied.

Joint stiffness   may be minimized by early activity, but transverse fractures (in which shoulder abduction is dangerous) may limit shoulder movement for several months.

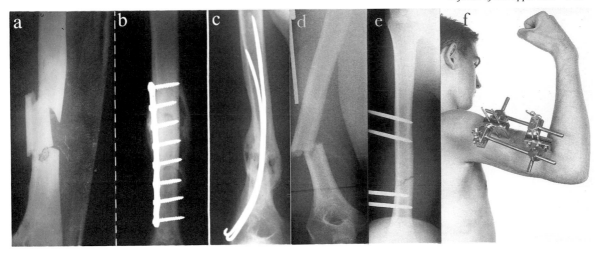

24.12 Fractured shaft of humerus – treatment   (a) This segmental fracture was treated by (b) plating. Rush nails (c) are still sometimes used for internal fixation. (d) Fractures that are difficult to hold reduced can be treated by (e) external fixation, with only moderate loss of function during healing (f).

Special features in children

Fractures of the humerus are uncommon; in children under 3 years of age the possibility of child abuse should be considered. The fracture is treated by simply bandaging the arm to the body for 2–3 weeks. Older children require a short plaster splint.

II. The elbow and forearm

Supracondylar fractures

Supracondylar fractures are usually seen in children. The distal fragment may be displaced either *posteriorly* or *anteriorly*.

Mechanism of injury

Posterior displacement   suggests an extension injury, usually due to a fall on the outstretched hand. The humerus breaks just above the condyles. The distal fragment is pushed backwards and (because the forearm is usually in pronation) twisted inwards. The jagged end of the proximal fragment pokes into the soft tissues anteriorly, sometimes injuring the brachial artery or median nerve.

Anterior displacement   – a much rarer occurrence – is thought to be due to direct violence (e.g. a fall on the elbow) with the elbow in flexion.

Clinical features

Following a fall, the child is in pain and the elbow is swollen; nevertheless the S-deformity of the elbow is usually obvious and the bony landmarks are abnormal. It is essential to feel the pulse and check the circulation. And the hand should be examined for evidence of nerve injury.

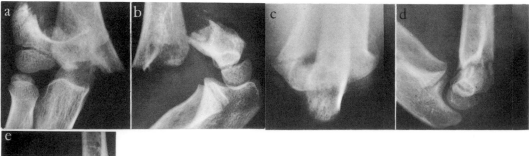

24.13 Supracondylar fractures (a, b) This considerably displaced supracondylar fracture was reduced (c, d) by the method shown in Fig. 24.14. (e) The much rarer variety, with anterior displacement.

X-RAY

The fracture is seen most clearly in the lateral view. In the common *posteriorly displaced fracture* the fracture line runs obliquely downwards and forwards and the distal fragment is shifted backwards and tilted backwards. In the *anteriorly displaced fracture* the fracture line is oblique and lower posteriorly; the fragment is tilted forwards.

An anteroposterior view is often difficult to obtain without causing pain and may need to be postponed until the child has been anaesthetized. It may show that the distal fragment is shifted or tilted sideways, and rotated (usually medially).

Treatment of posteriorly displaced fractures

If there is no displacement, reduction is unnecessary; the child merely wears a sling for 2–3 weeks.

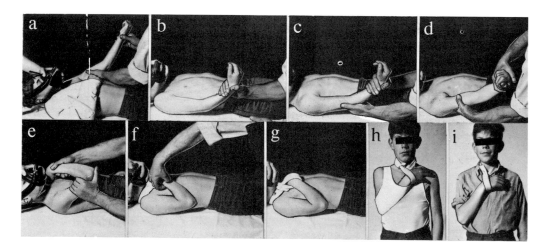

24.14 Supracondylar fractures – treatment of displaced fracture (a) The uninjured arm is examined first; (b) traction on the fractured arm; (c) correcting lateral shift and tilt; (d) correcting rotation; (e) correcting backward shift and tilt; (f) feeling the pulse; (g) the elbow is kept well flexed while x-ray films are taken. (h) For the first 3 weeks the arm is kept under the vest; after this (i) it is outside the vest.

Displaced fractures must be reduced as soon as possible, under general anaesthesia. This is done in a methodical, step-wise manoeuvre: (1) traction for 2–3 minutes in the length of the arm with counter-traction above the elbow; (2) correction of any sideways tilt, shift or twist (in comparison with the other arm); (3) gradual flexion of the elbow while traction is maintained; (4) finger pressure behind the distal fragment to correct posterior tilt. THEN FEEL THE PULSE; if it is absent, relax the amount of elbow flexion until it reappears. X-rays are taken to confirm reduction, checking carefully to see that there is no varus or valgus angulation and no rotational deformity (these features are revealed by noting Baumann's angle) (MacNicol, 1987).

Following reduction, the arm is held in a collar and cuff, continuously, for 3 weeks. After that, active elbow flexion is permitted but the arm is supported in a sling and extension is avoided for another 3 weeks.

Skeletal traction through the olecranon, with the arm held overhead, can be used in special situations: (1) when the fracture cannot be reduced by manipulation; (2) when, with the elbow flexed 90 degrees, the pulse is obliterated; or (3) for severe compound injuries or multiple injuries of the limb. Once the

swelling subsides, a further attempt can be made at closed reduction. Alternatively, the child may be treated by skin traction with the elbow almost straight and the arm in a small Thomas' splint (Dunlop traction) (Piggot, Graham and McCoy, 1986).

Open reduction is sometimes preferred for irreducible fractures. The fracture is exposed (preferably through two incisions, one on each side of the elbow), the haematoma is evacuated and the fracture is reduced and held by two Kirschner wires.

Treatment of anteriorly displaced fracture

This is a rare injury. However, 'posterior' fractures are sometimes converted to 'anterior' ones by excessive traction and manipulation.

The fracture is reduced by pulling on the forearm with the elbow semi-flexed, applying thumb pressure over the front of the distal fragment and then extending the elbow fully. A posterior slab is bandaged on and retained for 3 weeks. Thereafter, the child is allowed to regain flexion gradually.

Complications

EARLY

Vascular injury The great danger of supracondylar fracture is injury to the brachial artery. Peripheral ischaemia may be immediate and severe; more commonly it is complicated by forearm oedema and a mounting compartment syndrome which leads to necrosis of the muscle and nerve without causing peripheral gangrene. Undue pain plus one positive sign (pain on passive extension of the fingers, tense tender forearm, absent pulse or blunted sensation) demands urgent action (p. 544).

Nerve injury The median nerve may be injured, but loss of function is usually temporary and recovery can be expected in 6–8 weeks.

LATE

Myositis ossificans is feared but rarely occurs. If, at 3–4 weeks, movement is decreasing instead of increasing, the elbow should be rested in a plaster gutter.

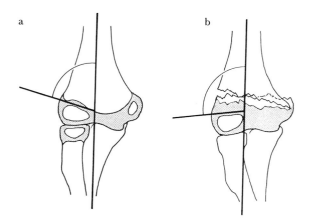

24.15 Baumann's angle In a child it is sometimes difficult to be sure that the distal fragment is reduced. Baumann's angle is subtended by the longitudinal axis of the humeral shaft and a line through the coronal axis of the capitellar physis. This is normally less than 80 degrees (a). If the distal fragment is tilted in varus, the increased angle is readily detected (b).

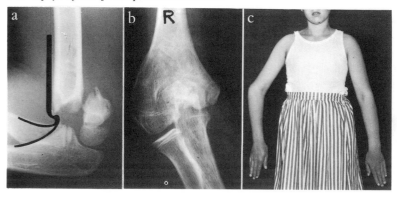

24.16 Supracondylar fractures The most serious complication is arterial damage (a) leading to Volkmann's ischaemia. (b, c) Varus deformity of the right elbow following poor reduction (rotation was never corrected).

Elbow stiffness even without myositis, is common, and extension in particular may take months to return. It must not be hurried. Passive movements (which include carrying weights) or forced movements are prohibited.

Malunion is common. With backward or sideways shift, the humerus gradually grows straight. Foward or backward tilt may limit flexion or extension, but consequent disability is slight.

Uncorrected sideways tilt or rotation is more important. It may lead to a varus deformity, which is ugly and sometimes requires osteotomy, or rarely to a valgus deformity, which may cause late ulnar palsy. Epiphyseal damage is often blamed for these deformities but usually faulty reduction is responsible.

If deformity is marked, it will need correction by supracondylar osteotomy.

Bicondylar fractures (T- and Y-fractures)

Bicondylar fractures are rare and usually confined to adults aged over 50.

Mechanism of injury

A fall on the point of the elbow drives the olecranon process upwards, splitting the condyles apart. The associated soft-tissue injury is usually severe.

Clinical features

Swelling is considerable, but if the bony landmarks can be felt the elbow is found to be wider than normal and the olecranon tip is too high.

X-RAY

The fracture extends from the lower humerus into the elbow joint; it may be T-shaped, Y-shaped or comminuted. Often the condyles are separated, and either may be tilted in any direction.

Treatment

These are severe injuries associated with joint damage; prolonged immobilization will almost certainly result in a stiff elbow. Early movement is therefore a prime objective.

Undisplaced fractures require only a posterior slab with the elbow flexed almost 90 degrees; movements are commenced after 2 weeks.

Moderately displaced fractures, if treated conservatively, will almost always result in a stiff elbow. Therefore, open reduction and internal fixation is preferred.

Through a posterior approach the ulnar nerve is identified and the fracture exposed. The fragments are reduced and held temporarily with Kirschner wires. Then plates or screws or both are used for fixation and the wires removed. This sounds straighforward and is the only method capable of giving a near-perfect result. But, if there is comminution, the technical difficulties are great, and unless the surgeon

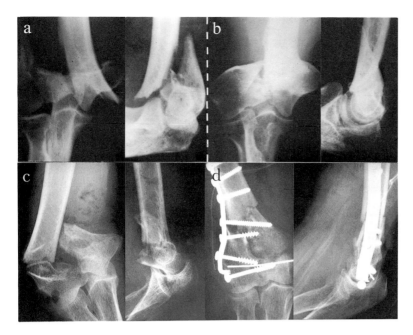

24.17 Bicondylar fractures (a) Before and (b) after treatment in a collar-and-cuff plus activity; reasonable movement was obtained by this method but a hinged brace would have been better. (c) Before and (d) after open reduction and internal fixation; the result was very good, though this is not always the case.

is more than usually skilful, the elbow may end up stiffer than if treated by activity (see below).

Severely comminuted fractures may be technically 'fixable', but the end result is usually disappointing. It is better to go for early movement. The arm is held in a collar and cuff or, better, a hinged brace, with the elbow flexed above a right angle; active movements are encouraged as soon as the patient is willing. The fracture usually unites within 6–8 weeks, but exercises are continued for another 3 months. A useful range of movement (45–90 degrees) is often obtained (Brown and Morgan, 1971).

An alternative method of treating either moderately displaced or severely comminuted fractures is by skeletal traction through the olecranon (beware the ulnar nerve!); the patient remains in bed with the humerus held vertical, and elbow movements are encouraged.

Complications

EARLY

Vascular injury may occur; vigilance is required to make the diagnosis and institute treatment as early as possible.

Nerve injury There may be damage to either the median or the ulnar nerve. It is vital to (1) examine the hand and (2) record the findings before treatment is commenced.

LATE

Myositis ossificans Severe soft-tissue damage may lead to heterotopic ossification. Forced movement should be avoided.

Stiffness Comminuted intercondylar fractures always result in some degree of stiffness. However, the disability may be reduced by encouraging an energetic exercise programme. Late operations to improve elbow movement are usually unrewarding.

Fracture-separation of the lateral condylar epiphysis

The lateral condylar epiphysis begins to ossify during the first year of life and fuses with the shaft at 12–16 years. Between these ages it may be sheared off or avulsed by forceful traction.

Mechanism of injury

The child falls on the hand with the elbow stressed in varus. A large fragment, which includes the lateral condyle, breaks off and is pulled upon by the attached wrist extensors. In severe injuries probably the elbow dislocates posterolaterally; the condyle is 'capsized' by muscle pull and remains capsized while the elbow reduces spontaneously.

The extent of this injury is often not appreciated. Because the capitellar epiphysis is largely cartilaginous, the bone fragment may look deceptively small on x-ray. Displacement can be quite marked due to muscle pull. The fracture is important for two reasons: (1) it may damage the growth plate; and (2) it always involves the joint, thus making accurate reduction desirable.

Clinical features

The elbow is swollen (but not deformed) and there is tenderness over the lateral condyle. Passive flexion of the wrist (pulling on the extensors) may be painful.

X-RAY

With so-called incomplete fractures, displacement is slight; comparison with films of the normal elbow is useful. The more common complete fracture is often grossly displaced and capsized, and it may carry with it a triangular piece of the metaphysis. Remember that the fragment is much larger than it looks on x-ray.

Treatment

If there is no (or only minimal) displacement the arm can be splinted in a backslab with the elbow flexed 90 degrees, the forearm pronated and the wrist extended. However, it is essential to repeat the x-ray after 5 days to make sure that the fracture has not displaced. The splint is removed after 2 weeks and exercises are encouraged.

A displaced fracture requires accurate reduction and internal fixation. If the fragment is only

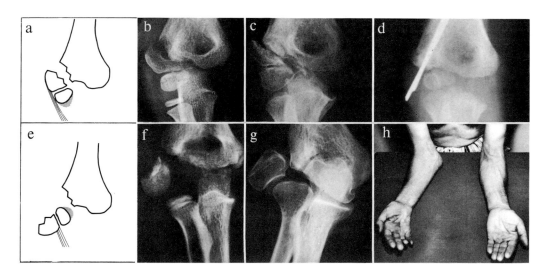

24.18 Fractured lateral condyle (a, b) A large fragment of bone and cartilage is avulsed; even with reasonable reduction, union is not inevitable (c), and open reduction with fixation (d) is often wise. (e, f) Sometimes the condyle is capsized; if left unreduced non-union is inevitable (g) and a valgus elbow with delayed ulnar palsy (h) the likely sequel.

moderately displaced (hinged), it may be possible to manipulate it into position by extending the elbow and pressing upon the condyle, and then fixing the fragment with percutaneous pins. If this fails, and for all widely separated fractures, open reduction and internal fixation with pins or screws is required.

Complications

Non-union and malunion   If the condyle is left capsized, non-union is inevitable; with growth the elbow becomes increasingly valgus, and ulnar nerve palsy is then likely to develop. Even minor displacements sometimes lead to non-union, and even slight malunion may lead to ulnar palsy; it is for these reasons that open reduction (and internal fixation) is often preferred.

Recurrent dislocation   Occasionally condylar displacement results in posterolateral dislocation of the elbow. The only effective treatment is reconstruction of the bony and soft tissues on the lateral side.

Separation of the medial epicondylar epiphysis

Mechanism of injury

The medial epicondylar epiphysis begins to ossify at the age of about 5 years and fuses to the shaft at about 16; between these ages it may be avulsed by a fall on the hand with the wrist in extension. The epiphysis is pulled distally by the attached wrist flexors. With more severe injuries the joint dislocates laterally and the epiphysis is pulled into the joint. The elbow may remain dislocated, or may reduce spontaneously and trap the epicondyle.

Clinical features

If the elbow is still dislocated, deformity is of course obvious. But even without dislocation the diagnosis should be suspected if injury is followed by pain and swelling on the medial side. Sensation in the ulnar fingers should be tested to exclude nerve damage.

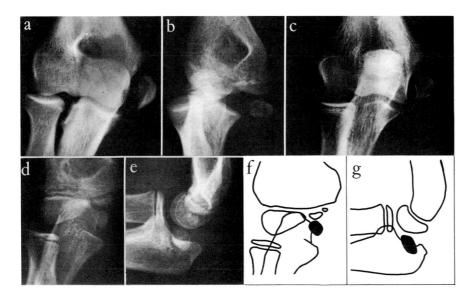

24.19 Fractured medial epicondyle   (a) Avulsion of the medial epicondyle following valgus strain. (b) Avulsion associated with dislocation of the elbow – (c) after reduction.
Sometimes the epicondylar fragment is trapped in the joint (d, e); the serious nature of the injury is then liable to be missed unless the surgeon specifically looks for the trapped fragment, which is emphasized in the tracings (f, g).

X-RAY

In the anteroposterior view the medial epicondylar epiphysis may be tilted or shifted downwards; if the joint is dislocated the epiphysis lies distal to the lower humerus. A lateral view may show the epicondyle looking like a loose body in the joint.

Treatment

Minor displacement may be disregarded but an epicondyle trapped in the joint must be freed. Manipulation with the elbow in valgus and the wrist hyperextended (to pull on the flexor muscles) may be successful; if it fails, the joint must be opened (the ulnar nerve must be visualized) and the fragment retrieved and sutured back in position.

Complications

EARLY

Ulnar nerve damage is not uncommon, but recovery is usual unless the nerve is left kinked in the joint.

LATE

Stiffness of the elbow is common and extension often limited for months; but, provided movement is not forced, it will eventually return.

Late ulnar nerve palsy may follow friction in the roughened bony groove.

Fracture-separation of the entire distal humeral epiphysis

Up to the age of 7 years the distal humeral epiphysis is a solid cartilaginous segment with maturing centres of ossification. With severe injury it may separate *en bloc*. This is likely to occur with fairly severe violence; for example, in birth injuries or child abuse (DeLee et al., 1980).

Clinical features

The child is in pain and the elbow is markedly swollen. The history may be deceptively uninformative.

X-RAY

In a very young child, in whom the bony outlines are still unformed, the x-ray may look normal. All that can be seen of the epiphysis is the pea-like ossification centre of the capitulum; its position should be compared with that of the normal side. Medial displacement of either the capitellar ossification centre or the proximal radius and ulna is very suspicious. In the older child the deformity is usually obvious.

Treatment

The injury is treated like a supracondylar fracture (p. 578). If the diagnosis is uncertain, the elbow is merely splinted in flexion for 2 weeks; any resulting deformity (which is rare) can be dealt with at a later age.

Fractured capitulum

This is an articular fracture which occurs only in adults. The patient falls on the hand, usually with the elbow straight. The anterior half of the capitulum and the trochlea are broken off and displaced proximally.

Clinical features

Fullness in front of the elbow is the most notable feature. Flexion is grossly restricted.

X-RAY

In the lateral view the capitulum (or part of it) is seen in front of the lower humerus, and the radial head no longer points directly towards it.

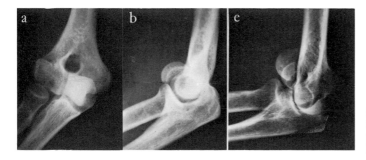

24.20 Fractured capitulum (a, b) Anteroposterior and lateral views showing proximal displacement and tilting; in (c) the capitulum has been sheared off vertically.

Treatment

Undisplaced fractures can be treated by simple splintage for 2 weeks.

Displaced fractures should be either reduced or excised. Closed reduction is feasible, but prolonged immobilization may result in a stiff elbow. Operative treatment is therefore preferred. The fragment is always larger than expected. If it can be securely replaced, it is fixed in position with a small screw. If this proves too difficult, the fragment is best excised. Movements are commenced as soon as discomfort permits.

Fractured head of radius

Radial head fractures are common in adults but are hardly ever seen in children (probably because the proximal radius is mainly cartilaginous).

Mechanism of injury

A fall on the outstretched hand forces the elbow into valgus and pushes the radial head against the capitulum. The radial head may be split or broken. In addition, the articular cartilage of the capitulum may be bruised or chipped; this cannot be seen on x-ray but is an important complication.

Clinical features

This fracture is sometimes missed, but painful rotation of the forearm and tenderness on the lateral side of the elbow should suggest the diagnosis.

X-RAY

The films may show: (1) a vertical split in the radial head; or (2) a single fragment of the lateral portion of the head broken off and usually displaced distally; or (3) the head broken into several fragments. The wrist also should be x-rayed, to exclude a concomitant injury of the distal radioulnar joint.

Treatment

With an undisplaced split the arm is held in a collar and cuff for 3 weeks; active flexion and extension may be encouraged, but rotation should be left to return by itself.

A single large fragment may be pinned back with a Kirschner wire.

A comminuted fracture is best treated by excising the radial head. If there are associated forearm injuries or disruption of the distal radioulnar joint, the risk of proximal migration of the radius is considerable; in such cases, if the head is excised it should be replaced by a Silastic prosthesis. Following the operation, early movement is encouraged.

Complications

Joint stiffness is common and may involve both the elbow and the radioulnar joints. Occasionally myositis ossificans develops. Stiffness may occur whether the radial head has been excised or not. Probably, however, the prognosis with a comminuted fracture is better after operation.

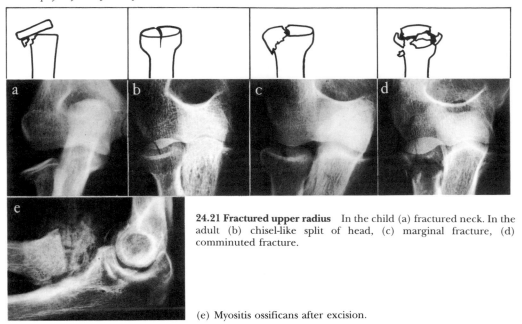

24.21 Fractured upper radius   In the child (a) fractured neck. In the adult (b) chisel-like split of head, (c) marginal fracture, (d) comminuted fracture.

(e) Myositis ossificans after excision.

Fractured neck of radius

A fall on the outstretched hand forces the elbow into valgus and pushes the radial head against the capitulum. In adults the radial head may be split or broken; in children the bone is more likely to fracture through the neck of the radius.

Clinical features

Following a fall, the child complains of pain in the elbow. There may be tenderness over the radial head and pain on rotating the forearm.

X-RAY
The fracture line is transverse. It is either situated immediately distal to the growth disc or there is true separation of the epiphysis with a triangular fragment of shaft. The proximal fragment is tilted distally, forwards and outwards. Sometimes the upper end of the ulna is also fractured.

Treatment

Up to 20 degrees of radial head tilt is acceptable. The arm is rested in a collar and cuff, and exercises are commenced after a week.

Displacement of more than 20 degrees requires reduction. The arm is pulled into extension and slight varus. With his thumb the surgeon pushes the displaced radial fragment into position. If this fails, open reduction is performed. The radial head tilt is corrected but internal fixation is unnecessarily meddlesome. The head of the radius must never be excised in children because this will interfere with the synchronous growth of radius and ulna.

Fractures that are seen a week or longer after injury should be left untreated (except for light splintage).

Following operation the elbow is splinted in 90 degrees of flexion for a week or two and then movements are encouraged.

Fractures of the olecranon

Mechanism of injury

Two types of injury are seen: (1) a comminuted fracture which is due to a direct blow or a fall on the elbow; and (2) a clean transverse break, due to traction when the patient falls onto the hand while the triceps muscle is contracted.

The fracture enters the elbow joint and therefore also damages the articular cartilage. With transverse fractures, the triceps aponeurosis may remain intact, in which case the fracture fragments stay together.

Clinical features

A graze or bruise over the elbow suggests a comminuted fracture; the triceps is intact and the elbow can be extended against gravity. With a transverse fracture there may be a palpable gap and the patient is unable to extend the elbow against resistance.

X-RAY

A properly orientated lateral view is essential to show details of the fracture, as well as the associated joint damage. The position of the radial head should be checked; it may be dislocated.

Treatment

A comminuted fracture with the triceps intact should be treated as a 'bruise'. Many of these patients are old and osteoporotic, and im-mobilizing the elbow will lead to stiffness. The arm is rested in a sling for a week; a further x-ray is obtained to ensure that there is no displacement and the patient is then encouraged to start active movements.

An undisplaced transverse fracture that does not separate when the elbow is x-rayed in flexion can be treated closed. The elbow is immobilized by a cast in about 60 degrees of flexion for 2–3 weeks and then exercises are begun.

Displaced fractures can be held only by splinting the arm absolutely straight – and stiffness in that position would be disastrous. The extensor mechanism should be repaired operatively. The fracture is reduced and held by a long screw or by tension band wiring. If the fragment is very small it may be excised and the triceps re-attached to the ulna. A sling is worn for 3 weeks and movements are then encouraged.

Complications

Stiffness used to be common, but with secure internal fixation and early mobilization the residual loss of movement should be minimal.

Non-union sometimes occurs after inadequate reduction and fixation of a transverse fracture. If elbow function is good, it can be ignored; if not, rigid internal fixation will be needed.

Osteoarthritis The fracture involves the elbow joint, so secondary osteoarthritis may occur if reduction is less than perfect. This can usually be treated symptomatically.

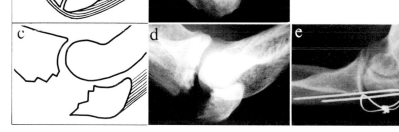
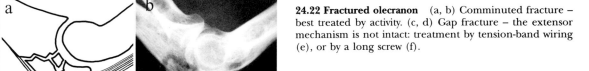
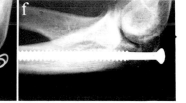

24.22 Fractured olecranon (a, b) Comminuted fracture – best treated by activity. (c, d) Gap fracture – the extensor mechanism is not intact: treatment by tension-band wiring (e), or by a long screw (f).

Dislocations of the elbow

Dislocation of the elbow is fairly common – more so in adults than in children. Injuries are usually classified according to the direction of displacement. However, in 90% of elbow dislocations the radioulnar complex is displaced posteriorly or posterolaterally, often together with fractures of the restraining bony processes.

Mechanism of injury

The cause of posterior dislocation is usually a fall on the outstretched hand with the elbow in extension. Once posterior dislocation has taken place, lateral shift may also occur. Soft tissue disruption is considerable: the anterior capsule and brachialis muscle are torn, the collateral ligaments are stretched or ruptured, and surrounding nerves and vessels may be damaged.

Clinical features

The patient supports his forearm with the elbow in slight flexion. Unless swelling is severe, the deformity is obvious. The bony landmarks (olecranon and epicondyles) are abnormal. It is important to exclude damage to vessels and nerves.

X-RAY

Even though the dislocation is clinically obvious, x-ray films must be taken to exclude an associated fracture.

Treatment

The patient should be fully relaxed under anaesthesia. The surgeon pulls on the forearm while the elbow is slightly flexed. With one hand, sideways displacement is corrected, then the elbow is further flexed while the olecranon process is pushed forward with the thumbs. Unless almost full flexion can be obtained, the olecranon is not in the trochlear groove. After reduction, the elbow should be put through a full range of movement to see whether it is stable. In addition, an x-ray is obtained (1) to confirm that the joint is reduced and (2) to disclose any associated fractures.

The arm is held in a collar and cuff with the elbow flexed above 90 degrees. After 1 week the patient gently exercises his elbow; at 3 weeks he discards the collar and cuff. Elbow movements are allowed to return spontaneously and are never forced.

Complications

Complications are fairly common; some are potentially so serious that the patient with a

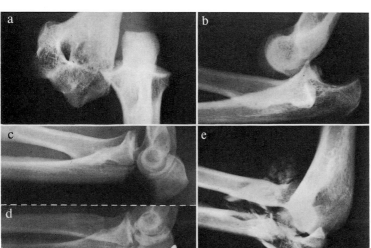

24.23 Elbow dislocations   (a, b) The usual uncomplicated dislocation.

(c) Forward dislocation with fractured olecranon; this needs (d) reduction, with stabilization of the olecranon. (e) Sideswipe fracture-dislocation.

dislocation or a fracture-dislocation of the elbow must be observed with the closest attention.

EARLY

Vascular injury The brachial artery may be damaged. Absence of the radial pulse is a warning. If there are other signs of ischaemia, this should be treated as an emergency. Splints must be removed and the elbow should be straightened somewhat. If there is no improvement, an arteriogram is performed; the brachial artery may have to be explored.

Nerve injury The median or ulnar nerve is sometimes injured. Spontaneous recovery usually occurs after 6–8 weeks.

Associated fractures are fairly common:

1. Small flakes off the coronoid need no special treatment.
2. An avulsed medial epicondyle may become trapped in the joint; this usually requires operative retrieval of the fragment and fixation with a Kirschner wire.
3. Head of radius. The dislocation should first be reduced; 3 weeks later, unless the fragments are in satisfactory position, the radial head is best excised.
4. Olecranon process. This fractures with the rare forward dislocation of the elbow; 2 cm of the olecranon is left behind as a separate fragment. Open reduction with internal fixation is the best treatment.
5. Side-swipe fracture-dislocation. Typically, this occurs when a car-driver's elbow, protruding through the window, is struck by another car. The result is forward dislocation with fractures of any or all of the bones. It is best to reduce the dislocation first, then hold it reduced in a split plaster, and treat the fractures when the joint becomes stable.

LATE

Myositis ossificans Heterotopic bone formation may occur in the damaged soft tissues in front of the joint. In former years this was a fairly common complication, usually associated with forceful reduction and overenthusiastic passive movement of the elbow (Kini, 1940). Nowadays it is rarely seen, but it is as well to be alert for signs such as excessive pain and tenderness, and tardy recovery of active movements. X-ray may show soft-tissue ossification 4–6 weeks after injury. If the condition is suspected, exercises are stopped and the elbow is splinted in comfortable flexion until pain subsides; gentle active movements are then begun. Anti-inflammatory drugs may help to reduce stiffness.

Calcification of the capsule or ligaments is fairly common. It occurs much later than myositis and is not painful, but it does restrict movement somewhat.

Unreduced dislocation A dislocation may not have been diagnosed; or only the backward displacement corrected, leaving the olecranon process still displaced sideways. Up to 6 weeks from injury, manipulative reduction is worth attempting but care is needed to avoid fracturing one of the bones. Other than this, there is no satisfactory treatment. Either the condition can be left, in the hope that the elbow will regain a useful range of movement, or the patient can be offered an arthrodesis or an arthroplasty.

Recurrent dislocation If this occurs, any loose bodies in the elbow should first be removed; then the lateral ligament and capsule are repaired or reattached to the lateral condyle. A plaster with the elbow at 90 degrees is worn for 4 weeks.

Dislocation of the radial head

Isolated dislocation of the radial head is rare in adults; when it is seen, one should always suspect a concurrent fracture of the ulna. If x-rays show that the proximal radius is dome-shaped instead of flat, the dislocation is of long standing; it may be congenital or associated with a short ulna.

If the condition is post-traumatic and the ulna is normal, the dislocation can be reduced by direct pressure over the radial head while the forearm is supinated. The arm is held supine in plaster for 6 weeks.

If there is concomitant shortening of the ulna (e.g. in diaphyseal aclasis), reduction will be impossible, and the abnormality must be accepted.

Pulled elbow

In young children the elbow may be injured by pulling on the arm, usually with the forearm pronated. It is sometimes called subluxation of the radial head; more accurately, it is a subluxation of the orbicular ligament which slips up over the head of the radius into the radio-capitellar joint.

A child aged 3 or 4 years is brought with a painful, dangling arm: there is usually a history of the child being jerked by the arm and crying out in pain. The forearm is held in pronation and any attempt to supinate it is resisted. There are no x-ray changes.

Spontaneous recovery sometimes occurs if the arm is rested in a sling for a few days. A more dramatic cure can be achieved by force-fully supinating and then flexing the elbow; the ligament slips back with a snap.

Fractures of the radius and ulna

Mechanism of injury

Fractures of the shafts of both forearm bones occur quite commonly in road accidents. A twisting force (usually a fall on the hand) produces a spiral fracture with the bones broken at different levels. A direct blow or an angulating force causes a transverse fracture of both bones at the same level. Additional rotation deformity may be produced by the pull of muscles attached to the radius: they are the biceps and supinator muscles to the upper third, the pronator teres to the middle third, and the pronator quadratus to the lower third. Bleeding and swelling of the muscle compartments of the forearm may cause circulatory impairment.

Clinical features

The fracture is usually quite obvious, but the pulse must be felt and the hand examined for circulatory or neural deficit.

X-RAY
Both bones are broken, either transversely and at the same level or obliquely with the radial fracture usually at a higher level. In children, the fracture is often incomplete (greenstick) and only angulated. In adults, displacement may occur in any direction – shift, overlap, tilt or twist.

Treatment

In children closed reduction is usually success-ful and the fragments can be held in a full-length cast, from axilla to metacarpal shafts; this

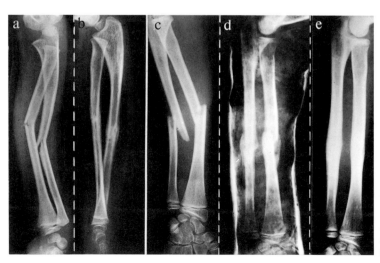

24.24 Fractured radius and ulna in children Green-stick fractures (a) only need correction of angulation (b), and plaster. Complete fractures (c) are harder to reduce; but provided alignment is corrected and held in plaster (d), slight lateral shift remodels with growth (e).

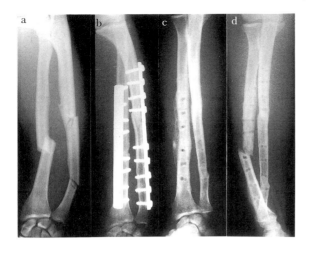

24.25 Fractured radius and ulna in adults (a, b) These fractures are usually treated by internal fixation with sturdy plates and screws. However, removal of the implants is not without risk. (c, d) In this case the radius fractured through one of the screw holes.

is applied with the elbow at 90 degrees and the forearm in the neutral position. The position is checked by x-ray at 2 weeks and, if it is satisfactory, splintage is retained until both fractures are united (usually 6–8 weeks). Throughout this period hand and shoulder exercises are encouraged.

In adults, unless the fragments are in close apposition, reduction is difficult and redisplacement in the cast almost invariable. So predictable is this outcome that most surgeons opt for open reduction and internal fixation from the outset. The fragments are held by plates and screws or intramedullary rods. The deep fascia is left open to prevent a build-up of pressure in the muscle compartments, and only the skin and subcutaneous tissue is sutured. After the operation the arm is kept elevated until the swelling subsides, and during this period active exercises are encouraged. At the end of 10 days the sutures are removed and a full-length cast is applied with the elbow in 90 degrees of flexion. This is retained for at least 6 weeks, mainly to protect against rotary strains. Fracture consolidation is not hastened by internal fixation and the bones still take about 12 weeks to attain strong union.

Open fractures

The forearm and the leg are the commonest sites of compound fractures.

A small wound due to perforation by one of the fragments should be debrided and sutured. Following this, the safest approach is to attempt gentle closed reduction of the fractures and to immobilize the arm in a full-length cast for 2 weeks. If, by then, the wound has healed and there is no sign of infection, open reduction and plating can be carried out in the usual way. Open fractures with significant tissue damage are best treated by immobilization with an external fixator.

Complications

EARLY

Nerve injury Nerve injuries are rarely caused by the fracture, but they may be caused by the surgeon! Exposure of the radius in its proximal third risks damage to the posterior interosseous nerve where it is covered by the superficial part of the supinator muscle. Surgical technique is particularly important here.

Vascular injury Injury to the radial or ulnar artery seldom presents any problem, as the collateral circulation is excellent.

Compartment syndrome Fractures (and operations) of the forearm bones are always associated with swelling of the soft tissues, with the attendant risk of a compartment syndrome. The threat is even greater, and the diagnosis more difficult, if the forearm is wrapped up in plaster. The byword is 'watchfulness'; if there are any signs of circulatory embarrassment, treatment must be prompt and uncompromising (see pp. 544–545).

LATE

Delayed union and non-union Delayed union of one or other bone (usually the ulna) is not uncommon; immobilization may have to be continued beyond the usual time. Non-union will require bone grafting and internal fixation (if this has not already been applied).

Malunion With closed reduction there is always a risk of malunion, resulting in angulation

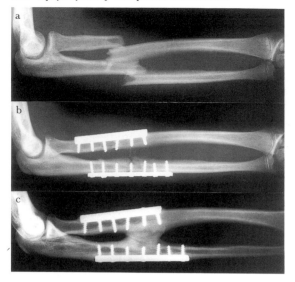

24.26 Fractured radius and ulna – cross-union If the interosseous membrane is severely damaged, even successful plating (a, b) cannot guarantee that cross-union will not occur (c).

or rotational deformity of the forearm, cross-union of the fragments, or shortening of one of the bones and disruption of the distal radio-ulnar joint. If pronation or supination is severely restricted, and there is no cross-union, mobility may be improved by excising the distal end of the ulna.

Iatrogenic Plating the radius and ulna is reasonably straightforward, but removing the plates may be quite difficult; if left to a junior the complication rate is considerable (Langkamer and Ackroyd, 1990).

Fractures of one forearm bone only

Fracture of the radius alone or the ulna alone is uncommon and usually caused by a direct blow. It is important for two reasons. (1) An associated dislocation may be undiagnosed; if only one forearm bone is broken and there is displacement, one or other radioulnar joint must be dislocated; as a precaution the entire forearm must always be x-rayed. (2) Non-union

is liable to occur unless it is realized that one bone takes just as long to consolidate as two.

Clinical features

Ulnar fractures are easily missed – even on x-ray. If there is local tenderness, a further x-ray a few days later is wise.

X-RAY
The fracture may be anywhere in the radius or ulna. The fracture line is transverse and displacement is slight. In children, the intact bone sometimes bends without actually breaking (Borden, 1975).

Treatment

Ulnar fractures are rarely displaced. With radial fractures there may be rotary displacement; to achieve reduction the forearm usually needs to be supinated for upper third fractures, neutral for middle third fractures and pronated for lower third fractures.

With an isolated fracture of the ulna, a forearm brace leaving the elbow free is usually sufficient (Pollock et al., 1983). However, with an isolated radial fracture a complete plaster, to include the elbow and the wrist joints, is needed, exactly as though both forearm bones were broken. It may be 12 weeks before consolidation is complete.

NOTE Because one bone is intact, the ends of the broken bone may be slightly sprung apart and union is liable to be delayed; for this reason many surgeons prefer internal fixation for single-bone fractures, though even then it is unsafe to resume manual work without the protection of an above-elbow splint which prevents rotation.

Fracture-dislocations of the forearm

When a single forearm bone is fractured, there is liable to be a dislocation of either the proximal or the distal radioulnar joint. These two types of injury are best known by their Italian eponyms, *Monteggia* and *Galeazzi*.

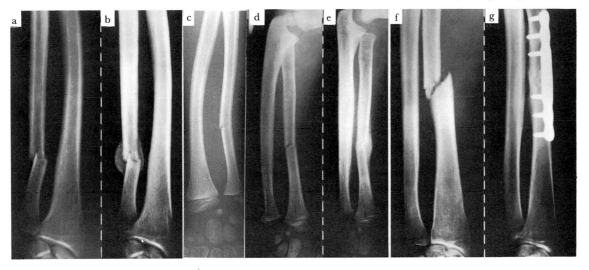

24.27 Fracture of one forearm bone A fracture of the ulna alone (a) usually joins satisfactorily (b). In children the intact radius may be bowed (c). Fracture of the radius alone in a child (d) may join in plaster (e), but in adults a fractured radius (f) is better treated by plating (g).

Monteggia fracture

The injury described by Monteggia in the early nineteenth century was a fracture of the proximal third of the ulna and dislocation of the radial head. Nowadays it is accepted that the ulnar fracture can be at any level.

Mechanism of injury

Usually the cause is a fall on the hand; if at the moment of impact the body is twisting, its momentum may forcibly pronate the forearm. The radial head dislocates forwards and the upper third of the ulna fractures and bows forwards. Sometimes the causal force is hyperextension.

Clinical features

The ulnar deformity is usually obvious but the dislocated head of radius is masked by swelling. A useful clue is pain and tenderness on the lateral side of the elbow,

The wrist and hand should be examined for signs of injury to the radial nerve.

X-RAY

In the usual case, the head of the radius (which normally points directly to the capitulum) is dislocated forwards, and there is a fracture of the upper third of the ulna with forward bowing. Sometimes radial dislocation is associated with an olecranon fracture. Occasionally the radial head dislocates posteriorly and the ulnar fracture bows backwards ('backward Monteggia').

With isolated fractures of the ulna, it is essential always to x-ray the elbow.

Treatment

The clue to successful treatment is to restore the length of the fractured ulna; only then can the dislocated joint be fully reduced. In children it is sometimes possible to do this by manipulation, but in adults open reduction and plating is preferable. If the radial head can be reduced closed, so much the better; if not, this too must be treated by operation. The arm is immobilized in plaster with the elbow flexed (to prevent redislocation of the radial head) for 6 weeks. Thereafter, active movements are encouraged.

Complications

Malunion of the ulna causes little disability but, unless the ulna has been perfectly reduced, the radial head remains dislocated and limits elbow flexion. In children, no treatment is advised. In adults, excision of the head of the radius may be needed.

Non-union of the ulna should be treated by bone grafting. If the radial head is dislocated it should be excised.

Galeazzi fracture

Mechanism of injury

The usual cause is a fall on the hand; probably a rotation force is superimposed. The radius fractures in its lower third and the inferior radioulnar joint subluxates or dislocates. The injury is an almost exact counterpart of the Monteggia fracture-dislocation.

Clinical features

The Galeazzi fracture is much more common than the Monteggia.

The prominent lower end of the ulna is the striking feature. It is important also to test for an ulnar nerve lesion, which is common.

X-RAY

A transverse or short oblique fracture is seen in the lower third of the radius, with angulation or overlap. The inferior radioulnar joint is subluxated or dislocated.

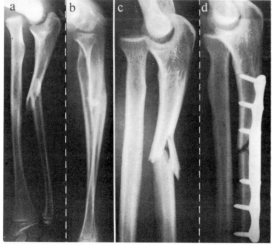

24.28 Fracture-dislocation – Monteggia (a) The ulna is fractured and the head of the radius no longer points to the capitulum; in the child closed reduction and plaster (b) is usually satisfactory. (c) In the adult open reduction and plating (d) is preferred.

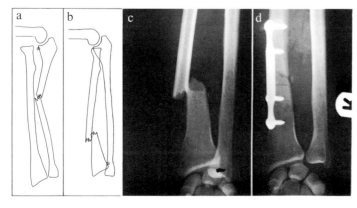

24.29 Fracture dislocation – Galeazzi The diagrams show the contrast between (a) Monteggia and (b) Galeazzi fracture-dislocations. (c, d) Galeazzi type before and after reduction and plating.

Treatment

As with the Monteggia fracture, the important step is to restore the length of the fractured bone. In children, closed reduction is often successful; in adults, reduction is best achieved by open operation and plating of the radius. An x-ray is taken to ensure that the radioulnar joint is reduced. The arm is immobilized in a cast for 6 weeks, after which active movements are encouraged.

III. The wrist and hand

Colles' fracture

The injury that Abraham Colles described in 1814 is a transverse fracture of the radius just above the wrist, with dorsal displacement of the distal fragment. It is the most common of all fractures in older people, the high incidence being related to the onset of postmenopausal osteoporosis. Thus the patient is usually a woman who gives a history of falling on her outstretched hand.

Mechanism of injury

Force is applied in the length of the forearm with the wrist in extension. The bone fractures at the corticocancellous junction and the distal fragment collapses into extension and dorsal displacement.

Colles' fractures are often classified according to whether the ulnar styloid process is also fractured, whether the radioulnar joint is involved and whether the radiocarpal joint is involved (Frykman, 1967). We prefer to consider separately those fractures which involve the radiocarpal joint; the remaining groups are, in the main, treated in the same way and are considered together.

Clinical features

We can recognize this fracture (as Colles did long before radiography was invented) by the 'dinner-fork' deformity, with prominence on the back of the wrist and a depression in front. In patients with less deformity there may only be local tenderness and pain on wrist movements.

X-RAY

There is a transverse fracture of the radius at the corticocancellous junction, and often the ulnar styloid process is broken off. The radial fragment is (1) shifted and tilted backwards, (2) shifted and tilted radially, and (3) impacted. Sometimes the distal fragment is severely comminuted or crushed.

Treatment

If the fracture is undisplaced (or only very slightly displaced), it is splinted in a plaster slab that is wrapped around the dorsum of the forearm and wrist and bandaged firmly in position.

Displaced fractures must be reduced under anaesthesia. The hand is firmly grasped and traction is applied in the length of the bone (sometimes with extension of the wrist to disimpact the fragments); the distal fragment is

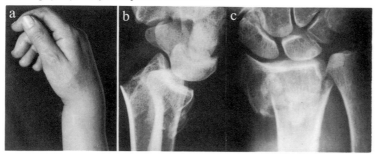

24.30 Colles' fracture   (a) Dinner-fork deformity. (b, c) The fracture is not into the wrist joint: the chief displacements are backwards and radially.

then pushed into place by pressing firmly on the dorsum while manipulating the wrist into flexion, ulnar deviation and pronation. The position is then checked by x-ray. If it is satisfactory, a dorsal plaster slab is applied, extending from just below the elbow to the metacarpal necks and two-thirds of the way round the circumference of the wrist. It is held in position by a crepe bandage. Extreme positions of flexion and ulnar deviation must be avoided; 20 degrees in each direction is adequate.

The arm is kept elevated for the next day or two; shoulder and finger exercises are started as soon as the patient is awake. If the fingers become swollen, cyanosed or painful, there should be no hesitation in splitting the bandage.

At 7–10 days fresh x-rays are taken; redisplacement is not uncommon and is usually treated by re-reduction; unfortunately, even if manipulation is successful, re-redisplacement is common.

The fracture unites in 6 weeks and, even in the absence of radiological proof of union, the slab may safely be discarded and replaced by a temporary crepe bandage.

Severely comminuted and unstable fractures may be impossible to hold in a plaster; for these, external fixation, with proximal pins transfixing the radius and distal pins the bases of second and third metacarpals, is advisable. A device such as the Pennig fixator has the advantage of permitting early wrist movement.

Whatever method of fixation is used, it is of the greatest importance for the patient to be drilled in exercising the free joints regularly.

Complications

EARLY

The circulation in the fingers must be checked; the bandage holding the slab may need to be split or loosened.

Nerve injury is rare, and even compression of the median nerve in the carpal tunnel is surprisingly uncommon. If it does occur, the transverse carpal ligament should be divided so that the carpal tunnel is decompressed.

Reflex sympathetic dystrophy is probably quite common, but fortunately it seldom progresses to the full-blown picture of *Sudeck's atrophy.*

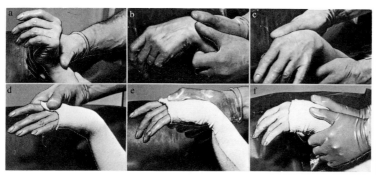

24.31 Colles' fracture   Reduction: (a) disimpaction (not always necessary), (b) pronation and forward shift, (c) ulnar deviation.

Splintage: (d) stockinette, (e) wet plaster slab, (f) slab bandaged on and reduction held till plaster set.

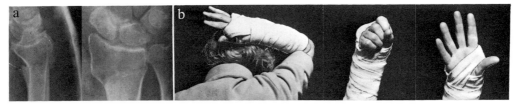

24.32 Colles' fracture   Same case as Fig. 24.30. (a) The post-reduction films are satisfactory. (b) Before going home she is taught these movement and persuaded to practise them regularly.

There may be swelling and tenderness of the finger joints, a warning not to neglect the daily exercises. In about 5% of cases, by the time the plaster is removed the hand is stiff and painful and there are signs of vasomotor instability. X-rays show osteoporosis and there is increased activity on the bone scan. Treatment is discussed on p. 240.

LATE

Malunion is common, either because reduction was not complete or because displacement within the plaster was overlooked. The appearance is ugly, and weakness and loss of rotation may persist. In most cases treatment is not

necessary. Where the disability is severe and the patient relatively young, the lower 2.5 cm of the ulna may be excised to restore rotation, and the radial deformity corrected by osteotomy.

Delayed union and non-union of the radius do not occur, but the ulnar styloid process often joins by fibrous tissue only and remains painful and tender for several months.

Stiffness of the shoulder, from neglect, is a common complication. Stiffness of the wrist may follow prolonged splintage.

Sudeck's atrophy, if it is not reversed, may lead to a stiff, wasted hand with severe trophic changes (see p. 240).

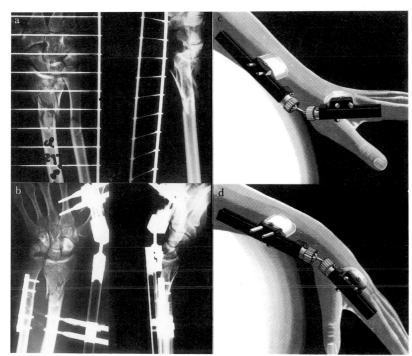

24.33 Comminuted fractures of lower forearm (a) Before and (b) after reduction and external fixation (there was also a fractured lower ulna which was plated). With the Pennig fixator (c, d) movements can be started with the fixator still in place after 2–3 weeks; this reduces the risk of stiffness which otherwise is liable to follow external fixation of these fractures.

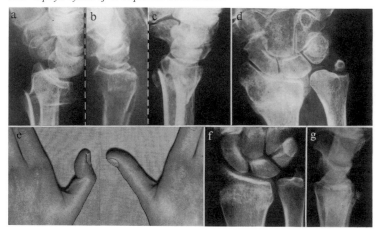

24.34 Colles' fracture Malunion: back-ward shift (a) was reduced (b), but re-curred (c). Slight malunion of radius with non-union of ulnar styloid (d). Delayed rupture of extensor pollicis longus (e) is not a complication of a true Colles' frac-ture, but of this apparently trivial fracture (f, g).

Tendon rupture (of extensor pollicis longus) occasionally occurs a few weeks after an apparently trivial undisplaced fracture of the lower radius. The patient should be warned of the possibility and told that operative treatment is available.

Smith's fracture

Smith (a Dubliner, like Colles) described a similar fracture about 20 years later. However, in this injury the distal fragment is displaced *anteriorly* (which is why it is sometimes called a 'reversed Colles'). It is caused by a fall on the back of the hand.

Clinical features

The patient presents with a wrist injury, but there is no dinner-fork deformity.

X-RAY
There is a fracture through the distal radial metaphysis; a lateral view shows that the distal fragment is displaced and tilted anteriorly – the very opposite of a Colles' fracture.

Treatment The fracture is reduced by traction and extension of the wrist, and the forearm is immobilized in a cast for 6 weeks.

24.35 Smith's fracture (a, b) Note that the displacement of the lower radial fragment is forwards – not backwards as in a Colles' fracture.

Distal forearm fractures in children

The distal radius and ulna are among the commonest sites of childhood fractures. The break may occur through the distal radial physis or in the metaphysis of one or both bones. Metaphyseal fractures are often incomplete or greenstick.

Mechanism of injury

The usual injury is a fall on the outstretched hand with the wrist in extension; the distal fragment is forced posteriorly (this is often called a 'juvenile Colles' fracture'). However, sometimes the wrist is in flexion and the fracture is angulated anteriorly. Lesser force may do no more than buckle the metaphyseal cortex (a type of compression fracture, or torus fracture).

Clinical features

There is usually a history of a fall, though this may be passed off as one of many childhood spills. The wrist is painful, and often quite swollen; sometimes there is an obvious 'dinner-fork' deformity.

X-RAY
The precise diagnosis is made on the x-ray appearances.

Physeal fractures are almost invariably Salter–Harris type 1 or 2, with the epiphysis shifted and tilted backwards and radially (the juvenile counterpart of Colles' fracture). Type V injuries are sometimes diagnosed in retrospect when premature epiphyseal fusion occurs.

Metaphyseal injuries may appear as mere *buckling* of the cortex (easily missed unless appropriate views are obtained), as angulated *greenstick fractures* or as *complete fractures* with

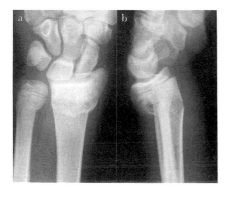

24.36 Distal forearm fractures – children
Fractures are usually greenstick; however, sometimes there is displacement resembling that of a Colles' fracture.

displacement and shortening. If only the radius is fractured, the ulna may be bent though not fractured.

Treatment

Physeal fractures are reduced, under anaesthesia, by pressure on the distal fragment. The arm is immobilized in a full-length cast with the wrist slightly flexed and ulnar deviated, and the elbow at 90 degrees. The cast is retained for 4 weeks. These fractures do not interfere with growth. Even if reduction is not absolutely perfect, further growth and modelling will obliterate any deformity within a year or two. Patients seen more than 2 weeks after injury are best left untreated.

Buckle fractures require no more than 2 weeks in plaster, followed by another 2 weeks of restricted activity.

Greenstick fractures are usually easy to reduce – but apt to redisplace in the cast! Angulation of less than 10 degrees can be accepted. If the deformity is greater, the fracture is reduced by thumb pressure and the arm is immobilized in a full-length cast with the wrist neutral, the forearm supinated (to relax brachioradialis) and the elbow flexed 90 degrees. The cast is changed and the fracture re-x-rayed at 2 weeks; if it has redisplaced a further manipulation can be carried out. The cast is finally discarded after 6 weeks.

Complete fractures can be embarrassingly difficult to reduce – especially if the ulna is intact. The fracture is manipulated in much the same way as a Colles' fracture; the reduction is checked by x-ray and a full-length cast is applied with the wrist neutral and the forearm supinated. After 2 weeks, a check x-ray is obtained; the cast is kept on for 6 weeks.

Complications

EARLY

Forearm swelling and a threatened *compartment syndrome* are prevented by avoiding overforceful or repeated manipulations, splitting the plaster, elevating the arm for the first 24–48 hours and encouraging exercises.

LATE

Malunion as a late sequel is uncommon in children under 10 years of age. Deformity of as much as 30 degrees will straighten out with further growth and remodelling over the next 5 years. This should be carefully explained to the worried parents.

Radioulnar discrepancy Premature fusion of the radial epiphysis may result in bone length disparity and subluxation of the radioulnar joint. If this is troublesome, the distal end of the ulna can be excised.

a starting handle 'kicks back'. The fracture line is transverse, extending laterally from the articular surface of the radius; the fragment, much more than the radial syloid, is often undisplaced.

If there is displacement it is reduced, and the wrist is held in ulnar deviation by a plaster slab round the outer forearm extending from below the elbow to the metacarpal necks. Imperfect reduction may lead to osteoarthritis; therefore if closed reduction is imperfect the fragment should be screwed back, or held with Kirschner wires.

Radiocarpal fractures

Fractures of the distal radius may enter the wrist joint, causing (1) a simple osteoarticular fracture, (2) a comminuted osteoarticular fracture or (3) a fracture-subluxation of the wrist.

Fractured radial styloid

This injury is caused by forced radial deviation of the wrist and may occur after a fall, or when

Comminuted fractures

Instead of the lower radius breaking transversely above the wrist as in a Colles' fracture, there may be a T-shaped fracture into the joint, or the lower radius may be comminuted. Accurate closed reduction is seldom possible, but an attempt should be made to restore the length and alignment of the lower forearm. This is best achieved by ligamentotaxis (traction on the ligaments) using an external fixator. Once the fracture is firm (usually 6–8 weeks) the fixator is removed and wrist movements are

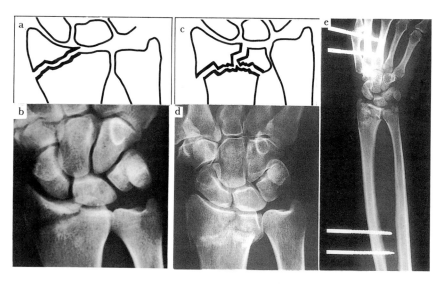

24.37 Other fractures of lower radius   (a, b) Radial styloid fracture (which used to be called a chauffeur's fracture); this needs to be reduced accurately. (c, d) Here the lower ulna is intact (unlike the lower forearm fracture shown in Fig. 24.33 – this is the more usual variety of comminuted lower radial fracture); because it extends into the joint, accurate reduction is important, hence (e) traction via an external fixator.

encouraged; with the Pennig appliance, wrist movements can begin while the fixator is still in place.

Volar fracture-subluxation (Barton's fracture)

This injury, sometimes mistaken for a Smith's fracture, differs from the latter in that the fracture line runs obliquely across the volar lip of the radius into the wrist joint; the distal fragment is displaced anteriorly, carrying the carpus with it. Because the fragment is small and unsupported, the fracture is inherently unstable.

Treatment The fracture can be easily reduced, but it is just as easily redisplaced. Internal fixation, using a small anterior buttress plate, is recommended.

Dorsal fracture-subluxation

This is sometimes called a 'dorsal Barton's fracture'. Here the line of fracture runs obliquely across the dorsal lip of the radius and the carpus is carried posteriorly.

Treatment The fracture is easier to control than the volar Barton's. It is reduced closed and the forearm is immobilized in a cast for 6 weeks. If it redisplaces, open reduction and plating is advisable.

Complications

EARLY

Associated injuries of the carpus must be excluded by careful x-ray examination.

Redisplacement There is a strong tendency for Barton's fracture to redisplace if it is held in a cast; hence our preference for internal fixation.

LATE

Carpal instability Chronic carpal instability may occur after a fracture-subluxation. The diagnosis and management are described on p. 301.

Secondary osteoarthritis may occur long afterwards, but disability is usually not severe.

Carpal injuries

Fractures and dislocations of the carpal bones are common. They vary greatly in type and severity. *It is a mistake to imagine that an isolated fracture is the only injury; the entire carpus suffers,* and, sometimes, long after the fracture has healed, the patient still complains of pain and weakness in the wrist.

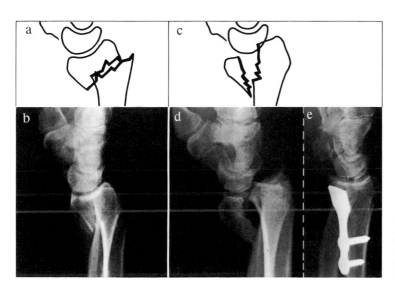

24.38 Fractures with forward displacement (a, b) True reversed Colles' fracture. (c, d) Fracture-dislocation (Barton's fracture), reduced and held (e) with a small anterior plate.

The commonest injuries are: (1) a sprain of the wrist; (2) fracture of a carpal bone (usually the scaphoid); (3) dislocations of the lunate or around it; and (4) subluxations and 'carpal collapse', which may be acute or chronic.

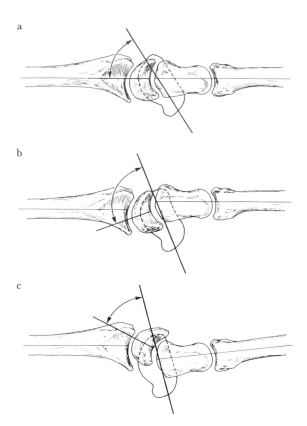

24.39 Carpal instability   (a) The normal wrist. (b) Dorsal intercalated segmental instability (DISI). (c) Volar intercalated segmental instability (VISI).

Clinical features

Following a fall, the patient complains of pain in the wrist. There may be swelling or well-marked deformity of the joint. Tenderness should be carefully localized; undirected prodding will confuse both the patient and the examiner. For scaphoid fractures, the 'jump spot' is in the anatomical snuffbox; for scapholunate injuries, just below Lister's tubercle; for lunate dislocation, in the middle of the wrist; for triquetral injuries, below the head of the ulna; and for hamate fractures, at the base of the hypothenar eminence. Movements are often limited (more by pain than by stiffness) and they may be accompanied by a palpable catch or an audible click.

X-RAYS

X-rays are the key to diagnosis. There are three golden rules: (1) accept only high-quality films; (2) if the initial x-rays are 'normal', treat the clinical diagnosis; and (3) repeat the x-rays 2 weeks later. At the first pass three standard views are obtained: anteroposterior and lateral with the wrist neutral, and an oblique 'scaphoid' view. If these are normal and clinical features suggest a carpal injury, four further views are obtained: anteroposterior x-rays with the wrist in maximum ulnar and maximum radial deviation, and lateral x-rays with the wrist in maximum flexion and extension.

In the anteroposterior x-rays note the shape of the carpus, whether the individual bones are clearly outlined and whether there are any abnormally large gaps suggesting disruption of the ligaments. The scaphoid may be fractured; or it may look squat and foreshortened, with an

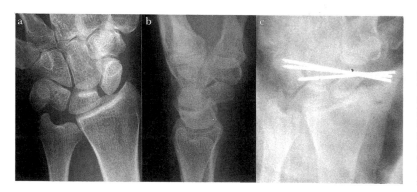

24.40 Carpal injuries Following a 'sprained wrist', this patient developed persistent pain and weakness. X-rays showed (a) radiolunate dissociation and (b) dorsal rotation of the lunate (the characteristic features of DISI). (c) Carpal stability was restored by open reduction and internal fixation with Kirschner wires.

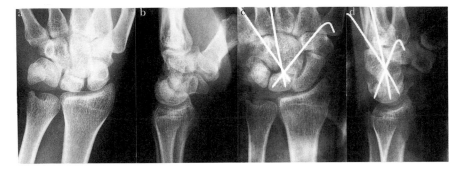

24.41 Carpal injuries This patient, too, had a sprained wrist. The anteroposterior and lateral x-rays (a, b) show foreshortening of the scaphoid and volar rotation of the lunate (VISI). The anatomy was completely restored by open reduction and internal fixation (c, d).

inner circular density (the cortical ring sign) – features of an end-on view when the bone is tilted or subluxated. The lunate is normally quadrilateral in shape, but if it is dislocated it looks triangular.

In the lateral x-ray the axes of the radius, lunate, capitate and third metacarpal are co-linear, and the scaphoid projects at an angle of about 45 degrees to this line. With traumatic instability the linked carpal segments collapse (like the buckled carriages of a derailed train). Two patterns are recognized: dorsal inter-calated segment instability (DISI), in which the lunate is torn from the scaphoid and tilted backwards; and volar intercalated segment instability (VISI), in which the lunate turns towards the palm and the capitate shows a complementary dorsal tilt.

In addition, there may be a flake fracture off the back of a carpal bone (usually the trique-trum).

Special studies are sometimes helpful: a *carpal tunnel view* may show a fractured hook of hamate; *motion studies* in different positions may reveal a subluxation; and a *radioisotope scan* may pinpoint a recent fracture.

Diagnosis and management

'Wrist sprain' should not be diagnosed unless a more serious injury has been definitely ex-cluded. Even with apparently trivial injuries, ligaments are sometimes torn and the patient may later develop carpal instability.

If the x-rays are normal but the clinical signs strongly suggest a carpal injury, a splint or plaster should be applied for 3 weeks, after which time *the x-rays are repeated.* A fracture or dislocation may become more obvious after a few weeks, but a second negative x-ray still does not exclude a serious injury (Dias et al., 1990). The patient should not be released from observation until the symptoms settle down completely.

The more common lesions are dealt with below.

Fractured carpal scaphoid

Scaphoid fractures account for almost 75% of all carpal injuries, but they are rare in the elderly and in children. With unstable fractures there may also be disruption of the scapho-lunate ligaments and dorsal rotation of the lunate.

Mechanism of injury

The scaphoid lies obliquely across the two rows of carpal bones, and is also in the line of loading between the thumb and forearm. The combination of forced carpal movement and compression, as in a fall on the dorsiflexed hand, exerts severe stress on the bone and it is liable to fracture. Most scaphoid fractures are stable; with unstable fractures the fragments may become displaced and this is often associated with carpal instability and dorsal tilting of the lunate (Cooney, Dobyns and Linscheid, 1980).

The blood supply of the scaphoid diminishes proximally (Gelberman and Menon, 1980). This may account for the fact that 30% of middle third fractures, and twice as many of the more proximal fractures, result in avascular necrosis of the proximal fragment.

Clinical features

The appearance may be deceptively normal, but the astute observer can usually detect fullness in the anatomical snuffbox; precisely localized tenderness in the same situation is an important diagnostic feature. Proximal pressure along the axis of the thumb may be painful (Chen, 1989).

X-RAY

Anteroposterior, lateral and oblique views are all essential; often a recent fracture shows only in the oblique view. Usually the fracture line is transverse, and through the narrowest part of the bone (waist), but it may be more proximally situated (proximal pole fracture). Sometimes only the tubercle of the scaphoid is fractured.

It is very important to look for subtle signs of displacement or instability: opening of the fracture line, angulation of the distal fragment, foreshortening of the scaphoid and, sometimes, a DISI pattern in the lateral x-ray.

A few weeks after the injury the fracture may be more obvious; if union is delayed, cavitation appears on either side of the break. Old, un-united fractures have 'hard' borders, making it seem as if there is an extra carpal bone. Abnormal sclerosis of the proximal fragment is pathognomonic of avascular necrosis.

Treatment

Fracture of the scaphoid tubercle needs no splintage and should be treated as a wrist sprain by a crepe bandage and encouraging early movement. Other scaphoid fractures are treated as follows.

An undisplaced fracture needs no reduction and is treated in plaster (see below). But displacement, often minimal, is not uncommon and, though treatment in plaster may be successful, it is better to reduce the fracture openly and to fix it with a compression screw (Cooney, Dobyns and Linscheid, 1980; Herbert, 1990).

Whether or not open reduction is needed, the carpus must be completely immobilized.

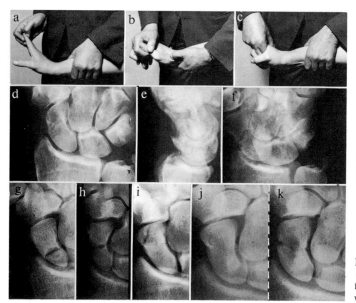

24.42 Scaphoid fractures – diagnosis Clinical signs: (a) pain on dorsiflexion, (b) localized tenderness, (c) pain on gripping.

X-ray signs: the anteroposterior view (d) and the lateral (e) often fail to show the fracture; even in an oblique view (f) it may be difficult to see.

Fracture may be through (g) the proximal pole, (h) the waist, or (i) the tubercle. Even when no fracture is seen at first (j), a repeat film at 2 weeks (k) is worthwhile.

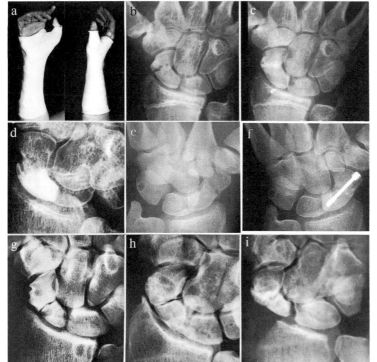

24.43 Scaphoid fractures – treatment and complications (a) Scaphoid plaster – position and extent. (b, c) Before and after treatment: in this case radiological union was visible at 10 weeks.

(d) Avascular necrosis of proximal half; (e) early non-union, treated successfully by (f) inserting a screw.

(g) Established non-union with sclerosis; (h) non-union with localized osteoarthritic changes; (i) osteoarthritis treated by excising the radial styloid.

Plaster is applied from the upper forearm to just short of the metacarpophalangeal joints of the fingers, but incorporating the proximal phalanx of the thumb. The wrist is held dorsiflexed and the thumb forwards in the 'glass-holding' position. The plaster must be carefully moulded into the hollow of the hand, and is not split. It is retained (and if necessary repaired or renewed) for 6 weeks.

After 6 weeks the plaster is removed and the wrist examined clinically and radiologically. If there is no tenderness and the x-ray shows signs of healing, the wrist is left free; complete radiographic union may take several months.

If the wrist is tender, or the fracture still visible on x-ray, the cast is reapplied for a further 6 weeks. At that stage, one of three pictures may emerge. (1) The wrist is painless and the fracture has healed – the cast can be discarded. (2) The x-ray shows bone resorption and cavitation around the fracture – this is delayed healing; union can be hastened by bone grafting. This is done by the palmar approach (Russe, 1960), so as to stabilize the collapsing volar surface. (3) There is established non-union – see below.

Complications

Avascular necrosis The proximal fragment may die, especially with proximal pole fractures, and then at 2–3 months it appears dense on x-ray. Although revascularization and union are theoretically possible, they take years. Bone grafting, as for delayed union (see above) may be successful, in which case the bone, though abnormal, is structurally intact. If the wrist becomes painful, the dead fragment and the radial styloid should be excised.

Non-union By 6 months it may be obvious that the fracture will not unite. Bone grafting may still be attempted, especially in the younger, more vigorous type of patient. If the scaphoid has collapsed, the graft should be so applied as to restore the length and position of the bone;

stability may be enhanced by also inserting a screw.

In older patients, and those who are cometely asymptomatic, non-union may be left untreated. Sometimes a patient is seen for the first time with a 'sprain', but x-rays show an old, un-united fracture with sclerosed edges; 3–4 weeks in plaster may suffice to make him comfortable once again, and no further treatment is required.

Old, established non-union associated with carpal collapse and pain may be treated by (1) periodic splintage of the wrist (if the patient is willing); (2) excision of the radial styloid, to reduce stresses on the scaphoid; or (3) arthrodesis of the wrist.

Osteoarthritis of the wrist may be a sequel to non-union of the scaphoid, especially when there has been avascular necrosis. If the arthritis is localized, excising the radial styloid may help. But once the entire radiocarpal joint is involved this is useless, and if a wrist strap or polythene splint fails to relieve symptoms, the wrist may need to be arthrodesed.

Carpal dislocations, subluxations and instability

The wrist functions as a system of intercalated segments or links, stabilized by the intercarpal ligaments and the scaphoid which acts as a bridge between the proximal and distal rows of the carpus. Fractures and dislocations of the carpal bones, or even simple ligament tears and sprains, may seriously disturb this system so that the links collapse into one of several well-recognized patterns (see p. 301 and p. 602).

Lunate and perilunar dislocations

A fall with the hand forced into dorsiflexion may tear the tough ligaments that normally bind the carpal bones. The lunate usually remains attached to the radius and the rest of the carpus is displaced backwards (*perilunar dislocation*). Usually the hand immediately snaps forwards again but, as it does so, the lunate may be levered out of position to be displaced anteriorly (*lunate dislocation*). Sometimes the scaphoid remains attached to the radius and the force of the perilunar dislocation causes it to fracture through the waist (*trans-scaphoid perilunar dislocation*).

CLINICAL FEATURES   The wrist is painful and swollen and is held immobile. If the carpal tunnel is compressed there may be paraesthesia or blunting of sensation in the territory of the median nerve, and difficulty in flexing the fingers actively.

X-RAY   Most dislocations are perilunar. In the anteroposterior view the carpus is diminished in height and the bone shadows overlap abnormally. One or more of the carpal bones may be fractured (usually the scaphoid). If the lunate is dislocated, it has a characteristic triangular shape instead of the normal quadrilateral appearance.

In the lateral view it is easy to distinguish a perilunar from a lunate dislocation. The *dislocated lunate* is tilted forwards and is displaced in front of the radius, while the capitate and metacarpal bones are in line with the radius. With a perilunar dislocation the lunate is tilted only sightly and is not displaced forwards, and the capitate and metacarpals lie behind the line of the radius (DISI pattern); if there is an associated *scaphoid fracture*, the distal fragment may be tilted anteriorly.

TREATMENT   The surgeon pulls strongly on the dorsiflexed hand. While maintaining traction he slowly palmarflexes the wrist, at the same time squeezing the lunate backwards with his other thumb. These manoeuvres usually effect reduction; they also prevent conversion of a perilunar to a lunate dislocation. A plaster slab is applied holding the wrist neutral.

Reduction is imperative, and if closed reduction fails, or if a later x-ray shows that the wrist has collapsed into the familiar DISI pattern, open reduction is performed. The carpus is exposed by an anterior approach which has the advantage of decompressing the carpal tunnel. While an assistant pulls on the hand, the lunate is levered into place and kept there by a Kirschner wire which is inserted through the

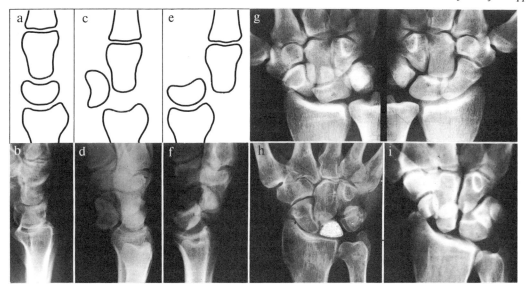

24.44 Lunate and perilunar dislocations (a, b) Lateral view of normal wrist; (c, d) lunate dislocation; (e, f) perilunar dislocation. (g) Anteroposterior view of both wrists with dislocated left lunate – note the triangular appearance. (h) Avascular necrosis following reduction. (i) Associated fracture of scaphoid.

radial styloid, transfixing the lunate and any adjacent carpal bone. If the scaphoid is fractured, this too can be reduced and fixed with a second Kirschner wire. Where possible, the torn soft tissues should be repaired. At the end of the procedure, the wrist is splinted in a plaster slab, which is retained for 3 weeks. Finger, elbow and shoulder exercises are practised throughout this period. The Kirschner wires are usually removed at 6 weeks.

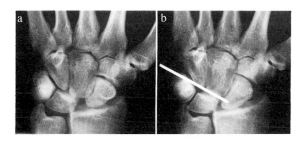

24.45 Subluxation of the scaphoid After a fall this patient had pain and tenderness in the anatomical snuffbox. The scaphoid is intact but (a) there is an obvious gap between the lunate and scaphoid. After open reduction the scaphoid was held in position with a Kirschner wire (b) until capsular healing was complete.

Scapholunate dissociation

A wrist sprain may be followed by persistent pain and tenderness over the dorsum just distal to Lister's tubercle. *X-rays* show an excessively large gap between the scaphoid and the lunate. The scaphoid may appear foreshortened, with a typical cortical ring sign. In the lateral view, the lunate is tilted dorsally and the scaphoid anteriorly (DISI pattern).

TREATMENT Scapholunate instability causes weakness of the wrist and recurrent discomfort. Once recognized, it should be treated by open reduction of the subluxation and Kirschner wire fixation of the scapholunate alignment; the wrist is splinted for 3 weeks.

Triquetrolunate dissociation

A medial sprain followed by weakness of grip and tenderness distal to the head of the ulna should suggest disruption of the triquetrolunate ligaments. *X-rays* show a noticeable gap between the triquetrum and the lunate, with a VISI carpal collapse pattern in the lateral view.

TREATMENT consists of open reduction and Kirschner wire fixation, followed by 3 weeks of splintage.

Complications of traumatic instability

Nerve injury The median nerve may be compressed in the carpal tunnel. This usually improves after reduction but it may still be necessary to divide the transverse carpal ligament in order to decompress the nerve.

Unreduced dislocation of the lunate This presents as a painful stiffish wrist, with median paraesthesia. The lunate should be excised through an anterior incision; it is worth seeing if a Silastic replacement can be fitted into the gap.

Avascular necrosis The lunate may be detached from its blood supply and undergo necrosis. There are no helpful signs until the x-ray shows increased bone density. Treatment is required only if the bone collapses or if secondary osteoarthritis ensues. If wrist movement is good, excision of the lunate and replacement by a Silastic prosthesis is advised; if the wrist is painful and stiff, arthrodesis may be preferable.

Chronic carpal instability Long after a wrist injury – perhaps no more than a 'sprain' – the patient may develop increasing ache and weakness in the wrist. Chronic instability is discussed in Chapter 15.

Fractures and dislocations in the hand

Hand injuries – the commonest of all injuries – are important out of all proportion to their apparent severity, because of the need for perfect function. Nowhere else do painstaking evaluation, meticulous care and dedicated rehabilitation yield greater rewards.

Assessment

If there is skin damage the patient should be examined in a clean environment with the hand displayed on sterile drapes.

A brief but searching history is obtained; often the mechanism of injury will suggest the type and severity of the trauma. The patient's age, occupation and 'handedness' also are important.

Superficial injuries and severe fractures are obvious, but deeper injuries are often poorly disclosed. What is important in the initial examination is to assess: (1) the degree of mutilation; (2) the presence or absence of any deformity; (3) the state of the circulation; (4) nerve function; and (5) tendon function.

X-rays should include at least three views (posteroanterior, lateral and oblique), and with finger injuries the individual digit must be x-rayed.

Treatment

Closed injuries and small wounds can often be treated under regional block anaesthesia. Large wounds and multiple fractures are better dealt with under general anaesthesia.

The guiding principles of treatment are as follows.

SWELLING Swelling must be controlled by elevating the hand and by early and repeated active exercises.

SPLINTAGE Splintage must be kept to a minimum. If it is essential, it is best to attach the injured finger to its neighbour (by strapping or by a double Tubigrip) so that both move as one. Apart from this, only the injured finger should be splinted. In the hand, splintage must always be in the 'position of safety' – with the knuckle joints flexed at least 70 degrees and the finger joints almost straight (James, 1970) (see p. 327). Sometimes an external splint, to be effective, would need to immobilize undamaged fingers; if so, it is preferable to use internal splintage with Kirschner wires. The wires can conveniently be cut short enough to close the skin and are subsequently removed under local anaesthesia.

SKIN DAMAGE Skin damage demands wound toilet followed by suture or skin grafting. Treatment of the skin takes precedence over treatment of the fracture. (Open injuries of the hand are discussed in full on p. 328.)

Metacarpal fractures

The metacarpal bones are vulnerable to blows and falls upon the hand, or the longitudinal force of the boxer's punch. Injuries are common and the bones may fracture at their *base*, in the *shaft* or through the *neck*.

Angular deformity is usually not very marked, and even if it should persist it does not interfere much with function. Rotational deformity, however, is serious. Close your hand with the distal phalanges extended, and look: the fingers converge across the palm to a point above the thenar eminence; malrotation of the metacarpal (or proximal phalanx) will cause that finger to diverge and overlap one of its neighbours. Thus, with a fractured metacarpal it is important to regain normal rotational alignment.

The fourth and fifth metacarpals are more mobile than the second and third, and therefore are better able to compensate for residual angular deformity.

Fractures of the thumb metacarpal usually occur near the base and pose special problems. They are dealt with separately below.

Fractures of the metacarpal shafts

A direct blow may fracture one or several metacarpal shafts transversely, often with associated skin damage. A twisting or punching force may cause a spiral fracture of one or more shafts. There is local pain and swelling, and sometimes a dorsal 'hump'.

TREATMENT Spiral fractures or transverse fractures with slight displacement require no reduction. Splintage also is unnecessary, but a firm crepe bandage may be comforting; this should not be allowed to discourage the patient from active movements of the fingers, which should be practised assiduously.

Transverse fractures with considerable displacement are reduced by traction and pressure. Reduction can be held by a plaster slab extending from the forearm over the fingers (only the damaged ones). The slab is maintained for 3 weeks and the undamaged fingers are exercised. A more elegant method is percutaneous insertion of Kirschner wires across the fracture; alternatively, the distal fragment, after reduction, may be transfixed to the neighbouring undamaged metacarpal by transverse wires.

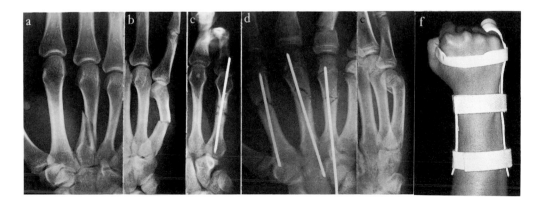

24.46 Metacarpal fractures (a) A spiral fracture of a single metacarpal (especially an 'inboard' one) is adequately held by neighbouring bones and muscles; (b) a displaced fracture (especially an 'outboard' one) is often best held by a wire (c). With several adjacent metacarpals fractured (d), internal fixation may be the only safe way to avoid stiffness. If splintage is used (f), only the damaged ray should be immobilized.

If the fracture is stable, no external splint is necessary and early movements are encouraged.

Oblique fractures are liable to rotate; they should be perfectly reduced (preferably open) and fixed with transverse wires.

Fractures of the metacarpal neck

A blow may fracture the metacarpal neck, usually of the fifth finger (the 'boxer's fracture') and occasionally one of the others. There may be local swelling, with flattening of the knuckle. X-rays show a transverse fracture with volar angulation of the distal fragment.

TREATMENT   In the fifth metacarpal, angulation of up to 20 degrees can be accepted but rotation must be fully corrected. The finger is held in flexion in a gutter plaster extending from below the elbow to the proximal finger joint; splintage can usually be removed after 10 days.

In the index finger, deformity should always be reduced; so, too, for the ring and little fingers if deformity is greater than 20 degrees. The reduction can be held by a plaster slab which extends from the forearm to the proximal finger joint; however, if the fracture tends to redisplace, it is better treated by percutaneous Kirschner wire fixation.

Fractures of the metacarpal base

Excepting fractures of the thumb metacarpal, these are stable injuries which can usually be treated by ensuring that rotation is correct and then splinting the digit in a volar slab extending from the forearm to the proximal finger joint. The splint is retained for 3 weeks and exercises are then encouraged.

Fractured base of thumb

A boxer may, while punching, sustain a fracture of the first metacarpal base. Localized swelling and tenderness are found, and x-ray shows a transverse fracture about 6 mm distal to the carpometacarpal joint, with outward bowing and usually impaction.

TREATMENT   To reduce the fracture, the surgeon pulls on the abducted thumb and, by levering the metacarpal outwards against his own thumb, corrects the bowing. A firm crepe bandage usually suffices to prevent redisplacement, but if the fracture feels unstable a plaster slab is applied, extending from the forearm to just short of the interphalangeal thumb joint; the thumb is in the position of function where the index finger can make pulp-to-pulp contact with it. The slab is removed after 3 weeks and movement usually recovers rapidly.

Bennett's fracture-dislocation

This fracture, too, occurs at the base of the first metacarpal bone and is commonly due to punching; but the fracture is oblique, extends into the carpometacarpal joint and is unstable. The thumb looks short and the carpometacarpal region swollen. X-rays show that a small triangular fragment has remained in contact with the medial half of the trapezium, while the remainder of the thumb has subluxated proximally.

TREATMENT   It is widely supposed (with little evidence) that perfect reduction is essential. It should, however, be attempted and can usually be achieved by pulling on the thumb, abducting it and extending it. Reduction can then be held in one of two ways: plaster or internal fixation.

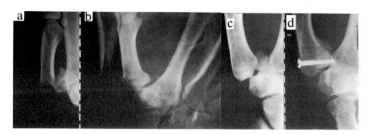

24.47 Fractures of the first metacarpal base A transverse fracture (a) can be reduced and held in plaster (b). Bennett's fracture-dislocation (c) is best held with a small screw (d).

Plaster may be applied with a felt pad over the fracture, and the first metacarpal held abducted and extended (usually best achieved by *flexing* the metacarpophalangeal joint). If x-ray shows that perfect reduction is being held, the plaster is worn for 4 weeks; otherwise the method is abandoned.

Internal fixation is usually the method of choice; it can be achieved by inserting a small screw, or by driving short lengths of Kirschner wire through the metacarpal base (bypassing the fracture) into the carpus; the protruding ends are incorporated in a small plaster slab. After 3 weeks the slab is removed and the wires are pulled out.

Metacarpal fractures in children

Metacarpal fractures are less common in children than in adults. In general they also present fewer problems: the vast majority can be treated by manipulation and plaster splintage; angular deformities will almost always be remodelled with further growth. However, rotational alignment is as important as it is in adults.

Bennett's fracture is rare; but when it does occur it usually requires open reduction. This is, by definition, a Salter–Harris type III frac-ture-separation of the physis; it must be accurately reduced and fixed with a Kirschner wire.

Fractures of the phalanges

The fingers are usually injured by direct violence, and there may be considerable swelling or open wounds. Injudicious treatment may result in a stiff finger – which, in some cases, can be worse than no finger.

Fractures of the proximal and middle phalanges

The phalanx usually fractures transversely, often with forward angulation which may damage the flexor tendon sheath. Fractures at either end of the phalanx may enter the joint; stiffness is the main threat, and if the fracture is displaced the finger may also be deformed.

TREATMENT   Undisplaced fractures can be treated by 'functional splintage'. The finger is strapped to its neighbour ('buddy strapping')

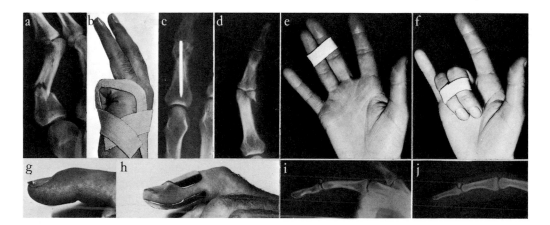

24.48 Phalangeal fractures   Fractured proximal phalanx (a) held reduced by strapping in flexion (b), or with a wire (c). A fracture into a joint (d) can be treated either by internal fixation or by movement with the finger strapped to its neigbour (e, f).
Mallet finger (g) treated by a splint (h); this is adequate when the bony fragment (if any) is small (i), but a large fragment (j) needs fixation.

and movements are encouraged from the outset. Splintage is retained for 2–3 weeks, but during this time it is wise to check the position by x-ray in case displacement has occurred.

Displaced fractures must be reduced and immobilized. The fracture is reduced by pulling on the bent finger and thumbing the phalanx straight. *Above all, it is essential to check for rotational correction* by (1) noting the convergent position of the finger when the metacarpophalangeal joint is flexed, and (2) checking to see that the fingernails are all in the same plane. The flexed position must be maintained to hold reduction, and this is best achieved by applying a forearm cast which ends in the palm but has a distal outrigger splint that supports the finger in about 80 degrees of flexion at the metacarpophalangeal joint and enough flexion at the interphalangeal joints to prevent redisplacement of the fracture. In this way, none of the other fingers is immobilized unnecessarily. The splint is retained for 3 weeks, and buddy strapping is continued for another 3 weeks. An alternative method (not quite as good, because it immobilizes the other fingers) is simply to place a rolled bandage in the palm and hold the flexed finger over it with a crepe bandage; after 10 days the bandage is removed and a removable posterior slab is substituted; it is taken off several times a day while the patient exercises the finger (protecting the fracture with his other hand).

Unstable phalangeal fractures (some experts would say all displaced phalangeal fractures) may be treated by internal fixation using crossed Kirschner wires or AO miniscrews.

Fractures of the terminal phalanx

The terminal phalanx may be struck by a hammer, or caught in a door, and the bone shattered. The fracture is disregarded and treatment is focused on controlling swelling and regaining movement.

Fractures into joints

Any finger joint may be injured by a direct blow (often the overlying skin is damaged), or by an angulation force, or by the straight finger being forcibly stubbed. The affected joint is swollen, tender and too painful to move. X-rays may show that a fragment of bone has been sheared off or avulsed.

TREATMENT   If the fragment is not displaced, it is best to disregard the fracture, to strap the finger to its neighbour and to concentrate on regaining movement.

If the fracture is displaced, there is a risk of permanent angular deformity. The fracture should be anatomically reduced by open operation (through a dorsal incision, splitting the extensor tendon) and fixed with small Kirschner wires. The finger is splinted for only a few days and then carefully supervised movements are commenced.

Mallet finger (see also Chapter 16)

The extensor tendon may avulse a fragment from the base of the terminal phalanx, thus eliminating active extension of the distal interphalangeal joint.

TREATMENT   With the bedmaking type of injury only a tiny flake is avulsed and treatment in a splint for 6 weeks is satisfactory. With a stubbing injury, such as mis-catching a cricket ball, the avulsed fragment is much larger; unless it reduces accurately with hyperextension, the fragment should be fixed back with a small piece of Kirschner wire; otherwise, painful stiffness is likely to develop.

Dislocations in the hand

Carpometacarpal

The thumb is most frequently affected and clinically the injury then resembles a Bennett's fracture-dislocation; but x-rays reveal proximal subluxation of the first metacarpal bone without a fracture. The dislocation is easily reduced by traction, but reduction is unstable and can be held only by one of the methods used for a Bennett's fracture-dislocation: plaster, or Kirschner wires driven through the metacarpal into the carpus. Splintage is discontinued after 3 weeks.

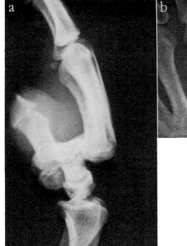
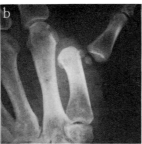
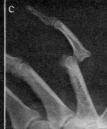
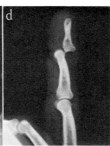

24.49 Dislocations (a) The motorcyclist's injury – carpometacarpal dislocation; (b) metacarpophalangeal dislocation in the thumb occasionally buttonholes and needs open reduction; (c, d) interphalangeal dislocations are easily reduced and easily missed if not x-rayed.

Dislocations at the other carpometacarpal joints occur typically when a motorcyclist, holding the handlebars, strikes an object; one hand is driven backwards, leaving the carpus, thumb and forearm projecting forwards. Closed manipulation is usually successful and a protective slab for 6 weeks restores stability.

Metacarpophalangeal

Usually the thumb is affected, sometimes the fifth finger, and rarely the other fingers. A hyperextension force may dislocate the phalanx backwards, and the capsule and muscle insertions in front of the joint may be torn. If the metacarpal head has been forced like a button through the hole, closed reduction may be impossible.

Closed reduction is first attempted by pulling on the thumb and levering the phalanx forwards. If this fails, the joint is exposed from behind and, while strong traction is applied, the metacarpal head is levered into place. The joint is then strapped in the flexed position for 1 week.

Interphalangeal

Backward dislocation at the distal joint is common and is easily reduced by pulling. The joint may be strapped flexed for a few days.

Sprains of the finger joints

Partial or complete tears of the ligaments are common and usually due to forced angulation at the joint. Healing is often slow and the joint remains slightly thickened for months.

Milder injuries require no treatment; with more severe sprains the finger should be splinted for a week or two. But the patient should be warned that the joint is likely to remain swollen and slightly painful for 6–12 months.

'Gamekeeper's thumb' (or 'skier's thumb')

In former years, gamekeepers who twisted the necks of little animals ran the risk of tearing the ulnar collateral ligament of the thumb metacarpophalangeal joint. Nowadays this injury is seen in skiers who fall onto the extended thumb, forcing it into hyperabduction. A small flake of bone may be pulled off at the same time.

If the ulnar collateral ligament ruptures completely (usually at its proximal attachment) it may not repair even with several weeks in plaster. If examination shows that the tear is complete, immediate operative repair is advised. A partial tear can be treated by plaster splintage for 2–3 weeks.

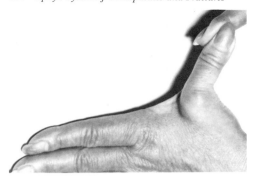

24.50 Gamekeeper's thumb The ulnar collateral ligament of the metacarpophalangeal joint is completely ruptured; immediate repair is advisable.

A neglected tear leads to weakness of pinch, which is probably best treated by arthrodesis, although, in early cases without articular damage, stability may be restored by advancing the insertion of adductor pollicis to the base of the phalanx, or by using a free tendon graft, or by reinforcing the ligament with the tendon of extensor pollicis brevis.

References and further reading

Bannister, G.C., Wallace, W.A., Stableforth, P.G. and Hutson, M.A. (1989) The management of acute acromioclavicular dislocation. *Journal of Bone and Joint Surgery* **71B**, 848–850

Barton, N. (1977) Fractures of the phalanges of the hand. *Hand* **9**, 1–10

Borden, S. (1975) Roentgen recognition of acute plastic bowing of the forearm in children. *American Journal of Roentgenology* **125**, 524–530

Brown, R.F. and Morgan, R.G. (1971) Intercondylar T-shaped fractures of the humerus. *Journal of Bone and Joint Surgery* **53B**, 425–428

Burrows, H.J. (1951) Tenodesis of subclavius in the treatment of recurrent dislocation of the sterno-clavicular joint. *Journal of Bone and Joint Surgery* **33B**, 240–243

Chen, S.C. (1989) The scaphoid compression test. *Journal of Hand Surgery* **14B**, 323–325

Cooney, W.P. III, Dobyns, J.H. and Linscheid, R.L. (1980) Fractures of the scaphoid: a rational approach to management. *Clinical Orthopaedics and Related Research* **149**, 90–97

DeLee, J.C., Wilkins, K.E., Rogers, L.F. and Rockwood, C.A. (1980) Fracture-separation of the distal humeral epiphysis. *Journal of Bone and Joint Surgery* **62A**, 46–51

Dias, J.J., Thompson, J., Barton, N.J. and Gregg, P.J. (1990) Suspected scaphoid fractures. *Journal of Bone and Joint Surgery* **72B**, 98–101

Fisk, G.R. (1980) An overview of injuries of the wrist. *Clinical Orthopaedics and Related Research* **149**, 137–144

Frykman, G. (1967) Fracture of the distal radius incuding sequelae. *Acta Orthopaedica Scandinavica* **38**, suppl. 108, 1–155

Gelberman, R.H. and Menon, J. (1980) The vascularity of the scaphoid bone. *Journal of Hand Surgery* **5**, 508–513

Herbert, T.J. (1990) *The Fractured Scaphoid*, Quality Medical Pubishing, St Louis MO

Hill, H.A. and Sachs, M.D. (1940) The grooved defect of the humeral head. A frequently unrecognized complication of dislocations of the shoulder joint. *Radiology* **35**, 690–700

James, J.I.P. (1970) Common single errors in the management of hand injuries. *Proceedings of the Royal Society of Medicine* **63**, 69–71

Kini, M.G. (1940) Dislocation of the elbow and its complications. *Journal of Bone and Joint Surgery* **22**, 107–117

Kristiansen, B. and Kofoed, H. (1987) External fixation of displaced fractures of the proximal humerus. *Journal of Bone and Joint Surgery* **69B**, 643–646

Kristiansen, B., Ulrich, L.S., Andersen, M.D. et al. (1988) The Neer classification of fractures of the proximal humerus. *Skeletal Radiology* **17**, 420–422

Langkamer, V.G. and Ackroyd, C.E. (1990) Removal of forearm plates. *Journal of Bone and Joint Surgery* **72B**, 601–604

MacNicol, M.F. (1987) Elbow injuries in children. *Current Orthopaedics* **1**, 412–419

Mikic, Z. (1975) Galeazzi fracture-dislocation. *Journal of Bone and Joint Surgery* **57A**, 1071–1080

Neer, C.S. II (1970) Displaced proximal humeral fractures. I. Classification and evaluation. *Journal of Bone and Joint Surgery* **52A**, 1077–1089

Neer, C.S. II and Foster, C.R. (1980) Inferior capsular shift for involuntary inferior and multidirectional instability of the shoulder. *Journal of Bone and Joint Surgery* **62A**, 897–908

Piggot, J., Graham, H.K. and McCoy, G.F. (1986) Supracondylar fractures of the humerus in children. *Journal of Bone and Joint Surgery* **68B**, 577–583

Pollock, F.H., Pankovich, A.M., Prieto, J.J. and Lorenz, M. (1983) The isolated fracture of the ulnar shaft. *Journal of Bone and Joint Surgery* **65A**, 339–342

Rosson, J.W., Petley, G.W. and Shearer, J.R. (1991) Bone structure after removal of internal fixation plates. *Journal of Bone and Joint Surgery* **73B**, 65–67

Rowe, C.R., Pierce, D.S. and Clark, J.G. (1973) Voluntary dislocation of the shoulder. *Journal of Bone and Joint Surgery* **55A**, 445–460

Russe, O. (1960) Fracture of the carpal navicular: diagnosis, non-operative treatment and operative treatment. *Journal of Bone and Joint Surgery* **42A**, 759–768

Smith, R.J. (1977) Post-traumatic instability of the metacarpophalangeal joint of the thumb. *Journal of Bone and Joint Surgery* **59A**, 14–21

Stableforth, P.G. (1984) Four-part fractures of the neck of the humerus. *Journal of Bone and Joint Surgery* **66B**, 104–108

Injuries of the spine   25

Spinal injuries carry a double threat: damage to the vertebral column and damage to the neural tissues. The full extent of the injury may appear from the outset as a *fait accompli*. However, there is always the fear that movement may cause or aggravate the neural lesion; hence the importance of defining these injuries as stable or unstable.

Stable and unstable injuries

As applied to the acute lesion, these terms have specific meanings: a stable injury is one in which the vertebral components will not be displaced by normal movements so that an undamaged cord is not in danger; an unstable injury is one in which further displacement may occur.

In assessing spinal stability, three structural elements must be considered (Denis, 1983): the posterior osseoligamentous complex consisting of the pedicles, facet joints, posterior bony arch, and interspinous and supraspinous ligaments; a middle component consisting of the posterior third of the vertebral body, the posterior part of the intervertebral disc and the posterior longitudinal ligament; and the anterior column made up of the anterior two-thirds of the vertebral body, the anterior part of the intervertebral disc and the anterior longitudinal ligament. Denis has suggested that, for instability to occur, both posterior and middle elements have to be disrupted; this is true particularly of the thoracolumbar spine.

Fortunately, only 10% of spinal fractures are unstable and less than 5% are associated with cord damage,

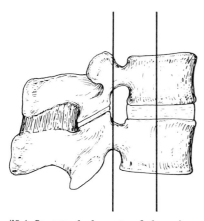

25.1 Structural elements of the spine
The vertical lines show Denis' classification of the structural elements of the spine. The three elements are: the posterior complex, the middle component and the anterior column. This concept is particularly useful in assessing the stability of lumbar injuries.

Mechanism of injury

In the lumbar spine resisted muscle effort may avulse transverse processes; in the cervical spine usually the seventh spinous process is avulsed ('clay-shoveller's fracture'). Avulsion fractures should alert the doctor to inspect the x-ray films with more than usual care so as to exclude other and more important injuries; but in themselves these 'muscle injuries' require no splintage and are best treated by activity.

Indirect injuries usually occur when the spinal column collapses in its vertical axis, typically in a fall from a height or when someone is trapped under a cave-in; the direction of force at any level of the spine is determined by the position of the vertebral column at the moment of impact. The flexible cervical and lumbar segments may also be injured by violent free movements of the neck or trunk. The important types of displacement are: (1) hyperextension; (2) flexion; (3) axial compression; (4) flexion and compression combined with posterior distraction; (5) flexion combined with rotation and shear; and (6) horizontal translation.

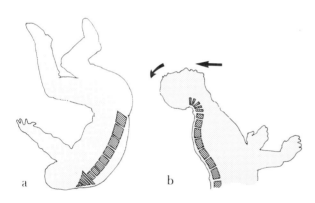

25.2 Mechanism of injury   The spine is usually injured in one of two ways: (a) a fall onto the head or the back of the neck; and (b) a blow on the forehead, which forces the neck into hyperextension.

Fractures may occur with minimal force in osteoporotic or pathological bone.

Hyperextension (combined distraction and extension)

Hyperextension is rare in the thoracolumbar region but quite common in the neck; a blow on the face or the forehead forces the head backwards and there is nothing to restrain the occiput until it strikes the upper part of the back. The anterior ligaments and the disc may be damaged or the neural arch may be fractured. Usually the injury is stable, but fracture of the pedicle of C2 ('hangman's fracture') is often unstable.

Flexion

If the posterior ligaments remain intact, forced flexion will crush the vertebral body into a wedge; this is a stable injury and is far the most common type of vertebral fracture. If the posterior ligaments are torn the injury is unstable and the upper vertebral body may tilt forward on the one below; this type of subluxation is often missed in the neck because by the time an x-ray is taken the vertebrae have fallen back into place.

Axial displacement (compression)

A vertical force acting on a straight segment of the cervical or lumbar spine will produce axial compression. The nucleus pulposus splits the vertebral end-plate and fractures the vertebra vertically; with greater force, disc material is forced into the vertebral body, causing a 'burst' fracture. Because the posterior elements are intact, this is by definition a stable injury. However, bony fragments may be driven backwards into the spinal canal and it is this that makes these fractures dangerous; there is a high incidence of neurological damage.

Flexion, compression and posterior distraction

The combination of flexion with anterior compression and posterior distraction may disrupt the middle vertebral complex as well as the posterior complex. Bony fragments and disc material may be displaced into the spinal canal. In contrast to pure compressive fractures, this is an unstable injury with a high risk of progression (Ferguson and Allen, 1984).

Excessive lateral flexion may cause compression of one half of the vertebral body and distraction of the lateral and posterior elements on the opposite side. If the facet and pedicle are crushed, the lesion is unstable.

Flexion-rotation

Most serious injuries of the spine are due to a combination of flexion, rotation and shear. The ligaments and joint capsules are strained to the limit; they may tear, the facets may fracture or the top of one vertebra may be sliced off. The result is a forward shift or dislocation of the vertebra above, with or without concomitant bone damage. All fracture-dislocations are unstable and there is a high risk of neurological damage.

Horizontal translation

The vertebral column is 'sliced through' and the upper or lower segments may be displaced anteroposteriorly or laterally. The lesion is unstable and there is a high incidence of neural damage.

Healing

Fracture-dislocations heal by the formation of new bone and fusion of the damaged vertebrae. Thus, the spine will eventually stabilize itself. However, in pure ligamentous injuries some degree of instability may persist. Flexion injuries in which there is both compression of the vertebral body and disruption of posterior ligaments may result in progressive deformity.

Diagnosis

Every patient who has suffered a major accident should be fully examined for spinal injury. In order to do this, his clothes may have to be cut from his body with the least possible disturbance of position. With an unconscious patient, awareness is everything; the force producing a serious head injury may also injure the neck and such injury should always be assumed until the contrary is proved. Any complaint of pain or stiffness in the neck or back should be taken seriously, even if the patient is walking or moving without apparent difficulty. Enquire about numbness, paraesthesia or weakness in the limbs.

The history of the accident may contain important clues: a fall from a height, a diving injury, head-on collisions, a cave-in or a ceiling collapsing on the patient, or a sudden jerk of the neck following a rear-end collision (whiplash injury) – these are all common causes of spinal damage.

Bruising of the face or a superficial abrasion of the forehead suggest a hyperextension force. The neck may be held skew, or the patient may be supporting the head with his hands. With the patient supine, the chest and abdomen can be examined for associated injuries. Next the limbs are quickly examined for evidence of neurological damage. To examine the back, the patient is turned onto one side with extreme care using a log-rolling technique. Bruising indicates the probable level of injury.

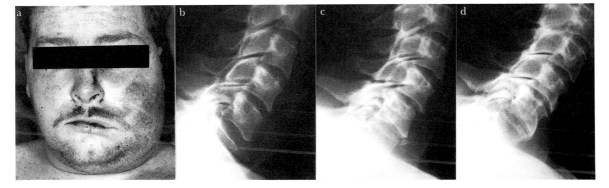

25.3 Cervical spine injuries (a) With severe facial bruising always suspect a hyperextension injury of the neck. (b) X-ray in this case showed a barely visible flake of bone anteriorly at the C6/7 disc space. (c) One month later the traction fracture at C6/7 was more obvious, as was the disc lesion at C5/6. (d) A year later C6/7 has fused anteriorly; he is left with chronic neck pain due to C5/6 disc degeneration.

The spinous processes are carefully palpated. Sometimes a gap can be felt where ligaments are torn; this, or a haematoma over the spine, is a sinister feature. The bones and soft tissues are gently tested for tenderness.

Movement of the spine can be dangerous – it may imperil the cord – so it is avoided until a diagnosis has been made.

A full neurological examination is carried out in every case; this may have to be repeated several times during the first few days. Initially, during the phase of spinal shock, there may be complete paralysis and loss of sensation below the level of injury. This may last for 48 hours or longer and during this period it is difficult to tell whether the neurological lesion is complete or incomplete. It is important to test for the primitive anal skin reflex and for perianal sensation. Once the primitive reflexes return, spinal shock has ended; if there is still loss of all motor and sensory function the neurological lesion is complete. Intact perianal sensation

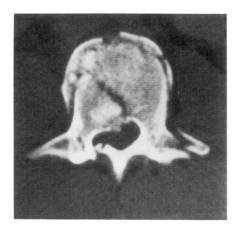

25.5 Spine injuries – x-ray diagnosis The plain x-ray showed the fracture but gave little indication of the amount of fragmentation and displacement. This CT scan revealed that one large fragment was encroaching dangerously on the spinal canal.

suggests an incomplete lesion, and further recovery may occur.

Imaging

The *x-ray examination* is crucial. It should be carried out with the least possible manipulation of the neck or back, yet it must be complete enough to provide the essential information. Lateral views of the cervical spine must include all the vertebrae from C1 to T1; unless the vertebrae are actually counted, a low injury may be missed. Anteroposterior views must include the odontoid process. Oblique views also may be necessary and it should be remembered that more than one area of the spine may be damaged. *CT* is invaluable for showing fractures of the vertebral body or the neural arch, or encroachment on the spinal canal.

MRI is helpful in displaying the soft tissues (intervertebral discs and ligamentum flavum) and lesions in the cord.

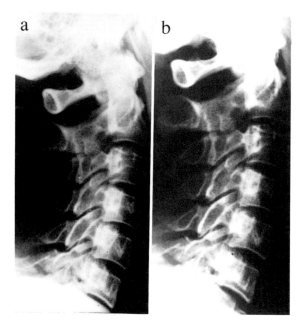

25.4 Spine injuries – x-ray diagnosis (a) Following a traffic accident this patient had a painful neck and consulted her doctor three times; on each occasion she was told 'the x-rays are normal'. But count the vertebrae! There are only six in this film. (b) When a strenuous effort was made to show the entire cervical spine a dislocation of C6 on C7 could be seen at the very bottom of the film.

Associated injuries

The patient should be carefully examined for associated injuries of the skull, thorax, abdomen or pelvis.

Principles of management

First aid

The first priority is to ensure that there is an adequate airway and ventilation. Patients with suspected spinal injuries should be moved as little as possible, and then only 'in one piece' so that there is no intervertebral movement. The neck should be supported in a collar during transport. Unconscious patients should be treated as if they had a spinal injury until this diagnosis is definitely excluded.

Early management in hospital

Management depends on the nature and severity of the injury, which cannot be judged by the superficial appearance. Some patients walk into the accident department, unaware of any cord-threatening fracture; some are obviously injured and in distress; some are unconscious.

A general assessment is carried out. Often there are severe associated injuries. If the patient needs resuscitation or tracheal intubation, beware the danger of flexing or extending the neck! Ventilation must be ensured, and shock and haemorrhage are treated. The patient is carefully assessed for spinal injury and a neurological examination is carried out; this will serve as an important baseline in future management. X-rays are taken.

The neck and back are held in the anatomical position with pillows and supports, and definitive treatment of the spinal injury is deferred until a full diagnosis has been made. The clinical examination is repeated some hours after admission; the signs may have changed.

General care of the face, the tracheal tube (if there is one), the chest, the abdomen, the bladder and the skin is important. Other fractures are splinted until the priorities have been decided.

Patients with cord damage need special attention to prevent pressure sores and bladder complications. A urethral catheter is inserted and urinary output is measured (it is reduced during the period of shock). If the bladder is paralysed the patient will need intermittent catheterization.

Definitive treatment

The objectives of treatment are: (1) to preserve neurological function; (2) to relieve any reversible nerve or cord compression; (3) to stabilize the spine; and (4) to rehabilitate the patient.

Patients with no bony damage and only mild soft-tissue injuries may be dealt with in the accident department and sent home, with instructions to return for assessment a week later. A firm collar may help to relieve neck pain and muscle spasm.

Severely injured patients must be admitted to hospital without delay and with the least possible disturbance of posture. Analgesics are given but narcotic drugs should be avoided. The patient should be nursed, unclothed, on a firm mattress. If there are neurological changes, special attention should be paid to the skin and bladder.

The principles of treatment are as follows.

PATIENTS WITH NO NEUROLOGICAL DEFECT

If the spinal injury is stable it can be left as it is and the patient treated by supporting the spine in a position that will cause no further strain; a firm collar or lumbar brace will usually suffice, but the patient may need to rest in bed until pain and muscle spasm subside. The exception is a burst fracture of the vertebral body: CT is advisable, and if this shows displaced fragments threatening the cord, decompression and spinal fusion should be considered. The decision will rest largely on whether specialized operative facilities are available; if they are not, the patient should be kept under observation for several weeks, reassessing the neurological state from time to time.

If the spinal injury is unstable it should be held secure until the tissues heal and the spine becomes stable. In the cervical spine this can be done (and should be done as soon as possible after admission) by traction, using tongs or a halo device attached to the skull. If the halo is attached to a body cast the combination can be used as an external fixator for prolonged immobilization (see below). Alternatively – particularly in the thoracolumbar spine – internal fixation can be carried out; spinal cord function should be monitored during the operation to ensure that the cord is not being injured. Dislocations and subluxations must be reduced, whether by adjusting the posture, by traction or by open operation.

During the first 48 hours the patient is in spinal shock. If there is no recovery after a week, the lesion is probably complete and permanent.

If the spinal injury is stable (which is rare), the patient can be treated conservatively and rehabilitated as soon as possible.

With the usual unstable injury, conservative treatment can be used; this is highly demanding and is best carried out in a special unit equipped for round-the-clock nursing, 2-hourly turning routines, skin toilet, bladder care and specialized physiotherapy and occupational therapy. After a few weeks the injury stabilizes spontaneously and the patient can be got out of bed for intensive rehabilitation. This approach is certainly applicable to high thoracic injuries with no associated rib or sternal fractures and minimal deformity. In most other situations the preference nowadays is for early operative stabilization: it facilitates nursing, reduces the risk of spinal deformity and persistent local pain, and speeds rehabilitation.

PATIENTS WITH INCOMPLETE NEUROLOGICAL LOSS

If the injury is stable, the patient can be treated conservatively with bed rest until pain subsides and then with some form of local support. Again the exception is the burst fracture, where CT may show fragments encroaching on the spinal canal and displacing the dura; in these cases decompression and stabilization are needed (see below).

If the injury is unstable, early operative reduction or decompression and stabilization may be indicated. However, cervical spine injuries, if they do not require open reduction, can be treated by traction followed by external fixation in a halo–body cast.

Treatment methods

The halo–body cast With the patient supine and his head supported by an assistant, the halo device is held in position just below the widest part of the skull. Under local anaesthesia, four sterilized pins are inserted through holes in the halo and screwed into the outer table of the skull; the halo is neatly centred by adjusting the screws. The pins are then locked in position on the halo. A plaster 'jacket' is applied, extending from the shoulders and moulded over the iliac crests. The halo is fixed to the body cast by outriggers. An alternative is to use a comfortably padded plastic jacket fitted to the halo.

Decompression and stabilization Decompression can be achieved from in front through a transthoracic or a transperitoneal approach, or from behind via a translaminar or a transpedicular approach. Anterior decompression is followed by fixation with bone grafts (strut grafts are often the best) supplemented by plates screwed to the intact vertebral bodies above and below the injured area.

From behind, reduction is first achieved by manual and postural repositioning, aided if necessary by Harrington distraction rods; these are attached well above and below the injured area, but are not biomechanically stable unless reinforced by sublaminar wires or spinous process wiring. Alternatively, a short segment can, after reduction, be fixed by a Hartshill rectangle, or by the Steffee VPS system in which special plates are attached by transpedicular screws (Gaines and Humphreys, 1988). Riska, Myllynen and Böstman (1987) advocate a two-stage procedure, first reducing and fixing the spine from behind and then, a few days later, achieving decompression (if necessary) through an anterolateral approach.

Cervical spine injuries

Neck pain and stiffness, or complaints of paraesthesia or weakness in the upper limbs, should never be regarded lightly. The force producing a serious head injury (e.g. a road traffic accident or a fall from a height onto the head) may also injure the neck. Consequently it should be a rule that in every patient unconscious from a head injury, a fractured cervical spine should be suspected.

An abnormal position of the neck may be suggestive, but palpation is rarely helpful. Move-

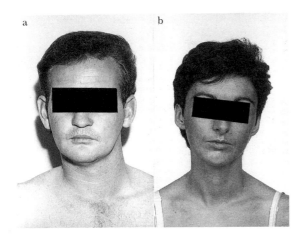

25.6 Cervical spine injuries A skew neck may be obvious, but even minor deformities are significant and call for x-ray examination. (a) This man had a fractured odontoid. (b) This woman had a hyperextension injury.

ments should be extremely gentle and, if painful, are best postponed until the neck has been x-rayed. Pain or paraesthesia in the limbs is significant, and the limbs should always be examined for evidence of cord or root damage.

X-ray films must be of high quality and should be inspected methodically. Note the following points.

1. In the anteroposterior view the lateral outlines should be intact, and the spinous processes and tracheal shadow in the midline. An open-mouth view is necessary to show C1 and C2 (for odontoid and lateral mass fractures).

2. The lateral view must include all seven cervical vertebrae and T1, otherwise a low injury will be missed. Count the vertebrae; if necessary, re-x-ray while applying downward traction to the arms. The smooth lordotic curve should be followed, tracing the four parallel lines formed by the front of the vertebral bodies, the back of the bodies, the lateral masses and the bases of the spinous processes; any irregularity suggests a fracture or displacement. An unduly wide interspinous space suggests anterior luxation. The trachea may be displaced by a soft-tissue haematoma.

3. The distance between the odontoid peg and the back of the anterior arch of the atlas should be no more than 4.5 mm in children or 3 mm in adults and does not vary with flexion.

4. To avoid missing a dislocation without fracture, lateral films in flexion and extension are occasionally necessary. Flexion should be guided by the doctor himself and must stop immediately if the patient experiences any arm or leg symptoms.

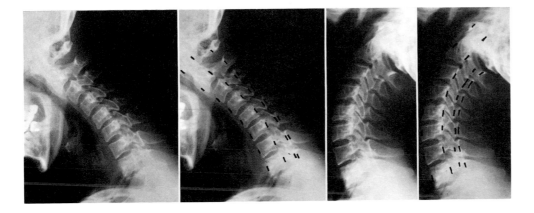

25.7 Cervical spine injuries – x-ray diagnosis In lateral films taken in both flexion and extension, four parallel lines can be traced unbroken from C1 to C7. They are formed by: (1) the anterior surfaces of the vertebral bodies; (2) the posterior surfaces of the bodies; (3) the posterior borders of the lateral masses; and (4) the bases of the spinous processes.

5. Forward shift of a vertebral body on the one below is important. Displacement of less than half the vertebral body width suggests unilateral facet dislocation and oblique views are needed to show the involved side; greater displacement suggests bilateral dislocation.

6. Unclear or doubtful lesions require CT.

MRI is particularly helpful in distinguishing between intrinsic lesions of the cord and cord compression by surrounding tissues such as a prolapsed disc or infolded ligamentum flavum.

Avulsion fractures

Fracture of the C7 spinous process may occur with severe muscle contraction ('clay-shoveller's fracture'). This is painful but harmless. As soon as symptoms permit, neck exercises are encouraged.

Cervical strain ('whiplash')

The imaginative term 'whiplash' is applied to a soft-tissue injury that occurs when the neck is suddenly jerked into hyperextension. Usually this follows a rear-end collision; the body is thrown forwards and the head jerked backwards. There is disagreement about the exact pathology but it is likely that the anterior longitudinal ligament is strained or torn and discs also may be damaged.

Patients complain of pain and stiffness in the neck, which may be quite intractable and persist for a year or longer. This is often accompanied by other, more ill-defined, symptoms such as headache, dizziness, depression, blurring of vision and numbness or paraesthesia in the arms. There are usually no physical signs, and x-rays show only minor postural changes. No form of treatment has been shown to be of much value. Analgesics will relieve pain and physiotherapy is soothing. Patients need to be encouraged to bear the discomfort until the symptoms subside.

Many patients recover completely within 4–8 weeks, but in the remainder the long-term prognosis is at best uncertain, at worst somewhat gloomy. More than half of the victims continue to suffer some discomfort 10 years after injury, and almost a third have symptoms that interfere significantly with daily activities (Gargan and Bannister, 1990; Hildingsson and Toolanen, 1990).

Fracture of C1

Sudden severe load on the top of the head may cause a 'bursting' force which fractures the ring of the atlas behind and in front of the lateral masses (Jefferson's fracture). There is no encroachment on the neural canal and, usually, no neurological damage. X-rays – and CT even better – will show the fracture. If it is undisplaced, the injury is stable and the patient needs only a collar. If there is sideways spreading of the lateral masses, the transverse ligament has ruptured; this injury is unstable and should be treated by 6 weeks' skull traction followed by a further 6 weeks in a firm collar; alternatively the skull traction can be discontinued once the acute pain subsides, and replaced by a halo–body cast for 6 weeks followed by another 6 weeks in a collar.

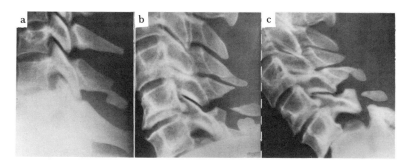

25.8 Avulsions (a) So-called clay-shoveller's fracture. (b) This patient might be thought to have a similar fracture, but a subsequent flexion film (c) shows the serious nature of the injury – a severe fracture-dislocation.

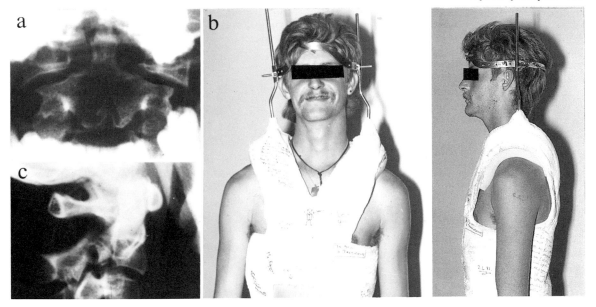

25.9 Fractures of C1 and C2 – neural arches   (a) Fracture of C1 with disruption of the arch (Jefferson fracture). The open-mouth view shows spreading of the lateral masses; the spine is unstable, and a halo–body cast (b) may be indicated. (c) Fracture of the pedicle or lateral pillar of C2 is usually due to a flexion injury ('hangman's fracture').

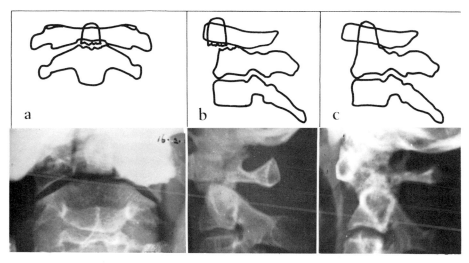

25.10 Odontoid fractures   (a, b) Fractured base of odontoid peg, permitting forward shift of the atlas and skull. (c) Similar forward shift follows rupture of the transverse ligament. The safest treatment is immobilization in a halo–body cast.

Fracture of the pedicle of C2

The '*hangman's fracture*' is seen in civilian life in motor accidents where the head strikes the windshield, forcing the neck into hyperextension. If both pedicles are fractured and severely displaced, the damage is lethal. Even undisplaced fractures are potentially dangerous and the patient is best treated by immobilization in a halo–body cast for 12 weeks. If, later, there is persistent instability, anterior fusion between C2 and C3 is advisable.

Fractures of the odontoid

Odontoid fractures result from high-velocity accidents or severe falls. A displaced fracture is really a fracture-dislocation of the atlantoaxial joint in which the atlas is shifted forwards or backwards, taking the odontoid process with it. Cord damage is rarely seen – perhaps because only the fortunate patients without damage survive!

Fractures of the tip and fractures extending into the vertebral body heal well; those between are prone to non-union (Ryan and Taylor, 1982).

Undisplaced fractures can be treated with a well-fitting cervical brace, which is worn for 12 weeks. Displaced fractures should be reduced and immobilized by applying a halo–body cast. The patient is allowed up, and if, at 12 weeks,

the fracture is still unstable, posterior fusion of C1 to C2 is advisable. An alternative approach to the upper cervical spine is by the transoral route (Ashraf and Crockard, 1990).

Hyperextension injuries – C3 to T1

The bone is undamaged, but the anterior longitudinal ligament may be torn. The history and facial bruising or lacerations often suggest the mechanism. Neurological damage is variable and probably due to compression between the disc and the ligamentum flavum; oedema and haematomyelia may cause the acute central spinal cord syndrome. X-rays show no fracture, but an extension film reveals a gap between the front of two vertebral bodies. These injuries are stable in the neutral position, in which they should be held by a collar for 6 weeks.

Sometimes no gap is seen, even in extension; instead the films show old spondylosis. Again there may be cord or root damage. The neck should be held in a collar in the neutral position for 6 weeks.

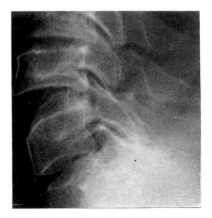

25.12 Hyperextension injury The anterior ligament has been torn; in the neutral position the gap will be closed and reduction will be stable, but a collar or brace will be needed until the soft tissues are healed. As the disc has been torn, its degeneration is inevitable.

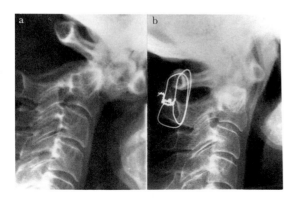

25.11 Odontoid fractures (a) A severely displaced odontoid fracture. (b) It has been reduced and held by fixing the spinous process of C1 to that of C2.

Wedge compression fractures – C3 to T1

Wedge compression is a flexion injury; the body is compressed but the posterior ligaments remain intact and the fracture is stable. No reduction is needed. A collar may be worn for comfort but can safely be removed to allow washing.

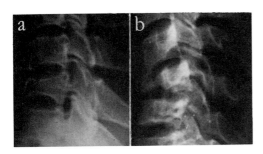

25.13 'Compression' fractures of the cervical spine A true wedge-compression fracture (a) is stable because the posterior ligaments remain intact. A comminuted fracture (b) is best regarded as unstable because the large posterior part of the vertebral body can be displaced backwards.

Burst fractures

These also are stable, but they are painful and the bony fragments may become displaced; it is

therefore prudent to restrict movement. A plaster collar is usually sufficient; after 6 weeks it can be replaced by a polythene collar which is worn until interbody fusion is seen on x-ray.

If CT scans show bone fragments encroaching on the spinal canal, more rigid fixation in a halo–body cast is advisable. If the cord is threatened, decompression and internal fixation may be needed.

Comminuted body fractures (teardrop fracture)

Comminution of the vertebral body is due either to severe axial compression or – a more sinister mechanism – to axial compression combined with flexion, as occurs most typically in diving injuries. The vertebral body ruptures and one or more fragments may be forced into the spinal canal, endangering the cord. Typically the anteroinferior corner of the body breaks off as a single fragment – the radiographic 'teardrop'. The lateral x-ray may show posterior displacement of the larger body fragment; spinal canal encroachment is best demonstrated by CT.

Displaced comminuted fractures are unstable and there is a high incidence of progressive neurological dysfunction. They are usually trea-

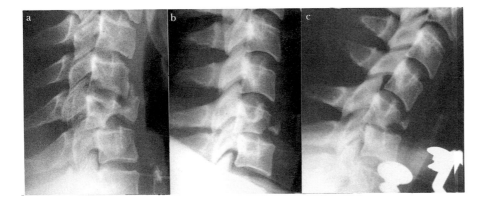

25.14 Teardrop fracture (a) This comminuted vertebral body fracture has produced a large anterior fragment and obvious posterior displacement of the posterior fragment. (b) In this case the anterior 'teardrop' was noted but the severity of the injury was underestimated and the patient was treated in a collar. Three weeks later (c) the fracture had collapsed, the large body fragment was tilted and displaced posteriorly and the patient complained of tingling and weakness in the right arm.

ted by skull traction for 8 weeks, followed by cervical bracing for a further 8 weeks. However, the period in hospital can be shortened by performing anterior spinal fusion after the first 4 weeks in traction; it is still necessary to use a cervical brace for 8–12 weeks.

If CT shows that the bony fragments are impinging on the cord, decompression and stabilization may be justified, through either an anterior or a posterior approach. Fixation can be achieved by plates and screws, by wires, or by rods combined with wires; bone grafts are added.

If there is no neurological abnormality and CT shows that the fracture is undisplaced, the patient can be treated in a halo–body cast for 6–8 weeks. It is important to do follow-up x-ray studies to disclose any tendency to late progressive deformity, which might require anterior cervical fusion.

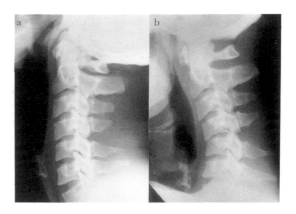

25.15 Cervical spine subluxation   (a) The film taken in extension shows no displacement of the vertebral bodies, but there is an unduly large gap between the spinous processes of C4 and 5. (b) With the neck slightly flexed the subluxation is obvious.

Subluxations – C3 to T1

Cervical subluxation is a pure flexion injury; the bones are intact but the posterior ligaments are torn. A vertebra tilts forward on the one below, opening up the interspinous space posteriorly. X-ray may reveal the increased gap between the spines; however, if the neck is held in extension this sign may be missed, so it is always advisable to obtain a lateral view with the cervical spine positioned gently in neutral position.

A collar for 6 weeks is usually adequate, but further x-rays at 6 weeks are essential; if flexion and extension films show persistent instability, a posterior spinal fusion may be necessary.

Dislocations and fracture-dislocations between C3 and T1

These are flexion-rotation injuries in which the articular facets ride forward over the facets below. Usually one or both of the articular masses is fractured but sometimes there is a pure dislocation ('jumped facets'). The posterior ligaments are ruptured and the spine is unstable. Often there is cord damage. X-ray shows the marked forward displacement of a vertebra on the one below.

Initial treatment   The displacement must be reduced. This can usually be achieved by heavy skull traction (10–15 kg) for several hours. If this fails (usually because of locked facets), gentle manipulation with relaxation may succeed. If this, too, is unsuccessful, open reduction from the back is essential.

Subsequent treatment   Once the displacement is reduced, there is a choice of further management. The easiest is simply to continue with traction (reduced to 5 kg) for 6 weeks and then a collar for a further 6 weeks. More convenient for the patient is to immobilize the neck in a halo–body cast for 12 weeks. The third method, most applicable when open reduction is required, is to carry out a posterior fusion straight away; the patient is allowed up in a cervical brace which is worn for 6–8 weeks.

Unilateral facet dislocation

This, too, is a flexion-rotation injury but only one articular facet is dislocated. On x-ray the vertebral body appears to be partially displaced (less than one-half of its width) and the upper segment of spine is slightly rotated on the lower. Cord damage is unusual and the injury is stable.

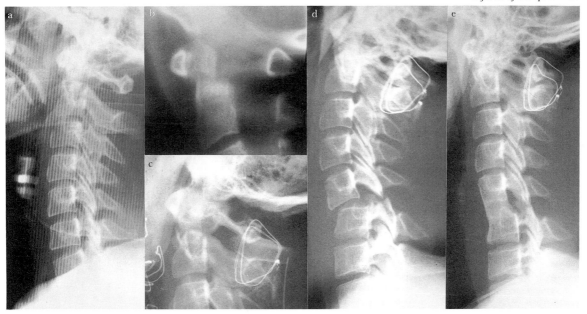

25.16 Subluxations – C3 to T1 (a) This patient with a neck injury was suspected of having an odontoid fracture. This was confirmed by tomography (b), and a posterior stabilization of C1/2 was performed (c). Only when the brace was removed and he started flexing his neck did the x-ray show an obvious subluxation lower down (d). This was treated by anterior fusion (e).

Reduction may occur spontaneously while the neck is being positioned for traction. In some cases, skull traction will unlock the single facet and reduce the dislocation. If so, traction is continued for a further 3 weeks; the patient is then allowed up in a collar which is worn for a further 6 weeks or, alternatively, the neck can be immobilized in a halo–body splint for 4 weeks.

If closed reduction fails, open reduction and internal fixation are advisable. Patients left with the hemi-dislocation unreduced are liable to develop pain (Rorabeck et al., 1987).

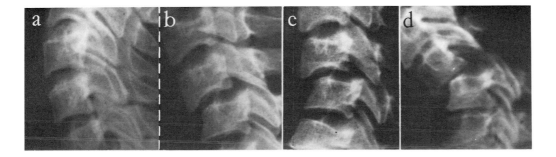

25.17 Unstable neck injuries In (a) the cervical spine looks normal, but the film in flexion (b) shows forward subluxation – the posterior ligaments are torn. (c) Fracture-dislocation with moderate forward shift signifying a unilateral facet dislocation; (d) another fracture-dislocation with severe forward shift.

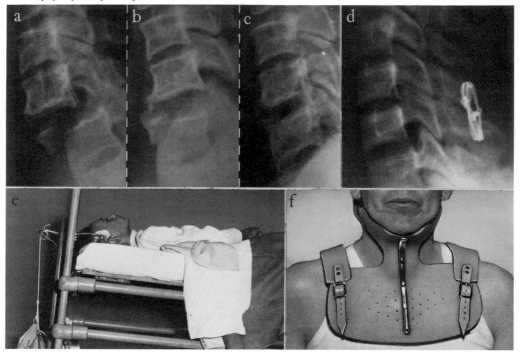

25.18 Treatment of cervical spine fractures (a, b, c) Stages in the reduction of a fracture-dislocation by skull traction; (d) subsequent wiring to ensure stability. (e) The patient was kept on skull traction until the wound was healed. A polythene collar as in (f) was then applied.

Thoracic spine injuries

Wedge-compression fractures (sometimes pathological) and fracture-dislocations both occur and, because of the rib cage, are usually stable. However, the spinal canal in this area is relatively narrow, and so cord damage is common; when this is present, in 5 out of 6 cases it is complete (Bohlman, 1985). Radiological diagnosis is usually adequate, but CT may be needed to differentiate paraspinal haemorrhage from a ruptured aorta and, with partial cord lesions, to identify the impingement of any bony fragments.

If there is complete paraplegia with no improvement after 48 hours, conservative management is adequate; the patient can be rested in bed for 5–6 weeks, then gradually mobilized in a brace. With severe bony injury, however, increasing kyphosis may occur and internal fixation should be considered.

If the paraplegia is partial, there is the potential for further recovery; decompression and stabilization are needed. Both can be performed simultaneously through a transthoracic approach, but Riska, Myllynen and Böstman (1987) advocate open reduction and fixation with Harrington rods followed, a few days later, by anterolateral decompression if this is indicated.

Thoracolumbar injuries

Management clearly depends upon precise diagnosis, but in one respect it must precede diagnosis. *When the patient is seen at the site of the accident it is essential that he is handled in such a way that, even if he has an unstable fracture,*

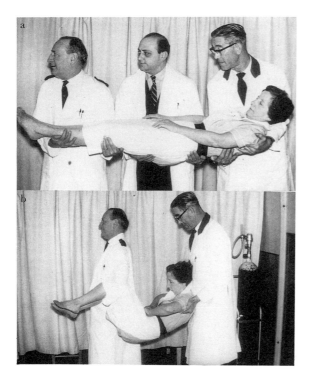

25.19 Thoracolumbar injuries (a) With even a remote possibility of spinal injury, displacement (or further displacement) must be prevented; this requires at least three people. (b) How not to do it; this is what may happen if only two people do the lifting.

displacement will not be increased. He must be moved onto the stretcher 'in one piece': the spine is kept straight.

Usually the patient is first seen lying supine on a stretcher or trolley. The opportunity should be taken to examine the chest and abdomen first for associated injuries. It must be remembered that, while abdominal pain and tenderness are suggestive of intra-abdominal damage, they can occur with a purely spinal injury. Next, the lower limbs are examined for evidence of neurological damage.

To examine the back, the patient is carefully turned (at least two and preferably three people are needed) onto one side; unless this can be done easily and painlessly, this stage of the examination should be postponed until x-ray films have been seen. The skin is inspected for abrasions or bruising; either indicates the probable level of injury. The spinous processes are palpated systematically. With unstable injuries a gap can be felt where the ligament has been torn; this important physical sign is surprisingly easy to elicit. Spinal movements should not be examined; the attempt may imperil the cord.

Next, x-rays are taken. As they must be of high quality, portable apparatus is quite inadequate. The minimum requirements are anteroposterior and lateral views, but two laterals are better – one centred over the vertebral bodies and the other over the spinous processes; oblique views and tomograms also may be helpful. Interpreting films is not always easy and it is important in both the anteroposterior and lateral views to inspect carefully: (1) the alignment of the vertebrae – is there any angulation or shift at any one point? (2) the shape of the individual vertebral bodies – is there any loss of the normal box-like appearance? (3) the neural arches – is there any evidence of fracture or of dislocation?

With unstable injuries, or comminuted fractures of the vertebral body, *CT* is invaluable. Occasionally, if there is a possibility that disc material is impinging, *MRI* also is needed.

Most injuries can be assigned to one of the following categories: extension injuries, wedge-compression fractures, burst fractures, jack-knife injuries, and various types of dislocation or fracture-dislocation. Stability is assessed on the basis of Denis' three-column concept.

Fractures of transverse processes

These are essentially 'soft-tissue injuries', often seen in association with fractures and dislocations of the spinal column or pelvis. If they are isolated injuries they need no treatment.

Extension injuries

Extension strains are fairly common but acute fractures are rare. Sudden back pain in a weight-lifter, gymnast or athlete – usually ascribed to a disc prolapse – may be due to fracture of the pars interarticularis ('traumatic spondylolysis'). This is best seen in the oblique x-rays, but a thin fracture line is easily missed;

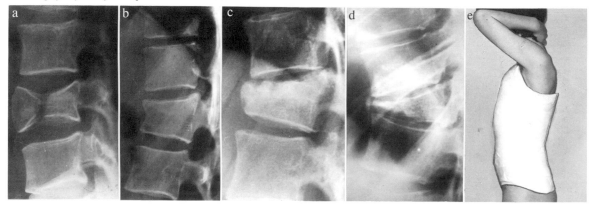

25.20 Thoracolumbar compression fractures   (a) Central compression fracture with intact posterior half of vertebral body. (b) Anterior wedge fracture with 20% loss of height. (c) Wedge fracture with 50% loss of height. (d) Severe wedge fracture with more than 50% loss of height. These are all stable injuries and lesser degrees of wedging can be treated by bracing or (e) a plaster jacket.

radioscintigraphy may show a 'hot' spot. Bilateral fractures occasionally lead to spondylolisthesis.

The fracture usually heals spontaneously – provided the patient is prepared to forego his (more often her) athletic passion for several months.

Wedge-compression fracture

This is by far the most common vertebral fracture and is due to spinal flexion with the posterior ligaments usually remaining intact; in these cases CT shows that the posterior part of the vertebral body is unbroken. Pain is usually quite marked but the fracture is stable. The best treatment is activity. The patient is kept in bed for a week or two until pain subsides but spinal exercises are encouraged from the outset. Once the patient gets up, a corset may lend additional comfort and security.

If loss of vertebral height is greater that 50% the mechanical force exerted on the front of the vertebral body is such that further collapse is then likely; in some cases this may lead to late neurological dysfunction. Although conservative treatment with a brace or plaster jacket is feasible, surgical correction and internal fixation is better.

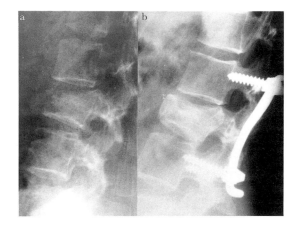

25.21 Wedge-compression fracture   (a) Left alone, the deformity in this case would almost certainly have increased. (b) Posterior fixation has prevented further collapse.

Burst fracture

Severe axial compression may 'explode' the vertebral body, causing failure of both the anterior and the middle columns. The posterior ligament complex is undamaged but the

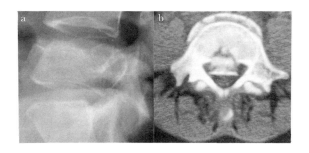

25.22 Lumbar burst fracture Severe compression may cause retropulsion of the vertebral body (a). The extent of spinal canal encroachment is best shown by CT (b).

fracture should be regarded as unstable. The posterior part of the vertebral body is shattered and fragments of bone and disc may be displaced into the spinal canal.

Anteroposterior x-rays show a pathognomonic spreading of the vertebral body with an increase of the interpedicular distance. CT will reveal posterior displacement of bone and soft-tissue fragments.

If there is no marked retropulsion of bone or neurological damage, the injury can be treated by immobilization in a plaster jacket, which is applied not with the spine hyperextended but in the neutral position. After 6 weeks it can safely be replaced by a polyethylene jacket which is taken off for washing and sleeping; at 12 weeks from injury it is discarded.

If there is neurological damage, or the CT suggests that the neural structures are in peril from displaced bone or discal fragments, decompression and stabilization are needed.

Jack-knife injuries

Combined flexion and distraction may cause the mid-lumbar spine to jack-knife around an axis that is placed anterior to the vertebral column. This is seen most typically in lap seat-belt injuries, where the body is thrown forward against the restraining strap. There is little or no crushing of the vertebral body, but the posterior and middle columns fail in tension; thus these fractures are unstable in flexion.

The tear passes transversely through the ligaments or the bony structures, or both. The most perfect example of tensile failure is the injury described by Chance (1948), in which the split runs through the spinous process, the lateral processes and the vertebral body. X-rays may show horizontal fractures in the pedicles or transverse processes, and in the anteroposterior

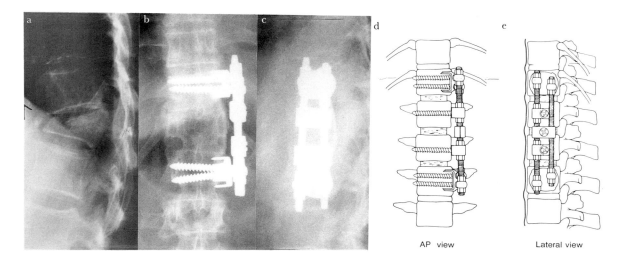

AP view   Lateral view

25.23 Burst fracture (a) Burst fracture in a 44-year-old man who fell from his horse; 3 months later he developed paraesthesia in both legs. (b–e) Internal fixation and grafting through a transthoracic transdiaphragmatic approach provided total stability (the Kaneda method).

a   b

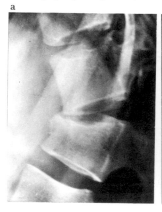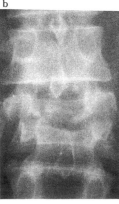

25.24 Jack-knife injuries (a) Whereas flexion usually crushes the vertebral body and leaves the posterior ligaments intact, the jack-knife injury disrupts the posterior ligaments causing only slight anterior compression. (b) The rare Chance fracture.

view the apparent height of the vertebral body may be increased. In the lateral view there may be opening up of the disc space posteriorly. Tomographs are helpful in showing the fractures.

Neurological damage is uncommon, though the injury is – by definition – unstable. The Chance fracture (being an 'all bone' injury) heals rapidly and requires no more than 6–8 weeks in a plaster jacket or well-fitting brace.

Severe ligamentous injuries are less predictable and posterior spinal fusion is advisable.

Fracture-dislocations

Segmental displacement may occur with various combinations of flexion, compression, rotation and shear. All three columns are disrupted and the spine is grossly unstable. These are the most dangerous injuries and are often associated with neurological damage.

X-rays may show fractures through the vertebral body, pedicles, articular processes and laminae, with varying degrees of subluxation or dislocation. Often there are associated fractures of transverse processes or ribs. CT is helpful in

demonstrating the degree of spinal canal occlusion.

The injury most commonly occurs at the thoracolumbar junction and is usually associated with damage to the lowermost part of the cord or the cauda equina. The patient should be examined with the greatest care so as not to jeopardize the cord or the nerve roots any further. Pelvic traction is applied while the patient's condition is assessed.

Treatment depends on whether or not the cord or nerve roots are damaged.

FRACTURE-DISLOCATION WITH PARAPLEGIA Traction alone may achieve reduction; with suitable facilities for nursing, patients with complete paraplegia can be treated conservatively. They require frequent turning (to prevent pressure sores), but the body must be moved in one piece ('log-rolling') and this requires a lot of assistance. The skin and soft tissues need constant attention. After 6–8 weeks the patient can be slowly mobilized out of bed; a spinal brace is usually necessary. In dedicated units it has been shown that 95% of paraplegic patients can be managed in this way; operation is reserved for the few who have locked facets or in whom the fracture-dislocation cannot be reduced for other reasons.

The alternative approach is to operate without delay and fix the unstable spine with metal implants. Nursing is made much easier, the patient often feels more comfortable and the period in bed can be significantly shortened. Furthermore, the risk of painful deformity is reduced by this approach.

If the paraplegia is partial, decompression and stabilization are required.

FRACTURE-DISLOCATION WITHOUT PARAPLEGIA These are definitely the minority. The unstable dislocation threatens to damage the cord, which has so far escaped injury. If the articular processes are fractured, the dislocation can usually be reduced by traction in extension; the spine is then immobilized, preferably by internal fixation.

If the articular processes are locked, reduction will be difficult and operation is advisable. Under direct vision the bones are carefully unlocked and the spine is fixed with plates or

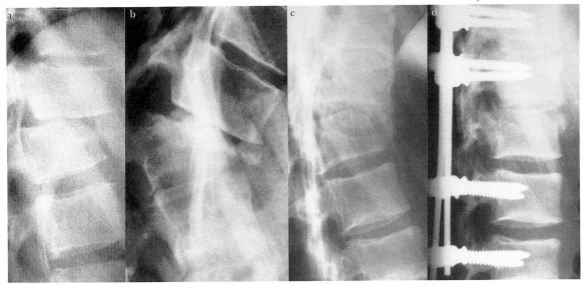

25.25 Thoracolumbar fracture-dislocation (a) Fracture-dislocation at T11/12 in a 32-year-old woman who was a passenger in a truck that overturned. She was completely paraplegic and operation was not thought worthwhile. (b) Four weeks later the deformity has increased, leaving her with a marked gibbus. (c, d) A similar injury in a 17-year-old man, treated by open reduction and internal fixation.

metal rods. Bone grafts should always be added because the implants alone cannot be relied upon to hold reduction indefinitely. A well-fitting brace is worn for at least 3 months.

If specialized operative facilities are not available, conservative treatment in plaster is both safe and effective. A reasonable routine is as follows. The patient is placed prone on an operating table and in that position re-x-rayed. Provided reduction has been achieved (and it often has), plaster is applied to the back half of the trunk and legs, as the first step towards making a plaster bed. When this is complete the patient lies in the back half, but for cleaning purposes he is turned over into the front half at least once a week. After 6 weeks the fracture is less unstable and a plaster jacket is applied with the spine in neutral position. The patient is then allowed up. He wears the jacket for a further 6–12 weeks, the precise time being determined by x-ray; the plaster is not discarded until bony fusion is seen between the fractured vertebra and its neighbour.

Neural injuries

In spinal injuries the displaced structures may damage the cord or the nerve roots, or both; cervical lesions may cause quadriplegia, thoracolumbar lesions paraplegia. The damage may be partial or complete. Three varieties of lesion occur: cord concussion, cord transection and root transection.

CORD CONCUSSION (NEURAPRAXIA)
Motor paralysis (flaccid), sensory loss and visceral paralysis below the level of the cord lesion may be complete, but within minutes or a few hours recovery begins and soon becomes full. The condition is most likely to occur in patients who, for some reason other than injury, have a small-diameter anteroposterior canal; there is, however, no radiological evidence of recent bony damage.

CORD TRANSECTION

Motor paralysis, sensory loss and visceral paralysis occur below the level of the cord lesion; as with cord concussion, the motor paralysis is at first flaccid. This is a temporary condition known as cord shock, but the injury is anatomical and irreparable.

After a time, however, the cord below the level of transection recovers from the shock and acts as an independent structure; that is, it manifests reflex activity. In a few hours the anal and penile reflexes return, and the plantar responses become extensor. In a few days or weeks the flaccid paralysis becomes spastic, with increased tone, increased tendon reflexes and clonus; flexor spasms and contractures may develop but sensation never returns. The presence of anal and penile reflexes in the absence of sensation in the legs is diagnostic of cord transection.

ROOT TRANSECTION

Motor paralysis, sensory loss and visceral paralysis occur in the distribution of the damaged roots. Root transection, however, differs from cord transection in two ways: (1) regeneration is theoretically possible; and (2) residual motor paralysis remains permanently flaccid.

Anatomical levels

CERVICAL SPINE

With cervical spine injuries the segmental level of cord transection nearly corresponds to the level of bony damage. Not more than one or two additional roots are likely to be transected. High cervical cord transection is fatal because all the respiratory muscles are paralysed. At the level of the C5 vertebra, cord transection isolates the lower cervical cord (with paralysis of the upper limbs), the thoracic cord (with paralysis of the trunk) and the lumbar and sacral cord (with paralysis of the lower limbs and viscera). With injury below the C5 vertebra, the upper limbs are partially spared and characteristic deformities result.

BETWEEN T1 AND T10 VERTEBRAE

The first lumbar cord segment in the adult is at the level of the T10 vertebra. Consequently, cord transection at that level spares the thoracic

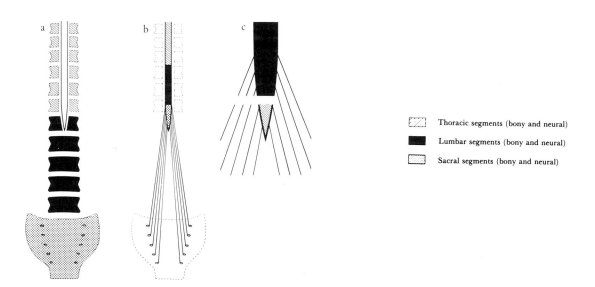

Thoracic segments (bony and neural)

Lumbar segments (bony and neural)

Sacral segments (bony and neural)

25.26 Traumatic paraplegia   (a) In the adult the cord ends at the lower border of L1. (b) The disposition of the nerve roots. (c) An injury to the T12 vertebra has transected the cord between the lumbar and sacral segments; on one side the roots also are transected, on the other there has been root escape.

cord but isolates the entire lumbar and sacral cord, with paralysis of the lower limbs and viscera. The lower thoracic roots may also be transected but are of relatively little importance.

BELOW T10 VERTEBRA
The cord forms a slight bulge (the conus medullaris) between the T10 and L1 vertebrae, and tapers to an end at the interspace between the L1 and L2 vertebrae. The L2 to S4 nerve roots arise from the conus medullaris and stream downwards in a bunch (the cauda equina) to emerge at successive levels of the lumbosacral spine. Therefore, spinal injuries above the T10 vertebra cause cord transection, those between the T10 and L1 vertebrae cause cord and nerve root lesions, and those below the L1 vertebra only root lesions.

The sacral roots innervate: (1) sensation in the 'saddle' area, a strip down the back of the thigh and leg, and the outer two-thirds of the sole; (2) motor power to the muscles controlling the ankle and foot; (3) the anal and penile reflexes, plantar responses and ankle jerks; and (4) control of micturition.

The lumbar roots innervate: (1) sensation to the entire lower limb other than that portion supplied by the sacral segment; (2) motor power to the muscles controlling the hip and knee; and (3) the cremasteric reflexes and knee jerks.

It is essential, when the bony injury is at the thoracolumbar junction, to distinguish between cord transection with root escape and cord transection with root transection. A patient with root escape is much better off than one with cord and root transection.

Signs

Clinical examination of the back nearly always shows the signs of an unstable fracture; however, a 'burst' fracture with paraplegia is stable. The nature and level of the bone lesion are demonstrated by x-ray, and that of the neural lesion by CT or MRI.

Neurological examination should be painstaking. Without detailed information, accurate diagnosis and prognosis are impossible; rectal examination is mandatory.

COMPLETE CORD LESIONS
Complete paralysis and anaesthesia below the level of injury suggest cord transection. During the stage of spinal shock when the anal reflex is absent (seldom longer than the first 24 hours) the diagnosis cannot be absolutely certain; if the anal reflex returns and the neural deficit persists, the cord lesion is complete. Any complete lesion lasting more than 72 hours will not recover.

INCOMPLETE CORD LESIONS
Persistence of any sensation distal to the injury (perianal pinprick is most important) suggests an incomplete lesion and therefore a favourable prognosis. Recovery may continue up to 6 months after injury (Tominaga, 1989). The commonest is the central cord syndrome where the initial flaccid weakness is followed by lower motor neuron paralysis of the upper limbs with upper motor neuron (spastic) paralysis of the lower limbs, and preservation of bladder control and perianal sensation (sacral sparing). With the less common anterior cord syndrome there is complete paralysis and anaesthesia but deep pressure and position sense are retained in the lower limbs (dorsal column sparing). The posterior cord syndrome is rare (only deep pressure and proprioception are lost), and the Brown-Séquard syndrome (cord hemisection, with ipsilateral paralysis and contralateral loss of pain sensation) is usually associated with thoracic injuries. Below the T10 vertebra discrepancies between neurological and skeletal levels are due to transection of roots descending from segments higher than the cord lesion.

Management of traumatic paraplegia and quadriplegia

With partial paralysis, decompression and stabilization offer the best chance of further recovery. With complete paralysis it is the overall management that is important, especially the early management.

The patient must be transported with great care to prevent further damage, and preferably taken to a spinal centre. The strategy is outlined below.

SKIN

Within a few hours anaesthetic skin may develop enormous pressure sores; these must be prevented by meticulous nursing. Immediate fixation of the spine enables these essential nursing procedures to be carried out much more easily and without discomfort to the patient. Creases in the sheets and crumbs in bed are not permitted. Every 2 hours the patient is gently rolled onto his side and his back is carefully washed (without rubbing), dried and powdered. After a few weeks the skin becomes a little more tolerant and the patient can turn himself. Later he should be taught how to relieve skin pressure intermittently during periods of sitting. If sores have been allowed to develop, they may never heal without excision and skin grafting.

BLADDER AND BOWEL

For the first 24 hours the bladder distends only slowly, but, if the distension is allowed to progress, overflow incontinence occurs and infection is probable. In special centres it is usual to manage the patient from the outset by intermittent catheterization under sterile conditions. If early transfer to a paraplegia centre is not possible, continuous drainage through a fine Silastic catheter is advised. The catheter drains in a closed manner into a disposable bag, and is changed twice weekly to prevent blockage. When infection supervenes, antibiotics are given.

Bladder training is begun at 1 week if possible. Although retention is complete to begin with, partial recovery may lead to either an automatic bladder which works reflexly or an expressible bladder which is emptied by manual suprapubic pressure.

A few patients are left with a high residual urine after emptying the bladder. They need special investigations, including cystography and cystometry; transurethral resection of the bladder neck or sphincterotomy may be indicated but should not be performed until at least 3 months of bladder training have been completed.

The bowel is more easily trained, with the help of enemas, aperients and abdominal exercises.

MUSCLES AND JOINTS

The paralysed muscles, if not treated, may develop severe flexion contractures. These are usually preventable by moving the joints passively through their full range twice daily. Later, splints become necessary.

With lesions below the cervical cord, the patient should be up within 3 months; standing and walking are valuable in preventing contractures.

Calipers are usually necessary to keep the knees straight and the feet plantigrade. The calipers are removed at intervals during the day while the patient lies prone, and while he is having physiotherapy. The upper limbs must be trained until they develop sufficient power to enable the patient to use crutches and a wheelchair.

If flexion contractures have been allowed to develop, tenotomies may be necessary. Painful flexor spasms are rare unless skin or bladder infection occurs. They can sometimes be relieved by tenotomies, neurectomies, rhizotomies or the intrathecal injection of alcohol.

Heterotopic ossification is a common and disturbing complication; it is more likely to occur with high lesions and complete lesions. It may restrict or abolish movement, especially at the hip. It is doubtful whether ossification can be prevented, but once the new bone is mature it can safely be excised.

MORALE

The morale of a paraplegic patient is liable to reach a low ebb, and the restoration of his self-confidence is an important part of treatment. Constant enthusiasm and encouragement by doctors, physiotherapists and nurses is essential. Their scrupulous attention to his comfort and toilet are of primary importance; the unpleasant smells associated with skin or urinary infection must be prevented. The earlier the patient gets up the better, and he must be trained for a new job as quickly as possible.

Injuries of the thorax

Rib fractures

Rib fractures are almost always due to direct injury. However, in osteoporotic patients ribs may fracture with minor stresses such as coughing or sneezing.

The patient complains of a sharp pain in the chest. This is markedly aggravated by deep breathing or coughing, or by anteroposterior compression of the chest wall. X-ray shows one or more fractures, usually near the rib angle.

Treatment

In most cases treatment is needed only for pain; an injection of local anaesthetic will bring immediate relief. Breathing exercises are encouraged.

Complications

Pulmonary injury   A rare but potentially serious complication is pneumothorax due to perfora-

tion of the lung by a jagged bone fragment. If tension develops, the chest should be promptly decompressed by inserting a needle into the upper part of the pleural cavity.

Fracture of the sternum

The sternum may be fractured by a direct blow to the chest, or indirectly during a flexion injury of the spine.

If displacement is minimal, no treatment is needed. If the sternum is severely displaced, it should be lifted forwards (under general anaesthesia) with the aid of a bone hook.

Stove-in chest

Violent injury to the thorax may cause multiple rib fractures on both sides of the sternum, thus

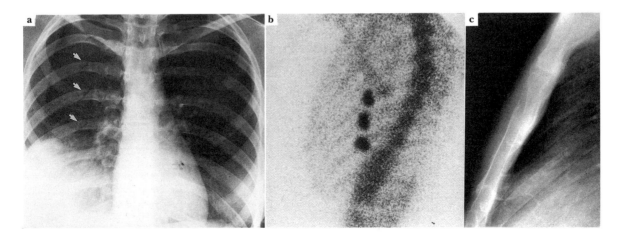

25.27 Thoracic cage fractures   (a) Rib fractures are usually obvious on plain x-ray. (b) Undisplaced fractures are sometimes difficult to see; a week later they show up clearly on the radionuclide scan. (c) Sternal fracture with minimal displacement.

producing a flail anterior segment of the thorax. Ventilation of the lungs is severely impaired and, if unrecognized or untreated, the condition may be fatal.

The quickest and most effective method of treatment is to anaesthetize the patient and apply positive pressure respiration. A clear airway is essential and this may require tracheotomy and intubation. The pleural cavity should be drained through an intercostal tube.

It is not essential to fix the fractures, provided positive pressure respiration is continued. If for some reason this cannot be done, the ribs should be stabilized with Kirschner wires.

References and further reading

Anderson, L.D. and D'Alonzo, R.T. (1974) Fractures of the odontoid process of the axis. *Journal of Bone and Joint Surgery* **56A**, 1663–1674

Ashraf, J. and Crockard, H.A. (1990) Transoral fusion for high cervical fractures. *Journal of Bone and Joint Surgery* **72B**, 76–79

Bohlman, H.H. (1985) Treatment of fractures and dislocations of the thoracic and lumbar spine – current concepts review. *Journal of Bone and Joint Surgery* **67A**, 165–169

Chance, C.Q. (1948) Note on a type of flexion fracture of the spine. *British Journal of Radiology* **21**, 452–453

Denis, F. (1983) The three column spine and its significance in the classification of acute thoracolumbar spinal injuries. *Spine* **8**, 817–831

Evans, D.K. (1966) Fractures and dislocations of the spine. In *Clinical Surgery*, vol. 12, *Fractures and Dislocations* (ed. R. Furlong), Butterworths, London

Evans, D.K. (1987) Editorial. Stabilisation of the cervical spine. *Journal of Bone and Joint Surgery* **69B**, 1–2

Ferguson, R.L. and Allen, B.L. (1984) A mechanistic classification of thoracolumbar spine fractures. *Clinical Orthopaedics and Related Research* **189**, 77–88

Gaines, R.W. and Humphreys, W.G. (1988) Thoracolumbar spinal injuries: role of operative treatment. *Current Orthopaedics* **2**, 231–235

Gargan, M.F. and Banister, G.C. (1990) Long-term prognosis of soft-tissue injuries of the neck. *Journal of Bone and Joint Surgery* **72B**, 901–903

Hardy, A.G. and Rossier, A.B. (1975) *Spinal Cord Injuries*, Georg Thieme, Stuttgart

Hildingsson, C. and Toolanen, G. (1990) Outcome after soft tissue injury of the cervical spine. A prospective study of 93 car-accident victims. *Acta Orthopaedica Scandinavica* **61**, 357–359

McAfee, P.G., Yuan, H.A., Frederickson, B.E. and Lubicky, J.P. (1983) The value of computed tomography in thoracolumbar fractures. *Journal of Bone and Joint Surgery* **65A**, 461–473

Riska, E.B., Myllynen, P. and Böstman, O. (1987) Anterolateral decompression for neural involvement in thoracolumbar fractures. *Journal of Bone and Joint Surgery* **69B**, 704–708

Rorabeck, C.H., Rock, M.G., Hawkins, R.J. and Bourne, R.B. (1987) Unilateral facet dislocation of the cervical spine: an analysis of the results of treatment in 26 patients. *Spine* **12**, 23–27

Ryan, M.D. and Taylor, T.K.F. (1982) Odontoid fractures. *Journal of Bone and Joint Surgery* **64B**, 416–421

Tominaga, S. (1989) Periodical, neurological–functional assessment of cervical cord injury. *Paraplegia* **27**, 227–236

Injuries of the pelvis 26

Fractures of the pelvis account for less than 5% of all skeletal injuries, but they are particularly important because of the high incidence of associated soft-tissue injuries and the risks of severe blood loss, shock, sepsis and adult respiratory distress syndrome (ARDS). Like other serious injuries, they demand a combined approach by experts in various fields.

About two-thirds of all pelvic fractures occur in road accidents involving pedestrians; over 10% of these patients will have associated visceral injuries, and in this group the mortality rate is probably in excess of 10% (Peltier, 1965; Eid, 1981).

Surgical anatomy

The pelvic ring is made up of the two innominate bones and the sacrum, articulating in front at the symphysis pubis (the anterior or pubic bridge) and posteriorly at the sacroiliac joints (the posterior or sacroiliac bridge). This basin-like structure transmits weight from the trunk to the lower limbs and provides protection for the pelvic viscera, vessels and nerves.

The stability of the pelvic ring depends upon the rigidity of the bony parts and the integrity of the strong ligaments that bind the three segments together at the symphysis pubis and the sacroiliac joints. The strongest and most important of the tethering ligaments are the sacroiliac and iliolumbar ligaments; as long as they are intact, loadbearing is unimpaired. This is an important factor in the differentiation between 'stable' and 'unstable' injuries of the pelvic ring.

The major branches of the common iliac arteries arise within the pelvis between the level of the sacroiliac joint and the greater sciatic notch. With their accompanying veins they are particularly vulnerable in fractures through the posterior part of the pelvic ring. The nerves of the lumbar and sacral plexuses, likewise, are at risk with posterior pelvic injuries.

The bladder lies behind the symphysis pubis. The trigone is held in position by the lateral ligaments of the bladder and, in the male, by the prostate. The prostate lies between the bladder and the pelvic floor. It is held laterally by the medial fibres of the levator ani, whilst anteriorly it is firmly attached to the pubic bones by the puboprostatic ligament. In the female the trigone is attached also to the cervix and the anterior vaginal fornix. The urethra is held by both the pelvic floor muscles and the pubourethral ligament. Consequently in females the urethra is much more mobile and less prone to injury.

In severe pelvic injuries the membranous urethra is damaged when the prostate is forced backwards whilst the urethra remains static. When the puboprostatic ligament is torn, the prostate and base of the bladder can become grossly dislocated from the membranous urethra.

The pelvic colon, with its mesentery, is a mobile structure and therefore not readily injured. However, the rectum and anal canal are more firmly tethered to the urogenital structures and the muscular floor of the pelvis and are therefore vulnerable in pelvic fractures.

Clinical assessment

Fracture of the pelvis should be suspected in every patient with serious abdominal or lower limb injuries. There may be a history of a road accident or a fall from a height or crush injury. Often the patient complains of severe pain and feels as if he has fallen apart, and there may be swelling or bruising of the lower abdomen, the thighs, the perineum, the scrotum or the vulva. All these areas should be rapidly inspected, looking for evidence of extravasation of urine. *However, the first priority, always, is to assess the patient's general condition and look for signs of blood loss. It may be necessary to start resuscitation before the examination is completed.*

The abdomen should be carefully palpated. Signs of irritation suggest the possibility of intraperitoneal bleeding. The pelvic ring can be gently compressed from side to side and back to front. Tenderness over the sacroiliac region is particularly important and may signify disruption of the posterior bridge.

A rectal examination is then carried out in every case. The coccyx and sacrum can be felt and tested for tenderness. If the prostate can be felt, which is often difficult due to pain and swelling, its abnormal position may indicate a urethral injury.

Enquire when the patient passed urine last and look for bleeding at the external meatus. An inability to void and blood at the external meatus are the classic features of a ruptured urethra. However, the absence of blood at the meatus does not exclude a urethral injury, because the external sphincter may be in spasm, halting the passage of blood from the site of injury. Thus every patient who has a pelvic fracture must be considered to be at risk.

The patient can be encouraged to void; if he is able to do so, either the urethra is intact or there is only minimal damage which will not be made worse by the passage of urine. *No attempt should be made to pass a catheter, as this could convert a partial to a complete tear of the urethra.* If the urethral injury is suspected, this can be diagnosed more accurately and more safely by retrograde urethrography.

A ruptured bladder should be suspected in patients who do not void or in whom a bladder is not palpable after adequate fluid replace-

ment. This palpation is often difficult because of abdominal wall haematoma. The physical findings initially can be minimal, with normal bowel sounds, as extravasation of sterile urine produces little peritoneal irritation. Only a very small proportion of patients with a ruptured bladder are hypotensive, so if a patient is hypotensive another cause must be sought.

Neurological examination is important; there may be damage to the lumbar or sacral plexus.

If the patient is unconscious, the same routine is followed. However, early x-ray examination is essential in these cases.

X-ray of the pelvis

As soon as the patient's condition will allow it, a plain anteroposterior x-ray of the pelvis should be obtained. In most cases this film will give sufficient information to make a preliminary diagnosis of pelvic fracture. The exact nature of the injury can be clarified by more detailed radiography once it is certain that the patient can tolerate an extended period of positioning and repositioning on the x-ray table. Five views are necessary: anteroposterior, an inlet view (tube cephalad to the pelvis and tilted 30 degrees downwards), an outlet view (tube caudad to the pelvis and tilted 40 degrees upwards), and right and left oblique views.

If any serious injury is suspected, a CT scan at the appropriate level is extremely helpful (some would say essential). This is particularly true for posterior pelvic ring disruptions and for complex acetabular fractures, which cannot be properly evaluated on plain x-rays.

Three-dimensional CT re-formation of the pelvic image gives the most accurate picture of the injury; this is the method of choice wherever the facilities are available (Fishman et al., 1989).

X-ray of the urinary tract

If there is evidence of upper abdominal injury, and the patient has haematuria, an intravenous urogram is performed to exclude renal injury. This will also show whether there is any ureteric or major bladder damage. In a case of urethral

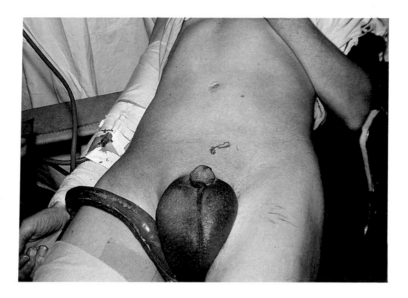

26.1 Fracture of the pelvis This young man crashed on his motorcycle and was brought into the accident and emergency department with a fractured femur. His perineum and scrotum were swollen and bruised, he was unable to pass urine and a streak of blood appeared at the external meatus. X-rays confirmed that he had a fractured pelvis.

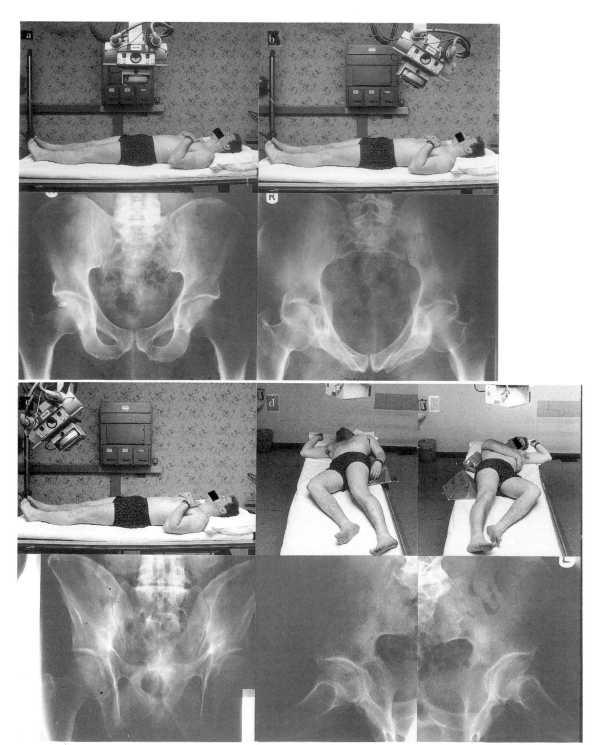

26.2 Pelvic fractures – x-ray diagnosis   Five views are ideal: (a) anteroposterior; (b) inlet view with the tube tilted 30 degrees downwards; (c) outlet view with the tube tilted 40 degrees upwards; (d, e) right and left oblique views. The corresponding x-rays are shown below.

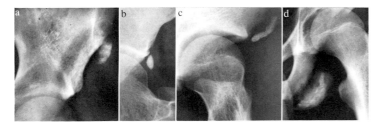

26.3 Avulsion injuries   These all result from powerful muscle action. (a) Avulsion of sartorius attachment; this should not be confused with (b) an os acetabuli, which is well-defined on all sides. (c) Avulsion of rectus origin. (d) Avulsion of hamstring origin – the clinical condition is much less alarming than the x-ray.

rupture, the base of the bladder may be riding high (dislocated prostate) or there may be a teardrop deformity of the bladder owing to compression by blood and extravasated urine (prostate-in-situ).

When a urethral injury is considered likely, a urethrogram should be undertaken using 25–30 ml of water-soluble contrast agent with suitable aseptic technique. A film must be taken during injection of the contrast agent to ensure that the urethra is fully distended. This technique will confirm a urethral tear and will show whether it is complete or incomplete.

In a patient with possible rupture of the bladder (so long as there is no evidence of a urethral injury) a cystogram should be performed.

Types of injury

Injuries of the pelvis fall into four groups: (1) isolated fractures with an intact pelvic ring; (2) fractures with a broken ring – these may be stable or unstable; (3) fractures of the acetabulum – although these are ring fractures, involvement of the joint raises special problems and therefore they are considered separately; and (4) sacrococcygeal fractures.

Isolated fractures

Avulsion fractures

A piece of bone is pulled off by violent muscle contraction; this is usually seen in sportsmen and athletes. The sartorius may pull off the anterior superior iliac spine, the rectus femoris the anterior inferior iliac spine, the adductor longus a piece of the pubis, and the hamstrings part of the ischium. All are essentially muscle injuries, needing only rest for a few days and reassurance.

Pain may take months to disappear and, because there is often no history of impact injury, biopsy of the callus may lead to an erroneous diagnosis of a tumour. Rarely, avulsion of the ischial apophysis by the hamstrings may lead to persistent symptoms, in which case open reduction and internal fixation is indicated (Wootton, Cross and Holt, 1990).

Direct fractures

A direct blow to the pelvis, usually after a fall from a height, may fracture the ischium or the iliac blade. Bed rest until pain subsides is usually all that is needed.

Stress fractures

Fractures of the pubic rami are fairly common (and often quite painless) in severely osteo-

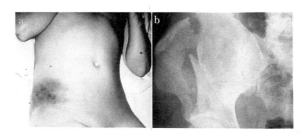

26.4 Fractured iliac blade   (a) The bruise points to the site of the fracture. (b) The fracture looks alarming and is certainly painful but, if the remainder of the bony pelvis is intact, it poses no threat to the patient.

porotic or osteomalacic patients. More difficult to diagnose are stress fractures around the sacroiliac joints; this is an uncommon cause of 'sacroiliac' pain in elderly osteoporotic individuals. Obscure stress fractures are best demonstrated by radioisotope scans.

Fractures of the pelvic ring

It has been cogently argued that, because of the rigidity of the pelvis, a break at one point in the ring must be be accompanied by disruption at a second point; exceptions are fractures due to direct blows (including fractures of the acetabular floor), or ring fractures in children, whose symphysis and sacroiliac joints are springy. Often, however, the second break is not visible – either because it reduces immediately or because the sacroiliac joints are only partially disrupted; in these circumstances the visible fracture is not displaced and the ring is stable. A

fracture or joint disruption that is markedly displaced, and all obvious double ring fractures, are unstable. This distinction has more practical value than pedantic classification into 'single' and 'double' ring fractures.

Mechanisms of injury

The basic mechanisms of pelvic ring injury are anteroposterior compression, lateral compression, vertical shear and combinations of these.

ANTEROPOSTERIOR COMPRESSION This injury is usually caused by a frontal collision between a pedestrian and a car. The pubic rami are fractured or the innominate bones are sprung apart and externally rotated, with disruption of the symphysis – the so-called 'open book' injury; posteriorly the sacroiliac ligaments are partially torn, or there may be a fracture of the posterior part of the ilium.

LATERAL COMPRESSION Side to side compression of the pelvis causes the ring to buckle and break. This is usually due to a side-on impact in a road accident or a fall from a height.

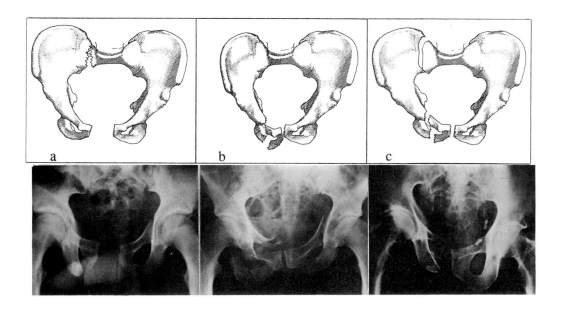

26.5 Pelvic ring fractures The three important types of injury are shown. (a) Anteroposterior compression with lateral rotation may cause the 'open book' injury. (b) Lateral compression causing the ring to buckle and break; the pubic rami are fractured, sometimes on both sides. (c) Vertical shear, with disruption of the sacroiliac region on one side.

Anteriorly the pubic rami on one or both sides are fractured, and posteriorly there is a severe sacroiliac strain or a fracture of the ilium, either on the same side as the fractured pubic rami or on the opposite side of the pelvis. If the sacroiliac injury is much displaced, the pelvis is unstable.

VERTICAL SHEAR The innominate bone on one side is displaced vertically, fracturing the pubic rami and disrupting the sacroiliac region on the same side. This occurs typically when someone falls from a height onto one leg. These are usually severe, unstable injuries with gross tearing of the soft tissues and retroperitoneal haemorrhage.

COMBINATION INJURIES In severe pelvic injuries there may be a combination of the above.

Stable and unstable fractures

Tile (1988) has classified pelvic fractures into those that are stable, those that are rotationally unstable and those that are rotationally and vertically unstable.

Table 26.1 Classification of pelvic fractures according to Tile (1988)

Type A	*Stable*
A1	Fractures of the pelvis not involving the ring
A2	Stable, minimally displaced fractures of the ring
Type B	*Rotationally unstable, vertically stable*
B1	Open book
B2	Lateral compression: ipsilateral
B3	Lateral compression: contralateral (bucket handle)
Type C	*Rotationally and vertically unstable*
C1	Unilateral
C2	Bilateral
C3	Associated with an acetabular fracture

Type A – stable: this includes avulsions (see above) and fracture of the pelvic ring with little or no displacement.

Type B – rotationally unstable, vertically stable: an external rotation force applied to one side of the pelvis may have sprung open the symph-

ysis ('open book' injury); or an internal rotation force – i.e. lateral compression – may have caused fractures of the ischiopubic rami on one or both sides, with posterior injuries also, but no opening of the symphysis ('closed book' injury).

Type C – rotationally and vertically unstable: there is disruption of the strong posterior ligaments with injuries on one or both sides and vertical displacement of one side of the pelvis; there may also be acetabular fractures.

Clinical features

In type A injuries the patient is not severely shocked but has pain on attempting to walk. There is localized tenderness but seldom any damage to pelvic viscera. Plain x-rays reveal the fractures.

In type B and C injuries the patient is severely shocked, in great pain and unable to stand; he may also be unable to pass urine. There may be blood at the external meatus. Tenderness may be localized but often it is widespread, and attempting to move one or both blades of the ilium is very painful. One leg may be partly anaesthetic because of sciatic nerve injury, and pulling or pushing may reveal the vertical instability (though this may be too painful). These are extremely serious injuries, carrying a high risk of associated visceral damage, intra-abdominal and retroperitoneal haemorrhage, shock, sepsis and ARDS; the mortality rate is considerable (Dalal et al., 1989).

X-RAY
This may show fractures of the pubic rami, ipsilateral or contralateral fractures of the posterior elements, separation of the symphysis, disruption of the sacroiliac joint or combinations of these injuries. The films are often difficult to understand and CT scans are much the best way of visualizing the nature of the injury, especially if three-dimensional CT is available.

Management

EARLY MANAGEMENT Treatment should not await full and detailed diagnosis. It is vital to keep a sense of priorities and to act on any

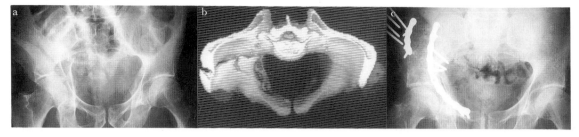

26.6 Pelvic fractures – imaging (a) The plain x-ray gives useful but limited information. (b) In this case the three-dimensional CT scan was much better and enabled the operative treatment (c) to be planned with precision. (Courtesy of Mr R. N. Brueton and Dr R. L. Guy.)

information that is already available while moving along to the next diagnostic hurdle. 'Management' in this context is a combination of assessment and treatment.

Six questions must be asked and the answers acted upon as they emerge:

1. Is there a clear airway?
2. Are the lungs adequately ventilated?
3. Is the patient losing blood?
4. Is there an intra-abdominal injury?
5. Is there a bladder or urethral injury?
6. Is the pelvic fracture stable or unstable?

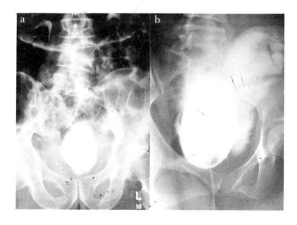

26.7 Pelvic fractures – complications (a) Intravenous urogram outlining the bladder and showing the typical globular appearance due to compression by blood and extravasated urine. There is also marked gastric dilatation suggesting retroperitoneal bleeding. (b) Cystogram showing extravasation of radio-opaque material. This patient had a ruptured bladder.

With any severely injured patient, the first step is to make sure that the airway is clear and ventilation is unimpaired. Resuscitation must be started immediately and active bleeding controlled. The patient is rapidly examined for multiple injuries and, if necessary, painful fractures are splinted. A single anteroposterior x-ray of the pelvis is obtained.

A more careful examination is then carried out, paying attention to the pelvis, the abdomen, the perineum and the rectum. The urethral meatus is inspected for signs of bleeding. The lower limbs are examined for signs of nerve injury.

If the patient's general condition is stable, further x-rays can then be obtained. If a urethral tear is suspected, a urethrogram is gently performed. The findings up to that stage may dictate the need for an intravenous urogram.

By now the examining doctor will have a good idea of the patient's general condition, the extent of the pelvic injury, the presence or absence of visceral injury and the likelihood of continued intra-abdominal or retroperitoneal bleeding. Ideally, a team of experts will be on hand to deal with the individual problems or undertake further investigations.

MANAGEMENT OF SEVERE BLEEDING The treatment of shock is described in Chapter 22. Additional measures which may be needed to deal with massive haemorrhage include the use of pneumatic antishock garments and the rapid application of an external fixator (Evers, Cryer and Miller, 1989).

The diagnosis of persistent bleeding is often difficult, and even when it seems clear that continuing shock is due to haemorrhage, it is not easy to determine the source of the bleeding. Patients with suspicious abdominal signs should be further investigated by peritoneal aspiration or lavage. If there is a positive diagnostic tap, the abdomen should be explored in an attempt to find and deal with the source of bleeding. However, if there is a large retroperitoneal haematoma, it should not be evacuated as this may release the tamponade effect and lead to uncontrollable haemorrhage.

MANAGEMENT OF THE URETHRA AND BLADDER Urological injury occurs in about 10% of patients with pelvic ring fractures. As these patients are often seriously ill from other injuries, a urinary catheter may be required to monitor urinary output, and therefore the urologist is placed under pressure to make a rapid diagnosis of urethral damage.

There is no place for passing a diagnostic catheter as this will most probably convert any partial tear to a complete tear. For an incomplete tear, the insertion of a suprapubic catheter as a formal procedure is all that is required. Around half of all incomplete tears will heal and require little long-term management.

The treatment of a complete urethral tear is controversial. Primary realignment of the urethra may be achieved by performing suprapubic cystostomy, evacuating the pelvic haematoma and then threading a catheter across the injury to drain the bladder. If the bladder is floating high it is repositioned and held down by a sling suture passed through the lower anterior part of the prostatic capsule, through the perineum on either side of the bulbar urethra and anchored to the thighs by elastic bands. An alternative – and much simpler – approach is to perform the cystostomy as soon as possible, making no attempt to drain the pelvis or dissect the urethra, and to deal with the resulting stricture 4–6 months later. The latter method is contraindicated if there is severe prostatic dislocation or severe tears of the rectum or bladder neck. With both methods there is a significant incidence of late stricture formation, incontinence and impotence.

TREATMENT OF THE FRACTURE For patients with very severe injuries, early external fixation is one of the most effective ways of reducing haemorrhage and counteracting shock (Evers, Cryer and Miller, 1989). If there are no life-threatening complications, definitive treatment is as follows.

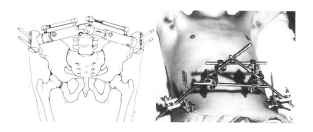

26.8 Pelvic fractures – external fixation Displaced fractures can often be reduced and held by external fixation.

Type A fractures Minimally displaced fractures and isolated fractures of the pelvis need only bed rest, possibly combined with lower limb traction. Within 4–6 weeks the patient is usually comfortable and may then be allowed up using crutches.

Type B fractures Provided it is certain that there are no displaced posterior injuries, open-book injuries with a gap of less than 2.5 cm can usually be treated satisfactorily by bed rest; a posterior sling or an elastic girdle helps to 'close the book'. A gap of more than 2.5 cm can often be closed by lying the patient on one side and pressing on the blade of the ilium. The most efficient way of maintaining reduction is by external fixation with pins in both iliac blades connected by an anterior bar; 'closing the book' may also reduce the amount of bleeding. Placing the pins is made easier if two temporary pins are first inserted hugging the medial and lateral surfaces of each iliac blade and then directing the fixing pins between them. Internal fixation by attaching a plate across the symphysis should be performed: (1) during the first few days after injury only if the patient needs a laparotomy; and (2) later on if the gap cannot be closed by less radical methods.

With closed-book injuries a sling or girdle is inappropriate. Bed rest for 6 weeks or so without any fixation is usually adequate, but, if leg length discrepancy exceeds 1.5 cm or there is gross pelvic deformity, reduction via pins in one iliac crest may be attempted and, if successful, maintained by connecting them to pins on the other side forming an external fixator. The fixation frame is usually needed for 6–8 weeks but in the later stages the patient may, if comfortable, be allowed to get up and walk about.

Type C fractures These are the most dangerous and the most difficult to treat. It may be possible to reduce some or all of the vertical displacement by skeletal traction combined with an external fixator; even so, the patient needs to remain in bed for at least 10 weeks. If reduction has not been achieved it is possible to reduce the fracture-dislocation openly and fix it with one or more dynamic compression plates. The operation is hazardous (the dangers include massive haemorrhage and infection) and should be attempted only by surgeons with considerable experience in this field (Matta and Sancedo, 1989; Leung et al., 1992). Persisting with skeletal traction and external fixation is probably safer, though the malposition is likely to leave a legacy of posterior pain. It should be emphasized that more than 60% of pelvic fractures need no fixation.

Open pelvic fractures are managed by external fixation. A diversion colostomy may be necessary.

Late complications

Persistent sacroiliac pain is fairly common after unstable pelvic fractures and may occasionally necessitate arthrodesis of the sacroiliac joint. *Sciatic nerve injury* usually recovers but sometimes exploration proves necessary. Severe urethral injuries may result in *urethral stricture, incontinence* or *impotence.*

Fractures of the acetabulum

Fractures of the acetabulum occur when the head of the femur is driven into the pelvis. This is caused either by a blow on the side (as in a fall from a height) or by a blow on the front of the knee, usually in a dashboard injury when the femur also may be fractured.

Acetabular fractures combine the complexities of pelvic fractures (notably the frequency of associated soft-tissue injury) with those of joint disruption (namely, articular cartilage damage, malcongruent loading and secondary osteoarthritis).

The classic work on this subject is the paper by the Judet brothers and Letournel (1964).

Patterns of fracture

There are four major types of acetabular fracture; though they are distinguished on

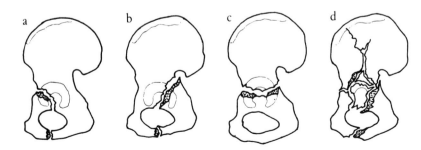

26.9 Acetabular fractures The four types of injury: (a) simple fracture of the anterior pillar; (b) fracture of the posterior pillar; (c) transverse fracture, which usually lies just above the cotyloid notch; and (d) a composite fracture. The transverse fractures (occasionally) and the composite fractures (almost always) damage the weightbearing surface and may cause post-traumatic osteoarthritis.

anatomical grounds, it is important to recognize that they also differ in their ease of reduction, their stability after reduction and their long-term prognosis.

ANTERIOR COLUMN FRACTURE The fracture runs through the thin anterior part of the acetabulum separating a segment between the anterior inferior iliac spine and the obturator foramen. It is uncommon, does not involve the weightbearing area and has a good prognosis.

POSTERIOR COLUMN FRACTURE This fracture runs upwards from the obturator foramen into the sciatic notch, separating the posterior ischiopubic column of bone and breaking the weightbearing part of the acetabulum. It is usually associated with a posterior dislocation of the hip and may injure the sciatic nerve. Treatment is more urgent and usually involves internal fixation to obtain a stable joint.

TRANSVERSE FRACTURE This is an uncomminuted fracture running transversely through the acetabulum and separating the iliac portion above from the pubic and ischial portions below. It is usually fairly easy to reduce and to hold reduced.

COMPLEX FRACTURES Most acetabular fractures are complex injuries which damage either the anterior or the posterior segments (or both) as well as the roof or the walls of the acetabulum. There is no value in precise subdivision of these complex fractures, because the differences between the various types are less important than their similarities. They all share the following features: (1) the injury is severe; (2) the joint surface is disrupted; (3) they usually need operative reduction and internal fixation; and (4) the end result is likely to be less than perfect.

Clinical features

There has usually been a severe injury – either a traffic accident or a fall from a height. Associated fractures are not uncommon and, because they may be more obvious, are liable to divert attention from the more urgent pelvic injuries. Whenever a fractured femur, a severe knee injury or a fractured calcaneum is diagnosed, the hips also should be x-rayed.

The patient may be severely shocked, and the complications associated with all pelvic fractures should be sought. Rectal examination is essential. There may be bruising around the hip and the limb may lie in internal rotation (if the hip is dislocated). No attempt should be made to move the hip.

Careful neurological examination is important, testing the function of the sciatic, femoral, obturator and pudendal nerves.

X-RAY
At least four views should be taken in every case: a standard anteroposterior view, the pelvic inlet view and two 45-degree oblique views (to show the anterior and posterior columns separately). The type of fracture, degree of comminution and the amount of displacement are noted. CT scans and three-dimensional re-formations are added refinements.

Treatment

EMERGENCY TREATMENT should consist only of counteracting shock and reducing a dislocation. Traction is then applied to the limb (10 kg will suffice) and during the next 3–4 days the patient's general condition is brought under control. Definitive treatment of the fracture is delayed until he is fit and operation facilities are optimal; but the delay should not exceed 7 days.

NON-OPERATIVE TREATMENT In recent years opinion has moved in favour of operative treatment for displaced acetabular fractures (Matta and Merritt, 1988). However, conservative treatment is still preferable in certain well-defined situations: (1) acetabular fractures with minimal displacement; (2) displaced fractures that do not involve the superomedial weightbearing segment of the acetabulum; (3) fractures in elderly patients, where closed reduction seems feasible; (4) patients with 'medical' contraindications to operative treatment (including local sepsis). Comminution in itself is not a contraindication to operative treatment, provided adequate facilities and expertise are available.

Matta and Merritt (1988) have listed certain criteria which should be met if conservative treatment is expected to succeed: (1) when traction is released, the hip should remain congruent; (2) the weightbearing portion of the acetabular roof should be intact; and (3) associated fractures of the posterior wall should be excluded by CT. Non-operative treatment is more suitable for patients aged over 50 years than for adolescents and young adults.

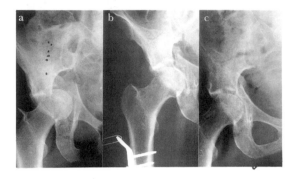

26.10 Fractured acetabulum – conservative treatment This severely displaced acetabular fracture (a) was almost completely reduced by (b) longitudinal and lateral traction. (c) The fracture healed and the patient regained a congruent joint with a fairly good range of movement.

If there are medical contraindications to operative treatment, closed reduction under general anaesthesia is attempted. In all patients treated conservatively, longitudinal traction, if necessary supplemented by lateral traction, is maintained for 6–8 weeks; this will unload the articular cartilage and will help to prevent further displacement of the fracture. During this period, hip movement and exercises are encouraged. The patient is then allowed up, using crutches with minimal weightbearing for a further 6 weeks.

OPERATIVE TREATMENT Patients with isolated posterior wall fractures and dislocation of the hip may require immediate open reduction and stabilization. In other cases operation is usually deferred for 4 or 5 days.

Matta and Merritt have made the important point that open reduction is an operation on the pelvis and not merely the acetabular socket. Adequate exposure is essential, if possible through a single approach which is selected according to the type of fracture. The most useful techniques are described in the paper by Matta and Merritt. Posterolateral exposure is facilitated by using the AO femoral distractor and osteotomizing the greater trochanter (Bray, Esser and Fulkerson, 1987). The fracture (or fractures) may be fixed with lag screws or special buttressing plates which can be shaped in the operating theatre (Matta, 1991). It is useful to monitor somatosensory evoked potentials during the operation, in order to avoid damaging the sciatic nerve (separate electrodes are required for medial and lateral popliteal branches).

Prophylactic antibiotics are used, and post-operatively hip movements are started as soon as possible. The patient is allowed up, partial weightbearing with crutches, after 7 days. Exercises are continued for 3–6 months; it may take a year or longer for full function to return.

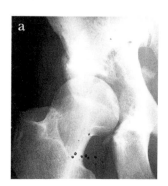
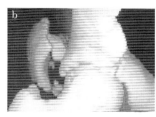
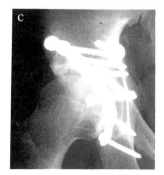

26.11 Acetabular fractures (a) Before and (c) after reduction and fixation. (b) The three-dimensional MRI shows the large posterior fragment which needed accurate repositioning. (Courtesy of Mr R. N. Brueton and Dr R. L. Guy.)

Complications

Iliofemoral venous thrombosis is fairly common and potentially serious. It is doubtful, however, whether routine prophylactic anticoagulation is warranted.

Sciatic nerve injury may occur either at the time of fracture or during the subsequent operation. Unless the nerve is seen to be unharmed during the operation, there can be no certainty about the prognosis. Intraoperative somatosensory monitoring is advocated as a means of preventing serious nerve damage. For an established lesion, it is worth waiting for 6 weeks to see if there is any sign of recovery. If there is none, the nerve should be explored in order to establish the diagnosis and ensure that the nerve is not being compressed.

Heterotopic bone formation is common after severe soft-tissue injury and extended surgical dissections. In cases where this is anticipated, prophylactic indomethacin is useful.

Avascular necrosis of the femoral head may occur even if the hip is not fully dislocated. The condition is probably overdiagnosed because of erroneous interpretation of the x-ray appearances following impacted marginal fractures of the acetabulum (Gruen, Mears and Tauxe, 1988).

Loss of joint movement and secondary osteoarthritis are common sequelae after displaced acetabular fractures involving the weightbearing portion of the joint. This may, ultimately, require joint replacement. However, the operation should be deferred until the fractures have consolidated; the acetabular implant is bound to work loose if there is any movement of the innominate segments.

Injuries to the sacrum and coccyx

A blow from behind, or a fall onto the 'tail' may fracture the sacrum or coccyx, or sprain the joint between them. Women seem to be affected more commonly than men.

Bruising is considerable and tenderness is elicited when the sacrum or coccyx is palpated

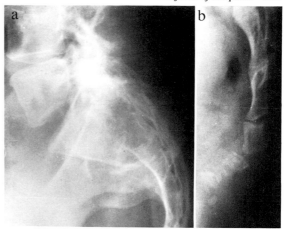

26.12 Sacrococcygeal fractures (a) Fractured sacrum; (b) fractured coccyx.

from behind or per rectum. Sensation may be lost over the distribution of sacral nerves.

X-rays may show: (1) a transverse fracture of the sacrum, in rare cases with the lower fragment pushed forwards; (2) a fractured coccyx, sometimes with the lower fragment angulated forwards; or (3) a normal appearance if the injury was a sprain of the sacrococcygeal joint.

If the fracture is displaced, reduction is worth attempting. The lower fragment may be pushed backwards per rectum. The reduction is stable, which is fortunate. The patient is allowed to resume normal activity, but is advised to use a rubber ring or Sorbo cushion when sitting. Occasionally, sacral fractures are associated with urinary problems, necessitating sacral laminectomy.

Persistent pain, especially on sitting, is common after coccygeal injuries. If the pain is not relieved by the use of a Sorbo cushion or by the injection of local anaesthetic into the tender area, excision of the coccyx may be considered.

References and further reading

Bray, T.J., Esser, M. and Fulkerson, L. (1987) Osteotomy of the trochanter in open reduction and internal fixation of acetabular fractures. *Journal of Bone and Joint Surgery* **69A**, 711–717

Dalal, S.A., Burgess, A.R., Siegel, J.H. et al. (1989) Pelvic fracture in multiple trauma. *Trauma* **29**, 981–1000

Eid, A.M. (1981) Non-urogenital abdominal complications associated with fractures of the pelvis. *Archives of Orthopedic and Traumatic Surgery* **98**, 35–40

Evers, B.M., Cryer, H.M. and Miller, S.B. (1989) Pelvic fracture hemorrhage. Priorities in management. *Archives of Surgery* **124**, 422–424

Fishman, E.K., Magid, D., Drebin, R.A. et al. (1989) Advanced three-dimensional evaluation of acetabular trauma: volumetric image processing. *Journal of Trauma* **29**, 214–218

Gruen, G.S., Mears, D.C. and Tauxe, W.N. (1988) Distinguishing avascular necrosis from segmental impaction of the femoral head following an acetabular fracture. *Journal of Orthopaedic Trauma* **2**, 5–9

Judet, R., Judet, J. and Letournel, E. (1964) Fractures of the acetabulum: classification and surgical approaches for open reduction. *Journal of Bone and Joint Surgery* **46A**, 1615–1646.

Letournel, E. (1981) *Fractures of the Acetabulum*, Springer, Berlin

Leung, K.S., Chien, P., Shen, W.Y. and So, W.S. (1992) Operative treatment of unstable pelvic fractures. *Injury* **23**, 31–37

Matta, J.M. (1991) Acetabulum. In *Manual of Internal Fixation*, 3rd edn (eds. M.E. Müller, M. Allgöwer, R, Schneider and H. Willeneger), Springer, Berlin, pp. 501–518

Matta, J.M. and Merritt, P.O. (1988) Displaced acetabular fractures. *Clinical Orthopaedics and Related Research* **230**, 83–97

Matta, J.M. and Sancedo, T. (1989) Internal fixation of pelvic ring fractures. *Clinical Orthopaedics and Related Research* **242**, 83–98

Peltier, L.F. (1965) Complications associated with fractures of the pelvis. *Journal of Bone and Joint Surgery* **47A**, 1060–1069

Perkins, G. (1966) Fractures of the pelvis. In *Clinical Surgery*, vol. 12, *Fractures and Dislocations* (ed. R. Furlong), Butterworths, London

Senegas, J., Liorzou, G. and Yates, M. (1980) Complex acetabular fractures: a transtrochanteric lateral surgical approach. *Clinical Orthopaedics and Related Research* **151**, 107–114

Tile, M. (1988) Pelvic ring fractures: should they be fixed? *Journal of Bone and Joint Surgery* **70B**, 1–12

Wootton, J.R., Cross, M.J. and Holt, K.W.G. (1990) Avulsion of the ischial apophysis. *Journal of Bone and Joint Surgery* **72B**, 625–627

I. The hip and femur

Dislocation of the hip

With the rise in the number of road accidents, dislocation of the hip has become more common. Often small fragments of bone are chipped off as the joint dislocates; if there is a major fragment, or comminution, it is regarded as a fracture-dislocation.

The injuries are classified according to the direction of dislocation: *posterior* (by far the commonest variety), *anterior* and *central* (a comminuted or displaced fracture of the acetabulum).

Posterior dislocation

Mechanism of injury

Four out of five traumatic hip dislocations are posterior. Usually this occurs in a road accident when someone seated in a truck or car is thrown forward, striking the knee against the dashboard. The femur is thrust upwards and the femoral head is forced out of its socket; often a piece of bone at the back of the acetabulum is sheared off (fracture-dislocation).

Clinical features

In a straightforward case the diagnosis is easy: the leg is short and lies adducted, internally rotated and slightly flexed. However, if one of the long bones is fractured – usually the femur – the hip injury can easily be missed. The golden rule is to x-ray the pelvis in every case of severe injury, and, with femoral fractures, to insist on an x-ray that includes the hip. The lower limb should be examined for signs of sciatic nerve injury.

X-RAY

In the anteroposteror film the femoral head is seen out of its socket and above the acetabulum. A segment of acetabular roof or femoral head may have been broken off and displaced; oblique films are useful in demonstrating the size of the fragment. If any fracture is seen, other bony fragments (which may need removal) must be suspected. A CT scan is the best way of demonstrating an acetabular fracture or any bony fragment.

Epstein (1973) suggested a classification which is helpful in planning treatment. Type I is a dislocation with no more than minor chip fractures. Type II is a dislocation with a single large fracture of the posterior acetabular lip. In type III there is comminution of the acetabular lip. Type IV has an associated fracture of the acetabular floor, and type V a fracture of the femoral head.

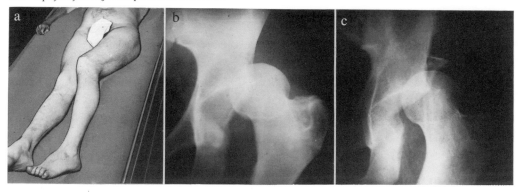

27.1 Posterior dislocation   (a, b) Uncomplicated posterior dislocation; reduction is usually straightforward, but it is important to be sure that no loose bony fragments remain in the joint. (c) Associated acetabular fracture which may need open reduction and fixation.

Treatment

The dislocation must be reduced as soon as possible under general anaesthesia. In the vast majority of cases this is performed closed. An assistant steadies the pelvis; the surgeon flexes the patient's hip and knee to 90 degrees and pulls the thigh vertically upwards. X-rays are essential to confirm reduction and to exclude a fracture. If there is the slightest suspicion that bone fragments have been trapped inside the joint, CT is needed.

Reduction is usually stable, but the hip has been severely injured and needs to be rested. The simplest way is to apply traction and maintain it for 3 weeks. Movement and exercises are begun as soon as pain allows. At the end of 3 weeks the patient is allowed to walk with crutches.

If the post-reduction x-rays or CT scan show the presence of intra-articular fragments, they should be removed and the joint washed out through a posterior approach. This is usually postponed until the patient's condition has stabilized.

Epstein type II fracture-dislocations are often treated by immediate open reduction and anatomical fixation of the detached fragment. However, if the patient's general condition is suspect, or the necessary surgical skills are not available, the hip is reduced closed, as described above. Only if the joint is unstable, or a large fragment remains unreduced, is open reduction and internal fixation essential. In type II cases, traction is maintained for 6 weeks.

Type III injuries are treated closed, but there may be retained fragments and these should be removed by open operation; traction is maintained for 6 weeks.

Type IV and V injuries are treated initially by closed reduction. A femoral head fragment may automatically fall into place, and this can be confirmed by post-reduction CT. If the fragment remains unreduced, operative treatment is indicated: a small fragment can simply be removed, but a large fragment should be replaced; the joint is opened, the femoral head dislocated and the fragment fixed in position with a countersunk screw. Postoperatively, traction is maintained for 4 weeks and full weight-bearing is deferred for 12 weeks.

Complications

EARLY

Sciatic nerve injury   The sciatic nerve is sometimes damaged but usually recovers. If, after reducing the dislocation, a sciatic nerve lesion and an unreduced acetabular fracture are diagnosed, the nerve should be explored and the fragment correctly replaced (and screwed in position). Recovery often takes months and in the meantime the limb must be protected from injury and the ankle splinted to overcome the foot drop.

Vascular injury Occasionally the superior gluteal artery is torn and bleeding may be profuse. If this is suspected, an arteriogram should be performed. The torn vessel may need to be ligated.

Associated fractured femoral shaft When this occurs at the same time as hip dislocation, the dislocation is commonly missed. It should be a rule that with every femoral shaft fracture the buttock and trochanter are palpated, and the hip clearly seen on x-ray. Even if this precaution has been omitted, a dislocation should be suspected whenever the proximal fragment of a transverse shaft fracture is seen to be adducted. Reduction of the dislocation is much more difficult, but a gentle closed manipulation should still be attempted. If this fails, open reduction should be performed, and at the same time the femur may be fixed with an intramedullary nail.

LATE

Avascular necrosis The blood supply of the femoral head is seriously impaired in at least 10% of traumatic hip dislocations; if reduction is delayed by more than a few hours, the figure rises to 40%. Avascular necrosis shows on x-ray as increased density of the femoral head; but this change is not seen for at least 6 weeks, and sometimes very much longer (up to 2 years), depending on the rate of bone repair. In the early weeks, radioscintigraphy may reveal signs of bone ischaemia. If the femoral head shows signs of fragmentation, an operation may be needed. If there is a small necrotic segment, realignment osteotomy is the method of choice. Otherwise, in younger patients, the choice is between femoral head replacement with a bipolar prosthesis or hip arthrodesis (never an easy procedure). In patients over the age of 50 a total hip replacement is better.

Myositis ossificans This is an uncommon complication, probably related to the severity of the injury. Being difficult to predict, it is difficult to prevent. But movements should never be forced and in severe injuries the period of rest and non-weightbearing may need to be prolonged.

Unreduced dislocation After a few weeks an untreated dislocation can seldom be reduced by closed manipulation and open reduction is needed. The incidence of stiffness or avascular necrosis is considerably increased and the patient may later need reconstructive surgery.

Osteoarthritis Secondary osteoarthritis is not uncommon and is due to (1) cartilage damage at the time of the dislocation, (2) the presence of retained fragments in the joint or (3) ischaemic necrosis of the femoral head. In young patients treatment presents a difficult problem (see p. 417).

Anterior dislocation

Anterior dislocation is rare compared with posterior. The usual cause is a road accident or air crash. Dislocation of one or even both hips may occur when a weight falls onto the back of a miner or building labourer who is working with his legs wide apart, knees straight and back bent forwards.

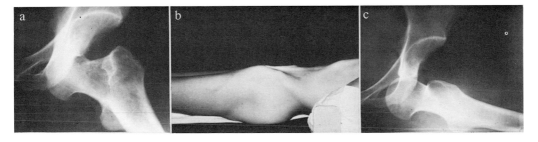

27.2 Anterior hip dislocations (a, b) The usual apearance of an anterior dislocation – the hip is only slightly abducted and the head shows clinically as a prominent lump. (c) Occasionally an anterior dislocation is in wide abduction.

Clinical features

The leg lies externally rotated, abducted and slightly flexed. It is not short, because the attachment of rectus femoris prevents the head from displacing upwards. Seen from the side, the anterior bulge of the dislocated head is unmistakable. Occasionally the leg is abducted almost to a right angle. The prominent head is easy to feel. Hip movements are impossible.

X-RAY

In the anteroposterior view the dislocation is usually obvious, but occasionally the head is almost directly in front of its normal position; any doubt is resolved by a lateral film.

Treatment and complications

The manoeuvres employed are almost identical with those used to reduce a posterior dislocation, except that, while the flexed thigh is being pulled upwards, it should be adducted. The subsequent treatment is similar to that employed for posterior dislocation. Avascular necrosis is the only complication.

Central dislocation (see also Chapter 26)

A fall on the side, or a blow over the greater trochanter, may thrust the femoral head into the floor of the acetabulum and fracture the pelvis.

Clinical features

The thigh is grazed or bruised but the leg lies in normal position. The trochanter and hip region are tender. Little movement is possible.

The patient should be carefully examined for pelvic and abdominal injuries.

X-RAY

The femoral head is displaced medially, and the acetabular floor fractured.

Treatment

An attempt should always be made to reduce the dislocation and restore the general shape of the hip. Even if secondary osteoarthritis is inevitable, a more or less normal anatomy will make reconstructive surgery easier.

Central dislocation with comminution of the acetabular floor can sometimes be reduced by manipulation under general anaesthesia. The surgeon pulls strongly on the thigh and then tries to lever the head outwards by adducting the thigh, using a firm bolster as a fulcrum. If this is successful, longitudinal skeletal traction is maintained for 4–6 weeks, checking by x-ray to see that the femoral head remains under the weightbearing part of the acetabulum.

If manipulation fails, combined longitudinal and lateral skeletal traction may reduce the dislocation over a period of 2–3 weeks. Should that not succeed it is wise to be content with even imperfect reduction.

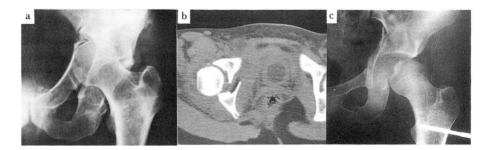

27.3 Central dislocation (a) The plain x-ray gives a good picture of the displacement, but (b) a CT scan shows the pelvic injury much more clearly. (c) Skeletal traction is an effective method of reduction.

With all these methods, it is important to commence movement as soon as possible. When traction is removed the patient is allowed up with crutches. Weightbearing is permitted after 8 weeks. The functional result is better than the x-ray appearances would suggest; but unless displacement was only trivial, all movements except flexion and extension remain considerably limited, and degenerative arthritis ultimately develops.

Displaced fractures of the anterior and posterior columns of the acetabulum are dealt with in Chapter 26.

Complications

EARLY

As with other pelvic fractures, visceral injury may be present and shock severe.

LATE

Joint stiffness, with or without osteoarthritis, is not uncommon. If total hip replacement is contemplated, it is essential to ensure that the acetabular fracture has united, otherwise the cup will inevitably work loose. In the young patient, arthrodesis may be wiser, though it is becoming more difficult to persuade patients to accept this option.

Fractures of the femoral neck

The femoral neck is the commonest site of fractures in the elderly. The vast majority of patients are women in the eight or ninth decade, and the association with osteoporosis is so manifest that the incidence of femoral neck fractures is used as a measure of age-related osteoporosis in population studies. Yet this is not merely a consequence of senescence: fractures tend to occur in people with above-average osteopenia, many of whom have bone-losing or bone-weakening disorders such as osteomalacia, diabetes, stroke (disuse), alcoholism and chronic debilitating disease (Solomon, 1973; Cooper, 1989); some of these conditions also contribute to an increased tendency to fall.

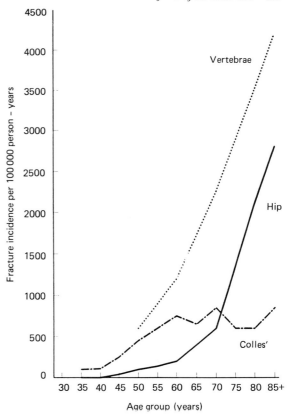

27.4 Fractures of the femoral neck The incidence of 'osteoporotic' fractures in women rises sharply from the menopause onwards.

By contrast, femoral neck fractures are unusual in negroid populations (Solomon, 1968) and in patients with osteoarthritis of the hip.

Mechanism of injury

A common injury is a fall (or a blow) on the greater trochanter. Or an elderly woman may merely catch her toe in the carpet and twist the hip into external rotation. Some patients have evidence of preceding stress fractures of the femoral neck.

Once fractured, the head and neck become displaced in progressively severe stages (Garden, 1961). Stage I is an incomplete impacted fracture. Stage II is a complete but undisplaced fracture. Stage III is a complete fracture with

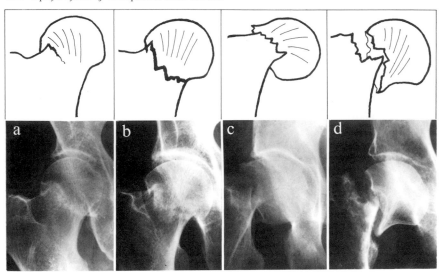

27.5 Garden's classification of femoral neck fractures (a) Stage I: incomplete (so-called abducted or impacted). (b) Stage II: complete without displacement. (c) Stage III: complete with partial displacement – fragments still connected by posterior retinacular attachment; the femoral trabeculae are malaligned. (d) Stage IV: complete with full displacement – the proximal fragment is free and lies correctly in the acetabulum so that the trabeculae appear normally aligned.

moderate displacement. And stage IV is a severely displaced fracture. Left untreated, a comparatively benign-looking stage I fracture may rapidly disintegrate to stage IV.

Pathology

The femoral head gets its blood supply from three sources: (1) intramedullary vessels in the femoral neck; (2) ascending cervical vessels in the capsular retinaculum; and (3) the vessels of the round ligament. The intramedullary supply is always interrupted by the fracture; the retinacular vessels, also, may be torn if there is much displacement. In elderly people, the remaining supply in the ligamentum teres is at best fairly meagre and, in 20% of cases, non-existent. Hence the high incidence of avascular necrosis in displaced femoral neck fractures.

Transcervical fractures are, by definition, intracapsular. They have a poor capacity for healing because: (1) by tearing the capsular vessels the injury deprives the head of its main blood supply; (2) intra-articular bone has only a

flimsy periosteum and no contact with soft tissues which could promote callus formation; and (3) synovial fluid prevents clotting of the fracture haematoma. Accurate apposition and impaction of bone fragments are therefore of more importance than usual. There is evidence that aspirating a haemarthrosis increases the blood flow in the femoral head by relieving tamponade (Harper, Barnes and Gregg, 1991).

Clinical features

There is usually a history of a fall, followed by pain in the hip. The patient lies with the limb in lateral rotation, and the leg looks short.

Beware, though: not all hip fractures are so obvious. With an impacted fracture the patient may still be able to walk; and debilitated or mentally handicapped patients may not complain at all – even with bilateral fractures.

X-RAY

Two questions must be answered: is there a fracture? and is it displaced? Usually the break

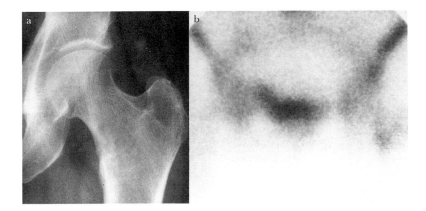

27.6 Fracture of the femoral neck – diagnosis (a) An elderly woman tripped on the pavement and complained of pain in the left hip. The plain x-ray showed no abnormality. Two weeks later she was still in pain; (b) a bone scan showed a 'hot' area medially at the base of the femoral neck, suggesting a stress fracture. Prophylactic fixation was performed.

is obvious, but an impacted fracture can be missed by the unwary. Displacement is judged by the abnormal shape of the bone shadows and the degree of mismatch of the trabecular lines in the femoral head and the stump of the femoral neck. This assessment is important because impacted or undisplaced fractures (Garden stages I and II) do well after internal fixation, whereas displaced fractures have a high rate of non-union and avascular necrosis (Barnes et al., 1976).

Diagnosis

There are three situations in which a femoral neck fracture may be missed – sometimes with dire consequences. (1) *Stress fracture* – the elderly patient with unexplained pain in the hip may have a stress fracture; the x-ray is normal but a bone scan will show the 'hot' lesion. (2) *Impacted fractures* – the fracture line is invisible, but the shape of the femoral head and neck is distorted; always compare the two sides. (3) *Painless fracture* – a bed-ridden patient may develop a 'silent' fracture.

Treatment

Operative treatment is almost mandatory. Displaced fractures will not unite without internal fixation, and in any case old people should be got up and active without delay if pulmonary complications and bed sores are to be prevented. Impacted fractures can be left to unite,

but there is always a risk that they may become displaced, even while lying in bed, so fixation is safer.

What if operation is considered dangerous? Lying in bed on traction may be even more dangerous, and leaving the fracture untreated too painful; the patient least fit for operation may need it most.

The principles of treatment are accurate reduction, secure fixation and early activity. With the patient under anaesthesia, the hip and knee are flexed and the fractured thigh is pulled upwards, then internally rotated, then extended and abducted; the foot is now tied to a footpiece. X-ray control (preferably with an image intensifier) is used to confirm reduction in anteroposterior and lateral views. Accurate reduction of stage III and IV fractures is

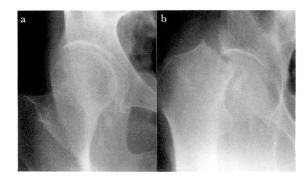

27.7 Femoral neck injuries (a) This fracture was thought to be securely impacted, but (b) a few days later it displaced completely. A pity it had not been fixed – the operation would have been easier and the prognosis better.

important; to fix an unreduced fracture is to invite failure. If a stage III or IV fracture cannot be reduced closed, and the patient is under 60 years of age, open reduction through an anterolateral approach is advisable. However, in older patients (and certainly in those over 70) this is seldom justified; if two careful attempts at closed reduction fail, prosthetic replacement is preferable.

Once the fracture is reduced, it is held with cannulated pins or screws or, sometimes, with a sliding compression screw ('dynamic hip screw') which attaches to the femoral shaft. A lateral incision is used to expose the upper femur. Guide wires, inserted under fluoroscopic control, are used to ensure correct placement of the fixing device. Two cannulated screws will suffice; they should lie parallel and extend into the subchondral bone plate; in the lateral view they are central in the head and neck, but in the anteroposterior view the distal screw lies against the inferior cortex of the neck (Olerud, Rehnberg and Hellquist, 1991).

From the first day the patient should sit up in bed or in a chair. She is taught breathing exercises, encouraged to help herself and to begin walking (with crutches or a walker) as soon as possible. To delay weightbearing may be theoretically ideal but is rarely practicable.

Prosthetic replacement Some argue that the prognosis for stage III and IV fractures is so unpredictable that prosthetic replacement is always preferable. This underestimates the morbidity associated with replacement. Our policy is therefore to attempt reduction and fixation in all patients aged under 75 and to reserve replacement for (1) the very old and the very frail, and (2) patients in whom closed reduction fails. The least traumatic replacement is an uncemented femoral prosthesis or a bipolar prosthesis inserted through a posterior ap-

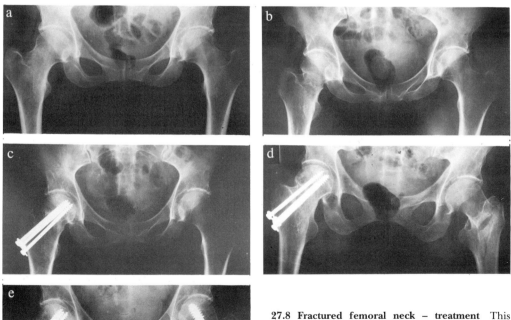

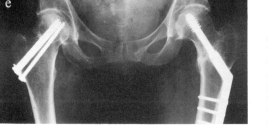

27.8 Fractured femoral neck – treatment This elderly woman was osteoporotic but otherwise well, until she stumbled and fractured the right femoral neck (b). The fracture was fixed with three long screws (c) and united soundly. Then, a year later, she tripped and sustained an intertrochanteric fracture on the left side (d). This needed more extensive fixation – a large screw fitted to a plate attached to the femoral shaft (e).

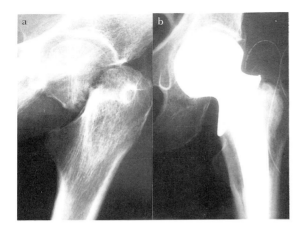

27.9 Fracture of the femoral neck – treatment (a) In a very old patient with a severely displaced fracture, prosthetic replacement (b) may be quicker and less traumatic than fixation and may also permit earlier rehabilitation.

proach. Total hip replacement may be better (1) if treatment has been delayed for some weeks and acetabular damage is suspected, or (2) in patients with metastatic disease or Paget's disease.

Complications

General complications such as follow any injury or operation in the elderly are liable to occur, especially calf vein thrombosis, pulmonary embolism, pneumonia and bed sores; not to mention disorders that might have been present before the fracture and which lead to death in a substantial proportion of cases. In some centres anticoagulants are used routinely.

Avascular necrosis occurs in about 30% of patients with displaced fractures and 10% of those with undisplaced fractures. There is no way of diagnosing this at the time of fracture. A few weeks later, the nanocolloid scan may show diminished vascularity. X-ray changes – increased density of the femoral head – may not become apparent for months or even years. Whether the fracture unites or not, collapse of the femoral head will cause pain and progressive loss of function. The treatment is total joint replacement.

Non-union More than one-third of all femoral neck fractures fail to unite, and the risk is particularly high in those that are severely displaced. There are many causes: poor blood supply, imperfect reduction, inadequate fixation, and the tardy healing that is characteristic of intra-articular fractures. The bone at the fracture site is ground away, the fragments fall apart and the nail or screw cuts out of the bone or is extruded laterally. The patient complains of pain, shortening of the limb and difficulty with walking. The x-ray shows the sorry outcome.

The method of treatment depends on the cause of the non-union and the age of the patient.

In the relatively young, three procedures are available. (1) If the fracture is unduly vertical but the head is alive, subtrochanteric osteotomy with nail-plate fixation changes the fracture line to a more horizontal angle. (2) If the reduction or fixation was faulty and there are no signs of necrosis, it is reasonable to remove the screws, reduce the fracture, insert fresh screws correctly and also to insert a fibular graft across the fracture (3) If the head is avascular, it may be

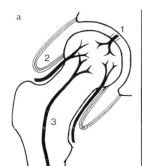

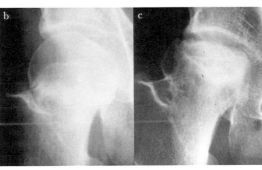

27.10 Fracture of the femoral neck – avascular necrosis (a) The blood supply to the femoral head comes from (1) a vessel in the ligamentum teres, (2) the retinacular vessels and (3) the nutrient artery. Fracture of the femoral neck interrupts at least one source of supply and may seriously compromise the others. Even (b) an impacted fracture, if it is displaced in marked valgus, can lead to avascular necrosis (c).

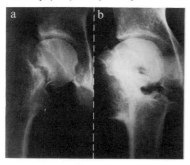

27.11 Fractures of the femoral neck – non-union (a, b) In this relatively young patient non-union has been treated successfully by osteotomy.

replaced by a metal prosthesis; if arthritis is already present, total replacement is necessary.

In elderly patients, only two procedures should be considered. (1) If the pain is not severe, a raised heel and a stout stick or elbow crutch are often sufficient. (2) If the pain is considerable, then, no matter whether the head is avascular or not, it is best removed; if the patient is reasonably fit, total joint replacement is performed.

Osteoarthritis Avascular necrosis or femoral head collapse may lead, after several years, to secondary osteoarthritis. If there is marked loss of joint movement and widespread damage to the articular surface, total joint replacement will be needed.

Femoral neck fractures in children

Hip fractures rarely occur in children but when they do they are potentially very serious.

The fracture is invariably due to severe trauma; for example, falling from a height or a car accident. There is a high risk of avascular necrosis – 42% in Ratliff's (1962) series – and particularly in displaced fractures.

TREATMENT Undisplaced fractures may be treated by immobilization in a plaster spica for 6 weeks. Displaced fractures – including 'doubtful' cases and those with mild displacement – should be treated by closed reduction and internal fixation using two threaded pins. Because of the risk of avascular necrosis, weight-bearing should be deferred until the fracture is firmly united and the femoral head appears normal.

COMPLICATIONS The main complication is avascular necrosis of the femoral head, which produces x-ray changes within a month or two of fracture. Treatment is problematic. Non-weightbearing, or 'containment splintage' in abduction and internal rotation, are usually advocated. The outcome is unpredictable: healing is sometimes excellent, but if the entire head is involved the child will end up with a stiff hip. Arthrodesis may be advisable, as a late salvage procedure.

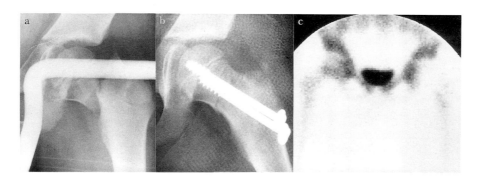

27.12 Femoral neck fractures – children (a) Fracture of the femoral neck in a child is particularly worrying because, even with perfect fixation (b), there is often ischaemia of the femoral head. (c) The scan shows deficient isotope uptake in the femoral head.

Intertrochanteric fractures

Intertrochanteric fractures are, by definition, extracapsular. As with femoral neck fractures, they are common in elderly, osteoporotic people; most of the patients are women in the 8th decade. However, in contrast to intracapsular fractures, extracapsular trochanteric fractures unite quite easily and seldom cause avascular necrosis.

Mechanism of injury

The fracture is caused either by a fall directly onto the greater trochanter or by an indirect twisting injury. The crack runs up between the lesser and greater trochanter and the proximal fragment tends to displace in varus. There may be comminution of the posteromedial cortex.

Intertrochanteric fractures are divided into stable and unstable varieties. Unstable fractures are mainly those in which the medial cortex is shattered, displacing a large fragment that includes the lesser trochanter; these are particularly difficult to hold with internal fixation.

Clinical features

The patient is usually old and unfit. Following a fall she is unable to stand. The leg is shorter and more externally rotated than with a cervical fracture (because the fracture is extracapsular) and the patient cannot lift her leg.

X-RAY

Undisplaced, stable fractures may show no more than a thin crack along the intertrochanteric line; indeed, there is often doubt as to whether the bone is fractured.

More often the fracture is displaced and there may be considerable comminution. If the lesser trochanter is separated and the medial cortex fragmented, internal fixation may not be stable and weightbearing should be delayed.

Treatment

Intertrochanteric fractures are almost always treated by early internal fixation – not because they fail to unite with conservative treatment (they unite quite readily), but (1) to obtain the best possible position and (2) to get the patient up and walking as soon as possible and thereby reduce the complications associated with prolonged recumbency.

Minimally displaced fractures are reduced by slight traction and internal rotation; the position is checked by x-ray and the fracture is fixed with an angled device – preferably a sliding nail or screw – that grips the femoral head and neck and is fixed to the shaft with screws.

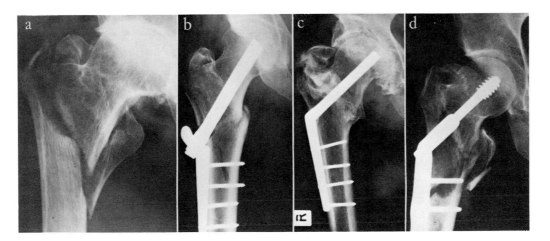

27.13 Intertrochanteric fractures (a) The medial femoral cortex just below the lesser trochanter is important for stability; (b) fixation with a McLaughlin pin and plate; (c) with a fixed-angle blade-plate; (d) with a sliding screw and plate.

If the fracture is comminuted and unstable, it is often better reduced in slight external rotation; a sliding device that allows the fragments to impact (e.g. a 'dynamic hip screw') is essential in these cases. An alternative approach is to evade the need for anatomical reduction and aim for stability instead, by displacing the distal shaft medially and/or valgus, impacting the fragments and then applying internal fixation. If the medial cortex seems grossly deficient it may be wise to add bone grafts.

Postoperatively, exercises are started on the day after operation and the patient is allowed up and partial weightbearing as soon as possible.

Complications

EARLY

Early complications are the same as with femoral neck fractures.

LATE

Deformity Varus and external rotation deformities are common. Fortunately they are seldom severe and rarely interfere with function.

Non-union is uncommon, but if the fracture is not firmly united by 6 months it probably will not join and further operation is advisable; the fracture is repositioned, the fixation device is applied more securely, and bone grafts are packed around the fracture.

Pathological fractures

Intertrochanteric fractures may be due to metastatic disease or myeloma. Unless patients are terminally ill, fracture fixation is essential in order to ensure an acceptable quality of life for their remaining years. In addition to internal fixation, methylmethacrylate cement may be packed in the defect to improve stability.

If there is involvement of the femoral neck, bone replacement with a cemented prosthesis may be preferable.

Fractures of the trochanters

In adolescents, the *lesser trochanter* apophysis may be avulsed by the pull of the psoas muscle;

the injury nearly always occurs during hurdling. Less commonly, part of the *greater trochanter* is avulsed by the abductor muscles. With either injury the patient needs to rest in bed for only 2–3 days and may then get up using crutches. As soon as he can balance on the affected leg, crutches may be discarded, but he is unlikely to resume athletic activities until the following season.

Occasionally the greater trochanter is fractured by a direct blow. A large, separated fragment should be fixed back in position with cancellous screws. Full weightbearing is prohibited for 6–8 weeks.

Subtrochanteric fractures

Subtrochanteric fractures may occur at any age if the injury is severe enough; but most occur with relatively trivial injury, in elderly patients with osteoporosis, osteomalacia or a secondary deposit. Blood loss is greater than with femoral neck or trochanteric fractures. The head and neck are abducted by the gluteal muscles, and flexed by the psoas.

Fracture healing is slow and, if an angled blade-plate is used, the implant may fail before the fracture unites.

Clinical features

The leg lies externally rotated, is short, and the thigh is markedly swollen. Movement is excruciatingly painful.

X-RAY

The fracture is through or below the lesser trochanter. It may be transverse, oblique or spiral, and is frequently comminuted. The upper fragment is flexed and appears deceptively short; the shaft is adducted and is displaced proximally.

Treatment

Open reduction and internal fixation is the treatment of choice. For fractures at the level of the

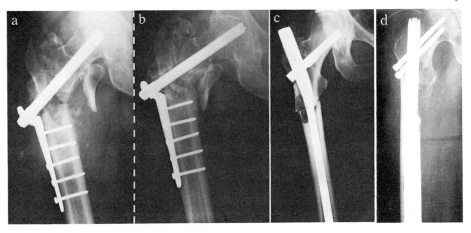

27.14 Subtrochanteric fractures   Fixation with a pin and plate (a) often fails (b). Intramedullary fixation (c) is better. (d) These fractures are not uncommonly through secondary deposits and need very secure fixation.

lesser trochanter, a compression (dynamic) hip screw and plate is satisfactory. With fractures lower than this, the bending forces are much more intense, and therefore it is better to use an intramedullary nail with a pin or locking screws entering the femoral neck and head. If the medial cortex is comminuted or deficient, bone grafts should be added. Postoperatively the patient is allowed partial weightbearing (with crutches) until union is secure – usually at 12 weeks.

Closed reduction is feasible and may be indicated for severely comminuted fractures where internal fixation is either impossible or unsafe, and for open fractures. Skeletal traction is applied through a distal femoral pin, thus permitting free knee movement. Because the proximal fragment is pulled into flexion and abduction, the patient must be nursed sitting, or else lying with the hip and knee flexed 90 degrees and slightly abducted. Traction needs to be maintained for 3 months, so the method is poorly suited to the elderly.

Complications

Non-union and *malunion* are quite common. They may require operative correction and bone grafting.

Femoral shaft fractures

The femoral shaft is well padded with powerful muscles – an advantage in protecting the bone from all but the most powerful forces, but a disadvantage in that fractures are often severely displaced by muscle pull, requiring powerful and prolonged traction for their reduction.

Mechanism of injury

This is essentially a fracture of young adults; if it occurs in an elderly patient it should be considered 'pathological' until proved otherwise.

A *spiral fracture* is usually caused by a fall in which the foot is anchored while a twisting force is transmitted to the femur. *Transverse* and *oblique fractures* are more often due to angulation or direct violence and are therefore particularly common in motorcycle accidents. With severe violence (often a combination of direct and indirect forces) the fracture may be *comminuted*, or the bone may be broken in more than one place (*segmental fractures*).

Although the soft tissues are always injured and bleeding may be severe (over a litre can be lost into the tissues), the muscles are still

capable of stabilizing a mid-shaft fracture treated by traction. Fractures at either end, on the
other hand, are usually difficult to control.

Clinical features

Most patients are young adults. Shock is severe,
and with closed fractures fat embolism is
common. The leg is rotated externally and may
be short and deformed. The thigh is swollen
and bruised.

X-RAY

The fracture may be situated in any part of the
shaft, but the middle third is the most common
site. It may be spiral or transverse, or there may
be a separate triangular ('butterfly') fragment
on one side. Displacement may occur in any
direction. Occasionally there are two transverse
fragments, such that a segment of the femur is
isolated.

The pelvis should always be x-rayed to avoid
missing an associated hip injury or pelvic
fracture.

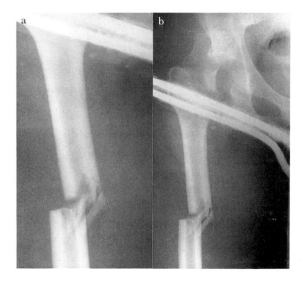

27.15 Femoral shaft fractures (a) The upper fragment of
this femur is adducted, which should alert the surgeon to
the possibility of (b) an associated hip dislocation. With this
combination of injuries the dislocation is frequently missed;
the safest plan is to x-ray the pelvis with every fracture of the
femoral shaft.

Emergency treatment

At the site of the accident, shock should be
treated and the fracture splinted before the
patient is moved. The injured limb may be tied
to the other leg or to any convenient splint. For
transport a Thomas' splint is ideal: the leg is
pulled straight and threaded through the ring
of the splint; the shod foot is tied to the cross-
piece so as to maintain traction, and the limb
and splint are firmly bandaged together.

Once in hospital and fit for operation the
patient is anaesthetized, the splint removed
(wound toilet is performed if the fracture was
open) and definitive treatment instituted.

Definitive treatment – choice of method

With open fractures internal fixaton should be
avoided, unless associated injuries dictate
otherwise.

With closed fractures there is a choice of four
methods: traction, traction followed by bracing,
open reduction with intramedullary nailing,
and closed intramedullary nailing. Closed treatment is safe but irksome; open treatment is
quick and convenient but not without risk.

Traction can reduce and hold most fractures
in reasonable alignment, and joint mobility can
be ensured by active exercises. The chief
drawback is the length of time spent in bed
(10–14 weeks for adults) with the attendant
problems of maintaining fracture alignment to
the end and reducing patient morbidity and
frustration. Some of these difficulties are overcome by reducing the time in traction and then
changing to *functional bracing*; indeed, for fractures in the lower half of the femur this is
regarded by some as the method of choice.
Some residual deformity is almost inevitable;
but up to 2 cm of shortening, 10 degrees of
angulation and 15 degrees of anterior bowing
can usually be tolerated without significant loss
of function.

However, non-operative treatment is unreliable for fractures in the upper half of the femur,
the very group in which internal fixation,
preferably by intramedullary nailing, is comparatively easy and dependable. Therefore, provided the necessary expertise and facilities are
available, *internal fixation* may (some would say
'should') be used for transverse fractures in the

proximal half of the bone, especially if closed reduction is difficult to maintain. Other indications are pathological fracture, multiple fractures, fracture associated with vascular injury and fracture in a patient presenting major nursing problems. In recent years, the method has been extended by the development of *closed medullary nailing*, which obviates the necessity to expose the fracture, and by the addition of *locking screws*, which allows internal fixation to be used for comminuted and unstable or lower third fractures.

A PLAN OF ACTION
Based on the above arguments, the following plan of action is advocated.

Prereduction   Initially all patients are placed on traction – skin traction for children, skeletal traction for adults. If this is to change, definitive treatment is commenced within a week.

Closed treatment   is continued if facilities are less than ideal, and the fracture is reduced (or almost reduced). This is the method of choice in children, who have a great capacity for healing and bone remodelling. Reduction is checked by x-ray at weekly intervals. After 3 weeks in children and 5–6 weeks in adults it may be possible to discontinue traction and hold the limb in a spica (for children) or a functional brace (for adults).

Internal fixation   is *strongly indicated* for pathological fractures and for patients with multiple injuries. It is also *preferable* for other closed fractures in adults, provided the facilities and the necessary expertise are available to perform *closed medullary nailing* (and interlocking screw fixation, if necessary). If such facilities are not available, elective internal fixation may still be preferable for upper third fractures that are difficult to hold reduced (malalignment of more than 10 degrees in the anteroposterior x-ray is the limit of acceptability).

External fixation   is sometimes used for open fractures that are unsuitable for internal fixation and difficult to hold by traction and splintage.

Definitive treatment – techniques

TRACTION AND SPLINTAGE   In children, *skin traction* without a splint is usually all that is needed,

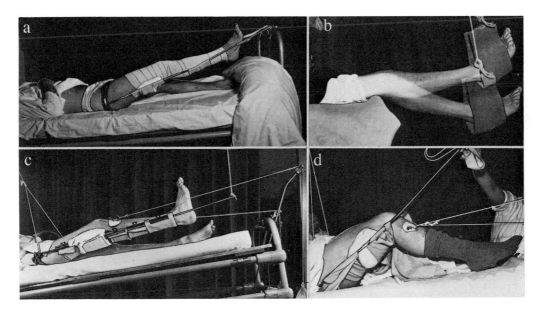

27.16 Femoral shaft fractures   (a) Fixed traction on a Thomas' splint: the splint is tied to the foot of the bed which is elevated. This method should be used only rarely because the knee may stiffen; (b) this was the range in such a case when the fracture had united. One way to minimize stiffness is to use skeletal balanced traction (c); the lower slings can be removed to permit knee flexion (d) while traction is still maintained.

Infants under 12 kg in weight are most easily managed by suspending the lower limbs from overhead pulleys ('gallows traction'), but no more than 2 kg weight should be used and the feet should be checked frequently for circulatory problems. Older children are better suited to *Russell's traction* (see p. 526). Fracture union occurs within 2–4 weeks (depending on the age of the child), and at that stage a *hip spica* is applied and the child is allowed up. Consolidation is usually complete by 4–8 weeks.

Adults (and older adolescents) require *skeletal traction* through a pin or a tightly strung Kirschner wire behind the tibial tubercle. Traction (8–10 kg for an adult) is applied over pulleys at the foot of the bed. The limb is usually supported on a *Thomas' splint*, and a flexion piece allows movement at the knee. However, a splint is not essential; indeed, *skeletal traction without a splint* (Perkins' traction) has the advantages of producing less distortion of the fracture and allowing freer movement in bed. Exercises are begun as soon as possible. Once the fracture is sticky (at about 6 weeks in adults) traction can be discontinued and the

patient allowed up and partial weightbearing in a *cast or brace*. For fractures in the upper half of the femur, a plaster spica is the safest, but it will almost certainly prolong the period of knee stiffness. For fractures in the lower half of the femur, cast-bracing is suitable. This type of protection is needed until the fracture has consolidated (16–24 weeks).

OPEN MEDULLARY NAILING   The operation is carried out under general anaesthesia with the patient positioned on his side. The fracture is exposed through a lateral incision and the fragments are grasped with bone-holders and brought into view. A guide rod is passed up the proximal fragment to emerge through a second, small incision over the buttock. The proximal fragment is then widened with reamers of increasing diameter (working either prograde or retrograde over the guide rod), if possible up to 12 or 14 mm. A nail of appropriate length, and 1 mm thinner than the largest reamer used, is then threaded over the guide rod (retrograde is easier) so that the distal end of the nail just reaches the fracture site. The nail is then fitted to the distal

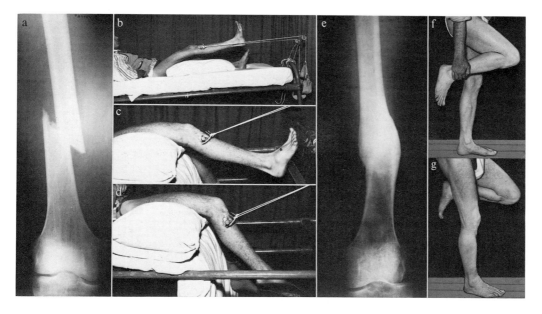

27.17 Femoral shaft fractures   Even in the adult, traction without a splint can be satisfactory, but skeletal traction is essential. The patient with this rather unstable fracture (a) can lift his leg and exercise his knee (b, c, d). At no time was the leg splinted, but clearly the fracture has consolidated (e), and the knee range (f) is only slightly less than that of the uninjured left leg (g).

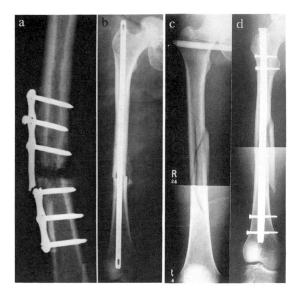

27.18 Femoral shaft fractures (a) This plate is absurdly inadequate to hold a fractured femur; longer and stronger plates can be used, but most surgeons nowadays prefer (b) intramedullary nailing. If the fracture is unstable (c) the nail should be anchored by locking screws (d).

even for subtrochanteric and distal third fractures.

The operation is performed with the patient on his side, the injured limb uppermost and skeletal traction still in place. The fracture is then reduced under x-ray control and the foot is fixed to extension bars on the table. The tip of the greater trochanter is identified through a gluteal muscle-splitting incision; slightly behind and medial to this is the piriform fossa, where the nail will be introduced. The cortex is perforated with a sharp 'bayonet' and then, under fluoroscopic control, a guide rod is passed down the femur crossing the fracture. Flexible reamers are used to widen the medullary canal. A pre-bent nail of suitable length and width (usually 1 mm smaller than the widest reamer used) is chosen; this is passed over the guide rod (or a second, stiffer, guide rod) and driven home under fluoroscopic control.

With proximal and distal third fractures, as well as with comminuted fractures, interlocking screws are needed. The proximal oblique screw is guided to its channel with the help of a jig fitted to the proximal end of the medullary nail; the distal transverse screws are inserted (usually with some difficulty) under fluoroscopic control. With both proximal and distal screws in place, load is taken through the nail; this form of *static loading* is necessary for comminuted and unstable fractures, at least until bone healing is advanced. *Dynamic loading* can be achieved by inserting only one transfixing system, either proximal or distal, depending on the site of fracture. This is ideal for non-comminuted fractures, as loading promotes more rapid healing of the fracture.

Postoperatively, the limb is left free and exercises are begun as soon as possible. Knee movement is more rapidly regained with a continuous passive motion (CPM) machine.

After a week or 10 days the patient is allowed up, partial weightbearing on crutches. Full weightbearing is usually achieved 4–6 weeks later, but comminuted fractures should be protected for longer than this. If static interlocking has been used for a comminuted fracture, one set of screws can be removed as soon as there are signs of fracture healing (usually by 8 weeks), thus converting the mechanism to a dynamic system.

fragment; the fracture is accurately reduced and the nail is driven across the fracture into the distal fragment. If there is comminution, one or two cerclage bands can be used to secure the fragments.

Immediately after operation, exercises to all the leg joints are begun. Within a fortnight the patient should have good muscle control of the limb and good movement of the hip and knee joints. He is then allowed up, partial weightbearing with crutches. For transverse fractures, full weightbearing is permitted after 4–6 weeks; for comminuted fractures, full weightbearing is postponed until the fixation afforded by the nail is reinforced by callus visible on x-ray.

CLOSED MEDULLARY NAILING This method can be used for almost any fracture of the femoral shaft. However, it should not be attempted unless the appropriate facilities and instruments are available. The basic implant system consists of an intramedullary nail (in a range of sizes) which is perforated near each end so that locking screws can be inserted transversely at the distal end and obliquely at the proximal end; this controls rotation and ensures stability

Open fractures

Open femoral fractures should be carefully assessed for (1) skin loss; (2) wound contamination; (3) muscle ischaemia; and (4) injury to vessels and nerves.

The immediate treatment is similar to that of closed fractures. Wound cleansing and debridement should be carried out with as little delay as possible. If there is tissue death or obvious contamination, the wound should be extended and dead tissue carefully excised. Wounds due to penetration by sharp bone fragments also need to be cleaned and excised, but a limited debridement will suffice. The major decision then is how to stabilize the fracture. With small, clean wounds and little delay from the time of injury, the fracture can be treated as for a closed injury, with the addition of prophylactic antibiotics. With large wounds, contaminated wounds, skin loss or tissue destruction, internal fixation should be avoided; after debridement the wound should be left open and the fracture stabilized by applying an external fixator. Some weeks later, once the wound has healed or has been successfully skin-grafted, a further decision can be made about the need for internal fixation.

Complications

All the complications described in Chapter 23, with the exception of visceral injury and avascular necrosis, are encountered in femoral shaft fractures. The more common ones are as follows.

EARLY

Shock One or two litres of blood can be lost even with a closed fracture, and shock may be severe. Prevention is better than cure; most patients will require a transfusion.

Fat embolism This is so common in young people with closed fractures of the femur that its presence should be assumed in every case. Blood gases should be measured soon after admission, and any suspicious signs such as shortness of breath, restlessness or a rise in temperature or pulse rate should prompt a search for petechiae. Treatment is supportive, with the emphasis on preventing hypoxia and maintaining blood volume.

Vascular injury The vascular lesion takes priority and the vessel must be repaired or grafted without delay. At the same operation the fracture is fixed by an intramedullary nail.

Thromboembolism Prolonged traction in bed predisposes to thrombosis. Movement and exercise are important in preventing this. Constant vigilance is needed and anticoagulant treatment is started immediately if thigh vein or pelvic thrombosis is diagnosed.

Infection In open injuries, and following internal fixation, there is always a risk of infection. Prophylactic antibiotics, and careful attention to the principles of fracture surgery, should keep the incidence below 2%. If the bone does become infected, it is essential to explore the wound, excise all dead tissue, and stabilize the fracture by fitting an external fixator. If a medullary nail is already in place, it should be left there. Even worse than an infected fracture is an infected unstable fracture. The long-term management of chronic osteomyelitis is discussed on p. 41.

LATE

Delayed union and non-union It is said that a fractured femur should unite in 100 days, plus or minus 20. If union is delayed much beyond this time, the fracture may need bone grafting. Certainly if the x-ray shows that the bone ends are becoming sclerotic, rigid internal fixation and the additon of cancellous bone grafts are needed.

Malunion Until the x-ray shows solid union the fracture is too insecure to permit weight-bearing; the bone will bend and what previously seemed a satisfactory reduction may end up with lateral or anterior bowing. This is more likely if the fragments were not straight to begin with: in an adult, no more than 15 degrees of angulation should be accepted. If malunion is marked, the mechanical effect on the hip or knee may predispose to secondary osteoarthritis. Shortening is seldom a major problem; if it occurs, the shoe can be built up. Malrotation is a consequence of faulty nailing.

Joint stiffness It is surprising how often the knee is affected after a femoral shaft fracture. The joint may be injured at the same time, or it stiffens due to soft-tissue adhesions during treatment; hence the importance of exercise and knee movements.

Special features in children

MECHANISM Fractures of the femur are quite common in older children and are usually due to *direct violence* (e.g. a road accident) or a *fall* from a height. However, in children under 2 years of age the commonest cause is *child abuse* (Anderson, 1982); if there are several fractures in different stages of healing, this is very suspicious. *Pathological fractures* are common in generalized disorders such as spina bifida and osteogenesis imperfecta, and with local bone lesions (e.g. a benign cyst or tumour).

TREATMENT The principles of treatment are discussed above. It should be emphasized that open treatment is very rarely necessary. The choice of closed method depends largely on the age and weight of the child.

Infants need no more than 1–2 weeks in balanced traction, followed by a spica cast for another 3–4 weeks. Angulation of up to 30 degrees can be accepted, as the bone remodels quite remarkably with growth.

Children between 2 and 10 years of age can be treated either with balanced traction (Russell's traction – see above) for 2–3 weeks followed by a spica cast for another 4 weeks, or by early reduction and a spica cast from the outset. Shortening of 1–2 cm and angulation of up to 20 degrees are acceptable.

Teenagers require somewhat longer (4–6 weeks) in balanced traction, and those aged over 15 (or even younger adolescents if they are large and muscular) may need skeletal traction. Once the fracture feels firm, traction is exchanged for either a spica cast (in the case of upper third and mid-shaft fractures) or a cast-brace (for lower third fractures), which is retained for a further 6 weeks. The position should be checked every few weeks; the limit of acceptable angulation in this age group is 15 degrees in the anteroposterior x-ray and 25 degrees in the lateral.

COMPLICATIONS *Shortening* is common but anything up to 1.5 cm is quite acceptable; indeed there is a tendency for the fractured bone to 'overgrow' and some surgeons prefer to end up with 1–2 cm of shortening. Unfortunately, this effect is unpredictable. *Malunion with angulation* can usually be tolerated within the limits mentioned above. However, the fact that bone modelling is excellent in children is no excuse for casual management; bone may be forgiving but parents are not.

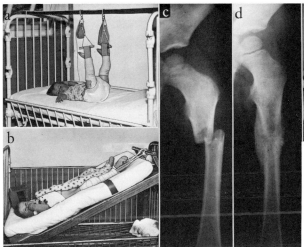

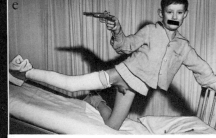

27.19 Femoral shaft fractures in children (a–d) Traction without a splint is certainly adequate in children, and skin traction is sufficient. (e) Clearly this fracture has united.

II. Injuries of the knee and leg

Supracondylar fractures

Supracondylar fractures resemble subtrochanteric fractures (p. 662) in two respects: (1) while they may occur in adults of any age who sustain a sufficiently severe injury, they often occur through osteoporotic bone in the elderly; (2) when the patient is young, continuous traction is a feasible method of treatment, but, for the elderly, early mobilization is so important that internal fixation is almost essential.

Direct violence is the usual cause. The fracture line is just above the condyles, but may extend between them. When the lower fragment is intact the pull of gastrocnemius may flex it, endangering the popliteal artery.

Clinical features

The knee is swollen and deformed; movement is too painful to be attempted. The tibial pulses should always be palpated.

X-RAY
The fracture is just above the femoral condyles and is transverse or comminuted. The distal fragment is often tilted backwards.

NOTE   The entire femur must be x-rayed so as not to miss a proximal fracture or dislocated hip.

Treatment

If the fracture is only slightly displaced, or if it reduces easily with the knee in flexion, it can be treated quite satisfactorily by traction through the proximal tibia; the limb is cradled on a Thomas' splint with a knee flexion piece, and movements are encouraged. If the distal fragment is displaced by gastrocnemius pull, a second pin above the knee, and vertical traction, will correct this.

At 4–6 weeks, when the fracture is beginning to unite, traction can be replaced by a cast-brace and the patient allowed up and partially weightbearing with crutches.

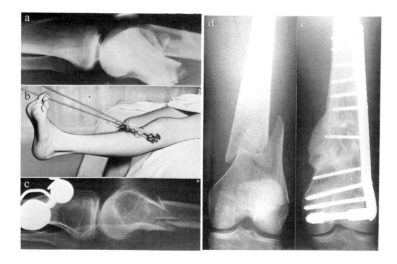

27.20 Supracondylar fractures   (a, b, c) These fractures can sometimes be treated successfully by skeletal traction through the upper tibia; if there is much posterior displacement (endangering the popliteal vessels) it may be corrected by vertical traction through a second pin above the knee. (d) If the bone is not too osteoporotic, (e) internal fixation is a good alternative.

If closed reduction fails, open reduction and internal fixation with an angled compression device, though difficult, may be successful. This does not necessarily lead to earlier mobilization because the bone is often osteoporotic and the patient may be old and frail, but nursing in bed is easier and knee movements can be started sooner. Unprotected weightbearing is not permitted until the fracture has consolidated (usually around 12 weeks).

Complications

EARLY

Skin damage is common and wound toilet is then necessary.

Arterial damage occasionally occurs, and there is danger of gangrene.

LATE

Knee stiffness is almost inevitable. A long period of exercise is necessary but full movement is rarely regained.

Non-union may be associated with knee stiffness and indeed may be due to forcing knee movement too soon. The fracture is difficult to treat and unless great care is exercised, the ultimate range of movement at the knee may be less than that at the fracture.

Fracture-separation of distal femoral epiphysis

In the childhood or adolescent equivalent of a supracondylar fracture, the lower femoral epiphysis may be displaced (1) to one side (usually laterally) by forced angulation of the straight knee or (2) forwards by a hyper-extension injury. Although not nearly as common as physeal fractures at the elbow or ankle, this injury is important because of its potential for causing abnormal growth and deformity of the knee.

The fracture is usually a Salter–Harris type 2 lesion – i.e. physeal separation with a large triangular metaphyseal bone fragment. Although this type of fracture usually has a good

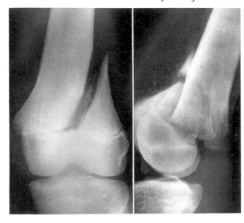

27.21 Fracture-separation of epiphysis These fractures are not difficult to reduce and can usually be held adequately in plaster, but they must be watched carefully for several weeks.

prognosis, asymmetrical growth arrest is not uncommon and the child may end up with a valgus or varus deformity. A type 4 or 5 injury may result in femoral shortening.

Clinical features

The knee is swollen and perhaps deformed. The pulses in the foot should be palpated because, with forward displacement of the epiphysis, the popliteal artery may be obstructed by the lower femur.

Treatment

The fracture can usually be perfectly reduced manually, but further x-ray checks will be needed over the next few weeks to ensure that reduction is maintained. If there is a tendency to redisplacement, the fragments may be stabilized with percutaneous Kirschner wires or Steinmann pins. The limb is immobilized in the plaster and the patient is allowed partial weight-bearing on crutches. The cast can be exchanged for a posterior splint after 4 weeks.

Complications

EARLY
There is danger of gangrene unless the hyper-extension injury is reduced without delay.

LATE

Damage to the physis is not uncommon and residual deformity may require corrective osteotomy at the end of the growth period. Shortening, if it is marked, can be treated by femoral lengthening.

Femoral condyle fractures

A direct injury or a fall from a height may drive the tibia upwards into the intercondylar fossa. One femoral condyle may be fractured and driven upwards or both condyles split apart.

Clinical features

The knee is swollen and may be deformed. There is a tender, 'doughy' feel characteristic of a haemarthrosis. The knee is too painful to move, but the foot should be examined to exclude nerve damage.

X-RAY

One femoral condyle may be fractured obliquely and shifted upwards, or both condyles may be split apart so that the fracture line is T-shaped or Y-shaped.

Treatment

Closed reduction is often successful; indeed, the fracture may not necessarily be severely displaced and the position may be almost acceptable. Skeletal traction is applied through the proximal tibia and the fracture is 'reduced' by manual compression. Traction is maintained for 4–6 weeks and is then exchanged for a cast-brace which is worn until the fracture is firmly united.

Open reduction is indicated if closed methods fail to bring the condylar fragments together. It may also be the preferred method of primary treatment in a young, fit patient who is anxious to be up and mobile as soon as possible. The fracture is exposed through a lateral incision; the fragments are reduced and held together

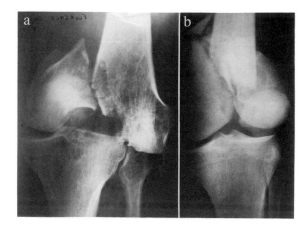

27.22 Femoral condyle fractures Closed reduction and skeletal traction through the upper tibia is often satisfactory for (a) unicondylar or (b) bicondylar fractures.

with a blade-plate or (better still) with a dynamic condylar screw and plate. Provided fixation is secure the patient can begin knee exercises and be got out of bed within a day or two, but very little weight should be taken through the leg until the fracture is consolidated.

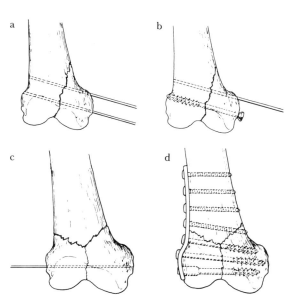

27.23 Femoral condyle fractures – treatment (a) A single condylar fracture can be reduced open and held with Kirschner wires preparatory to (b) inserting compression screws. (c) T- or Y-shaped fractures are best fixed with a dynamic condylar screw and plate (d).

Tibial plateau fractures

Mechanism of injury

Fractures of the tibial plateau are caused by a varus or valgus force combined with axial loading (a pure valgus force is more likely to rupture the ligaments). This is sometimes the result of a car striking a pedestrian (hence the term 'bumper fracture'); more often it is due to a fall from a height in which the knee is forced into valgus or varus. The tibial condyle is crushed or split by the opposing femoral condyle, which remains intact. Patients are usually between 50 and 60 years and somewhat osteoporotic, but the fracture can occur in adults of any age.

Clinical features

The knee is swollen and may be deformed. Bruising is usually extensive and the tissues feel 'doughy' because of haemarthrosis. Gentle examination (or examination under anaesthesia) may suggest medial or lateral instability. The leg and foot should be carefully examined for signs of vascular or neurological injury.

X-RAY

Anteroposterior, lateral and oblique x-rays will usually show the fracture, but the amount of comminution or plateau depression may not be appreciated without tomography. Stress views (under anaesthesia) are sometimes helpful in assessing the degree of joint instability. With a crushed lateral condyle the medial ligament is often intact, but with a crushed medial condyle the lateral ligament is often torn.

It is essential in planning treatment to separate the different types of fracture, which fall into six basic patterns:

Type 1 – a simple fracture of the lateral tibial condyle. In younger patients who are not severely osteoporotic, there may be a vertical split with separation of a single fragment. It may be virtually undisplaced, or quite markedly depressed and tilted. If the split is wide, loose fragments or the lateral meniscus may have become jammed in the crevice.

Type 2 – a comminuted crush of the lateral condyle with depression of the fragments. This is the commonest type of fracture and it usually occurs in older people with osteoporosis.

Type 3 – a comminuted crush with an intact outer fragment. This is similar to type 2, but the outer segment of bone offers an intact piece of articular surface. The depressed fragments may be wedged firmly into the subchondral bone.

Type 4 – fracture of the medial tibial condyle. This is sometimes the result of severe injury, with tearing of the lateral collateral ligament.

Type 5 – fracture of both condyles, with the tibial shaft wedged in between them.

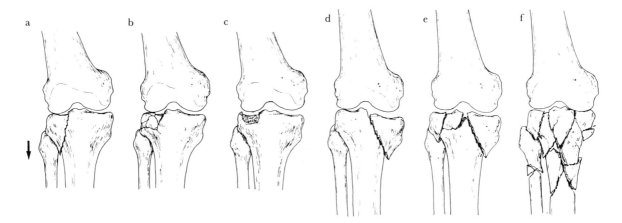

27.24 Tibial plateau fractures   (a) Type I – simple fracture of lateral condyle. (b) Type II – comminuted crush of lateral condyle with depression. (c) Comminuted crush with intact lateral fragment. (d) Fractured medial condyle. (e) Fractures of both condyles. (f) Combined condylar and subcondylar fractures.

Type 6 – combined condylar and subcondylar fractures, usually the result of severe axial force.

Treatment

Treatment by traction is simple and often produces a well-functioning knee, but slight residual angulation is not uncommon (Apley, 1979). On the other hand, obsessional surgery to restore the shattered surface may produce a good x-ray appearance – and a stiff knee.

Undisplaced or minimally displaced fractures The haemarthrosis is aspirated and a compression bandage is applied. The limb is rested on a continuous passive motion (CPM) machine and knee movements are begun. As soon as the acute pain and swelling have subsided (usually within a week), a hinged cast-brace is fitted and the patient is allowed partial weightbearing on crutches. Free weightbearing is delayed until the fracture has healed (6–8 weeks).

Type 1 – displaced fractures The large condylar fragment should be perfectly reduced and fixed in position. This is best done by open operation (see below).

Type 2 – comminuted fractures This is essentially a compression fracture, similar to a vertebral compression fracture. If depression is slight (less than 5 mm) and the knee is not unstable, or if the patient is old and frail or osteoporotic, the fracture is treated closed with the aim of regaining mobility and function rather than anatomical restitution. After aspiration and compression bandaging, skeletal traction is applied via a threaded pin passed through the tibia 7 cm below the fracture. An attempt is made to squeeze the condyle into shape; the knee is then flexed and extended several times to 'mould' the upper tibia on the opposing femoral condyle. The leg is cradled on pillows and, with 5 kg traction in place, active exercises are carried out every day. Alternatively, the knee can be treated from the outset on a CPM machine, increasing the range of movement progressively; after a week of this treatment the machine is removed and active exercises are begun. As soon as the fracture is 'sticky' (usually at 3–4 weeks), the traction pin is removed, a hinged cast-brace is applied and the patient is allowed up on crutches. Full weightbearing is deferred for another 6 weeks.

In younger patients with type 2 fractures this treatment may be regarded as unnecessarily conservative, and open reduction with elevation of the plateau and internal fixation is often preferred (see below). Postoperatively the knee is treated on a CPM machine; after a few days

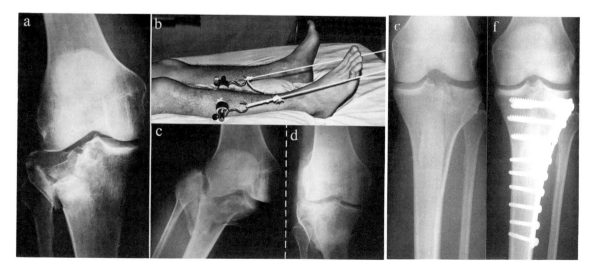

27.25 Tibial plateau fractures (a–d) Skeletal traction well below the knee is often effective in reducing these fractures, especially when combined with early movements. (e, f) The alternative is internal fixation, which certainly produces a satisfying x-ray.

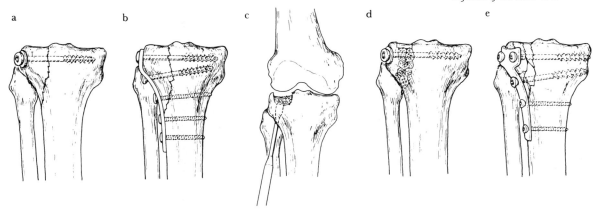

27.26 Tibial plateau fractures Fixation. (a) A single screw may be sufficient for a simple split, though (b) a buttress plate and screws is more secure. (c) Depression of more than 1 cm can be treated by elevation from below and (d) supported by bone grafts. (e) Complex fractures can be treated operatively, but, unless perfect reduction can be guaranteed, traction and movement is probably wiser; to fix a fragment which projects above the articular surface is to invite early osteoarthritis.

active exercises are begun and at 2 weeks the patient is allowed up in a cast-brace which is retained until the fracture has united.

Type 3 – comminution with intact lateral fragment The principles of treatment are similar to those applying to type 2 fractures. However, the lateral fragment with intact articular cartilage is a potential weightbearing surface, so perfect reduction is more important. This can sometimes be done closed by strong traction and lateral compression; if this is successful, the fracture is treated by traction or CPM. If closed

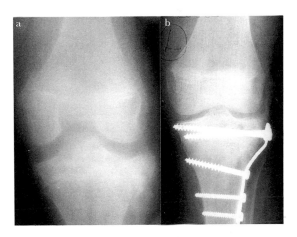

27.27 Tibial plateau fractures (a) A tomograph showed significant depression and some lateral displacement, so (b) open reduction and internal fixation was performed.

reduction fails, open reduction and fixation is worth while (see below). Postoperatively, exercises are begun as soon as possible and 2 weeks later the patient is allowed up in a cast-brace which is retained until the fracture has united.

Type 4 – fracture of the medial condyle Minimally displaced fractures can be treated in a cast-brace. If the fragment is markedly displaced or tilted, open reduction and fixation is indicated. If the lateral ligament is also torn, this should be repaired at the same time.

Type 5 and 6 fractures are severe injuries that carry the added risk of a compartment syndrome. A bicondylar fracture can often be reduced by traction and the patient is then treated as for a type 2 injury. More complex fractures with severe comminution are, likewise, better managed closed, though traction and exercises may have to be continued for 4–6 weeks before the fracture is 'sticky' enough to permit the use of a cast-brace. If there are several well-defined, displaced fragments, internal fixation (with plates applied medially and laterally) may be justified.

OPEN REDUCTION AND FIXATION Plateau fractures are difficult to reduce and fix; operative treatment should be undertaken only if the full range of implants (and the necessary surgical experience) are available.

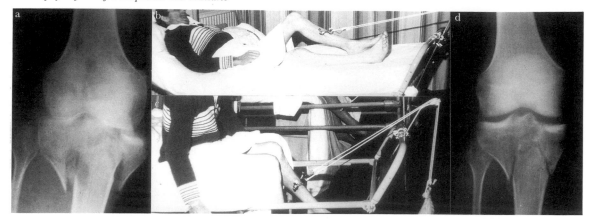

27.28 Tibial plateau fractures   (a) It seemed unlikely that this complex bicondylar fracture could be perfectly reduced and satisfactorily fixed by operation, so (b, c) a low traction pin was inserted and movements were practised assiduously. (d) The x-ray 10 days later shows very good reduction and the end result was excellent.

Through a longitudinal parapatellar incision the joint capsule is exposed. The aim is to preserve the meniscus while fully exposing the fractured plateau; this is best done by entering the joint through a transverse capsular incision beneath the meniscus. A single large fragment may be repositioned and held with cancellous screws and washers without too much difficulty. Comminuted, depressed fractures must be elevated by pushing the fragmented mass upwards from below; the osteoarticular surface is then supported by packing the subchondral area with cancellous grafts (obtained from either the femoral condyles or the iliac crest) and held in place by applying a suitably contoured buttress plate and screws to the side of the bone (Schatzker, 1987). Unless it is torn, the meniscus should be preserved and sutured back in place when the capsule is repaired.

Complex fractures of the proximal tibia are difficult to fix and many surgeons would prefer to treat these by traction and mobilization. If it is elected to operate, adequate exposure of the injuries is essential; Schatzker (1987) recommends dividing the patellar ligament and turning the patella upwards.

Postoperatively the limb is elevated and splinted until swelling subsides; movements are begun as soon as possible and active exercises are encouraged. At the end of 4 weeks the patient can usually be allowed up in a cast-brace, partial weightbearing with crutches; full weightbearing is resumed when healing is complete.

Complications

EARLY

Compartment syndrome   With closed bicondylar fractures there is considerable bleeding and a risk of developing a compartment syndrome. The leg and foot should be examined separately for signs of ischaemia.

LATE

Joint stiffness   With severely comminuted fractures, and after complex operations, there is a considerable risk of developing a stiff knee. This is prevented by (1) avoiding prolonged plaster immobilization and (2) encouraging movement as early as possible.

Deformity   Some residual valgus or varus deformity is quite common – either because the fracture was incompletely reduced or because, although adequately reduced, the fracture became redisplaced during treatment. Fortunately, moderate deformity is compatible with good function, although constant overloading of one compartment may predispose to osteoarthritis in later life.

Osteoarthritis   Contrary to popular belief, osteoarthritis is not a common long-term sequel of conservative treatment. Lansinger et al. (1986), in a 20-year follow-up of a large series of cases, reported 90% excellent or good results in the absence of ligamentous instability or marked depression. Even when the x-ray appearance suggests osteoarthritis the knee may well be painless. If, however, painful osteoarthritis has developed and the lateral condyle is depressed, reconstructive surgery may be considered.

Fractured tibial spine

Severe valgus or varus stress, or twisting injuries, may damage the knee ligaments and fracture the tibial spine.

Clinical features

The patient – usually a young adult or a child – presents with a swollen immobile knee. The joint feels tense, tender and 'doughy'; aspiration will reveal a haemarthrosis. Examination under anaesthesia may show that extension is blocked; there may also be associated ligament injuries.

X-RAY
The fracture is not always obvious and a small posterior fracture may be missed, unless the x-rays are carefully examined. The fragment –

often including part of the intercondylar eminence – may be undisplaced, tilted upwards or completely detached.

Treatment

Under anaesthesia the joint is aspirated and gently manipulated into full extension. Often the fragment falls back into position and the x-ray shows that the fracture is reduced. If there is a block to full extension, or if the bone fragment remains displaced, operative reduction is essential. The fragment – often larger than suspected – is restored to its bed and anchored by sutures.

After either closed or open reduction, a long plaster cylinder is applied with the knee almost straight; it is worn for 6 weeks and then movements are encouraged.

Fracture-separation of the proximal tibial epiphysis

This uncommon injury is caused by a severe hyperextension and valgus strain. The epiphysis displaces forwards and laterally, often taking a small fragment of the metaphysis with it (a Salter–Harris type 2 injury).

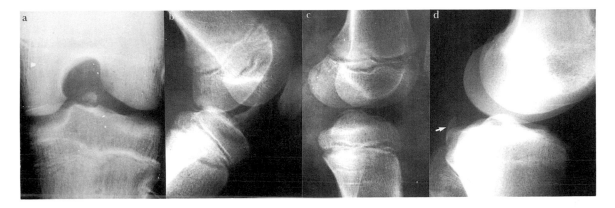

27.29 Tibial spine fracture   (a, b) This young man injured his knee while playing football; x-rays showed a large, displaced avulsion fracture of the tibial spine. (c) An undisplaced tibial spine fracture. (d) Posterior fractures, with avulsion of the posterior cruciate ligament, are often missed.

Clinical features

The knee is tensely swollen and extremely tender. If the epiphysis is displaced, there may be a valgus or hyperextension deformity. All movements are resisted.

X-RAY

The entire upper tibial epiphysis may be tilted forwards or sideways. Sometimes, when the ligament is attached to a small apophysis separate from the main epiphysis, this apophysis is avulsed and shifted upwards.

Treatment

Under anaesthesia, closed manipulative reduction can usually be achieved. If the small separate apophysis remains displaced it is operatively reduced and sutured in position. Occasionally, when the entire tibial epiphysis cannot be accurately reduced by closed manipulation, it is replaced at operation and held by a screw. The rare Salter–Harris 3 or 4 fractures also may need open reduction and fixation.

Following reduction, whether closed or open, a plaster tube is applied from the upper thigh to the malleoli with the knee straight. It is worn for 6 weeks.

Weightbearing is permitted at once. Knee flexion quickly returns when the plaster is removed.

Complications

Epiphyseal fractures in young children sometimes result in angular deformity of the proximal tibia. Ths may later require operative correction.

Fracture of the proximal end of the fibula

Fracture of the proximal end of the fibula may be caused by either direct injury or an indirect twisting injury of the lower limb.

The fracture itself is of little moment and it requires no treatment. However, complications are frequent and, if the injury is regarded too lightheartedly, they may cause prolonged disability.

Complications

Associated injuries are common and should be looked for in every case. These are (1) peroneal nerve injury, (2) collateral ligament injury and (3) injuries at the other end of the fibula – i.e. fractures or ligament strains around the ankle. An occasional late complication is (4) peroneal nerve entrapment. Each of these conditions may require specific treatment.

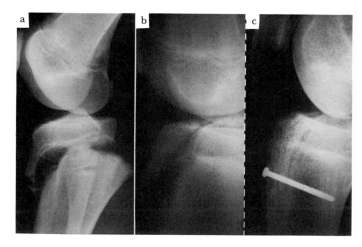

27.30 Fracture-separation of proximal tibial epiphysis   (a) A fracture like this needs urgent reduction because the popliteal vessels are endangered. (b) Avulsion of the patellar ligament insertion is rare; in this case reduction was held with internal fixation (c).

Instability of the proximal tibiofibular joint

A blow or twisting injury may cause subluxation or dislocation of the proximal tibiofibular joint; occasionally the condition is habitual and associated with generalized ligamentous laxity. The fibular head displaces upwards, anterolaterally or posteromedially. There is usually pain and local tenderness; the patient often prefers, when standing, to press the dorsum of the other foot against the fibular head as if to stabilize it. If manual reduction followed by a plaster cylinder for 3 weeks is unsuccessful, the head of the fibula can be excised.

Fractured patella

The key to the management of patellar fractures is the state of the extensor mechanism.

Mechanism of injury

The patella may be fractured, either by a *direct force* that cracks the bone like a tile under the blow of a hammer or by an *indirect traction force* that pulls the bone apart (and often tears the extensor expansions as well).

Direct injury – usually a fall onto the knee or a blow against the dashboard of a car – causes either an *undisplaced crack* or else a *comminuted ('stellate') fracture* without severe damage to the extensor expansions.

Indirect injuries occur, typically, when someone catches his foot against a solid obstacle and, to avoid falling, contracts the quadriceps muscle forcefully. This is a *transverse fracture* with a gap between the fragments.

Clinical features

Following one of the typical injuries, the knee becomes swollen and painful. There may be an abrasion or bruising over the front of the joint.

The patella is tender and sometimes a gap can be felt.

Active knee expansion should be tested. If the patient can lift the straight leg, the quadriceps mechanism is still intact.

X-RAY

The films may show: (1) one or more fine fracture lines without displacement (the appearance is not to be confused with a bipartite patella in which a smooth line extends obliquely across the superolateral angle of the bone); (2) multiple fracture lines with irregular displacement; or (3) a transverse fracture with a gap between the fragments.

Treatment

UNDISPLACED OR MINIMALLY DISPLACED FRACTURES
If there is a haemarthrosis it is aspirated. The extensor mechanism is intact and treatment is mainly protective. A plaster cylinder holding the knee straight is worn for 3–4 weeks, and during this time quadriceps exercises are practised every day.

COMMINUTED (STELLATE) FRACTURE The extensor expansions are intact and the patient may be able to lift the leg. However, the undersurface of the patella is irregular and there is a serious risk of damage to the patellofemoral joint. For this reason many people advocate patellectomy, whatever the degree of displacement. To others it seems reasonable to preserve the patella if the fragments are not severely displaced; a backslab is applied but removed several times daily for exercises to mould the fragments into position and to preserve mobility.

DISPLACED TRANSVERSE FRACTURE The lateral expansions are torn and the entire extensor mechanism is disrupted. Operation is essential: the fragments are held apposed by internal fixation and the extensor expansions are repaired.

Technique Through a transverse incision the fracture is exposed and the lateral expansions are repaired with strong catgut sutures. The patella is reconstituted by the tension-band principle. The fragments are reduced and transfixed with two stiff Kirschner wires; flexible

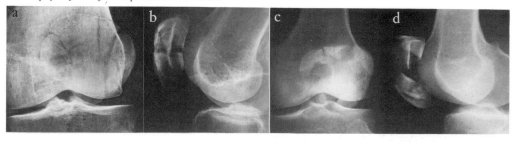

27.31 Fractured patella – stellate   (a, b) A fracture with little or no displacement can be treated conservatively by a posterior slab of plaster which is removed several times a day for gentle active exercises. (c, d) With severe displacement, patellectomy is probably the best treatment, though a 'purse-string' wire suture pulling the fragments together, combined with active movements, is a possibility; if necessary, the patella can be excised later.

wire is then looped tightly around the protruding Kirschner wires and over the front of the patella. Any irregularity of the articular surface may be smoothed away by active use; if patellofemoral signs develop later, the patella can then be excised and the knee recovers more quickly than it does after immediate post-traumatic patellectomy. A plaster backslab is worn until active extension of the knee is regained; the backslab may be removed every day to permit active knee-flexion exercises.

Prognosis

Patients usually regain good function but, depending on the severity of the injury, there is a significant incidence of late patellofemoral osteoarthritis.

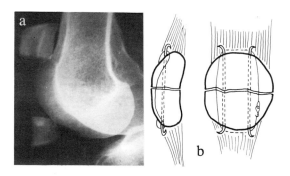

27.32 Fractured patella – transverse The separated fragments (a) are transfixed by Kirschner wires; malleable wire is then looped around the protruding ends of the Kirschner wires and tightened over the front of the patella (b).

Acute knee ligament injuries

The bony parts of the knee joint are inherently unstable and abnormal shifts are prevented mainly by the ligaments and muscles. These structures may be damaged if the tibia and femur are forcibly angulated or rotated upon each other. Such injuries are common in footballers, skiers, gymnasts and the victims of road accidents.

Mechanism of injury

Most ligament injuries occur while the knee is bent, relaxing the capsule and ligaments, and permitting rotation. The damaging force may be a straight thrust (e.g. a dashboard injury forcing the tibia backwards) or, more commonly, a combined rotation and impact injury to the bent weightbearing knee as in a football tackle. A wide variety of complex injuries may result (O'Donoghue, 1973; Hughston et al., 1976).

The medial ligaments are most commonly affected, the usual cause being a twisting injury with the knee rotated and thrust into valgus. The tissues rupture layer by layer: first the superficial capsular ligament, then the medial collateral ligament, and then – as the tibia rotates externally – the anterior cruciate ligament. Similar injuries occur (though much less often) on the lateral side when the knee is forced into varus, and to the posterior cruciate ligament when the tibia is thrust backwards in relation to the femur.

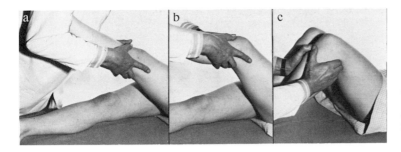

27.33 Knee ligaments Grips used in examination for abnormal movements. (a) Sideways tilting with the knee straight, and (b) with the knee flexed; (c) anteroposterior glide (this should also be tested flexed only 20 degrees).

Clinical features

The patient gives a history of a twisting or wrenching injury and may even claim to have heard a 'pop' as the tissues snapped. The knee is painful and (usually) swollen – and, in contrast to the story in meniscal injury, the swelling appears almost immediately. Tenderness is most acute over the torn ligament, and stressing one or other side of the joint may produce excruciating pain. The knee may be too painful to permit deep palpation or much movement.

For all the apparent consistency, the findings can be somewhat perverse: thus, with a complete tear the patient may have little or no pain, and can usually walk or even run; with a partial tear the knee is painful and the patient lame. Swelling also is worse with partial tears, because haemorrhage remains confined within the joint; with complete tears the ruptured capsule permits leakage and diffusion. With a partial tear attempted movement is always painful; the abnormal movement of a complete tear is often painless or prevented by spasm.

Abrasions suggest the site of impact, but bruising is more important and indicates the site of damage. The doughy feel of a haemarthrosis distinguishes ligament injuries from the fluctuant feel of the synovial effusion of a meniscus injury. Tenderness localizes the lesion, but the sharply defined tender spot of a partial tear (usually medial and 2.5 cm above the joint line) contrasts with the diffuse tenderness of a complete one. The entire limb should be examined for other injuries and for vascular or nerve damage.

The most important aspect of the examination is to test for ligamentous stability. Partial tears permit no abnormal movement, but the attempt causes pain. Complete tears permit abnormal movement which sometimes is painless. To distinguish between the two is critical because their treatment is different; so, *if there is doubt, examination under anaesthesia is mandatory.*

Sideways tilting is examined, first with the knee at 30 degrees of flexion and then with the knee straight. Movement is compared with the normal side. If the knee angulates only in slight flexion, there is probably an isolated tear of the collateral ligaments; if it angulates in full extension, there is almost certainly rupture of the cruciate ligaments as well as the collateral ligament.

Anteroposterior stability is assessed first by placing the knees at 90 degrees with the feet resting on the couch and looking from the side for posterior sag of the proximal tibia; when present, this is a reliable sign of posterior

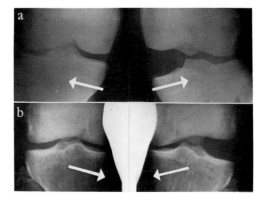

27.34 Ligament injuries Strain films show: (a) complete tear of medial ligament, left knee; (b) complete tear of lateral ligament, left knee. In both, the anterior cruciate also was torn.

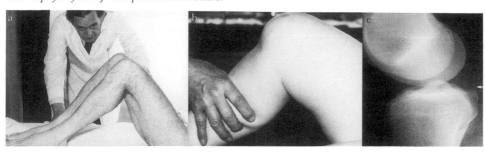

27.35 Posterior cruciate ligament tears   (a) Viewed from the side, any backward displacement of the upper tibia is plainly visible and can be confirmed by (b) pushing the tibia backwards. (c) X-ray may also show displacement and sometimes a small flake of bone pulled off the back of the tibia.

cruciate instability. Next, the drawer test is carried out in the usual way; a positive drawer sign is diagnostic of a tear, but a negative test does not exclude one. The Lachman test is more reliable; anteroposterior glide is tested with the knee flexed 15–20 degrees. Rotational stability can usually be tested only under anaesthesia.

X-RAY
Plain films may show that the ligament has avulsed a small piece of bone – the medial ligament usually from the femur, the lateral ligament from the fibula, the anterior cruciate ligament from the tibial spine and the posterior cruciate from the back of the upper tibia. Stress films (if necessary under anaesthesia) demonstrate if the joint hinges open on one side.

ARTHROSCOPY
With severe tears of the collateral ligaments and capsule, arthroscopy should not be attempted; fluid extravasation will hamper diagnosis and may complicate further procedures. The main indication for arthroscopy is in suspected 'isolated' cruciate ligament tears, and in lesser sprains to exclude other internal injuries such as meniscal tears, which (if present) can be dealt with then and there.

Treatment

PARTIAL TEARS
The intact fibres splint the torn ones and spontaneous healing will occur. The hazard is adhesions, so active exercise is prescribed from the start, facilitated by aspirating a tense effusion, applying ice-packs to the knee and, sometimes, by injecting local anaesthetic into the tender area. Weightbearing is permitted but the knee is protected from rotation or angulation strain by a heavily padded bandage or a posterior splint. A complete plaster cast is unnecessary and disadvantageous; it inhibits movement and prevents weekly reassessment – an important precaution if the occasional error is to be avoided. With a dedicated exercise programme, the patient can usually return to sports training by 6–8 weeks.

COMPLETE TEARS
In theory, healing can occur provided the torn ends are closely apposed and held still in plaster. But the outcome is uncertain. Operation is wiser and affords the best chance of avoiding future instability (Kannus, 1988). The guiding principles are: (1) operate early (the earlier the better and certainly within 14 days); (2) use a generous incision (if posterior structures also are torn and access is inadequate, a second, posterior, incision helps); (3) repair every torn structure tightly and, if possible, by reattachment to bone (staples, or sutures through drill holes, are necessary); (4) consider reinforcing the repair with an allograft or implant; (5) protect the repair for 6 weeks in an above-knee plaster.

With extensive tears the joint should be explored, and torn or detached pieces of meniscus removed. If the cruciate ligaments are torn, they too should be repaired.

The posteromedial capsule may have to be reattached by suturing it to drill holes in the bone. Frayed ligaments can be reinforced by using any of the tendinous structures in the vicinity (e.g. the pes anserinus or semimembranosus).

The anterior cruciate ligament may be avulsed at either end. It can be reattached by screw fixation or by sutures which are led out of the joint via suitably placed drill holes in the tibia or femur. Tears within the substance of the ligament are difficult to suture; the repair may be augmented by using one of the nearby tendons or a free implant (Alio, Letho and Kujala, 1986).

Posterior cruciate ligament repair or augmentation may be more easily carried out through a posterior approach.

Postoperatively the limb is immobilized in a full-length cast with the knee 40 degrees flexed (the leg should be medially rotated if medial structures mainly are involved, laterally rotated with lateral damage). This can usually be replaced by a hinged cast-brace after 3–4 weeks. Free weightbearing is not permitted until 8 weeks after ligament repair. Active muscle strengthening exercises are important and should continue for at least 6 months.

NON-OPERATIVE TREATMENT   If the patient is unathletic or no longer young (or if the diagnosis is in doubt), non-operative treatment may be preferable. Certainly, medial collateral ligament tears (i.e. where the knee is stable in full extension) can be treated quite effectively without operation (Ballmer and Jacob, 1988). The limb is immobilized in a plaster cylinder for 6–8 weeks, during which time the patient is allowed weightbearing with crutches. The results, though not as good as those following skilled operative repair by modern techniques, are nevertheless acceptable (Sandberg et al., 1987). Residual instability can be dealt with later, if necessary, by reconstructive surgery (see below).

Complications

Adhesions If the knee with a partial ligament tear is not actively exercised, torn fibres stick to intact fibres and to bone. The knee 'gives way' with catches of pain; localized tenderness is present, and pain on medial or lateral rotation.

The obvious confusion with a torn meniscus can be resolved by the grinding test (p. 442), or by manipulation and injection under anaesthesia, which is usually curative. If there is still doubt about the possibility of a torn meniscus, arthroscopy is indicated. Occasionally an abduction injury is followed by calcification near the upper attachment of the medial ligament (*Pellegrini–Stieda's disease*).

Instability As the sequel to an injury the knee may continue to give way. The instability tends to get worse and eventually degeneration may follow. This important subject is discussed under a separate heading, below.

Chronic ligamentous instability

Instability ('giving way') of the knee may be obvious soon after the acute injury has healed, or it may only become apparent much later. It is usually progressive (a meniscectomy is likely to make it worse) but, except in people engaged in strenuous sport, dancing or work activities, the disability is often tolerated without complaint. In the more severe cases, osteoarthritis may eventually supervene.

Functional pathology

Unstable tibiofemoral relationships may result in abnormal *sideways tilt* (valgus or varus), excessive *anteroposterior glide* (forwards or backwards), unnatural *rotation* (medially or laterally), or *combinations* of these unphysiological movements.

Seldom is only one ligament at fault. Stability is normally maintained by primary and secondary stabilizers (not to mention the dynamic forces of surrounding muscles). Thus, the medial collateral ligament is the primary stabilizer preventing valgus tilt, but the cruciate ligaments also play a part and they are therefore secondary stabilizers in this plane. *Medial instability* may become apparent only when the knee is held in 20–30 degrees of flexion; valgus tilt with the knee fully extended implies that both primary and secondary stabilizers are torn.

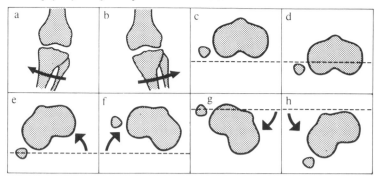

27.36 Knee ligaments – instability
Straight subluxations: (a) tilting into varus, (b) into valgus; (c) forward shift, (d) backward.

Rotary subluxations of tibia: (e) medial condyle forward; (f) lateral condyle forward; (g) medial condyle backward; (h) lateral condyle backward.

Anteroposteror and rotational shifts are even more complex. A positive *anterior drawer sign* means that both the anterior cruciate and the posteromedial structures are torn or lax. Disruption of the anterior cruciate ligament with minimal involvement of other ligaments (so-called 'isolated' anterior cruciate ligament deficiency) causes *anterolateral instability* – i.e. the lateral tibial condyle subluxates forwards and the tibia rotates on an axis through the medial condyles. This is the basis of the *lateral pivot shift phenomenon* (Losee, Johnson and Southwick, 1978; Galway and MacIntosh, 1980).

A positive *posterior drawer sign* means that the posterior cruciate ligament is torn. Soon after injury, however, this sign is difficult to elicit unless the arcuate and oblique ligaments also are torn. Chronic deficiency of the arcuate ligament complex causes a type of posterolateral rotational instability which is the counterpart of the pivot shift phenomenon. Complete tears of all the posterior structures also allow the knee to hyperextend.

Clinical features

The patient complains of a feeling of insecurity and of giving way. With collateral ligament instability the cause is obvious even to the patient. With the common anterior cruciate insufficiency, symptoms are more subtle. The knee suddenly 'gives out' as he pivots towards the affected side (the lateral pivot shift phenomenon). Trickey (1987) has noted how patients describe this jerking sensation by grinding the knuckles of clenched fists upon each other. The explanation is that, with the

knee just short of full extension, the lateral femoral condyle slips backwards; then, as the knee flexes, the iliotibial band pulls the subluxated condyle back into the reduced position. For a sportsman, 'cutting' is particularly troublesome. In the less common posterior cruciate insufficiency, symptoms are mild unless the arcuate ligament complex also is torn or stretched; instability is sometimes felt only on climbing stairs.

Locking is *not* a feature of instability and should always suggest an associated meniscal tear.

The joint looks normal, apart sometimes from slight wasting, and there is rarely any tenderness, but there is excessive movement in one or more directions. Comparison with the normal knee is essential.

A careful routine is to examine the knee first for dynamic instability, then for hyperextension, then for increased angulation at 0 degrees and 30 degrees, then for increased anteroposterior movement at 90 degrees and 20 degrees, and finally to perform the special tests for rotational instability.

Start by watching the patient walk and noting knee posture and movement in the stance phase. Then ask the patient to stand on one leg and try to reproduce the instability by twisting to one side or the other.

Hyperextension is tested with the patient supine and the knee straight; now try to lift each heel in turn.

To test lateral angulation, grasp the patient's thigh with one hand and his leg with the other and stress the knee in valgus and varus; or, if the limb is too large for your hands, tuck the leg between your trunk and your upper arm while

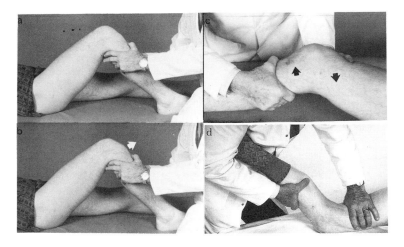

27.37 Testing for cruciate ligament tears   (a, b) Testing at 90 degrees may reveal a positive drawer sign but (c) Lachman's test is more sensitive. (d) For those with small hands, it is best performed with the patient prone.

your hands try to move the knee into valgus and varus. Perform the test, first with the knee straight and then flexed 30 degrees.

Next, place the knees at 90 degrees with the feet flat on the couch and the quadriceps completely relaxed; looking from the side, note if there is any posterior sag of the upper tibia – a sure sign of posterior cruciate laxity. Then ask the patient to slide the foot slowly down the couch; as the quadriceps contracts, the sag is pulled up and the proximal tibia shifts forward (Daniel et al., 1988).

Again with the knees flexed 90 degrees and both feet resting on the couch, grasp the upper tibia with both hands (making sure that the hamstrings are relaxed) and test for anterior and posterior laxity (the drawer signs).

A more reliable test for cruciate laxity is to examine for anteroposterior displacement with the knee almost straight (the Lachman test). Hold the calf with one hand and the thigh with the other, with the knee flexed 20 degrees; now try to displace the joint backwards and forwards. A positive test may be graded as mild (+), moderate (++) or severe (+++). Surgeons with small hands will find it easier to do the Lachman test with the patient prone (Feagin and Cooke, 1989).

Rotational stability is tested by taking advantage of the pivot shift phenomenon. This can be done in several ways, the aim being to try to reproduce the anterior subluxation and relocation of the lateral tibial condyle (Larson, 1983). The simplest method is to repeat the Lachman test while flexing and extending the knee, watching to see if the lateral tibial condyle slips forwards (subluxates) and backwards (reduces). This is similar to the 'jerk test' in which the examiner starts with the patient's knee flexed (the reduced position); the knee is gradually extended while the knee is stressed into valgus with internal rotation of the tibia, aiming to make the lateral tibial condyle subluxate. At about 20 degrees there is a sudden jerk as the tibial condyle 'slips out'. The test originally described by MacIntosh is quite difficult and is often more reliably performed with the patient anaesthetized. Start with the knee fully extended and locked in the reduced position; rotate the leg inwards, force the tibia into valgus and slowly flex the knee: as the joint unlocks, the lateral tibial condyle subluxates; with further flexion it suddenly jumps back into place.

IMAGING

MRI is a reliable method of diagnosing both cruciate ligament and meniscal injuries, providing almost 100% sensitivity and over 90% accuracy (Mink, Levy and Cruess, 1988).

ARTHROSCOPY

Arthroscopy is indicated if: (1) the diagnosis, or the extent of the ligament injury, remains in doubt; (2) other lesions, such as meniscal tears or cartilage damage, are suspected; or (3) surgical treatment is anticipated. Partial me-

niscectomy and removal of loose cartilage tags can be performed at the same time.

Treatment

Most patients with chronic instability have reasonably good function and will not require an operation. The first approach should always be a supervised, disciplined and progressively vigorous exercise programme to strengthen the quadriceps and the hamstrings. At the end of 6 months the patient is re-evaluated. The indications for operation are: (1) recurrent locking, with MRI or arthroscopic confirmation of a meniscal tear – arthroscopic meniscectomy alone may alleviate the patient's symptoms (though this may later lead to increased instability); (2) intolerable symptoms of giving way; (3) suboptimal function in a sportsman or others with similarly demanding occupations (even in this group, some patients will accept the use of a knee-brace for specific activities that are known to cause trouble); and (4) adolescents with ligament injuries (the long-term effects of chronic instability in this group are more marked). There is still much controversy about the need for surgery in partial tears of the anterior cruciate ligament. The decision should be made on the basis of symptoms and functional capacity rather than the appearance of the ligament. Young adults with chronic anterior cruciate insufficiency and proven partial tears show diminished activity and run the risk of developing secondary problems such as meniscal lesions, cartilage damage, increasing instability and – eventually – secondary osteoarthritis (Fruensgaard and Johannsen, 1989). With careful follow-up and reassessment, those most at risk can usually be identified and advised to undergo reconstructive surgery.

OPERATIVE TREATMENT

Medial collateral ligament insufficiency seldom causes much disability unless there is an associated anterior cruciate tear. However, if valgus instability is marked, and particularly if it is progressive, ligament reconstruction, by advancing the proximal or distal end and reinforcing the medial structures with the semimembranosus tendon, is justified. A varus osteotomy may be needed as well.

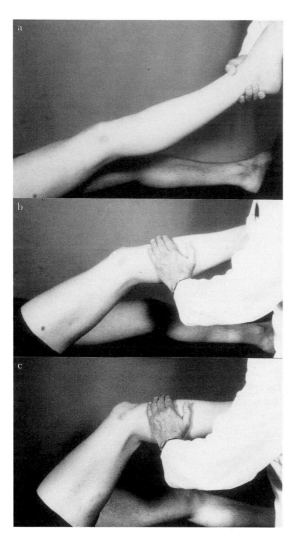

27.38 Cruciate ligament tears – MacIntosh's test (a) The leg is lifted with the knee straight. (b) The fibula is pushed forwards – if the anterior cruciate is torn the lateral tibial condyle is now subluxed forwards. (c) It is held forwards while the knee is flexed; at 30–40 degrees the condyle reduces with a jerk. This may be painful and an alternative method is to lift the straight leg by holding it with both hands just above the ankle, rotating the leg inwards, then flexing the knee – the jerk is often visible and usually painless.

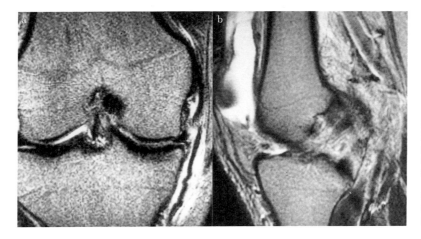

27.39 Torn knee ligaments – MRI (a) Coronal T_2-weighted image showing a medial collateral ligament tear with surrounding oedema and joint effusion. (b) Sagittal T_2-weighted image showing an intrasubstance tear of the anterior cruciate ligament with a large joint effusion.

Lateral instability is uncommon and ligament repair usually unsatisfactory. Reconstruction may be attempted but it should always be combined with a varus high tibial osteotomy.

Posterior cruciate insufficiency can be disabling when combined with posterolateral instability. Reconstruction using the medial head of gastrocnemius to augment the ligament is feasible but the results are unimpressive.

Anterior cruciate ligament insufficiency is the commonest reason for reconstructive surgery. Reattachment or repair alone is not enough; the ligament must be augmented by: (1) an internal graft or implant carefully placed so as to reproduce the attachments, the tension and the movements of the ligament; (2) an external structure (usually a long strip of the iliotibial tract routed deep to the lateral collateral ligament) that prevents rotatory subluxation of the lateral tibial condyle; or (3) a combination of these. The choice of material for the internal graft is controversial. Most surgeons prefer an autologous structure fashioned from local material (e.g. a central strip of quadriceps ligament and its attached slivers of bone). The ideal synthetic graft has yet to be developed.

Operative details of a standard 'internal' and a standard 'external' procedure are given in two excellent papers by Clancy (1982) and Ireland and Trickey (1980).

Postoperatively the knee is splinted in a castbrace for 6–8 weeks; exercises are continued for at least 6 months and a return to sport activities is postponed for 1 year.

Dislocation of the knee

The knee can be dislocated only by considerable violence, as in a road accident. The cruciate ligaments and one or both lateral ligaments are torn.

Clinical features

There is severe bruising, swelling and gross deformity. The circulation in the foot must be examined because the popliteal artery may be torn or obstructed. Distal sensation and movement should be tested to exclude nerve injury.

X-RAY

In addition to the dislocation, the films occasionally reveal a fracture of the tibial spine (cruciate ligament avulsion). If there is any doubt about the circulation, an arteriogram should be obtained.

Treatment

Reduction under anaesthesia is urgent; this is usually achieved by pulling directly in the line of the leg, but hyperextension must be avoided because of the danger to the popliteal vessels. If reduction is achieved, the limb is rested on a back-splint with the knee in 15 degrees of flexion and the circulation is checked re-

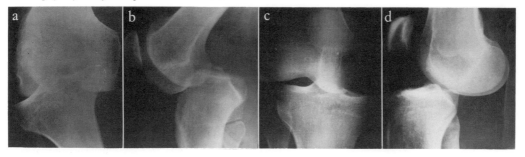

27.40 Dislocations of the knee   (a, b) Posterolateral dislocation; (c, d) anteromedial dislocation.

peatedly during the next week. Because of swelling, a plaster cylinder is dangerous.

Occasionally, closed reduction fails because the torn medial ligament lies between the femur and the tibial condyles; open reduction must then be performed, the ligament is sutured back into place and the capsule is repaired. Similarly, if there is an open wound, or vascular damage which needs operation, the opportunity is taken to repair the ligaments and capsule. Otherwise, these structures are left undisturbed.

When swelling has subsided, a plaster is applied and is worn for 12 weeks. Quadriceps muscle exercises are practised from the start. Weightbearing in the plaster is permitted as soon as the patient can lift his leg. Knee movements are regained when the plaster is removed.

Complications

EARLY

Arterial damage Popliteal artery damage is common, and early repair is important.

Nerve injury especially to the lateral popliteal nerve, may occur but usually recovers.

LATE

Joint instability (increased anteroposterior glide or lateral wobble) usually remains but, provided the quadriceps muscle is sufficiently powerful, the disability is usually not severe.

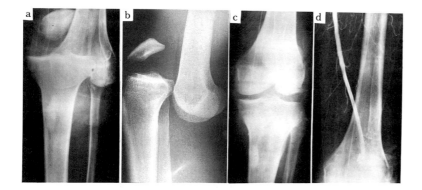

27.41 Knee dislocation and vascular trauma   (a, b) This patient was admitted with a dislocated knee. After reduction (c) the x-ray looked satisfactory, but the circulation did not. (d) An arteriogram showed vascular cut-off just above the knee; had this not been recognized and treated, amputation might have been necessary.

Dislocation of the patella

While the knee is flexed and the quadriceps muscle relaxed, the patella may be forced laterally by direct violence. It may perch temporarily on the ridge of the lateral femoral condyle and then either slip back into position or be displaced to the outer side, where it lies with its anterior surface facing laterally.

Clinical features

The knee usually collapses and the patient may fall to the ground. There is obvious (if somewhat misleading) deformity: the displaced patella is not easily noticed but the uncovered medial femoral condyle is unduly prominent and may be mistaken for the displaced patella. The patella can be felt on the outer side of the knee. Neither active nor passive movement is possible.

X-RAY
The patella is seen to be laterally displaced and rotated. In 5% of cases there is an associated osteochondral fracture.

Treatment

The patella is easily pushed back into place, and anaesthesia is not always necessary. If there is much bruising medially the quadriceps expansion is torn, and immediate operative repair may prevent later recurrent dislocation.

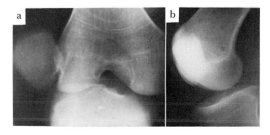

27.42 Dislocation of the patella   (a) Anteroposterior and (b) lateral films of traumatic dislocation of the patella.

With the knee straight, a plaster backslab is applied. It is worn for 3 weeks. Quadriceps muscle exercises are begun at once and practised assiduously. As soon as the patient can elevate his leg, walking is allowed. When the backslab has been removed, flexion is easily regained.

OPERATIVE TREATMENT   Operation reduces the likelihood of recurrence. The inevitable medial capsular tear is repaired and any osteochondral fragments are removed; if the lateral retinaculum is tight it is released. A plaster slab is worn for 3 weeks and quadriceps exercises are practised as with closed treatment.

Complications

The dislocation may recur, either because the quadriceps muscle has not been redeveloped or because the torn medial capsule has not healed securely.

Fractured tibia and fibula

Because of its subcutaneous position, the tibia is more commonly fractured, and more commonly sustains an open fracture, than any other long bone.

Mechanism of injury and pathology

A twisting force causes a spiral fracture of both leg bones at different levels; an angulatory force produces transverse or short oblique fractures, usually at the same level. With an indirect injury, one of the bone fragments may puncture the skin; a direct injury crushes or splits the skin over the fracture. Motorcycle accidents are the most common cause.

Many of the fractures are caused by blunt trauma, and the risk of complications is directly related to the amount and type of soft-tissue damage. Tscherne (1984) has emphasized the importance of assessing and grading the soft-tissue injury: C0 = minor soft-tissue damage with a simple fracture; C1 = superficial abrasion or contusion from within; C2 = deep abrasions, soft-tissue contusion and swelling, with severe fractures; and C3 = extensive soft-tissue damage with a threatened compartment syndrome.

For open fractures, Gustilo's grading is used (Gustilo, Merkow and Templeman, 1990). Type I is a simple fracture with a tiny, clean wound due to perforation by a spike of bone. Type II is a moderately severe fracture with a wound more than 1 cm long but no extensive soft-tissue damage. Type III is a severe injury with extensive soft-tissue damage and wound contamination; this group is further subdivided into those with adequate soft-tissue coverage (III A), those with skin loss (III B) and those associated with arterial injury (III C). Type III C usually requires multidisciplinary care. The incidence of infection ranges from 1% for type I to 30% for type III C.

The average time to union following immobilization ranges from 10 weeks for 'minor' fractures (open or closed) to 20 weeks for severe injuries (Ellis, 1958). However, these figures tend to obscure the fact that many tibial fractures take 6 months or longer to unite.

Clinical features

The skin may be undamaged or obviously divided; sometimes it is intact but is tented or has been crushed, and there is danger that it may slough within a few days. The foot is usually rolled outwards and deformity is obvious. The leg may be bruised and swollen. The pulses are palpated to assess the circulation, and the toes felt for sensation. Movement at the fracture should not be attempted, but the patient is asked to move his toes. It is important to grade the severity of the injury before planning treatment.

X-RAY

A spiral fracture is usually in the lower third of the tibial shaft; the fibular fracture also is spiral and usually at a higher level; often there is lateral shift, overlap and outward twist below the fracture.

With a transverse fracture both bones are broken at the same level, and there may be shift, tilt or twist in any direction; sometimes there is a separate triangular 'butterfly' fragment.

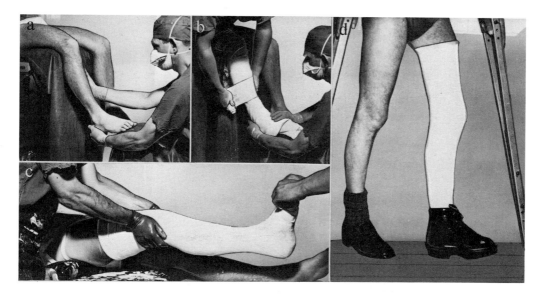

27.43 Fractured tibia and fibula – closed treatment   Reduction is facilitated by bending the knee over the end of the table, with the normal leg alongside for comparison (a). The surgeon holds the position while an assistant applies plaster from the knee downwards (b). When the plaster has set, the leg is lifted and the above-knee plaster completed (c); note that the foot is plantigrade, the knee slightly bent, and the plaster moulded round the patella. A rockered boot is fitted for walking (d).

Treatment of closed fractures

The principles of treatment are: (1) to limit soft-tissue damage and preserve skin cover; (2) to prevent – or at least recognize – compartment swelling; (3) to obtain fracture alignment; (4) to start early weightbearing (loading promotes healing); and (5) to start joint movements as soon as possible.

The first priority is to assess the degree of soft-tissue damage. Even though it is closed, a severe fracture with extensive soft-tissue contusion may require early external fixation and elevation of the limb. A threatened compartment syndrome needs urgent fasciotomy.

CLOSED TREATMENT Most fractures with minor or moderate soft-tissue damage (C0 and 1, and some C2 injuries) can be treated closed. If the fracture is *undisplaced or minimally displaced,* a full-length cast from upper thigh to metatarsal necks is applied with the knee slightly flexed and the ankle at a right angle (displacement of the fibular fracture is unimportant and can be ignored). If the fracture is *displaced,* it is reduced under general anaesthesia with x-ray control. Apposition need not be complete but alignment must be near-perfect (no more than 7 degrees of angulation) and rotation absolutely perfect. A full-length plaster is applied as for undisplaced fractures (note, however, that if

placing the ankle at 0 degrees causes the fracture to displace, a few degrees of equinus are acceptable). The position is checked by x-ray; minor degrees of angulation can still be corrected by making a transverse cut in the plaster and wedging it into a better position. The limb is elevated and the patient is kept under observation for 48–72 hours. If there is excessive swelling, the cast is split.

Patients with grade 0 or 1 injuries are usually allowed up (and home) on the second or third day, bearing minimal weight with the aid of crutches. Those with more severe injuries need to be observed for several days until it is certain that no complications are threatened; thereafter, partial weightbearing is allowed.

After 2 weeks the position is checked by x-ray. The cast is retained (or renewed if it becomes loose) until the fracture unites – which is around 8 weeks in children but seldom under 16 in adults.

The immediate application of plaster may be unwise if skin viability is doubtful, in which case a few days on skeletal traction is useful as a preliminary measure.

EXERCISE Right from the start, the patient is taught to exercise the muscles of the foot, ankle and knee. When he gets up, an overboot with a

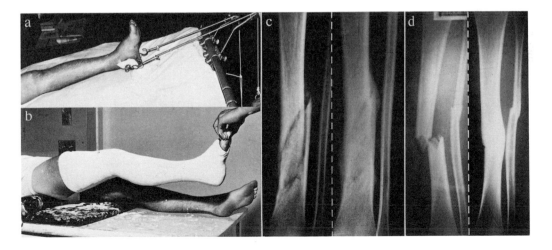

27.44 Fractured tibia and fibula – closed treatment (continued)   Skeletal traction is useful to reduce overlap, and also as provisional treatment when skin viability is doubtful (a). Plaster is applied 10–14 days later (b) using the technique shown in the previous illustration, except that the skeletal pin is retained until the plaster has set. (c, d) Examples of spiral and transverse fractures treated in this way.

rockered sole is fitted, and he is taught to walk correctly. When the plaster is removed, a crepe bandage is applied and the patient is told that he may either elevate and exercise the limb or walk correctly on it, but he must not let it dangle idly.

FUNCTIONAL BRACING With transverse fractures (which are relatively stable) the full-length cast may be changed after 3–4 weeks to a functional below-knee cast (or a brace) which is carefully moulded to bear upon the upper tibia and patellar tendon. This liberates the knee and allows full weightbearing (Sarmiento et al., 1989).

SKELETAL FIXATION If follow-up x-rays show unsatisfactory fracture alignment, and wedging fails to correct this, the plaster is abandoned and the fracture is reduced and fixed. Fractures with severe soft-tissue contusion or vascular injury, and severely comminuted fractures (C3 and some C2 injuries), are better treated by skeletal fixation from the outset.

External fixation is the method of choice for unstable fractures, long oblique or spiral fractures and severely comminuted fractures; in these cases, weightbearing must be delayed until fracture union is advanced.

Closed intramedullary nailing is preferable for transverse fractures that can be reduced and 'hooked-on' under the image intensifier. If interlocking screws are used, the indications can be extended to more unstable fractures.

Interfragmentary lag screws are sometimes useful to hold a long spiral fracture, but a neutralization plate should be added and the leg still needs to be immobilized in plaster.

Plate fixation is best for metaphyseal fractures that are unsuitable for nailing. However, with these open procedures the risk of infection is considerably greater; they should not be used for C2 or C3 injuries.

'Elective' nailing Whether closed intramedullary nailing should be used routinely for uncomplicated fractures is highly controversial. Protagonists claim that it significantly shortens the period of inactivity and diminishes the likelihood of angulation deformity and joint stiffness when compared with closed treatment.

Moreover, with modern methods of closed nailing, the complication rate is low (Hooper, Keddell and Penny, 1991). The fracture is reduced under fluoroscopic control. The tibia is broached at its proximal end through a small incision slightly above and medial to the tibial tubercle. A flexible, blunt-ended guide is inserted through the cortex into the medullary canal beyond the fracture (x-ray control is essential). Progressively larger reamers are threaded over the guide to attain the desired diameter. Then the chosen nail is inserted over the guide and driven home. The guide is, of course, withdrawn. Locking screws are added if necessary.

POSTOPERATIVE MANAGEMENT After the nailing of a transverse or short oblique fracture, weightbearing can be started within a few days, progressing to full weight when this is comfortable.

After plating, partial weightbearing only is permitted for 6–8 weeks; thereafter, full weight can be permitted if a protective plaster is used.

After external fixation only partial weight is allowed until a hint of callus is seen on x-ray. Then the device is dynamized and progressively increasing weight is taken, guided by comfort. After 6–8 weeks (occasionally more) the apparatus is removed and a patellar-tendon-bearing plaster or brace applied and worn until the fracture is consolidated. If there is no fracture healing by 8 weeks, it may be wise to remove the fixator and substitute some form of internal fixation with bone grafting.

Treatment of open fractures

The management of severe open fractures is embodied in the following words: (1) antibiotics, (2) debridement, (3) stabilization, (4) delayed closure and (5) rehabilitation.

Antibiotics are started immediately. The wound is debrided and thoroughly cleaned. Gustilo grade I injuries can be closed primarily and then treated as for closed injuries. More severe wounds are left open and inspected after 3 days; if necessary, a further debridement is carried out.

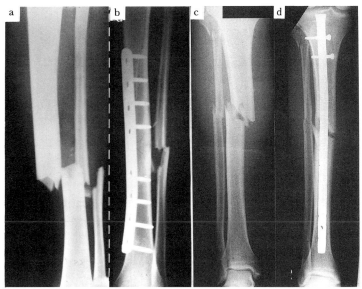

27.45 Fractured tibia and fibula – open treatment (a, b) Plating of this subcutaneous fracture is easily performed but it requires a long wound and stripping of soft tissues (with the attendant risk of infection). (c, d) 'Closed' intramedullary nailing (if necessary with interlocking screws) is preferable; active movements and weightbearing can be started soon after operation.

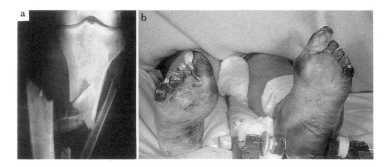

27.46 Fractured tibia and fibula – arterial injury (a) With this type of fracture, skin damage is inevitable and arterial damage not unlikely. (b) This patient, who fell down a mountain, had bilateral tibial fractures with vascular injury; he suffered the ultimate fate of delay – bilateral gangrene.

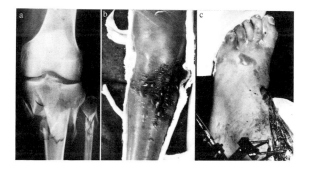

27.47 Fractured tibia and fibula – compartment syndrome (a) Although not as severely displaced as the fracture in Fig. 27.46, an injury at this level is always dangerous. This man was treated in plaster. Pain became intense, and when the plaster was split (which should have been done immediately after its application) the leg was swollen and blistered (b). A tibial compartment decompression was performed – but too late; 1 week later (c) the foot showed signs of irreversible ischaemia.

It is important to stabilize the fracture. This is best achieved by applying an external fixator, leaving the wound free to be inspected and treated as necessary. As soon as it is certain that the wound is clean and granulating, it can be closed by either direct suture (without tension) or a skin graft.

The external fixator is retained until the fracture is 'sticky' and may then be replaced by a cast. Partial weightbearing is permitted. The cast is removed only when the fracture is consolidated.

Complications

EARLY

Infection Open fractures are always at risk; even a small perforation should be treated with respect and debridement carried out before the wound is closed. Larger lacerations require wide excision, and the wound should be left open until the risk of infection has passed (see p. 542).

Vascular injury Fractures of the proximal half of the tibia may damage the popliteal artery (see p. 543). This is an emergency of the first order, requiring exploration and repair.

Compartment syndrome Proximal third fractures are inclined to cause bleeding and progressive soft-tissue expansion within the fascial compartments of the leg, thus precipitating muscle ischaemia (see p. 544). A tight plaster on a swollen leg may have the same effect. Operative decompression of all the affected compartments is essential. The fracture is then treated as a grade III open fracture requiring an external fixator and delayed wound closure.

LATE

Malunion Slight shortening (up to 1.5 cm) is usually of little consequence, but rotation and angulation deformity, apart from being ugly, are disabling, because the knee and ankle no longer move in the same plane. In the long run, the deformity may predispose to osteoarthritis of the knee or ankle.

Angulation should be prevented at all stages; anything more than 7 degrees in either plane is unacceptable; rotational alignment should be perfect.

Backward angulation (caused by allowing the fracture to sag while plaster is being applied) is common and, if accompanied by a stiff equinus ankle, is dangerous, for when the patient tries to force the foot up in walking the tibia is liable to refracture. This may occur insidiously and lead to non-union.

Late deformity, if marked, should be corrected by tibial osteotomy.

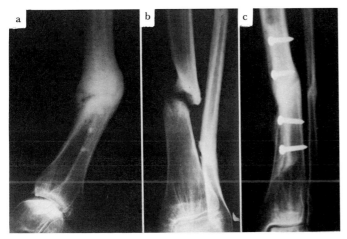

27.48 Fractured tibia and fibula – complications (a) Malunion: if the fracture is even slightly angulated in plaster, deformity is liable to increase when weightbearing begins. (b) Nonunion (atrophic) and (c) a similar case treated with a sliding bone graft.

Delayed union   Union is slow when the fracture is open (especially with infection), if the initial displacement was considerable, if the tibia is fractured in two places or if the fracture is comminuted. Union may be hastened by weightbearing (especially with bracing) but if delay seems unduly prolonged, bone grafting and intramedullary fixation are indicated.

If the fibular fracture has joined and is splinting the tibia apart, then 2.5 cm of fibula may be excised and a sliding bone graft screwed across the tibial fracture.

Non-union   may follow bone loss or deep infection, but a common cause is faulty treatment. Either delayed union has not been recognized and splintage has been discontinued too soon, or the patient with a recently united fracture has walked with a stiff equinus ankle.

Once non-union is established the patient must either wear a permanent splint or the fracture must be operated upon. Hypertrophic non-union can be treated by intramedullary nailing or compression plating; atrophic non-union needs bone grafting in addition. If the fibula has united, a small segment should be excised so as to permit compression of the tibial fragments.

Joint stiffness   is often due to neglect in treatment of the soft tissues; but with the prolonged splintage necessary, and especially in the presence of sepsis, some stiffness may be unavoidable. Limitation of movement at the ankle and foot may persist for 6–12 months after removal of the plaster, in spite of active exercises.

Osteoporosis   of the distal fragment, and sometimes the tarsal bones as well, is so common with all forms of treatment as to be regarded as a 'normal' concomitant of tibial fractures. Axial loading of the tibia is important and weightbearing should be re-established as soon as possible. After prolonged external fixation, special care should be taken to prevent a distal stress fracture.

Algodystrophy   With distal third fractures, algodystrophy is not uncommon. Exercises should be encouraged throughout the period of treatment. The management of established algodystrophy is discussed on p. 240.

Fracture of the fibula alone

Most spiral fibular fractures are associated with injuries of the ankle or knee; especially with a high fracture the ankle should be examined and x-rayed.

An isolated fracture of the fibula (usually transverse) may be due to stress or to a direct blow. There is local tenderness, but the patient is able to stand and to move the knee and ankle. Analgesics will control pain, and no other treatment is necessary.

Fracture of the tibia alone

In children a twisting injury may cause a spiral fracture of the tibia without fracture of the fibula; this is rare in adults. At any age a direct injury, such as a kick, may cause a transverse or slightly oblique fracture of the tibia alone at the site of impact.

Local bruising and swelling are usually evident, but knee and ankle movements are possible. The child with a spiral fracture may be able to stand on the leg, and, as the fracture may be almost invisible in an anteroposterior film, unless two views are taken the injury can be missed; a few days later an angry mother brings the child with a lump which proves to be callus. Transverse and slightly oblique fractures are easily seen on x-ray but displacement is slight.

Treatment

With displacement, reduction should be attempted. An above-knee plaster is applied as

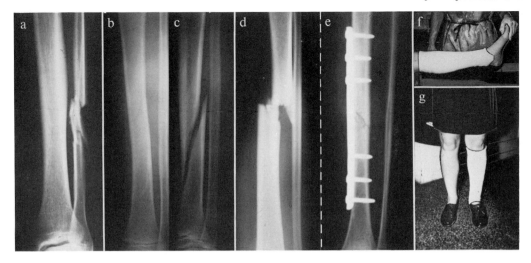

27.49 Fracture of one bone only   (a) Fracture of the fibula alone. (b, c) In this child's leg the spiral fracture of the tibia shows only in one view. (d) Transverse fracture of the tibia alone in the adult: it has been plated (e) and is now so stable that a plaster gaiter (f, g) is the only protection needed.

with a fracture of both bones; first a split plaster and then, when swelling has subsided, a complete one. A fracture of the tibia alone takes just as long to unite as if both bones were broken; so at least 12 weeks is needed for consolidation and sometimes much more. The child with a spiral fracture, however, can be safely released after 6 weeks; and with a mid-shaft transverse fracture the surgeon may (if he is a skilled plasterer and reduction is perfect) replace the above-knee plaster by a short plaster gaiter.

Complications

An open fracture will, of course, need wound excision; with infection, union will be slow. When closed, isolated tibial fractures, especially in the lower third, may be slow to join, and the temptation is to discard splintage too soon. Even slight displacement may delay union, so open reduction with internal fixation is often preferred. In managing delay, union can usually be hastened by excising 2.5 cm of the fibula, which allows the tibial fragments to impact.

Fatigue fracture of the tibia

Repetitive stress may cause a fatigue fracture of the tibia. This is seen in army recruits, runners and ballet dancers, who complain of pain in the front of the leg. There is local tenderness and slight swelling.

X-RAY
For the first 4 weeks there may be nothing abnormal about the x-ray, but a bone scan shows increased activity. After some weeks periosteal new bone may be seen, with a small transverse defect in the cortex. There is a danger that these appearances may be mistaken for those of an osteosarcoma, with tragic consequences. If the diagnosis of stress fracture is kept in mind, such mistakes are unlikely.

Treatment

The patient is told to avoid the stressful activity. Usually after 8–10 weeks the symptoms settle down.

III. Injuries of the ankle and foot

Ankle ligament injuries

The patient falls or stumbles and the foot inverts under him. As a rule, there is only a partial tear of the lateral ligament and the injury is an ankle sprain. Sometimes, however, the ligament is completely torn and the joint subluxates; the talus momentarily tilts into inversion, then snaps back into position.

Clinical features

Bruising may be severe (suggesting a complete tear) or may be faint and only appear a day or two after the injury (more likely with a sprain). The ankle is always swollen. Tenderness is usually maximal on the lateral aspect of the joint. Passive inversion is painful, but only with a complete tear of the ligament is the movement excessive. Pain may prevent excessive movement from being demonstrated and, if the injury is severe, inversion must be tested again under local or general anaesthesia.

X-RAY
The x-ray appearance of the resting ankle is normal whether the joint has been sprained or subluxed, for a subluxation reduces itself. X-ray films are taken with both ankles inverted (if necessary, using local or general anaesthesia); these 'stress films' show whether the talus tilts unduly on the affected side ('undue' tilting means 10 degrees more than on the normal side).

Treatment

PARTIAL TEAR
An ankle sprain should be treated by activity. A crepe bandage is applied and active exercises are begun immediately and persevered with until full movement is regained. The patient is not allowed to dangle the leg and the bandage is worn until swelling has disappeared. Weight may be taken as soon as the patient will walk, but he must be taught to walk correctly with the normal heel–toe gait. A common cause of prolonged pain is repeated stress due to unstable footwear or weak muscles.

COMPLETE TEAR
Operative repair of acutely ruptured ligaments may be advisable in athletes and dancers. In most patients, however, subluxation can be treated in plaster, which is applied from just below the knee to the toes, with the foot plantigrade. If there is swelling, the plaster is split and replaced when the swelling has subsided. Plaster is worn until the ligament may be expected to have repaired, which takes about 10 weeks. The patient is encouraged to walk normally with the aid of an overboot with a rockered sole. When plaster is removed, a crepe bandage is worn and movements are regained by active use.

Complications

Adhesions Following an ankle sprain, adhesions are liable to form unless the foot is actively and correctly used. The patient complains that the ankle 'gives way' and lets him down. Following such an incident, there is tenderness on the outer side and pain on inversion, but no excessive inversion. If active exercises fail to restore full painless movement, the joint should be manipulated under anaesthesia and full range maintained by activity.

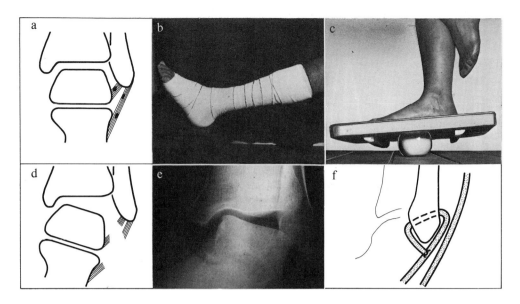

27.50 Ankle sprains The commonest is a partial tear of the lateral ligament (a). In treatment a crepe bandage (b) is more efficient than adhesive strapping. The balancing board (c) is a useful method of strengthening the muscles.
A complete tear of the lateral ligament (d) causes recurrent giving way; a strain film reveals talar tilt (e). The operation shown in (f) is simple and effective.

Recurrent subluxation If a complete tear of the lateral ligament was undiagnosed, and consequently unsplinted, the ligament fails to repair and subluxation becomes recurrent. The history is similar to that of adhesions following a sprain; the patient, after an injury, complains that the ankle gives way at intervals. The talus, however, can be inverted further than that of the normal ankle. If the diagnosis is in doubt, the patient should be anaesthetized and both ankles x-rayed in full inversion. If the talus tilts, the injury is a subluxation; if not, the adhesions should be broken down forthwith by manipulation.

Recurrent subluxation is usually treated quite satisfactorily by raising the outer side of the heel and extending its lower surface laterally ('floated-out heel'). However, if this fails to relieve the patient's symptoms, operation may be necessary.

A simple and effective procedure is to detach the peroneus brevis tendon from the muscle, thread it through a hole drilled in the fibula and then sew it back to itself, to the peroneus longus and to the ligamentous structures at the tip of the fibula. If, when the tendon has been threaded through the malleolus, tension is applied and the ankle tested for stability, this will show if the procedure is adequate; if not, the tendon is also threaded through a vertical hole drilled in the neck of the talus and sewn to the periosteum over the tip of the malleolus. In either case, plaster must afterwards be worn for 8 weeks.

Deltoid ligament tears

Rupture of the deltoid ligament is usually associated with either a fracture of the distal end of the fibula or tearing of the distal tibiofibular ligaments (or both). The diagnosis is made by x-ray: there is widening of the medial joint space in the mortise view; sometimes the talus is tilted, and diastasis of the tibiofibular joint may be obvious.

Treatment   Provided the medial joint space is completely reduced, the ligament will heal. The fibular fracture or diastasis must be accurately reduced, if necessary by open operation and internal fixation. Occasionally the medial joint space cannot be reduced; it should then be explored in order to free any soft tissue trapped in the joint. A below-knee plaster is applied with the foot plantigrade and is retained for 8 weeks.

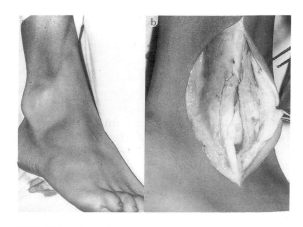

27.51 Dislocation of peroneal tendons   (a) On movement of the ankle, the peroneal tendons slip forward over the lateral malleolus. (b) The anterior part of the retinaculum is being reconstructed.

Recurrent dislocation of peroneal tendons

The condition is unmistakable, for the patient can demonstrate that the peroneal tendons dislocate forwards over the fibula during dorsiflexion and eversion. Treatment is operative and is based on the observation that the attachment of the retinaculum to the periosteum on the front of the fibula has come adrift, creating a pouch into which the tendons displace. Using Dexon sutures through drill holes in the bone, the normal anatomy is recreated (Das De and Balasubramaniam, 1985).

Tears of the inferior tibiofibular ligaments

The inferior tibiofibular ligaments may be torn, allowing partial or complete separation of the tibiofibular joint (diastasis). *Complete diastasis*, with tearing of both the anterior and posterior fibres, follows a severe abduction strain. *Partial diastasis*, with tearing of only the anterior fibres, is due to an external rotation force. These injuries may occur in isolation, but they are usually associated with fractures of the malleoli.

Clinical features

Following a twisting injury, the patient complains of pain in the front of the ankle. There is swelling and marked tenderness directly over the inferior tibiofibular joint.

X-RAY
With a partial tear the fibula usually lies in its normal position and the x-ray looks normal. With a complete tear the tibiofibular joint is separated and the ankle mortise is widened; sometimes this becomes apparent only when the ankle is stressed in abduction. There may be associated fractures of the distal tibia or fibula, or an isolated fracture more proximally in the fibula.

Treatment

Partial tears can be treated by strapping the ankle firmly for 2–3 weeks. Thereafter exercises are encouraged.

Complete tears are best managed by internal fixation with a transverse screw just above the joint. This must be done as soon as possible so that the tibiofibular space does not become clogged with organizing haematoma and fibrous tissue. If the patient is seen late and the ankle is painful and unstable, open clearance of the syndesmosis and transverse screw fixation may be warranted. The ankle is immobilized in plaster for 6 weeks, after which the screw is removed. However, some degree of instability usually persists.

Fractures around the ankle

Fractures and fracture-dislocatons of the ankle are common. One such injury was described by Percivall Pott in 1768, and the group as a whole is now referred to colloquially as Pott's fracture.

Mechanism of injury

Normally the talus is seated firmly in the mortise made up of the distal tibia and the medial and lateral malleoli. If it is twisted and tilted in the mortise, either the ligaments may rupture or the malleoli may be pushed off or pulled off by intact collateral ligaments. If a malleolus is pushed off, it usually fractures obliquely; if it is pulled off, it fractures transversely.

Usually the foot is anchored to the ground while the momentum of the body continues forwards; the patient may stumble over an unexpected obstacle or stair, or into a small depression in the ground, or he may have fallen from a height. The momentum of the body may impose any one of a variety of forces upon the ankle, the most important being external rotation, abduction and adduction; moreover external rotation may occur while the foot is pronated or supinated. In addition, if the patient has fallen from a height an upward thrust is added.

Lauge-Hansen (1950) classified these injuries on the basis of their supposed pathogenesis, which it is important to appreciate if displacement is to be corrected by manipulation. A simpler, and in some ways more useful, classification is that of Danis and Weber (Muller et al., 1991) who regarded the fibula as the key to ankle stability. There are three types of fibular fracture. *Type A* is a fracture below the tibiofibular syndesmosis, caused by adduction or abduction. The medial malleolus may be fractured, or the deltoid ligament torn, as well, but after reduction the ankle is stable. *Type B* is an oblique fibular fracture running upwards from the joint line, caused by external rotation. Usually the medial structures are disrupted too, but the syndesmosis is intact and the mortise has not sprung apart. *Type C* is a fibular fracture above the syndesmosis, caused either by abduction alone or by a combination of abduction and external rotation; the syndesmosis (and, with higher fractures, the interosseous membrane) is ruptured, the fibula is often tilted and the mortise is widened. This is an unstable fracture – stability is regained only by reducing the fracture, restoring the length of the fibula and closing the diastasis.

Clinical features

The ankle is swollen, and deformity may be obvious. The site of tenderness is important; if both sides are tender, an injury (bony or ligamentous) must be suspected on both sides.

X-RAY

At least three views are needed: anteroposterior, lateral and a half oblique 'mortise' view. The level of the fibular fracture is often best seen in the lateral view; diastasis may not be appreciated without the mortise view. Further x-rays may be needed to exclude a proximal fibular fracture. Several well-marked fracture patterns can be recognized.

External rotation injuries typically produce a spiral or oblique fracture of the fibula. If the

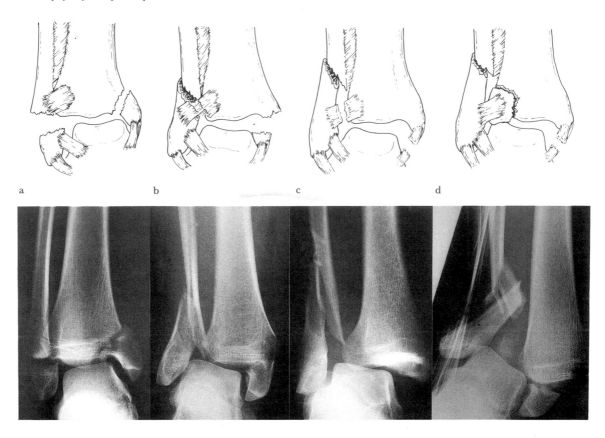

a   b   c   d

27.52 Ankle fractures – classification   The Danis–Weber classification is based on the level of the fibular fracture. (a) Type A – a fracture below the syndesmosis. (b) Type B – a fracture at the syndesmosis, often associated with disruption of the anterior fibres of the tibiofibular ligament. (c) Type C – the fibular fracture is above the syndesmosis; the tibiofibular ligament must be torn, or else (d) the ligament avulses a small piece of the tibia.

fracture is at or below the level of the tibial plafond (Danis–Weber type A or B), the syndesmosis is intact; if the fracture is above this level (type C), the syndesmosis must be ruptured. Diastasis is best seen in the mortise view; sometimes there is a telltale chip of bone torn from the tibial attachment of the ligament. If the distal fibular fragment and the talus are displaced and tilted, there must be either disruption of the medial structures or a diastasis or both. *It is vital to appreciate this point because one of the commonest causes of displacement (and a poor outcome) is failure to reduce the unseen syndesmotic and/or medial collateral rupture.* If the deltoid ligament does not rupture, the medial malleolus may be avulsed and fractured transversely; further rotation may lead to avulsion of a posterior fragment of the tibia, to which the tibiofibular ligament is attached.

A type C fracture with no widening of the tibiofibular joint on x-ray suggests a partial rupture of the syndesmotic ligaments and spontaneous reduction.

Abduction injuries   are recognized by the typical transverse or short oblique fibular fracture (either type A or type C) and avulsion of the medial malleolus or tearing of the deltoid ligament (the medial joint space opened up). With a high fibular fracture, there may be

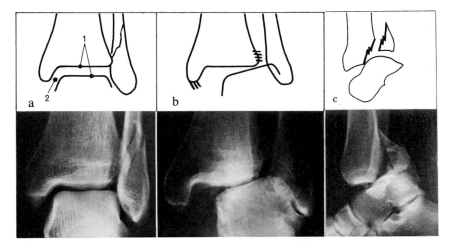

27.53 Ankle fractures – the talus The position of the talus is important. (a) Fracture without subluxation: 1, the surfaces of the tibia and talus are precisely parallel; 2, the distance of the talus from the medial malleolus is normal. (b) Subluxation – the talus is tilted and unduly separated from the medial malleolus; there is also diastasis (displacement was permitted by a high fracture of the fibula – the Maisonneuve injury). (c) If the posterior margin of the tibia is fractured, the talus may be displaced upwards.

obvious tibiofibular diastasis; the talus may be driven up between the two bones.

Adduction injuries cause a near-vertical fracture of the medial malleolus extending upwards from the medial angle of the mortise, and either avulsion of the lateral malleolus or rupture of the ligament. The entire distal complex (medial malleolus, talus and lateral malleolus) may be shifted medially, but the tibiofibular syndesmosis is intact. Tilting of the talus may crush the medial tibial articular surface and set the scene for secondary osteoarthritis no matter how perfect the reduction.

Vertical compression may drive the talus into the tibial articular surface and fracture the plafond (or pilon). There may be a vertical split with separation of a posterior or anterior triangular fragment; if it is displaced, there will be a step in the articular surface. More severe injuries can cause marked comminution of the distal tibial surface. Combined twisting and compression injuries can cause various combinations of malleolar and pilon fractures.

Treatment

Like other intra-articular injuries, ankle fractures must be accurately reduced and held if later mechanical dysfunction is to be prevented. Persistent displacement of the talus leads to increased stress and predisposes to secondary osteoarthritis (Ramsay and Hamilton, 1976).

In assessing the accuracy of reduction, four important objectives must be met: (1) the fibula must be restored to its full length; (2) the talus must sit squarely in the mortise, with the talar and tibial articular surfaces parallel; (3) the medial joint space must be restored to its normal width (about 4 mm); and (4) oblique x-rays must show that there is no tibiofibular diastasis. Unless closed reduction is perfect and the fracture will remain in place (both uncommon), open methods are needed.

Two further principles must be observed. Swelling is rapid and severe; if the fracture is not reduced within a few hours, definitive treatment may have to be deferred for several days while the leg is elevated so that the swelling can subside. After reduction – whether closed or open – the leg must be held in plaster for 6–8 weeks or until the fractures unite.

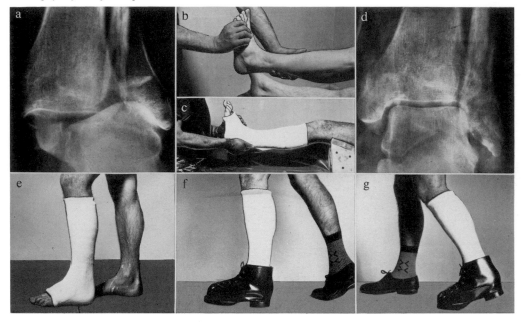

27.54 Ankle fractures – closed treatment An external rotation fracture (a) is reduced by traction followed by internal rotation (b); a below-knee plaster is applied, moulded and held till it has set (c). Reduction is checked by x-ray (d). The plaster must be plantigrade (e); a rockered boot permits an almost normal gait (f, g).

CLOSED TREATMENT

Undisplaced fractures, fractures below the tibio-fibular joint and fractures in the elderly can be treated closed.

Those with no trace of displacement clearly require no reduction and are sometimes treated without plaster, the patient being allowed to walk with the ankle in a crepe bandage. The method is safe only when it is certain that there has not been spontaneous reduction of a displacement. Fractures with displacement are treated as follows.

First manual traction is applied; then a force is added, the reverse of that which caused the injury. Unless the causal force has been correctly deduced and reversed by manipulation, accurate replacement of the talus is unlikely.

A padded plaster is applied from just below the knee to the toes, with the foot plantigrade; that is, with the foot at an angle of 90 degrees to the leg and neither in varus nor in valgus. (The tendency to apply the plaster with the foot inverted must be resisted.) The plaster may need to be split and, if so, it must be completed

or replaced when swelling has subsided. An x-ray to confirm reduction must be taken after the plaster has been applied and another after it has been changed. With an external rotation injury in which the fibular fracture is below the tibiofibular joint, 6 weeks in plaster is sufficient; all other fractures should be kept in plaster for 12 weeks.

An overboot is fitted and the patient is taught to walk correctly as soon as possible. Ankle and foot movements are regained by active exercises when the plaster is removed. As with any lower-limb fracture, the leg must not be allowed to dangle idly. It must be exercised or elevated. After removal of the plaster a temporary crepe bandage is necessary.

OPERATIVE TREATMENT

Open reduction and internal fixation is advisable (1) for all severe fracture-subluxations (Danis–Weber type C); (2) for displaced pilon fractures (see below); and (3) if closed reduction fails. Operation is best performed within a few hours of injury, before swelling is severe; if

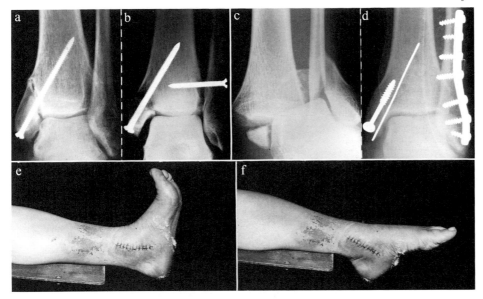

27.55 Ankle fractures – open treatment   (a) A large medial fragment needs a malleolar screw; (b) if diastasis is present, a tibiofibular screw may be added; (c, d) if the fibula is displaced its length must be restored and held by internal fixation; (e and f) show this patient exercising his ankle a few days after operation, and before the walking plaster was applied.

the optimal time has passed, the leg should be elevated and lightly splinted until swelling has subsided (usually for 1–2 weeks).

With unstable type C fracture-subluxations the first step is to reduce the fibula and restore it to full length; this reduction is best held with a plate and screws. Diastasis is then reduced and held with a transverse tibiofibular screw. By that stage the medial disruption will probably have been reduced; if there is a large medial malleo-lar fragment, it should be fixed in anatomical position with either a screw or semi-rigid pins and tension-band wiring; deltoid ligament rup-ture used not to be sutured, but if the medial joint space remains abnormally wide, it should be explored (in case the ligament has become snared in the joint), released and sutured.

Fracture-subluxations more than a week old may prove difficult to reduce because of clot organi-zation in the syndesmosis. Granulation tissue should be removed from the syndesmosis and transverse tibiofibular fixation secured, if neces-sary with a long bolt.

Type C fractures with minimal displacement and only partial diastasis can be treated closed, but it is safer to apply a small fibular plate to prevent late drifting into valgus which may pass undetected.

With adduction fractures the syndesmosis is usually stable. Fibular fixation is therefore less critical and an intramedullary screw or pin will suffice.

Pilon fractures require special attention. An undisplaced split can be treated closed by cast immobilization (see above). A single large displaced fragment (more than 25% of the articular surface) may lead to progressive anter-ior or posterior subluxation and it should therefore be reduced and fixed with one or two screws. Comminuted, impacted fractures are extremely difficult to reduce and it may be wiser to manage these by calcaneal traction and active exercises to maintain ankle movement. If there are associated malleolar fractures (which is usual), the fibula should be reduced to full length and plated; this may restore the plafond

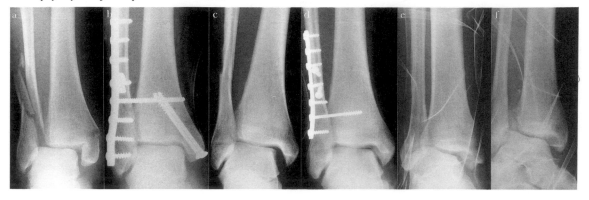

27.56 Ankle fractures with diastasis – treatment   (a) In this type B fracture there is partial disruption of the distal tibiofibular syndesmosis. Treatment (b) required medial and lateral fixation as well as a tibiofibular screw. (c) A type C fracture must, inevitably, disrupt the tibiofibular ligament; in this case the medial malleolus was intact but the deltoid ligament was torn. (d) By fixing the fibular fracture and using a tibiofibular screw, the ankle was completely reduced and it was therefore unnecessary to explore the deltoid ligament. (e) This patient presented 5 days after his injury; he, too, had a diastasis with disruption of the deltoid ligament (f). In this case the tibiofibular joint as well as the deltoid ligament had to be explored before the ankle could be reduced.

to some extent. If the appropriate facilities and skills are available, an attempt can be made to disimpact and reassemble the mortise and hold it with a buttress plate: the defect in the tibia is filled with cancellous bone grafts (Mast, Spiegel and Pappas, 1988).

POSTOPERATIVE MANAGEMENT

After open reduction and fixation of ankle fractures, movements should be regained before applying a below-knee plaster cast. The patient is then allowed partial weightbearing with crutches; the cast is maintained until the fractures have consolidated (anything from 6 to 12 weeks).

If a transverse tibiofibular screw or bolt has been inserted, the patient should be recalled to have this removed after 6–8 weeks.

Complications

EARLY

Vascular injury   With a severe fracture-subluxation the pulses may be obliterated. The ankle should be immediately reduced and held in a splint until definitive treatment has been initiated.

LATE

Malunion   Incomplete reduction is common and, unless the talus fits the mortise accurately, degenerative changes may occur. Sometimes degeneration can be halted or prevented by a corrective osteotomy. If osteoarthritis becomes severe, arthrodesis may prove necessary.

Secondary malunion from epiphyseal arrest in an adolescent is rare.

Non-union   of the medial malleolus occasionally occurs if a flap of periosteum is interposed between it and the tibia. It should be prevented by operative reduction and screw fixation.

Joint stiffness   and swelling of the ankle are usually the result of neglect in treatment of the soft tissues. The patient must walk correctly in plaster and, when the plaster is removed, he must, until circulatory control is regained, wear a crepe bandage and elevate the leg whenever he is not using it actively. Occasionally, several months after the fracture, manipulation under anaesthesia may be needed to restore full movement.

Algodystrophy   often follows fractures of the ankle. The patient complains of pain in the

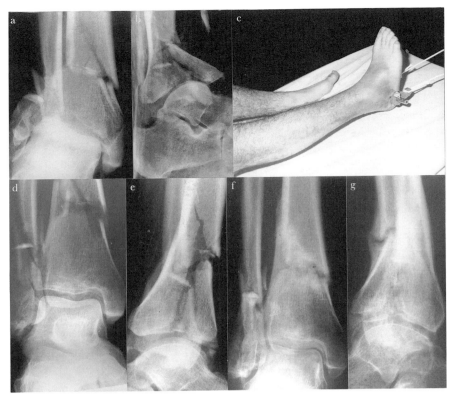

27.57 Pilon fractures (a, b) This complex pilon fracture was treated by (c) traction and movements. A calcaneal pin used for more than 3 weeks is very liable to loosen and become septic but if 'Simonis swivels' (hooks that contain ballbearings and are almost frictionless) are used, traction can safely be used for much longer. In this patient it was used for 8 weeks. (d, e) Movement moulded the fragments into position and (f, g) the end result was satisfactory. (By courtesy of R. B. Simonis, whose patient this was.)

foot; there may be swelling and diffuse tenderness, with gradual development of trophic changes and severe osteoporosis.

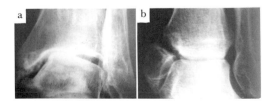

27.58 Ankle fractures – complications (a) Malunion following failure of reduction; with this degree of localized overload, osteoarthritis is a likely sequel. (b) Non-union of the medial malleolus; this could have been prevented by removing the interposed flap of periosteum and fixing the malleolus.

Fracture-separation of the distal tibial and fibular epiphyses

Physeal injuries are quite common in children and almost a third of these occur around the ankle.

Mechanism of injury

The foot is fixed to the ground or trapped in a crevice and the leg twists to one or the other side. The tibial (or fibular) physis is wrenched apart, usually resulting in a Salter–Harris type 1 or 2 fracture. With severe external rotation or abduction the fibula may also fracture more proximally. The tibial metaphyseal fragment comes off posterolaterally and the epiphysis tends to displace posteriorly or laterally. With adduction injuries the tip of the fibula may be avulsed.

Type 3 and 4 fractures are uncommon. The epiphysis is split vertically and one piece of the epiphysis may be displaced. In the notorious triplane fracture, there is both a vertical split posteromedially and a horizontal separation through the remaining physeal plate, thus creating three separate fragments – the split-off piece, the tibia and the lateral part of the epiphysis. Injury to the growth disc may result in either asymmetrical growth or arrested growth.

Clinical features

Following a sprain the ankle is painful, swollen, bruised and acutely tender. There may be an obvious deformity, but sometimes the injury looks deceptively mild.

X-RAY
Undisplaced physeal fractures – especially those in the distal fibula – are easily missed.

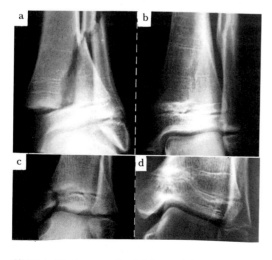

27.59 Ankle fractures in children (a) Salter–Harris type 2 injury; after reduction (b) growth has proceeded normally. (c) Salter–Harris type 3 injury; (d) the medial side of the physis has not grown – presumably it was bridged by bone.

Even a hint of physeal widening should be regarded with great suspicion and the child x-rayed again after a week. In an infant the state of the physis can sometimes only be guessed at, but a few weeks after injury there may be extensive periosteal new-bone formation.

Treatment

Salter–Harris type 1 and 2 injuries are treated closed. If it is displaced, the fracture is gently reduced under general anaesthesia; the limb is immobilized in a full-length cast for 3 weeks and then in a below-knee walking cast for a further 3 weeks.

Type 3 or 4 fractures, if undisplaced, can be treated in the same manner, but the ankle must be re-x-rayed after 5 days to ensure that the fragments have not slipped. Displaced fractures can sometimes be reduced closed by reversing the forces that produced the injury. However, unless reduction is near-perfect, the fracture should be reduced open and fixed with thin transverse or oblique cancellous screws (which will have to be removed after about 4 months). Postoperatively the leg is immobilized in a below-knee cast for 6 weeks.

Complications

Malunion Imperfect reduction may result in angular deformity of the ankle – usually valgus. In children under 10 years old, mild deformities may be accommodated by further growth and modelling. In older children the deformity should be corrected by a supramalleolar closing-wedge osteotomy.

Asymmetrical growth Fractures through the epiphysis (Salter–Harris type 3 or 4 may result in localized fusion of the physis. The bony bridge is usually in the medial half of the growth plate; the lateral half goes on growing and the distal tibia gradually veers into varus. Tomography or CT is helpful in showing precisely where physeal arrest has occurred. If the bony bridge is small (less than 30% of the physeal width) it can be excised and replaced by a pad of fat in the hope that physeal growth may be restored (Langenskiold, 1975). If more than half of the physis is involved, or the child is near the end of the growth period, supramalleolar closing-wedge osteotomy is indicated.

Shortening Early physeal closure occurs in about 20% of children with distal tibial injuries. Fortunately the resulting limb length discrepancy is usually mild. If it promises to be more than 2 cm and the child is under 14 years of age, proximal tibial epiphysiodesis in the opposite limb may restore equality. If the discrepancy is marked, or the child near the end of the growth period, leg lengthening is indicated.

Injuries of the talus

Talar injuries are rare and due to considerable violence, usually a car accident or falling from a height. The injuries include fractures (of the head, neck, body or lateral process of the talus), dislocations (mid-tarsal, subtalar or total dislocation of the talus) and fracture-dislocations (talar fractures combined with dislocation). Mid-tarsal injuries are often missed; they have been classified according to the deforming force: longitudinal compression, plantar and crush varieties are described, as well as medial or lateral displacements, sometimes of a 'swivel' type (Main and Jowett, 1975).

The talus receives a rich blood supply from the anterior tibial, posterior tibial and peroneal arteries, as well as anastomotic vessels from the surrounding capsule and ligaments. The intraosseous vessels run mainly from anterior to posterior. In fractures of the talar neck these vessels are divided; if the fracture is displaced, the extraosseous plexus too may be damaged and the body of the talus is at risk of ischaemic necrosis.

Clinical features

The foot is obviously deformed and swollen. The skin may have been split or may rapidly necrose. The dorsalis pedis artery should be palpated.

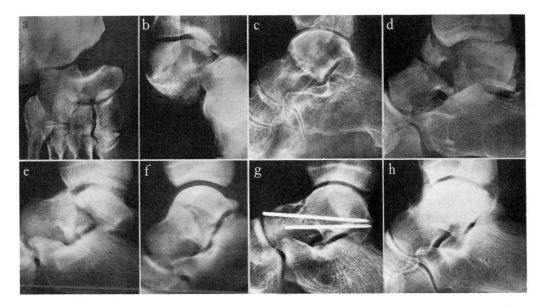

27.60 Talar fractures and dislocations (a, b) Two views of subtalar dislocation. (c) Talar fracture without displacement, and (d) with considerable displacement. (e, f) Talar fracture before and after reduction by forced plantarflexion. (g) Another method of treatment, by open reduction and internal fixation. (h) Avascular necrosis of the posterior half of the talus following fracture.

X-RAY

Anteroposterior, lateral and oblique views are needed. The talus is first identified (not always easy); then inspected to see if it is fractured (and, if so, how the fragments are displaced); next its relationship to the tibia, calcaneum and other tarsal bones is studied (to identify dislocation); finally the mid-tarsal joint is carefully inspected – the bones must fit precisely and comparison with the normal foot is useful.

The fracture usually crosses the neck of the talus and the fragments may be widely displaced; if so, there must inevitably be subluxation of the talocalcaneal joint. Sometimes the posterior fragment is completely dislocated from the ankle mortise.

Fractures of the talar head or body or processes are rare. But beware – an innocuous-seeming flake beneath the lateral malleolus may, on a 20 degree oblique view, prove to be a substantial fragment – the lateral process of the talus.

Treatment

UNDISPLACED FRACTURES OF THE TALUS
When displacement is no more than trivial, reduction is not needed. A split below-knee plaster is applied and, when the swelling has subsided, is replaced by a complete plaster in the plantigrade position. With fractures of the head, weightbearing is allowed; with body or neck fractures, it is avoided. At 8 weeks the plaster is removed and function regained by normal use.

DISPLACED FRACTURES AND FRACTURE-DISLOCATIONS
Reduction is urgent (because the stretched skin soon necroses), and should be perfect (to avoid the worst effects of avascular necrosis). Closed manipulation is tried first, and forced plantar-flexion is often the key manoeuvre. If this proves ineffective, a Steinmann pin through the calcaneum can be used to exert powerful traction while a second Steinmann pin trans-fixes the displaced bone and is used to reduce it. Should this also fail there must be no hesitation in performing open reduction; access can be obtained by osteotomizing the medial malleolus.

Once reduced, the fracture should be immobilized with Kirschner wires or a lag screw. If there is much swelling, the leg is elevated until this settles: a below-knee cast is then applied. Most of these injuries are stable only with the foot plantarflexed; this unpleasant position is maintained in a split plaster for 2–3 weeks. Then, without anaesthesia, the plaster is removed, and the patient is persuaded to dorsi-flex his foot gently; a complete below-knee plaster is then applied with the foot planti-grade, and this is worn for a further 6 weeks. When the plaster is removed, the patient is encouraged to exercise the leg and foot, but he should avoid weightbearing until x-rays show that the talus has not undergone avascular necrosis.

Fractures of the *body*, the *head* or the *talar processes* are treated in much the same way as those of the neck. Any substantial fragment that is displaced should be accurately reduced (and fixed with a screw or wires if necessary) in order to minimize distortion of the adjacent articular surface.

Complications

EARLY

Skin damage Skin damage is common either because the skin has been split or because it is tightly stretched and necroses. Skin tenting should be immediately relieved by reducing the fracture or dislocation. Open injuries and established skin necrosis should be treated by painstaking debridement in order to reduce the risk of infection; in these cases, the wound is best left open for 5–7 days and closed by delayed primary suture only when swelling subsides and it is certain that the wound is clean.

Talar detachment Sometimes, in open injuries, the talus is completely detached and lying in the wound. After adequate debridement and cleansing, the talus should be replaced in the mortise and stabilized, if necessary, with crossed Kirschner wires.

LATE

Malunion The importance of accurate reduction has been stressed. Malunion may lead to distortion of the joint surface, limitation of movement and pain on weightbearing. If early follow-up x-rays show redisplacement of the fragments, a further attempt at reduction is justified.

Avascular necrosis Avascular necrosis of the body (or the whole) of the talus occurs in over 50% of displaced fractures of the talar neck. The earliest x-ray sign (often present by the 6th week) is apparent increased density of the avascular segment; in reality it is the rest of the tarsus that has become slightly porotic with disuse, but the avascular portion remains unaffected. Later, sclerosis is due also to reactive new-bone formation, the only counter to progressive collapse of the avascular portion. Despite necrosis, the fracture may heal, so treatment should not be interrupted by this event; if anything, weightbearing should be delayed in the hope that the bone is not unduly flattened. Function may yet be reasonable. However, if the talus becomes flattened or fragmented, or pain and disability are marked, the ankle may need to be arthrodesed.

Secondary osteoarthritis Osteoarthritis of the ankle and/or subtalar joints may occur some years after injury. There are several causes: articular damage due to the initial trauma; malunion and distortion of the articular surface; and avascular necrosis of the talus.

Fractures of the calcaneum

Mechanism of injury

The patient usually falls from a height, often from a ladder, onto one or both heels. The calcaneum is driven up against the talus and is split or crushed. The same accident may also have damaged the spine, pelvis or hip, which must always be examined in calcaneal injuries.

Avulsion fractures occasionally follow traction injuries of the tendo Achillis or the ankle ligaments; and sometimes the bone is shattered by a direct blow.

Pathological anatomy

Based largely on the work of Palmer (1948) and Essex-Lopresti (1952), it has been customary to divide calcaneal fractures into extra-articular fractures (those involving the various calcaneal processes or the body posterior to the talocalca-neal joint) and intra-articular fractures (those that split the talocalcaneal articular facet).

EXTRA-ARTICULAR FRACTURES follow fairly simple patterns, with shearing or avulsion of the anterior process, the sustentaculum tali, the tuberosity, the inferomedial process or the posterior part of the body. They are usually easy to manage and have a good prognosis.

INTRA-ARTICULAR FRACTURES are much more complex and unpredictable in their outcome. They are best understood by imagining the impact of the talus cleaving the bone from above to produce a primary fracture line that runs obliquely across the posterior articular facet and the body from posteromedial to anterolateral; where it splits the articular facet depends upon the position of the foot at impact; if the heel is in valgus (abducted), the fracture is in the lateral part of the facet; if the heel is in varus (adducted), the fracture is more medial. This may occasionally be the entire extent of the injury, i.e. a two-part fracture with a larger posterolateral segment and a slightly smaller anteromedial segment. More frequently a secondary crack appears in the lateral wall, propagating in one of two ways: (1) the fracture line runs posteriorly along the superior crest of the body to split off a large tongue of bone consisting of the lateral wall and the lateral portion of the articular facet; more often (2) the secondary crack curves round just behind the articular facet to produce a small fragment consisting of the thalamic portion of the os calcis with the lateral portion of the articular facet. Essex-Lopresti called these two injuries 'tongue fractures' and 'joint depression fractures'. They are, in fact, three-part fractures in which the central segment of the bone is driven up between a large anteromedial buttress containing the sustentaculum tali and the medial portion of the posterior joint facet, and a smaller lateral segment of bone containing the lateral part of the joint facet. The articular facet is not so much depressed as split apart by the impact of the talus as the heel strikes the ground. Any one of the fragments may, in addition, be comminuted.

Clinical features

Unless the patient is unconscious, there will be a history of a fall from a height; in elderly

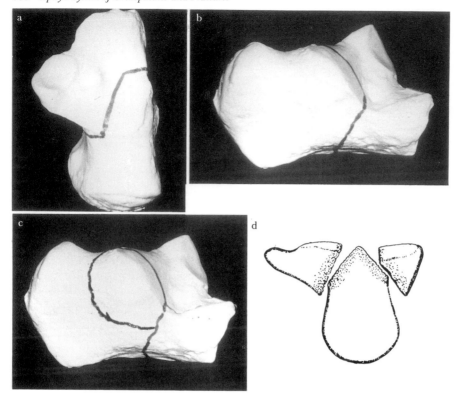

27.61 Intra-articular calcaneal fracture   (a, b) The primary fracture line runs obliquely across the articular facet from posteromedial to anterolateral. (c) A secondary fracture may split off a portion of the lateral wall. (d) Coronal section showing how the calcaneal body is driven upwards, splitting the articular surface asunder.

osteoporotic people even a comparatively minor injury may fracture the calcaneum.

The foot is painful and swollen, and a large bruise appears in the sole. The heel may look broad and squat. The surrounding tissues are thick and tender, and the normal concavity below the lateral malleolus is lacking. The subtalar joint cannot be moved but ankle movement is possible.

X-RAY

Plain x-rays should include lateral, oblique and axial views. Extra-articular fractures are usually fairly obvious. Intra-articular fractures, also, can often be identified in the plain films, and if there is displacement of the fragments the lateral view may show flattening of the tuber–joint angle (Böhler's angle). However, for accurate definition of intra-articular fractures, CT is essential; coronal views are obtained by

placing the foot in about 20 degrees of plantar-flexion and pointing the scanner towards the dorsal surface almost perpendicular to the sole (Lowrie et al., 1988). The fracture is categorized according to the patterns described above.

With severe injuries – and especially with bilateral fractures – it is essential to x-ray the spine and pelvis as well.

Treatment

For all except the most minor injuries, the patient is admitted to hospital so that the leg and foot can be elevated and treated with ice-packs until swelling subsides. This also gives time to obtain the necessary x-rays and CT scans.

EXTRA-ARTICULAR FRACTURES are treated closed – excepting the occasional instance of a markedly displaced avulsion fracture of the tuberosity. In the majority, exercises are encouraged from the outset. When the swelling subsides, a firm bandage is applied and the patient is allowed up non-weightbearing on crutches; with bilateral fractures, below-knee walking casts are applied and partial weightbearing is permitted. Displaced avulsion frac-

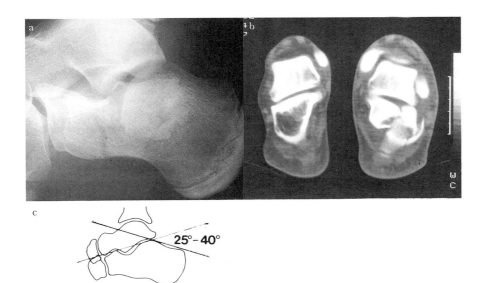

27.62 Fracture of the calcaneum – imaging   (a) The plain x-ray gives only an approximate idea of the nature and extent of the injury. (b) The CT scan in this case shows how the body of the calcaneum has split the articular fragments apart. (c) Böhler's angle is normally 25–40 degrees; compare the appearance in (a).

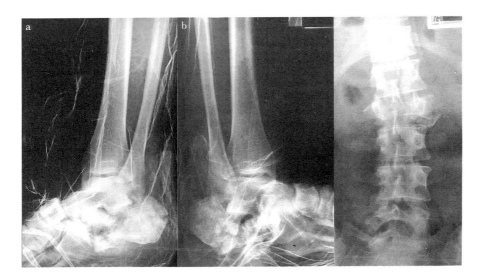

27.63 Calcaneal fractures   Bilateral calcaneal fractures (a, b) are caused either by a fall on the heels from a height or by an explosion from below. In either case the spine also may be fractured, as it was (c) in this patient. With bilateral heel fractures, always x-ray the spine.

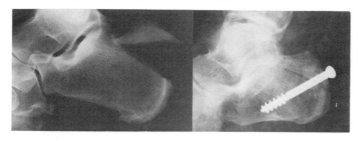

27.64 Calcaneal fractures   Avulsion fracture of posterosuperior corner fixed by screw.

tures of the tuberosity should be reduced and fixed with one or two screws; the foot is then immobilized in slight equinus to relieve tension on the tendo Achillis. In all cases, weightbearing can usually be permitted after 4–6 weeks.

UNDISPLACED, OR MINIMALLY DISPLACED, INTRA-ARTICULAR FRACTURES   are treated in the same way as extra-articular fractures: elevation followed by exercises and non-weightbearing for 4–6 weeks.

DISPLACED INTRA-ARTICULAR FRACTURES   are best treated by open reduction and internal fixation (as for intra-articular fractures generally). CT has greatly facilitated this approach; the medial and lateral fragments can be clearly defined and, with suitable drawings or models, the surgical procedure can be carefully planned and rehearsed. The operation can usually be performed through a single, wide lateral approach. It is essential, however, to ensure that the medial wall fracture is anatomically reduced – i.e. the upwardly displaced body is levered away from the sustentacular fragment – before

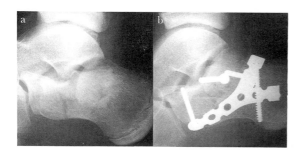

27.65 Fracture of the calcaneum – treatment   (a) In this displaced fracture of the calcaneum, Böhler's angle is completely flattened. (b) After open reduction and internal fixation, the normal anatomy is restored. (Courtesy of Mr R. M. Atkins.)

the lateral wall is reconstituted; this may be more easily achieved through a combined medial and lateral approach (Stephenson, 1987). The subtalar articular facet is reduced under vision and the various fragments are fixed with screws or staples. Bone grafts are used to fill any defects. If there is much bleeding from the bone, the wound should be drained. Postoperatively the foot is lightly splinted and elevated. Exercises are begun as soon as pain subsides and after 2–3 weeks the patient can be allowed up non-weightbearing on crutches. Partial weightbearing is permitted only when the fracture has healed (seldom before 8 weeks), and full weightbearing about 4 weeks after that. Restoration of function may take 6–12 months.

Complications

EARLY

Intense swelling and blistering may jeopardize operative treatment. The limb should be elevated with the minimum of delay.

LATE

Malunion   Closed treatment of displaced fractures, or injudicious weightbearing after open reduction, may result in malunion. Usually the foot is in valgus and walking may be impaired. Varus deformity causes pain and instability of the ankle.

Peroneal tendon impingement   Flattening and abduction of the calcaneum may cause painful compression of the peroneal tendons against the lateral malleolus. Treatment consists of operative paring down of protuberant bone on the lateral wall of the calcaneum.

Broadening of the heel is quite common and may cause problems with shoe fitting.

Talocalcaneal stiffness and osteoarthritis Displaced intra-articular fractures may lead to joint stiffness and, eventually, osteoarthritis. This can usually be managed conservatively, but persistent or severe pain may necessitate subtalar arthrodesis. If the calcaneocuboid joint is also involved, a triple arthrodesis is better.

Mid-tarsal and tarsometatarsal injuries

Falls in which the foot is twisted or forced into equinus may cause a variety of injuries, from a relatively benign ligamentous strain to fracture-dislocation of the tarsal or tarsometatarsal joints. Crushing injuries are worse, because they are accompanied by severe soft-tissue damage; bleeding into the fascial compartments of the foot may cause a typical ischaemic compartment syndrome.

Clinical features

The foot is bruised and swollen. With a strain, pain is elicited by moving the forefoot; with a fracture or dislocation, all attempts at movement will be resisted. The foot should be carefully examined for signs of ischaemia.

X-RAY
Multiple views are necessary to determine the extent of the injury. Tarsometatarsal dislocation may be missed if the forefoot falls back into place; fractures of the tarsal bones or bases of the metatarsals should alert the surgeon to this possibility.

Treatment

Ligamentous strains The foot may be bandaged until acute pain subsides. Thereafter, movement is encouraged.

Undisplaced fractures The foot is elevated to counteract swelling. After 3 or 4 days a below-knee cast is applied and the patient is allowed up on crutches with limited weightbearing. The plaster is retained for 4–6 weeks.

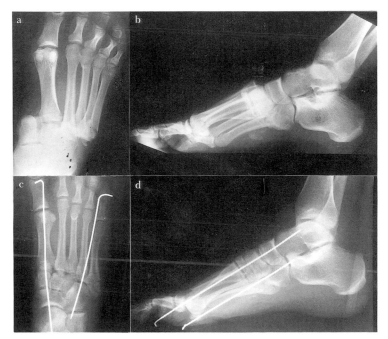

27.66 Tarsometatarsal injuries (a, b) X-ray of the foot showing fracture-dislocation of the tarsometatarsal joints. This injury was treated by open reduction and fixation with Kirschner wires (c, d).

Displaced fractures A cuboid fracture is sometimes displaced and, if so, may need open reduction and screw fixation.

Fracture-dislocation These are severe injuries. Under general anaesthesia, the dislocation can usually be reduced by closed manipulation, but holding it is a problem. If there is the least tendency to redisplacement, stout Kirschner wires or Steinmann pins are run across the joints to fix them in position. The foot is immobilized in a below-knee plaster for 6–8 weeks. Exercises are then begun and should be practised assiduously; it may be 6–8 months before function is regained.

Complications

Compartment syndrome A tensely swollen foot may hide a serious compartment syndrome which could result in ischaemic contractures. If this is suspected, intracompartmental pressures can be measured (see p. 545). Treatment should be prompt and effective: through a medial longitudinal incision, all the compartments can be reached and decompressed; the wound is left open until swelling subsides and the skin can be closed without tension.

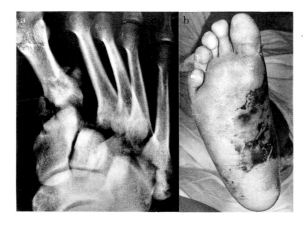

27.67 Tarsometatarsal injuries – complications (a) A severe injury such as this inevitably causes bleeding into the soft tissues of the foot. (b) This patient developed a compartment syndrome and threatened Volkmann's ischaemia. Prompt incision and decompression of the plantar compartment prevented a disaster.

Unreduced tarsometatarsal dislocation Patients who present more than 4 weeks after injury are best left without any attempt at reduction. The foot may be somewhat deformed and painful, but this can usually be helped by fitting suitable footwear or an orthotic support.

Injuries of the metatarsal bones

Metatarsal fractures are relatively common and are due either to a direct blow (a heavy object falling on the foot), a severe twisting injury, traction or repetitive stress.

Crush injury

Any or all of the metatarsal bones may be fractured by crush injuries. Usually the metatarsal necks fracture and often the overlying skin is damaged. The orthodox treatment is to reduce the fractures by manipulation and to hold them in plaster for a few weeks.

The functional method is as follows. Unless displacement is gross, which is rare, it may be ignored. The leg is elevated and active movements are started immediately. As soon as swelling has subsided, and the patient is comfortable, he is encouraged to walk normally. (A well-padded shoe or boot will feel more comfortable.) Malunion rarely results in disability when mobility has been regained.

In the unlikely event of severe displacement of a first or fifth metatarsal fracture, reduction and Kirschner wire fixation may be justified.

Twisting injury

If the forefoot is violently twisted, abducted or plantarflexed, tarsometatarsal dislocation may occur. The first metatarsal is either dislocated or fractured near its base; the other metatarsal bones are fractured more distally. Minor degrees of displacement are easily missed but are serious, and severe displacement may endanger the circulation of the foot.

Reduction is urgent and is maintained by a padded split plaster. The leg is kept elevated until it is certain that the circulation is satisfactory. After 3 weeks, plaster is discarded, active exercises are started, and weightbearing is resumed at 6 weeks.

Traction injury

Forced inversion of the foot (the 'pot-hole injury') may cause avulsion of the base of the fifth metatarsal. Pain due to a sprained ankle may overshadow pain in the foot. Examination will disclose a point of tenderness directly over the prominence at the base of the fifth metatarsal bone.

X-ray shows a transverse fracture near the tip of the metatarsal base; the small fragment is usually only slightly displaced. (Occasionally a normal peroneal ossicle in this area may be mistaken for a fracture; x-ray of the other foot will show a symmetrical opacity.)

If pain is severe, the foot should be rested and elevated for a few days. Thereafter, activity is encouraged and the patient walks as normally as possible in an ordinary shoe. Full painless function is rapidly regained.

Stress injury (march fracture)

In a young adult (often a recruit or a nurse) the foot may become painful after overuse. A tender lump is palpable just distal to the mid-shaft of a metatarsal bone. Usually the second metatarsal is affected, especially if it is much longer than an 'atavistic' first metatarsal. The x-ray appearance may at first be normal but a radioisotope scan will show an area of intense activity in the bone. Later a hairline crack may be visible, and later still a mass of callus is seen.

Unaccountable pain in elderly osteoporotic people may be due to the same lesion; x-ray diagnosis is more difficult because callus is minimal and there may be no more than a fine linear periosteal reaction along the metatarsal.

No displacement occurs and neither reduction nor splintage is necessary. The forefoot may be supported with an elastic bandage and normal walking is encouraged.

Injuries of the metatarsophalangeal joints

Sprains and dislocations of the metatarsophalangeal joints are common in dancers and athletes. A simple sprain requires no more than light splinting; strapping the toe to its neighbour for a week or two is the easiest way. If the toe is dislocated, it should be reduced by traction and manipulation; the foot is then protected in a short walking cast for a few weeks.

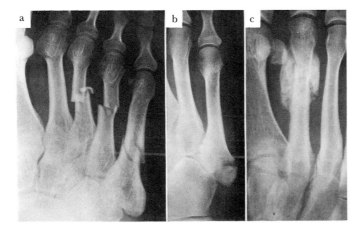

27.68 Metatarsal injuries (a) Transverse fractures of three metatarsal shafts. (b) Avulsion fracture of the base of the fifth metatarsal – the pot-hole injury, or Robert Jones fracture. (c) Florid callus in a stress fracture.

Fractured toes

A heavy object falling on the toes may fracture phalanges. If the skin is broken it must be covered with a sterile dressing. The fracture is disregarded and the patient encouraged to walk in a suitably mutilated boot. If pain is marked, the toe may be splinted by strapping it to its neighbour for 2–3 weeks.

Fractured sesamoids

One of the sesamoids (usually the medial) may fracture from either a direct injury (landing from a height on the ball of the foot) or sudden traction; chronic, repetitive stress is more often seen in dancers and runners.

The patient complains of pain directly over the sesamoid. There is a tender spot in the same area and sometimes pain can be exacerbated by passively hyperextending the big toe. X-rays will usually show the fracture (which must be distinguished from a smooth-edged bipartite sesamoid).

Treatment is often unnecessary, though a local injection of lignocaine helps for pain. If discomfort is marked, the foot can be immobilized in a short-leg walking cast for 2–3 weeks. Occasionally, intractable symptoms call for excision of the offending ossicle.

References and further reading

Alio, A.J., Letho, M.U.K. and Kujala, U.M. (1986) Repair of the anterior cruciate ligament: augmentation versus conventional suture of fresh rupture. *Acta Orthopaedica Scandinavica* **57**, 354–357

Anderson, W.A. (1982) The significance of femoral fractures in children. *Annals of Emergency Medicine* **11**, 174–177

Apley, A.G. (1979) Fractures of the tibial plateau. *Orthopedic Clinics of North America* **10**, 61–74

Ballmer, P.M. and Jacob, R.P. (1988) The non-operative treatment of isolated complete tears of the medial collateral ligament of the knee: a prospective study. *Archives of Orthopedic and Traumatic Surgery* **107**, 273–276

Barnes, R., Brown, J.T., Garden, R.S. and Nicoll, E.A. (1976) Subcapital fractures of the femur. A prospective review. *Journal of Bone and Joint Surgery* **58B**, 2–24

Clancy, W.G. (1982) Anterior cruciate functional instability. *Clinical Orthopaedics and Related Research* **172**, 102–106

Cooper, C. (1989) Osteoporosis – an epidemiological perspective: a review. *Journal of the Royal Society of Medicine* **82**, 753–757

Daniel, D.M., Stone, M.L., Barnett, P. and Sachs, R. (1988) Use of the quadriceps active test to diagnose posterior cruciate ligament disruption and measure posterior laxity of the knee. *Journal of Bone and Joint Surgery* **70A**, 386–391

Das De, S. and Balasubramaniam, P. (1985) A repair operation for recurrent dislocation of the peroneal tendons. *Journal of Bone and Joint Surgery* **67B**, 585–587

Ellis, H. (1958) The speed of healing after fracture of the tibial shaft. *Journal of Bone and Joint Surgery* **40B**, 42–46

Epstein, H.C. (1973) Traumatic dislocations of the hip. *Clinical Orthopaedics and Related Research* **92**, 116–142

Essex-Lopresti, P. (1952) The mechanism, reduction technique and results in fractures of the os calcis. *British Journal of Surgery* **39**, 395–419

Feagin, J.A. and Cooke, T.D.V. (1989) Prone examination for anterior cruciate ligament insufficiency. *Journal of Bone and Joint Surgery* **71B**, 863

Fruensgaard, S. and Johannsen, H.V. (1989) Incomplete ruptures of the anterior cruciate ligament. *Journal of Bone and Joint Surgery* **71B**, 526–530

Galway, H.R. and MacIntosh, D.L. (1980) The lateral pivot shift: a symptom and sign of anterior cruciate ligament insufficiency. *Clinical Orthopaedics and Related Research* **147**, 45–50

Garden, R.S. (1961) Low-angle fixation in fractures of the femoral neck. *Journal of Bone and Joint Surgery* **43B**, 647–663

Gustilo, R.B., Merkow, R.L. and Templeman, D. (1990) The management of open fractures. *Journal of Bone and Joint Surgery* **72A**, 299–304

Harper, W.M., Barnes, M.R. and Gregg, P.J. (1991) Femoral head blood flow in femoral neck fracture. *Journal of Bone and Joint Surgery* **73B**, 73–75

Hooper, G.J., Keddell, R.C. and Penny, I.D. (1991) Conservative management or closed nailing for tibial shaft fractures. A randomised prospective trial. *Journal of Bone and Joint Surgery* **73B**, 83–85

Hughston, J.C., Andrews, J.R., Cross, M.J. and Moschi, A. (1976) Classification of knee ligament instabilities. *Journal of Bone and Joint Surgery* **58A**, 159–172; 173–179

Ireland, J. and Trickey, E.L. (1980) MacIntosh tenodesis for anterolateral instability of the knee. *Journal of Bone and Joint Surgery* **62B**, 340–345

Kannus, P. (1988) Long-term results of conservatively treated medial collateral ligament injuries of the knee joint. *Clinical Orthopaedics and Related Research* **226**, 103–111

Langenskiold, A. (1975) An operation for partial closure of an epiphyseal plate in children, and its experimental basis. *Journal of Bone and Joint Surgery* **57B**, 325–330

Lansinger, O., Bergman, B., Korner, L. and Andersson, G.B.J. (1986) Tibial condylar fractures. *Journal of Bone and Joint Surgery* **68A**, 13–19

Larson, R.L. (1983) Editorial. The knee – the physiological joint. *Journal of Bone and Joint Surgery* **65A**, 143–144

Lauge-Hansen, N. (1950) Fractures of the ankle. II. Combined experimental-surgical and experimental-roentgenologic investigations. *Archives of Surgery* **60**, 957–985

Losee, R.E., Johnson, T.R. and Southwick, W.D. (1978) Anterior subluxation of the lateral tibial plateau. A diagnostic test and operative repair. *Journal of Bone and Joint Surgery* **60A**, 1015–1030

Lowrie, I.G., Finlay, D.B., Brenkel, I.J. and Gregg, P.J. (1988) Computerised tomographic assessment of the subtalar joint in calcaneal fractures. *Journal of Bone and Joint Surgery* **70B**, 247–250

Main, B.J. and Jowett, R.L. (1975) Injuries of the midtarsal joint. *Journal of Bone and Joint Surgery* **57B**, 89–97

Mast, J.W., Spiegel, P.G. and Pappas, J.N. (1988) Fractures of the tibial pilon. *Clinical Orthopaedics and Related Research* **230**, 68–82

Mink, J.H., Levy, T. and Cruess, J.V. III (1988) Tears of the anterior cruciate ligament and menisci of the knee: MR imaging evaluation. *Radiology* **167**, 769–774

Muller, M.E., Allgöwer, M., Schneider, R. and Willeneger, H. (1991) *Manual of Internal Fixation*, 3rd edn, Springer, Berlin, pp. 598–600

O'Donoghue, D.H. (1973) Reconstruction for medial instability of the knee. *Journal of Bone and Joint Surgery* **55A**, 941–955

Olerud, C., Rehnberg, L. and Hellquist, E. (1991) Internal fixation of femoral neck fractures. *Journal of Bone and Joint Surgery* **73B**, 16–19

Palmer, I. (1948) The mechanism and treatment of fractures of the calcaneus. *Journal of Bone and Joint Surgery* **30A**, 2–8

Ramsay, P.L. and Hamilton, W. (1976) Changes in tibio-fibular area of contact caused by lateral talar shift. *Journal of Bone and Joint Surgery* **58A**, 356–357

Ratliff, A.H.C. (1962) Fractures of the neck of the femur in children. *Journal of Bone and Joint Surgery* **44B**, 528–542

Sandberg, R., Balkfors, B., Nilsson, B. and Westlin, N. (1987) Operative versus non-operative treatment of recent injuries to the ligaments of the knee: a prospective randomized study. *Journal of Bone and Joint Surgery* **69A**, 1120–1126

Sarmiento, A., Gersten, L.M., Sobol, P.A., Shankwiler, J.A. and Vangsness, C.T. (1989) Tibial shaft fractures treated with functional braces. *Journal of Bone and Joint Surgery* **71B**, 602–609

Schatzker, J. (1987) Fractures of the tibial plateau. In *The Rationale of Operative Fracture Care* (eds. J. Schatzker and M. Tile), Springer, Berlin, pp. 279–296

Solomon, L. (1968) Osteoporosis and fracture of the femoral neck in the South African Bantu. *Journal of Bone and Joint Surgery* **50B**, 2–13

Solomon, L. (1973) Fracture of the femoral neck in the elderly. Bone ageing or disease? *South African Journal of Surgery* **11**, 269–279

Stephenson, J.R. (1987) Treatment of displaced intra-articular fractures of the calcaneus using medial and lateral approaches, internal fixation, and early motion. *Journal of Bone and Joint Surgery* **69A**, 115–130

Trickey, E.L. (1987) Soft tissue injuries of the knee – clinical evaluation. *Current Orthopaedics* **1**, 135–139

Tscherne, H. (1984) The management of open fractures. In *Fractures with Soft Tissue Injuries* (eds. H. Tscherne and L. Gotzen), Springer, Berlin, pp. 10–32

Overuse injuries

Whereas most injuries are a consequence of some obvious event, those due to overuse are elusive and insidious. They are seen mainly in athletes (hence the unfortunate term 'sporting injuries') and in dancers, but may occur in anyone after overactivity without adequate training. Some are listed as occupational injuries and have acquired diagnostic labels such as 'cumulative trauma disorder' and 'repetitive strain injury'.

Pathology

There are three main causes of overuse trauma: *friction, stress* and *ischaemia.*

FRICTION   A tendon or bursa may, during joint movement, be subjected to excessive friction within a fibrous sheath or over a bony prominence. An inflammatory reaction starts up ('peritendinitis' or bursitis); swelling occurs and gliding movement is further restricted. With time the sheath may become fibrosed and thickened ('tenovaginitis').

STRESS   Repeated or unguarded stress may result in tears of muscle or tendon fibres, incomplete fracture of bone, or impact lesions of articular cartilage (usually of the patella). Occasionally a sudden, excessive force causes a complete rupture of tendon or muscle.

ISCHAEMIA   This usually occurs in muscles that are firmly enclosed in fascial compartments (e.g. in the forearm or leg). Ischaemia may be relative, arising only when excessive activity makes demands on the blood supply which cannot be met; or absolute, when intramuscular

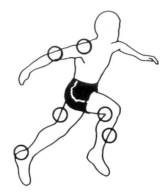

28.1 Overuse injuries The areas commonly affected are the shoulder, the elbow, the hamstrings, the posterior band of the fascia lata, the tendo Achillis and the tibial compartments.

oedema causes swelling in a tight compartment.

The sites most commonly affected are the shoulder, elbow, wrist and knee.

Clinical syndromes

ROTATOR CUFF INJURIES
Sporting activities involving throwing or pitching (and, sometimes, overarm swimming) may result in chronic or recurrent shoulder pain. There are a number of causes and more than one may be present in any particular patient. In throwing, the arm moves from extension, abduction and external rotation to flexion, adduc-

tion and internal rotation. Such forceful movement in the 'impingement position', if repeated often enough, may give rise to a typical rotator cuff syndrome (see p. 264). In addition, however, sudden acceleration and deceleration movements may cause stretching or tears of the posterior capsule, the anterior capsule or the glenoid labrum. With recurrent subluxation of the shoulder there is a feeling of sudden pain and weakness as the arm sweeps into full circumduction (the tennis serving position). Each of these disorders should be looked for during the clinical examination and special investigations. They are described in Chapter 13.

TENNIS ELBOW AND GOLFER'S ELBOW
Pain and tenderness below the lateral humeral epicondyle ('tennis elbow') or the medial epicondyle ('golfer's elbow') is thought to be due to repetitive strains on the common tendon of origin of the wrist extensors or flexors. Thus, these syndromes are seen most typically in patients whose activities involve repeated, forceful extension or flexion of the wrist. In tennis players the condition is aggravated by using a racquet that is too heavy, or has too large a grip, or simply by employing poor technique. The pathological lesion may be microscopic tearing of the aponeurosis followed by a local inflammatory reaction, or vascular congestion, or crystal deposition. The condition usually responds to rest and local injection of corticosteroids, but it frequently recurs when activity is resumed (see also p. 292).

TROCHANTERIC 'BURSITIS'
A ballet dancer or runner complains of pain around the greater trochanter of the femur. There is local tenderness and crepitus in the bursa. Sometimes the tender spot is behind the trochanter, and an x-ray may show calcification in this region; the diagnosis in these cases is probably tendinitis of the gluteus medius – a condition similar to supraspinatus tendinitis of the shoulder. It may respond to treatment with non-steroidal anti-inflammatory drugs; if it does not, local injection with corticosteroids is usually effective.

ILIOTIBIAL BAND FRICTION
This usually occurs in long-distance runners who increase their distance too quickly; it is thought to be due to rubbing of the posterior part of the iliotibial band against the lateral femoral condyle. Pain is felt when the knee reaches about 20 degrees of flexion; the patient walks with a stiff-knee gait and tenderness is localized to a point just behind the lateral condyle. Tensing the iliotibial band by pressing it against the femur and then flexing the knee produces sharp pain at the point of irritation.

PATELLAR TENDINITIS ('JUMPER'S KNEE')
The word 'tendinitis' is customary but inaccurate, because it is the patellar ligament which is affected. The condition is common in both dancers and athletes (especially long-jumpers and high-jumpers). Repeated sudden contraction of the quadriceps at take-off may cause tiny ruptures of fibres at or near the attachment of the ligament to the lower pole of the patella; there is an associated vascular reaction. Pain and tenderness are maximal at the site of the lesion.

CHONDROMALACIA PATELLAE ('RUNNER'S KNEE')
The symptoms and signs are those of chondromalacia, though, unlike the usual case which involves adolescent girls, the 'overuse' injury occurs in fit runners. It has been attributed to weakness of the vastus medialis, or to postural abnormalities such as pes valgus and internal rotation of the tibia; whether due to the quadriceps weakness or to mild malalignment of the knee, the patella tends to subluxate during active knee extension, damaging the articular cartilage. A similar condition occurs in truck drivers.

PAINFUL TENDO ACHILLIS
Three syndromes are recognized, though it is doubtful whether they are completely distinct entities.

Peritendinitis (or paratendinitis) is an inflammation around the tendon, which gives rise to pain, diffuse swelling over the tendon, crepitus on moving the foot, and tenderness which remains in one spot regardless of the position of the foot.

Achillis tendinitis causes similar features, except that the tenderness is more clearly in the tendon and shifts as the tendon moves with dorsi- and plantarflexion. It is attributed to small ruptures of tendon fibres.

Calcaneal bursitis presents as a painful heel; tenderness is anterior to the tendo Achillis and more directly on the underlying bone.

All three disorders tend to occur in young athletes who increase their activity, or in older individuals (those over 40) who overstress the tendon by using unaccustomed force in sprinting, climbing or uphill running.

Occasionally, after a period of pain and moderate swelling, the tendon may rupture. This is especially likely after injudicious injection of local anaesthetic or corticosteroids into the substance of the tendon.

MUSCLE TEARS

The clinical picture is similar, whether the area involved is the calf, the quadriceps or the hamstrings. During muscular exertion the patient feels a sharp pain, and sometimes a 'snapping' or 'tearing' sensation. Later, bruising appears and the affected area is tender. Complete muscle tears have been reported, but are very rare.

'SHIN SPLINTS'

This term is used for pain and tenderness along the posteromedial border of the lower half of the tibia; the symptoms characteristically increase with activity and subside with rest. They may be due to tendinitis of the tibialis posterior, but more serious conditions such as a mild posterior compartment syndrome or a stress fracture of the tibia must be excluded.

Stress fractures are quite common in runners; they tend to occur either in the proximal half of the tibia or the distal third of the fibula. Tenderness is localized to the fracture site. X-rays may show a fringe of periosteal reaction, but even before that radionuclide scintigraphy will reveal the area of increased bone activity.

METATARSALGIA

Pain in the forefoot may accompany any disorder that causes a change in pedal mechanics. Similar aching may result from overuse – long stretches of walking on hard surfaces, hiking in unsuitable footwear or standing with poor balance for long periods. Simple forms of treatment, such as rest and foot-baths followed by intrinsic muscle exercises, usually suffice. However, it is important to exclude any underlying stress lesion.

Stress fracture of the second or third metatarsal is common in overactive army recruits (the 'march fracture') and in elderly osteoporotic individuals. The x-ray and scintigraphic signs are diagnostic.

Osteochondritis of the head of the second metatarsal sometimes occurs (or perhaps is merely brought to light) after a period of stressful walking or running (see p. 495).

Management of overuse injuries

Prevention is better than cure and most overuse injuries can be avoided by adhering to a few simple rules: increases in activity must be graded; training before races must be adequate; changes in activity must be gradual; and warning signals of mild pain at the characteristic sites must be heeded.

Treatment is usually non-specific and consists of reducing activity (rather than complete rest), relieving stress (e.g. on the tendo Achillis, by elevating the heel), and counteracting inflammation (usually by giving anti-inflammatory drugs, occasionally by injecting local anaesthetic and corticosteroids around – but not into – the affected tendon).

Operation may be necessary in resistant cases – to incise the iliotibial band, to release a constricted tendon, or to decompress a tight fascial compartment. In all cases physiotherapy is important and is aimed at graded muscle stretching combined with strengthening exercises.

Musician's problems

String players, keyboard performers and occasionally woodwind players may be affected by a wide variety of upper limb disorders, any of which may threaten their livelihood (Lambert, 1992). The weight of the instrument, the player's posture and technique, as well as repetitive movements, may be aetiological factors. Characteristically, symptoms are produced by playing and relieved by rest; there are seldom any abnormal physical signs.

The player's posture and technique should be studied, preferably in conjunction with an experienced teacher of the instrument, because the first step in treatment is the correction of any faults. Other possibilities are the administration of non-steroidal anti-inflammatory tablets, a period of rest (if the patient will tolerate this) as well as relaxation training. Occasionally, gentle physiotherapy to strengthen particular muscle groups is helpful. Only rarely, in the most severe and resistant cases, is a change of career indicated.

Repetitive strain injury

The term 'repetitive strain injury' (RSI) refers to a painful condition in the upper limb which follows frequent repetition of a particular movement; thus typists and other keyboard operators tend to be affected. The disorder has many synonyms (overuse syndrome, cumulative trauma disorder) but in few cases is there any recognizable pathology (Semple, 1991). The modern increase in frequency, which has sometimes reached epidemic proportions (Ferguson, 1987), has been attributed to the possibility of attracting industrial compensation, but this cannot be the whole story since professional musicians also may be affected.

The present confused situation would be clarified if RSI were diagnosed only when the following features were present.

1. The onset followed a substantial increase of a particular activity, or a recent change of activity.
2. The pain occurs whenever the offending activity is performed and is relieved by discontinuing that activity, or (temporarily)

by injecting local anaesthetic into the tender area.
3. There are definite physical signs such as localized tenderness, pain on contracting the appropriate muscles and creptius.

The commonest site is the dorsum of the forearm in the line of the radial extensors of the wrist, where there may also be a tender fusiform swelling. The term 'tenosynovitis' should not be used in the absence of crepitus and certainly not when there is no tendon sheath at the affected site (Barton, 1989).

If there is sufficient evidence to justify the diagnosis, treatment is worthwhile. The provoking activity is stopped for 3–4 weeks and the painful area treated by elastic support and physiotherapy (ultrasound). If this fails or pain recurs as soon as the activity is resumed, a change of occupation is desirable. Sometimes, however, the occupation is not only repetitive but also boring, in which case psychological factors play a part and treatment is unlikely to succeed; nor is success likely when medicolegal considerations predominate.

References and further reading

Barton, N. (1989) Editorial. Repetitive strain disorder. *British Medical Journal* **299**, 405–406

Ferguson, D.A. (1987) Editorial. 'RSI': putting the epidemic to rest. *Medical Journal of Australia* **147**, 213–214

Lambert, C.M. (1992) Hand and upper limb problems of instrumental musicians. *British Journal of Rheumatology* **31**, 265–271

Semple, J. (1991) Editorial. Tenosynovitis, repetitive strain injury, etc. *Journal of Bone and Joint Surgery* **73B**, 536–538

Index